Handbook of Gynecologic Surgery

Handbook of Gynecologic Surgery

Edited by Vivian Stone

hayle
medical

New York

Hayle Medical,
750 Third Avenue, 9th Floor,
New York, NY 10017, USA

Visit us on the World Wide Web at:
www.haylemedical.com

ISBN: 978-1-63241-768-8

Trademark Notice: Registered trademark of products or corporate names are used only for explanation and identification without intent to infringe.

Cataloging-in-Publication Data

Handbook of gynecologic surgery / edited by Vivian Stone.
    p. cm.
Includes bibliographical references and index.
ISBN 978-1-63241-768-8
1. Generative organs, Female--Surgery. 2. Gynecology. 3. Generative organs, Female--Diseases.
I. Stone, Vivian.
RG104 .H35 2019
618.105 9--dc23

Table of Contents

Permissions

List of Contributors

Index

Preface

The medical specialty that studies the functioning and health of the breasts and the female reproductive organs, including the vagina, uterus and ovaries is called gynecology. Infertility, menorrhagia, incontinence of urine, vaginitis and prolapse of pelvic organs are some of the common medical conditions which come under the scope of gynecology. Antibiotics, antihypertensives, diuretics and gynecological surgery are some of the common ways to treat gynecologic disorders. Gynecological surgery is usually performed in case of infertility, cancer, benign conditions and incontinence. It is generally performed by gynecologists. This book unfolds the innovative aspects of gynecological surgery which will be crucial for the progress of this discipline in future. It is a valuable compilation of topics, ranging from the basic to the most complex advancements in this field. As this field is emerging at a rapid pace, the contents of this book will help the readers understand the modern concepts and applications of the subject.

The researches compiled throughout the book are authentic and of high quality, combining several disciplines and from very diverse regions from around the world. Drawing on the contributions of many researchers from diverse countries, the book's objective is to provide the readers with the latest achievements in the area of research. This book will surely be a source of knowledge to all interested and researching the field.

In the end, I would like to express my deep sense of gratitude to all the authors for meeting the set deadlines in completing and submitting their research chapters. I would also like to thank the publisher for the support offered to us throughout the course of the book. Finally, I extend my sincere thanks to my family for being a constant source of inspiration and encouragement.

Editor

A hybrid technique of combined conventional and robotic-assisted laparoscopy for staging and debulking of early, advanced, and recurrent ovarian, fallopian tube, and primary peritoneal cancer

Farr R. Nezhat · Susan S. Khalil · Tamara N. Finger · Patrick F. Vetere

Abstract This study aims to describe a hybrid laparoscopic and robotic-assisted laparoscopic technique to access all four abdominal quadrants during pelvic procedures. This technique was utilized in the surgical management of select cases that included early, advanced, and recurrent ovarian, fallopian tube, and peritoneal cancer. A retrospective analysis of a prospectively maintained database was used to extract cases that this surgical method was utilized in. This included 20 patients that underwent 21 surgical procedures using this hybrid technique of conventional laparoscopy and robotic-assisted laparoscopy. Ten were early stage, and 11 were advanced and/or recurrent (six advanced, five recurrent). In the early-stage group, mean age was 42.3 years (range, 29–55), average BMI was 32.1 kg/m^2 (range, 17–65 kg/m^2), mean blood loss was 212.5 ml (range, 50–1,000 mL), operating room time (ORT) was 306.1 min (range, 87–639), and average length of stay (LOS) was 1.6 days (range, 1–2). There were no intraoperative complications and two grade 1 postoperative complications. Of the 11 for advanced and/or recurrent disease, mean age was 63.9 years (range, 39–92), average BMI was 29.7 kg/m^2 (range, 22.1–37.2), mean blood loss was 129.1 ml (range, 20–400), ORT was 238 min (range, 103–477), and LOS was 3.8 days (range, 1–17). There were no intraoperative complications. Three cases had postoperative grade 1–3 complications. There was one second look, nine cytoreductions to no visible disease, and 1 to <0.5 cm. Use of this hybrid technique, combining conventional laparoscopy and the present robotic platform, is effective in the surgical management of early, advanced and recurrent ovarian, fallopian tube, and peritoneal cancer in accessing all four abdominal quadrants with pelvic surgery.

Keywords Hybrid technique · Conventional laparoscopy · Robotic-assisted laparoscopy · Ovarian cancer Staging and Cytoreduction

F. R. Nezhat
Division of Gynecologic, Oncology and Minimally Invasive Surgery, Department of Obstetrics and Gynecology, Columbia University, New York, NY 10019, USA

F. R. Nezhat (✉)
Department of Obstetrics and Gynecology, St. Luke's-Roosevelt Medical Center, 10th Floor, 1000 10th Avenue, New York, NY 10019, USA
e-mail: fnezhat@chpnet.org

F. R. Nezhat
e-mail: frn2103@columbia.edu

F. R. Nezhat · S. S. Khalil · T. N. Finger
Division of Minimally Invasive Surgery, Department of Obstetrics and Gynecology, St. Luke's-Roosevelt Medical Center, New York, NY, USA

F. R. Nezhat · P. F. Vetere
Division of Minimally Invasive Gynecologic Surgery, Department of Obstetrics and Gynecology, Winthrop University Hospital, Mineola, NY, USA

Introduction

Advances in minimally invasive surgical techniques now make it feasible to accomplish comprehensive surgical staging, using conventional or robotic-assisted laparoscopy in select patients [1]. The present computer enhanced telesurgery (Intuitive Surgical, Sunnyvale, CA, USA), called robot-assisted surgery, was approved by the Food and Drug Administration for gynecological surgery in 2005 and has been increasingly applied to complex gynecologic procedures, such as surgical staging for gynecologic malignancies including endometrial, cervical, and ovarian cancers [2–5].

Limitations exist with the present robotic platform for staging and cytoreduction in ovarian cancer. Once the robot is docked for pelvic surgery, it is more difficult to access the upper abdomen, without having to undock and reposition the robot, or add additional ports to be able to perform the procedure. The Society of Gynecologic Oncology's consensus statement on robotic-assisted surgery commented on its utility in ovarian cancer as poorly suited for advanced ovarian cancer due to its limitation, with conventional port placement for pelvic surgery, in gaining upper abdominal access [6].

In the USA, ovarian cancer will affect approximately 22,280 women in 2012 with 15,500 estimated deaths. Currently, the lifetime risk of developing ovarian cancer in the USA is approximately 1 in 70 with more than 65 % given the diagnosis of advanced stage disease [7]. The standard treatment of ovarian cancer includes upfront surgery with intent to properly diagnose, stage, and to achieve maximal cytoreduction preferably to no visible disease followed by taxanes and platinum-based combination chemotherapy in majority of cases [8]. Traditionally, a comprehensive surgical staging procedure for ovarian, fallopian tube, and primary peritoneal cancers include total abdominal hysterectomy, bilateral salpingo-oophorectomy, peritoneal washings, biopsies of adhesions and peritoneal surfaces, omentectomy, and retroperitoneal lymph node sampling from the pelvic and para-aortic regions through a generous vertical midline laparotomy incision.

There have been attempts to strategize the utility of the robot for such cases in order to gain upper abdominal access without difficulty. Magrina et al. described their technique for approaching debulking procedures in patients with epithelial ovarian cancer that require upper abdominal access and for infrarenal aortic lymphadenectomy. This method involves undocking the robotic arms, then rotating the operating table 180°, insertion of additional ports, and then redocking [5, 9].

We describe our surgical method, a hybrid technique, in which both conventional laparoscopy and the robot are utilized in gynecologic malignancies in all four abdominal quadrants and the pelvic cavity. This surgical technique and its use in select patients with early and advanced ovarian cancer will be described for laparoscopic management of both pelvic and upper abdominal disease.

Materials and methods

A retrospective analysis of a prospectively maintained database was performed to extract select cases where this hybrid technique combining conventional laparoscopy (CL) and robotic-assisted laparoscopic surgery (RALS) was utilized. These cases included early, advanced, and recurrent ovarian, fallopian tube, and peritoneal cancer. Institutional review board approval was obtained and data was collected from two urban university affiliated community hospitals. All patients underwent preoperative evaluation including history, physical examination, medical assessment, computed tomography imaging of the chest or abdomen and pelvis, or positron emission tomography scan, and tumor marker assays, and were counseled extensively preoperatively and appropriate informed consent was obtained. Patients with significant perioperative morbidity who were not candidates for any surgical procedures, either laparoscopy or laparotomy, or who had significant metastatic disease involving chest or solid organs, such as liver, were excluded. The same board-certified gynecologist oncologist, assisted by a minimally invasive gynecological surgical fellow and resident performed the surgeries. Early stage disease included patients that were in stages I to II. This group also included patients referred for restaging after prior ovarian cystectomy or oophorectomy. Advanced disease was classified as International Federation of Gynecology and Obstetrics stages III to IV. Postoperative complications were graded using the Memorial Sloan-Kettering Cancer Center severity grading system [10].

Technique

Under general endotracheal anesthesia, the patients were positioned in dorsal lithotomy position, bilateral sequential compression devices were placed on both lower extremities and arms were padded and tucked. Egg crate foam was also placed across the chest to protect patients and they were secured to the operating table with tape or a gel pad underneath them. They were draped in a sterile manner, and given preoperative antibiotic prophylaxis with 1–2 g of cefazolin or 80 mg or gentamycin and 900 mg of clindamycin if they were allergic to penicillin. A Foley catheter was inserted into the bladder, and a uterine manipulator was placed if the uterus was in situ. An incision is made in either the left upper quadrant or 4–5 cm above the umbilicus, using a Veress needle to introduce carbon dioxide gas and establish pneumoperitoneum. After adequate pneumoperitoneum is obtained, a 5 or 8 mm primary port is inserted into the left upper quadrant. If pneumoperitoneum is established supraumbilically, then a 12-mm trocar and sleeve are introduced into the supraumbilical port. After assessing the abdominopelvic cavity, either a 10- or 12-mm port is introduced into the right upper quadrant or two 8-mm robotic ports are introduced 8–10 cm lateral to the umbilicus bilaterally (Fig. 1). Further peritoneal inspection is performed by conventional laparoscopy and peritoneal washings or aspiration of existing ascites are obtained and sent for cytology. Decision to proceed with laparoscopic/robotic-assisted surgical or laparotomy staging or debulking was made based on the extent of the disease and patients comorbidity for lengthy operation. In advanced stages, the goal was to achieve cytoreduction to preferably no visible or at least <1 cm disease either via robotic-assisted laparoscopy, conventional laparoscopy, or laparotomy.

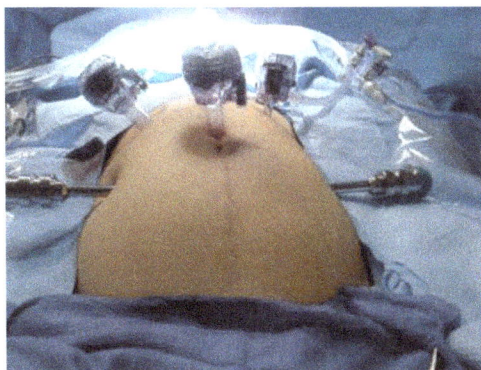

Fig. 1 Port placement

Thorough four-quadrant abdominopelvic cavity evaluation was performed by inserting additional ports, when necessary, to implement the choice of treatment. If surgical debulking to no visible disease is not possible, then biopsies are taken and salpingo-oophorectomy is performed if feasible [11, 12]. The procedure is terminated and the patient is given neoadjuvant chemotherapy to achieve higher rate of optimal cytoreductive surgery and decrease morbidity [13]. The patient is then reoperated on after reducing the load of the disease, which has been shown in randomized trials not to compromise oncological outcomes. Only patients in whom this hybrid technique was utilized were included in this study.

If disease is present in the upper abdomen and pelvis, surgery begins with conventional laparoscopy to perform an omentectomy and upper abdominal debulking (Fig. 2). This is performed via use of the supraumbilical port for the camera and ports for introduction of instruments. The surgeon stands between the patient's legs with two assistants on either side of the patient and an additional monitor placed towards the patient's head. A combination of various conventional laparoscopic instruments such as the Harmonic shears, the 5- or 10-mm LigaSure™ (Covidien, Boulder, CO) or other blood vessel sealant devices including surgical clips and staples can be used. The infracolic omentum is transected from the transverse colon and the gastrocolic omentum is transected all the way towards the spleen and stomach by coagulating and transecting the short gastric vessels. The specimen(s) is removed confined to a laparoscopic bag. Metastatic lesions noted on the hepatic flexure or transverse colon are mobilized. Using a combination of Harmonic shears (Ethicon Endo-Surgery, Cincinnati, OH, USA), PlasmaJet (Plasma Surgical Limited, Oxfordshire, UK), and bipolar electrocoagulation, all diaphragmatic lesions are removed in the form of stripping, ablation, and coagulation (Fig. 2a,b). This same approach can be applied if there is no upper abdominal disease and only infracolic omentectomy is performed as part of surgical staging for presumed early ovarian cancer.

Any abdominal and pelvic adhesions which interfere with proper application of the robotic platform are lysed using conventional laparoscopy. After the upper abdominal portion is performed, the robotic apparatus is side docked on the patient's left side, using the supraumbilical port for the camera and the bilateral robotic 8-mm ports. The posterior parietal peritoneum over the right common iliac is incised and retroperitoneal dissection is completed cephalad to above inferior mesenteric artery. We use the electrosurgical spatula or scissors as a cutting modality and bipolar forceps for achieving hemostasis. The left and right upper assist ports are utilized for introduction of ancillary instruments for traction, tissue removal, as well as suction and irrigation. After para-aortic lymphadenectomy is completed, pelvic lymphadenectomy, hysterectomy, bilateral salpingo-oophorectomy, and any pelvic tumor debulking are performed (Fig. 3). The same

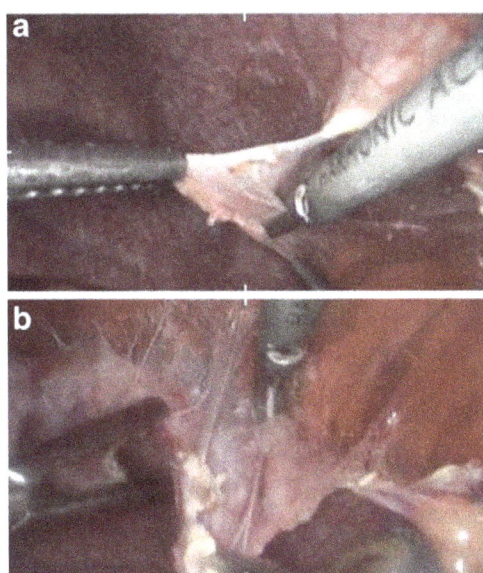

Fig. 2 a Diaphragmatic stripping of peritoneum with grasper and Harmonic scalpel (Ethicon Endosurgery, Cincinnati, OH, USA). b Diaphragmatic stripping showing stripped-away peritoneum and the underlying muscle fibers

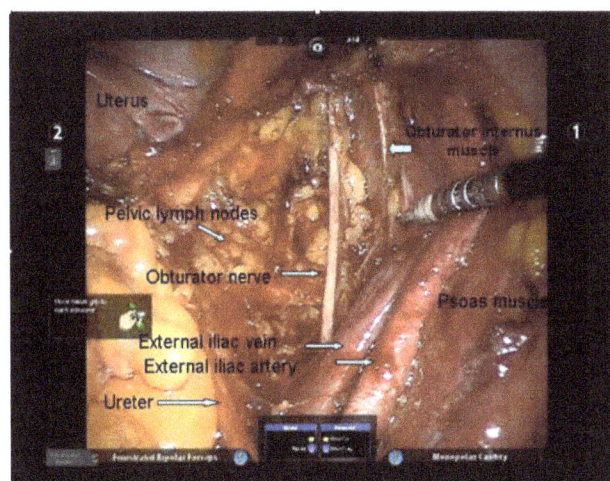

Fig. 3 Right pelvic sidewall exposing the iliac vessels and obturator fossa for robotic-assisted laparoscopic pelvic lymphadenectomy

instrumentation utilized is as before, or at times, standard blood vessel sealing devices such as the LigaSure(Covidien, Boulder, CO, USA), etc. can be employed for ligation of the infundibular ligaments and performing hysterectomy. If access to the para-aortic lymph nodes above the inferior–mesenteric artery is not possible using the robotic platform setup, this portion of the operation is performed using a conventional laparoscopic approach after undocking the robot or the camera is moved from supraumbilical port to the right upper quadrant one. After the uterus is transected, it is removed from the vagina along with the omentum and any other specimens, which are confined to a laparoscopic specimen bag. The vaginal cuff is closed in two layers. After complete hemostasis is achieved, the robotic apparatus is undocked.

Bowel resections can be performed with conventional laparoscopy and robotically using the appropriate port and robot placement. In case of the need for mid-abdominal debulking, such as appendectomy or ileocecal resection, mobilization of the bowel is performed using the robotic platform, and appendectomy or bowel resection is performed using a stapling device introduced in the right upper abdominal port. Anastomosis can be performed either in situ or extracorporeally by extending the supraumbilical incision after pelvic tumor debulking and undocking the robot. This approach can be utilized for segmental transverse colon resection and reanastomosis to achieve optimal cytoreduction to no visible disease. For rectosigmoid colon resection and anastomosis, we use a 12-mm port in the right lower abdomen for introduction of the stapling device. This is especially true for a bulky lesion involving the rectosigmoid colon. Using a laparoscopic 60 mm GIA stapler, a rectosigmoid resection can be performed proximally and distally. Once the proximal sigmoid colon is appropriately mobilized, this end can be brought out through a widened incision in the right lower quadrant, lower middle incision, or transvaginally along with the specimen. An anvil can then be placed and secured with a purse string suture. The anvil and proximal sigmoid colon is then brought back into the pelvis and an end-to-end anastomosis can be performed with an end-to-end anastomosis stapler passed through the rectum. Once the device is properly activated, it is important to test the integrity of the anastomosis. This can be accomplished by clamping the proximal colon with a bowel grasper, filling the pelvis with saline, and insufflating the rectum with air while observing laparoscopically. The anastomosis can be alternatively or additionally examined by filling the rectum with indigo carmine and observing for leakage. Cystoscopy is routinely performed to ensure that there is no damage to the bladder or ureters. Ports are removed and port sites are closed in a routine manner.

In the case of recurrences that occur primarily in the upper abdomen, debulking can be performed with the robotic apparatus. In this situation, after exploratory laparoscopy and peritoneal washings are performed using conventional laparoscopy, the robot is side docked from above the patient on the right side using the same port placement as above (Fig. 1) and instrumentation is as described previously.

Results

There were 20 women that underwent 21 surgical procedures for the management of early, advanced, and recurrent ovarian, fallopian tube, or peritoneal cancer using our hybrid technique of conventional laparoscopy and RALS. There were 10 surgical procedures performed for early stage disease and 11 for advanced and/or recurrent disease (six advanced and five recurrent). The early group consisted of three cases that were stage IA (Table 1; cases 1–3), six that were stage IC (Table 1; cases 4–9), and one case that was stage IIC (Table 1, case 10). The advanced and recurrent group consisted of seven cases that were advanced, with six cases that were stage IIIC (Table 2: cases 1,2,3,5,7 and 11), one case that was stage IV (Table 2: case 4). The remainder in this group had recurrent disease (Table 2: cases 6,8,9, 10). There were no conversions to laparotomy in either group.

Of the 10 surgeries for early stage disease, the mean age was 42.3 years (range, 29–55), average BMI was 32.1 kg/m^2 (range, 17–65 kg/m^2), average estimated blood loss (EBL) was 212.5 ml (range, 50–1,000 mL), surgical time was 306.1 min (range, 87–639), and average length of stay (LOS) was 1.6 days (range, 1–2). In this group, the surgical procedures performed included five hysterectomies, eight oophorectomies, one cystectomy, eight omentectomies, five pelvic lymph node dissections (average, 10.3; range, 5–18), four para-aortic lymph node dissections (average, 8.6; range, 3–12), four appendectomies, and seven upper abdominal and diaphragmatic biopsies. None of these patients were upstaged after surgical and pathological staging.

There were no intraoperative complications or intraoperative transfusions, and two grade 1 postoperative complications. One patient was readmitted on postoperative day 9 with a wound infection. The other was readmitted with fever of unknown origin that resolved with IV antibiotics.

Three patients in this group underwent fertility sparing surgery (Table 1; cases 6, 8, and 9) [14]. In the first case listed (Table 1), the para-aortic lymphadenectomy was performed laparoscopically as there was difficulty with adequate visualization when the robotic apparatus was docked. Four patients in the early ovarian cancer group had prior surgical intervention and presented for restaging (Table 1; cases 3, 5, 8, and 9). Two patients in this group did not have an omentectomy (Table 1; cases 2 and 6). Case 2 was a double primary that was initially staged for endometrial cancer with final pathology that showed ovarian cancer as a second primary. Case 6 presented for restaging, after prior left salpingo-oophorectomy and staging.

Table 1 Early stage ovarian cancer cases

Case	Age	BMI	Procedure		Pathology	EBL	ORT	LOS	Complications
			Laparoscopic	Robotic					
1	52	17	Infracolic omentectomy, para-aortic lymphadenectomy, diaphragmatic biopsy, right upper abdominal peritoneal biopsy, peritoneal washings	LAVH, left oophorectomy, pelvic lymphadenectomy, appendectomy, peritoneal biopsies	Grade 3 serous carcinoma of the fallopian tube	200	n/a	2	None
2	53	21	Exploratory laparoscopy, peritoneal washings	Pelvic and para-aortic lymphadenectomy, hysterectomy, BSO	Grade 3 endometrioid adenocarcinoma of the ovary	150	366	2	None
3	54	40	Infracolic omentectomy, peritoneal biopsies, diaphragmatic biopsy and upper abdominal peritoneal biopsies, peritoneal washings	Lysis of extensive small bowel and pelvic adhesions, bilateral pelvic lymphadenectomy, peritoneal biopsies, total hysterectomy	Grade 3 serous carcinoma of the ovary	150	361	2	Admission on POD#21 for FUO
4	38	25	Infracolic omentectomy, appendectomy, upper abdominal peritoneal biopsies, peritoneal washings	Para-aortic lymphadenectomy, pelvic lymphadenectomy, hysterectomy, LSO, peritoneal biopsies	Mucinous low malignant potential tumor of the ovary	100	338	2	Wound infection
5	55	27	Upper abdominal peritoneal biopsies, peritoneal washings	Infracolic omentectomy, hysterectomy, LSO	Serous low malignant potential tumor of the ovary	50	178	1	None
6	34	23	Upper abdominal biopsies, peritoneal washings	Pelvic and para-aortic lymphadenectomy, RSO, peritoneal biopsies, lysis of pelvic adhesions	Grade 3 mucinous adenocarcinoma of the ovary	125	271	1	None
7	30	53	Infracolic omentectomy, peritoneal washings	Right ovarian cystectomy, resection of pelvic endometriosis, appendectomy, myomectomy, peritoneal biopsies	Serous low malignant potential tumor of the ovary	50	87	1	None
8	29	22	Infracolic omentectomy, resection of diaphragmatic lesions, peritoneal biopsies, peritoneal washings	Resection of pelvic lesions, LSO, peritoneal biopsies, LOA	Grade 2 immature ovarian teratoma	200	172	1	None
9	31	28	Infracolic omentectomy, diaphragmatic biopsies, upper abdominal peritoneal biopsies, peritoneal washings	LSO, resection of pelvic lesions and endometriosis, pelvic and para-aortic lymphadenectomy, peritoneal biopsies, LOA	Grade 2 endometrioid adenocarcinoma of the ovary	100	343	1	None
10	47	65	Infracolic omentectomy	Radical hysterectomy, BSO, tumor debulking, resection of endometriosis, appendectomy, peritoneal biopsies, , extensive LOA	Grade 1 endometrioid adenocarcinoma of the ovary	1000	639	3	None

BMI body mass index, *EBL* estimated blood loss, *ORT* operating room time, *LOS* length of stay, *LAVH* laparoscopic-assisted vaginal hysterectomy, *BSO* bilateral salpingo-oophorectomy, *LSO* left salpingo-oophorectomy, *D&C* dilation and curettage, *POD* postoperative day, *LOA* lysis of adhesions

Table 2 Advanced and recurrent ovarian cancer cases

Case	Age	BMI	Disease status	Procedure Laparoscopic	Robotic	Other	Pathology	Status of cytoreduction	EBL	ORT	LOS	Complications
1	92	24.7	Advanced	Total omentectomy, lysis of extensive adhesions, enterolysis	Hysterectomy, BSO, pelvic tumor debulking	Cystoscopy	Grade 3 serous carcinoma of the fallopian tube	Optimal to no visible disease	200	362	2	None
2	54	37.2	Advanced	Total omentectomy, lysis of pelvic and upper abdominal adhesions	Hysterectomy, BSO, resection of pelvic implants	Cystoscopy	Grade 3 serous carcinoma, primary peritoneal	Optimal to no visible disease	100	306	2	None
3	50	36.2	Advanced	Total omentectomy, upper abdominal tumor debulking including tumor of hepatic flexure, and transverse colon, diaphragmatic stripping and ablation, appendectomy	Hysterectomy, BSO, pelvic tumor debulking, metastatic lymph node debulking	Cystoscopy, sigmoidoscopy	Grade 3 serous carcinoma of the ovary	Optimal to no visible disease	20	103	3	None
4	75	29.3	Advanced	Total omentectomy, diaphragmatic biopsy	Hysterectomy, BSO, resection of pelvic tumor metastasis, anterior and posterior cul de sac tumor debulking and culdectomy, resection of rectal tumor	Cystoscopy, sigmoidoscopy, inguinal lymph node dissection	Grade 3 serous carcinoma of the ovary	Optimal to no visible disease	400	477	6	None
5	70	27	Advanced	Supracolic omentectomy, upper abdominal and diaphragmatic debulking	Tumor debulking of anterior cul-de-sac and rectosigmoid, hysterectomy, LOA, enterolysis, peritoneal biopsies	Cystoscopy sling procedure	Grade 3 serous carcinoma of the ovary	Optimal to no visible disease	150	454	17	Bowel perforation
6	55	29.1	Recurrent	Aspiration of ascites, lysis of adhesions, enterolysis	Appendectomy, para-aortic lymphadenectomy, tumor debulking		Grade 3 clear cell carcinoma of the ovary	Optimal to no visible disease	100	252	1	None
7	53	32.9	Recurrent	Diaphragmatic biopsy (second look)	Pelvic and para-aortic lymphadenectomy, lysis of adhesions, peritoneal biopsies.	Cystoscopy	Grade 3 serous carcinoma of the ovary	N/A	100	226	2	None
8	39	25	Recurrent	Peritoneal biopsies, diaphragmatic biopsy, aspiration of ascites, upper abdominal tumor and diaphragmatic tumor debulking	Pelvic tumor debulking, lysis of adhesions.	Cystoscopy, sigmoidoscopy, insertion of IP port	Grade 1 mucinous adenocarcinoma of the ovary	Optimal to less than 0.5 cm	100	317	3	port-site cellulitis, peritoneal vaginal fistula

Table 2 (continued)

Case	Age	BMI	Disease status	Procedure Laparoscopic	Robotic	Other	Pathology	Status of cytoreduction	EBL	ORT	LOS	Complications
9	70	35.4	Recurrent	Omentectomy, appendectomy	Lysis of extensive pelvic adhesions, upper vaginectomy, pelvic tumor debulking, peritoneal biopsies	Cystoscopy	Grade 3 serous carcinoma of the ovary	Optimal to no visible disease	100	212	1	None
10	63	27.5	Recurrent	Lysis of severe upper abdominal adhesions, resection of porta hepatis mass, cholecystectomy, supracolic omentectomy	Pelvic and para-aortic lymphadenectomy, lysis of adhesions, peritoneal biopsies	Cystoscopy	Grade 3 serous carcinoma of the ovary	Optimal to no visible disease	50	322	3	None
11	82	22.1	Advanced	Infracolic omentectomy	Hysterectomy, BSO, bilateral pelvic lymphadenectomy, appendectomy	Cystoscopy	Grade 3 serous carcinoma of the ovary	Optimal to no visible disease	100	238	2	None

BMI body mass index, EBL estimated blood loss, ORT operating room time, LOS length of stay, BSO bilateral salpingo-oopherectomy, IP port intraperitoneal port, FIGO International Federation of Gynecology and Obstetrics

Among the 11 cases operated for advanced and/or recurrent ovarian cancer, the mean age was 63.9 years (range, 39–92), average BMI was 29.7 kg/m^2 (range, 22.1–37.2), EBL was 129.1 ml (range, 20–400), operating room time was 238 min (range, 103–477), and LOS was 3.8 days (range, 1–17). In this group, surgical procedures consisted of six hysterectomies, five oophorectomies, eight omentectomies, three pelvic lymph node dissections (average, 10.7; range, 4–18), three para-aortic lymph node dissections (average, 5; range, 1–9), four appendectomies, five diaphragmatic biopsies, four upper abdominal debulking or diaphragmatic debulking, and one resection of a porta hepatis mass (Table 2; case 10; Fig. 4). Five patients had received neoadjuvant chemotherapy (Table 2; cases 2, 3, 4, 5, and 11). Of the 11 procedures, there was one second look (Table 2, case 7), 9 were cytoreduced to no visible disease and 1 to less than <0.5 cm. There were no intraoperative complications.

There were three postoperative complications; two were grade 1 and one was grade 3. Two complications (both grade 1) occurred in the same patient; one being port-site cellulitis and the other a peritoneal vaginal fistula. Both were managed conservatively with antibiotic therapy and observation. The peritoneal vaginal fistula was revealed by leakage of peritoneal ascites. The other patient was reoperated on postoperative day 3 for a sigmoid colon perforation which required reoperation and was discharged home on day 17 (Table 2; case 5). This case was the only Intensive Care Unit admission in both early and advanced groups.

Of all the patients operated on, there were no trocar site metastases within the follow-up period. However, one patient developed trocar metastasis beyond 30 days postoperatively and had recurrent intraperitoneal disease.

Discussion

Laparoscopy offers multiple advantages over laparotomy such as better visualization, smaller incisions, shorter hospital

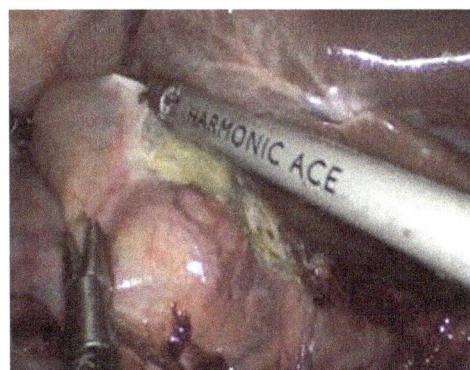

Fig. 4 Porta hepatis mass attached to the gallbladder that has been resected laparoscopically, with cholecystectomy

stays, decreased blood loss, less need for analgesics, more rapid recovery, and shorter interval to chemotherapy and radiation when indicated. In the assessment of an adnexal mass and early-stage ovarian cancer, laparoscopy can be both diagnostic and therapeutic. The combination of laparoscopic visualization and frozen section analysis is the most reliable method for the detection of malignancy [15]. Once malignancy is diagnosed, comprehensive surgical staging can be performed laparoscopically, which has been shown to be feasible, safe, and accurate in tumors of low malignant potential and invasive early-stage disease [16–19]. Furthermore, in select cases of localized disease, it can be used to perform fertility-sparing surgical staging [14].

Minimally invasive surgery has emerged as an option in the management of advanced or recurrent ovarian cancer with multiple applications that have been presented in the literature [5, 20–22]. This includes a triage tool for resectability, primary and secondary cytoreduction, second-look evaluation, and placement of intraperitoneal catheters for chemotherapy [23].

In the early 1990s, the pioneers of laparoscopic surgery applied minimally invasive surgical techniques to gynecologic cancers for the staging of early and select cases of advanced or recurrent ovarian cancer cytoreduction [24, 25]. Since that time, the role of minimally invasive surgery in gynecologic oncology has been continuously expanding and has even been further applied to other disease sites in the female genital tract.

The advent of computer enhanced telesurgery or robotic-assisted surgery has seemingly presented itself as a new alternative to conventional laparoscopy. It offers the benefits of improving the learning curve associated with conventional laparoscopy, and other additional features, such as optimal visualization and a wider range of motion for more precise surgical manipulation. Yet, this innovation currently presents with limitations in the surgical management of patients with malignancy. Conventional laparoscopy offers a better understanding of the status of the disease, while robotic-assisted laparoscopy presents as an innovation in offering precise surgical motion and visualization of the disease process. However, this comes at the cost of some key elements required with surgical management, which are possible with conventional laparoscopy.

One such limitation is the lack of haptics, which may lead to missing tumor entirely or the ability to discern between normal tissue and tissue that is involved with carcinoma. Further limitations are in accessing all four abdominal quadrants simultaneously in one surgical setting and completing comprehensive surgical evaluation and treatment for patients with ovarian malignancy. This hybrid technique is presented to overcome these challenges, and the limited manipulation that exists with robotic-assisted surgery with the current platform. This is particularly true with limitations encountered when manipulating bulky tumor and tissue, such as that of the rectosigmoid with the present robotic platform and instruments.

The hybrid technique described offers advantages that are inherent to conventional laparoscopy for management of ovarian cancer. One limitation is the need for a second setup of a conventional laparoscopy in addition to the robotic platform. In our experience, it is customary to use this setup as an adjunct to robotic-assisted surgery. Conventional laparoscopy is used for port placement, in preparation of robotic-assisted laparoscopic surgery, thus making this setup not an additional component. Thus, using this method offers an extension of the use of conventional laparoscopy, while retaining the same port setup for pelvic surgery and utilizing conventional laparoscopy to operate cephalad to the pelvis.

Another inherent benefit is that conventional laparoscopy can also be used as an initial checkpoint in triaging for resectability based on the extent of disease and surgeon experience with robotic-assisted surgery versus other conventional methods. The conventional laparoscopy setup can also be further utilized after completion of robotic-assisted surgery to survey the abdomen and pelvis for any potential injury caused by the robotic instruments not detected due to the blind spot of the robotic camera and lack of haptics. Studies are lacking with innovative methods or strategies to counter this limitation of upper abdominal access with pelvic surgery when using the robotic platform. With advanced laparoscopic skills, this method facilitates the limitations of the robotic platform. An added advantage of using this method is enhanced visualization of surgical planes that require fine dissection in the pelvis due to prior surgery or disease involvement in the pelvis. In the upper abdomen, conventional laparoscopic methods can be utilized for limited disease, with this as the initial portion of the surgery, thus reducing surgeon fatigue (of the primary surgeon).

This technique also extends to novice surgeons who are aided by tactile feedback that conventional laparoscopy extends. However, it has its limitations in more challenging skills that are more easily afforded with robotic assistance (i.e., suturing, controlling bleeding, etc.). In comparison to other described techniques for accessing the upper abdomen, this method is less cumbersome and can be used in settings with residency and fellowship training programs that have bedside assistants who are less experienced. One complication reported with use of the alternate technique of placing the robot tower at the patient's head was conversion to laparotomy in order to access bleeding from the descending branch of the inferior mesenteric artery that could not be reached by the bedside assistant or the surgeon [9]. The access afforded in operating cephalad with use of this technique is not hindered in our experience. This technique has widespread application for use, and is versatile with the level of experience required by surgical assistants.

Minimally invasive surgical staging, more specifically cytoreductive surgery, are time-consuming procedures that are associated with surgeon fatigue that ensues with the course of the procedure. This method offers the benefit of conventional laparoscopy at the beginning of the case followed by the robotic-assisted portion of the procedure, which can help in the reduction of surgeon fatigue during the course of these lengthy procedures. This is an added benefit when the skill of an expert laparoscopist is needed for challenging initial portions of the procedure in the upper abdomen and then for more difficult portions with pelvic disease site affection in the latter portion of the procedure.

One issue that has to be addressed is the cost-effectiveness of the initial investment in the robotic platform relative to the cost of performing laparotomy, conventional laparoscopy, or robotic hybrid technique. Although only well-designed randomized studies will be able to adequately address this issue, presently, it is rather difficult to establish such a study in early and advanced ovarian cancer. In Wright et al. [26], the cost of robotic-assisted radical hysterectomy was least expensive comparative to laparotomy and even laparoscopy, due to shorter hospital stay. We believe that the use of this modality will allow more patients to be managed by a minimally invasive approach and thus reduce the number of laparotomies.

In summary, minimally invasive surgical techniques are consistently furthered from conventional laparoscopy to computer-enhanced telesurgery (also known as robotic surgery), and eventually to more compact devices that provide greater surgical precision with versatility in accessing all four abdominal quadrants more readily. Our technique serves as an interim improvisation to counter the limitations that exist with the present robotic platform.

Successful maximum cytoreductive interperitoneal metastatic disease in advanced ovarian cancer has been associated with the best outcomes [23]. However, this technique is not always possible and it carries significant morbidity. In randomized clinical trials, neoadjuvant chemotherapy followed by cytoreductive surgery has been shown much more effective in decreasing morbidity without compromising oncological outcomes [13]. Another benefit of neoadjuvant chemotherapy is that by reducing the bulky tumor, the chance of achieving optimal cytoreductive surgery by minimally invasive approach is greatly increased.

It has been our experience that using this hybrid technique, of a combination of conventional laparoscopy and the present robotic platform has been effective in the management of early, advanced, and recurrent ovarian, fallopian tube and peritoneal cancer while gaining the advantages of both technical approaches.

References

1. Sternchos J, Finger T, Mahdavi A, Nezhat F (2013) Laparoscopic management of ovarian, fallopian tube and primary peritoneal cancer. In: Nezhat C, Nezhat F, Nezhat C (eds) Nezhat's video-assisted and robotic-assisted laparoscopy and hysteroscopy, 4th edn. Cambridge University Press, Cambridge, pp 508–525
2. Nezhat FR, Shoma D, Liu C, Chuang L, Zakashansky K (2008) Robotic radical hysterectomy versus total laparoscopic radical hysterectomy with pelvic lymphadenectomy for treatment of early cervical cancer. JSLS 12:227–237
3. Cho JE, Nezhat FR (2009) Robotics and gynecologic oncology: review of the literature. J Minim Invasive Gynecol 16(6):669–681
4. Lim PC, Kang E, Park DH (2011) A comparative detail analysis of the learning curve and surgical outcome for robotic hysterectomy with lymphadenectomy versus laparoscopic hysterectomy with lymphadenectomy in treatment of endometrial cancer: a case-matched controlled study of the first one hundred twenty-two patients. Gynecol Oncol 120:413–418
5. Magrina JF, Zanagnolo V, Noble BN et al (2011) Robotic approach for ovarian cancer: perioperative and survival results and comparison with laparoscopy and laparotomy. Gynecol Oncol 121(1):100–105
6. Ramirez PT, Adams S, Boggess JF, Burke WM, Frumovitz MM, Gardner GJ, Havrilesky LJ, Holloway R, Lowe MP, Magrina JF, Moore DH, Soliman PT, Yap S (2012) Robotic-assisted surgery in gynecologic oncology: a Society of Gynecologic Oncology consensus statement. Developed by the Society of Gynecologic Oncology's Clinical Practice Robotics Task Force. Gynecol Oncol 124(2):180–184
7. Siegel R, Deepa N, Ahmedin AJ (2012) Cancer statistics 2012. Cancer J 62(10):10–29
8. Katz VL, Lentz GM, Lobo RA, Gershenson DM (2007) Comprehensive gynecology, 5th edn. Elsevier, Philadelphia
9. Magrina JF, Long JB, Kho RM et al (2010) Robotic transperitoneal infrarenal aortic lymphadenectomy. Int J Gynecol Cancer 20(1):184–187
10. Dindo D, Demartines N, Clavien PA (2004) Classification of surgical complications: a new proposal with evaluation in a cohort of a 6336 patients and results of a survey. Ann Surg 240:205–213
11. Nezhat FR, Denoble SM, Cho JE, Brown DN, Soto E, Chuang L, Gretz H, Saharia P (2012) The safety and efficacy of video laparoscopic surgical debulking of recurrent ovarian, fallopian tube, and primary peritoneal cancers. JSLS 16:511–518
12. Nezhat FR, DeNoble SM, Liu CS, Cho JE, Brown DN, Chuang L, Gretz H, Saharia P (2010) The safety and efficacy of laparoscopic surgical staging and debulking of apparent advanced stage ovarian, fallopian tube, and primary peritoneal cancers. JSLS 14:155–168
13. Vergote I, Tropè C, Amant F et al (2010) Neoadjuvant chemotherapy or primary surgery in stage IIIC and IV ovarian cancer. N Engl J Med 363:943–953
14. Finger T, Nezhat F (2013) Robotic-assisted fertility sparing surgery for early ovarian cancer. JSLS (in press)
15. Nezhat F, Nezhat C, Welander CE, Benigno B (1992) Four ovarian cancers diagnosed during laparoscopic management of 1011 women with adnexal masses. Am J Obstet Gynecol 167:790–796
16. Liu CS, Nagarsheth NP, Nezhat FR (2009) Laparoscopy and ovarian cancer: a paradigm change in the management of ovarian cancer? J Min Inv Gynecol 16(3):250–262

17. Park JY, Bae J, Lim MC, Lim SY, Seo SS, Kang S et al (2008) Laparoscopic and laparotomic staging in stage I epithelial ovarian cancer: a comparison of feasibility and safety. Int J Gynecol Cancer 18:1202–1209

18. Tozzi R, Kohler C, Ferrara A, Schneider A (2004) Laparoscopic treatment of early ovarian cancer: surgical and survival outcomes. Gynecol Oncol 93:199–203

19. Nezhat FR, Ezzati M, Chuang L, Shamshirsaz AA, Rahaman J, Gretz H (2009) Laparoscopic management of early ovarian and fallopian tube cancers: surgical and survival outcome. Am J Obstet Gynecol 200(1):e1–e6

20. Nezhat FR, Datta MS, Lal N (2008) Laparoscopic cytoreduction for primary advanced or recurrent ovarian, fallopian tube, and peritoneal malignancies. Gynecol Oncol 108:S60

21. Fanning J, Yacoub E, Hojat R (2011) Laparoscopic-assisted cytoreduction for primary ovarian cancer: success, morbidity and survival. Gynecol Oncol 123:47–49

22. Krivak TC, Elkas JC, Rose GS, Sundborg M, Winter WE, Carlson J, MacKoul PJ (2005) The utility of hand-assisted laparoscopy in ovarian cancer. Gynecol Oncol 96:72–76

23. Nezhat F, Lavie O (2013) The role of minimally invasive surgery in ovarian cancer. Int J Gynecol Cancer 23(5):782–783

24. Querleu D, Leblanc E (1994) Laparoscopic infrarenal para-aortic lymph node dissection for restaging of carcinoma of the ovary or fallopian tube. Cancer 73:1467–1471

25. Amara DP, Nezhat C, Teng N, Nezhat F, Nezhat C, Rosati M (1996) Operative laparoscopy in the management of ovarian cancer. Surg Laparoscop Endosc 6:38–45

26. Wright JD, Herzog TJ, Neugut AI et al (2012) Comparative effectiveness of minimally invasive and abdominal radical hysterectomy for cervical cancer. Gynecol Oncol 127:11–17

2

Laparoscopic management of an 11-week rudimentary uterine horn pregnancy using extracorporeal Roeder knot to secure the dilated vascular pedicle

Vasileios Minas · Elizabeth Shaw · Thomas Aust

Abstract Pregnancy in a uterine rudimentary horn carries a high risk of uterine rupture with severe and potentially lethal intra-abdominal haemorrhage. There is now growing evidence that this condition can be safely managed by minimally invasive surgery. We report a case of an unruptured 11-week rudimentary horn pregnancy that was diagnosed and treated laparoscopically. We have performed a literature review using PubMed, Embase and Cochrane Database of Systematic Reviews to identify relevant cases and draw conclusions with regards to their management. We have collated 20 published cases of rudimentary horn pregnancies that were managed by laparoscopy. The surgical technique appears consistent among these cases with few variations. In advanced gestations, feticide may need to be performed. Morcellation has been shown to be possible without compromising patient safety from trophoblast spill. The possibility of uncommon presentations such as duplicated or absent ureter should be taken into account. Extracorporeal Roeder knot can be used safely to secure unusually dilated vascular pedicles. Overall, laparoscopy appears to be as safe as and potentially superior to laparotomy for the management of rudimentary horn pregnancies.

Keywords Rudimentary horn pregnancy · Uterine malformations · Laparoscopy · Extracorporeal knot

V. Minas (✉) · E. Shaw · T. Aust
Minimal Access Centre, Department of Obstetrics and Gynaecology, Wirral University Teaching Hospital, Arrowe Park Rd, Wirral, Merseyside CH49 5PE, UK
e-mail: billminas@gmail.com

Introduction

A rudimentary uterine horn results from incomplete embryological development of one of the two Müllerian duct systems. More than 500 cases of rudimentary horn pregnancies (RHPs) have been reported to date [1]. This is a rare form of ectopic pregnancy with reported incidence that ranges from 1:76,000 to 1:140,000 pregnancies [1]. The natural course of such pregnancies is rupture either in the first or mid-second trimester. Only 10 % reaches a term with a fetal survival rate ranging from 0 to 13 % and maternal mortality rates up to 0.5 % [1, 2]. Accurate diagnosis and appropriate management are therefore crucial to prevent risk to the mother from the current and future pregnancies.

Case report

A 29-year-old woman, with one previous normal delivery at term, presented to our unit for her routine dating ultrasound scan (USS). She was amenorrhoeic for 12 weeks and had a positive urine pregnancy test. Trans-abdominal and trans-vaginal USS revealed an 11^{+6}-week live extra-uterine pregnancy (Fig. 1). We suspected either a RHP or an abdominal pregnancy, and plans were made for a laparoscopy to accurately diagnose the location of the pregnancy and potentially remove it at the same time. At laparoscopy, a left RHP was diagnosed (Fig. 2). A small band of fibromuscular tissue approximately 3-cm long and 0.5-cm thick was seen connecting the rudimentary horn with the uterus. There was no hemoperitoneum. A decision to proceed with horn excision was made. The rudimentary horn was excised intact using a combination of LigaSure™ (Valleylab, Colorado, USA) and extracorporeal knot tying (Roeder knots) (Biosyn 1 suture) [3] (Fig. 2). The course of the left ureter was first identified. A left salpingectomy was performed to prevent future ipsilateral

Fig. 1 Ultrasonographic findings of the presented case. **a** Transabdominal ultrasound showing an extra-uterine live pregnancy of 11^{+6}-week gestational age. **b** Transvaginal ultrasound scan confirming the above findings. *u* uterus, *f* fetus

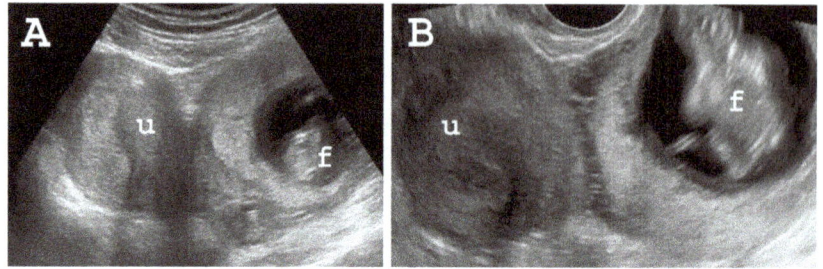

tubal ectopic pregnancies. The left round ligament was then transected, and the anterior leaf of the broad ligament and the bladder were dissected off the uterine horn. A fenestration was made to the posterior leaf of the left broad ligament and used to pass a suture and tie an extracorporeal Roeder knot around the large dilated vessels of the ovarian ligament pedicle. The pedicle was secured with two ties, and the rudimentary horn was thus separated from the left ovary. The remaining fibromuscular connection between the rudimentary horn and the unicornuate uterus was secured with a Roeder knot and

Fig. 2 Intra-operative findings and procedures: **a, b** A left RHP was diagnosed at laparoscopy. The structures associated with the rudimentary horn (left ovary, fallopian tube and round ligament) were identified. **c** A fibromuscular band of tissue connecting the rudimentary horn with the unicornuate uterus was seen (the probe is resting on the tissue). **d** A left salpingectomy is done. **e** The round ligament (*black arrow*) is transected, and the anterior leaf of the broad ligament and bladder flap are dissected. A fenestration was made in the posterior leaf of the broad ligament. **f** The ovarian ligament is seen containing large dilated vessels of approximately 15–20 mm in diameter. The pedicle is tied with extracorporeal Roeder knot and transected. **g, h** The connection between the rudimentary horn and the unicornuate uterus is tied with an extracorporeal knot, and the horn is finally separated (the knot is secured with a knot pusher). *r* round ligament, *f* fallopian tube, *o* ovary, *rh* rudimentary horn, *u* unicornuate uterus

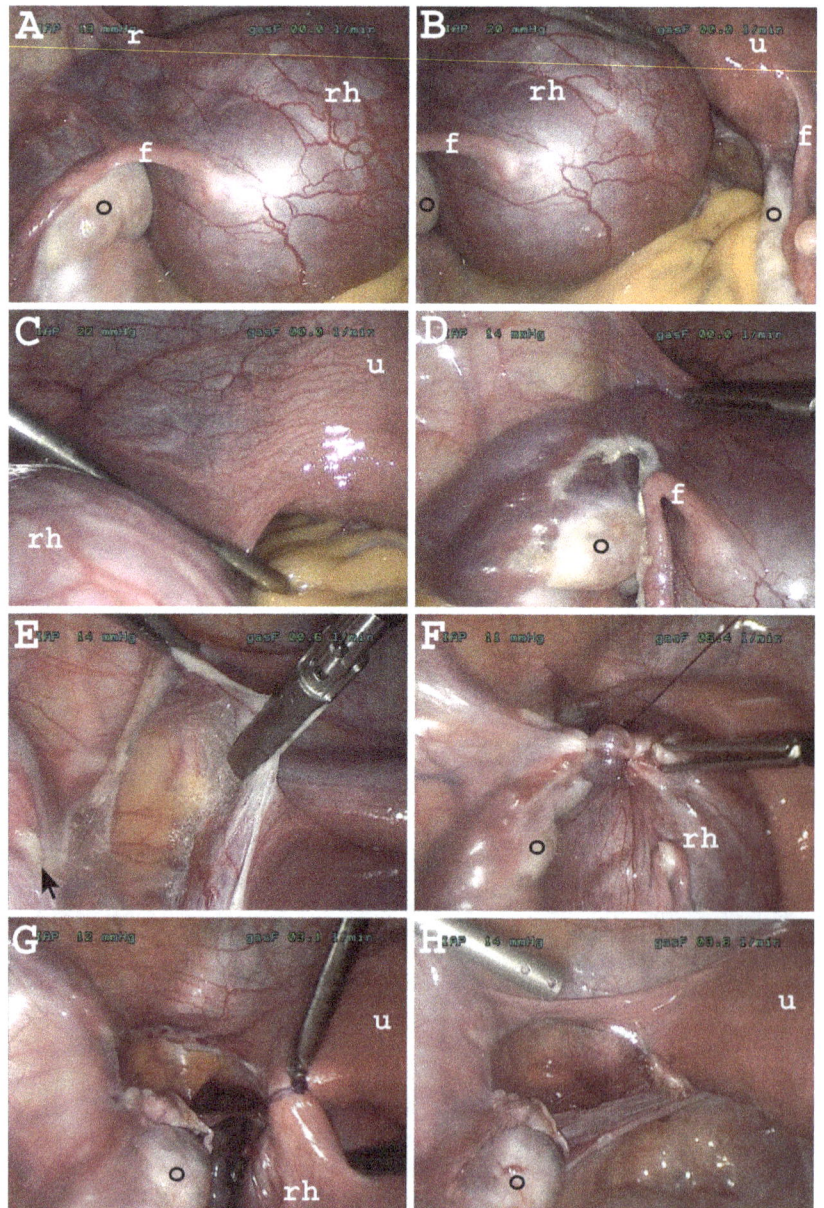

transected with LigaSure™ to complete the horn excision. The suprapubic laparoscopic incision was extended to 3 cm, and the specimen was extracted in a nylon bag. At the conclusion of the procedure, a hysteroscopy was performed which revealed a normal vagina, single cervix with a single cervical canal leading to a right-sided non-gravid unicornuate uterus with no communication with the rudimentary horn. The procedure took 57 min. Estimated blood loss was less than 50 ml, and the patient went home on the first post-operative day.

Discussion

Women with a unicornuate uterus associated with a rudimentary horn may experience various pregnancy and non-pregnancy-related complications. These include endometriosis, hematometra, infertility, recurrent miscarriages, uterine rupture and abnormally adherent placenta [4]. Renal tract anomalies also occur in 38 % of such patients [5]. Pregnancies occurring in non-communicating rudimentary horns are thought to result from transperitoneal migration of either spermatozoa or the fertilized ovum which reaches the peritoneal cavity via the contralateral tube [6].

The diagnosis of RHP can be difficult. Jurkovic et al. reported an USS sensitivity for the diagnosis of RHP of 26 % [7]. Subsequently, other authors have attempted, through short series of cases, to develop specific USS criteria to facilitate preoperative diagnosis [8]. A recent literature review showed that only 5 % of the reported RHPs were diagnosed pre-operatively [9], whereas our search of laparoscopically managed RHP revealed that 9/20 (45 %) were confidently diagnosed pre-operatively. Jihong et al. reported that their case was misdiagnosed by USS as missed miscarriage at 5, 7 and 8 weeks of gestational age. An endometrial curettage was eventually performed that yielded no pregnancy tissue. They finally diagnosed a RHP at 12 weeks by laparoscopy, following a repeat USS which suggested a tubal ectopic pregnancy [10]. In the present case, our differential diagnosis pre-operatively included both abdominal pregnancy and RHP, and we conclusively diagnosed the RHP at laparoscopy. Missed diagnoses at laparoscopy have also been reported. A case of a 16-week ruptured RHP was initially thought to be an intra-uterine pregnancy developing in a bicornuate uterus at laparoscopy performed at 7 weeks for abdominal pain [11]. Magnetic resonance imaging (MRI) can help differentiate between a RHP and a pregnancy in a bicornuate uterus which can be potentially viable [9].

Due to the thin and poorly developed myometrium, most RHPs rupture between 10 and 20 weeks of gestational age [2]. Therefore, once diagnosed, management of such pregnancies includes excision of the rudimentary horn together with the ipsilateral fallopian tube to prevent future ectopic pregnancies [15]. Similarly, planned removal of rudimentary horns is advised when those are diagnosed pre-pregnancy in women who desire future pregnancies [12].

The majority of reported RHPs (>97 %) have been managed by laparotomy. That is usually due to either lack of advanced laparoscopic skills by the involved surgeons or because the clinicians encountered a haemodynamically unstable patient with a ruptured horn. We have collated 20 reported RHPs which have been managed laparoscopically in Table 1 (including the current case). A number of different instruments have been used to achieve excision of the rudimentary horn, including bipolar forceps and scissors, LigaSure™, Harmonic® scalpels, Endoloops® and stapling devices. The surgical technique is consistent among most of these reports and includes the steps described in our case. Few variations have been reported. Yan injected vasopressin into the fibromuscular band to reduce its vascularity prior to transection [13], whereas other authors used Endoloops® to secure their vascular pedicles [14].

We used extracorporeal Roeder knots to secure our vascular pedicles. This type of knot has been shown to be one of the strongest laparoscopic slip knots [15], and we have found it consistently safe when performing laparoscopic hysterectomies. The uterine blood supply in pregnancy rises gradually until the end of week 9 and thereafter rapidly with concomitant dilatation of the uterine vasculature [16]. In particular, in our case, the ovarian ligament was seen containing large dilated vessels with the whole pedicle measuring 20–25 mm in diameter (Fig. 2f). Therefore, suture ligation was preferred over coagulation.

When planning such a procedure, there are a few important points to be kept in mind. Pre-operative intravenous urography and/or intra-operative ureterolysis may be necessary particularly in cases associated with urinary tract malformations (such as ureteric duplication and absent kidney/ureter) or significant endometriosis [17]. Nevertheless, very few of the authors shown in Table 1 endorsed the above two measures. Still, the ureter must be confidently identified before the excision of the rudimentary horn [18]. An ipsilateral salpingectomy should be performed in all cases to prevent future tubal ectopic pregnancies [18]. The type of connection between the unicornuate uterus and the rudimentary horn must be defined [19]. Thin connections are relatively easy to deal with and can be transected either by coagulation or by suture ligation. In our case, we coagulated the uterine artery with bipolar diathermy and secured the connecting tissue pedicle with an extracorporeal Roeder knot. When the rudimentary horn is firmly attached to the unicornuate uterus, haemostasis may be more difficult. In these cases, the myometrium of the remaining uterus should be repaired by suturing following horn excision to reduce the risk of rupture in future pregnancies [20].

Table 1 Twenty cases of rudimentary horn pregnancies managed laparoscopically

author	Patient age (years)	Gestational age (weeks)	Parity	Imaging tools	Pre-operative diagnosis	Pre-operative rupture	Medical treatment	Horn excision technique	Tissue/fetus extraction technique
Dulemba et al (1996) (24)	26	13		USS	Right isthmic tubal pregnancy	no	no	Bipolar forceps	
Dicker et al (1998) (17)	31	8	P0	USS	Right cornual pregnancy	no	no	Bipolar forceps	15mm suprapubic incision
Yahata et al (1998) (25)	22	7	P0	USS	RHP/isthmic/cornual pregnancy	no	no	Stapling device	
Yoo et al (1999) (26)	23	8	P0	USS	RHP/tubal pregnancy	no	no	Bipolar forceps	Endobag through 11mm incision
Adolph and Gilliland (2002) (27)	25	6	P0	USS	Right RHP	no	no	Stapling device	Bag through 12mm incision
Edelman (2003) (22)	24	6	P0	USS; MRI	RHP	no	MTX		Morcellation
Chakravarti and Chin (2003) (28)	23	9		USS	Left adnexal pregnancy	no	no		
Cutner et al (2004) (23)	32	12	P0	3D USS	Right RHP	no	KCL;MTX; GnRHa	Harmonic scalpel; bipolar forceps	Morcellation
Cutner et al (2004) (23)	32		P0	USS; MRI	Right RHP	no	KCL;MTX; GnRHa	Harmonic scalpel; bipolar forceps	Morcellation
Sonmezer et al (2006) (20)	28	6	P0	USS	Right RHP	no	no	Bipolar forceps	Endobag through 10mm incision
Park and Dominguez (2007) (5)	36	8	P1	USS; MRI	Right RHP	no	KCL;MTX	LigaSure	Endobag through 10mm incision
Henriet et al (2008) (12)	28	7	P0	USS	Left RHP	no	no	Bipolar forceps	
Kadan and Romano (2008) (18)	37	11		USS	Left RHP	no	no	Bipolar forceps	Horn placed in Endobag, incised and contents suctioned; right incision slightly enlarged for extraction
Contreras et al (2008) (21)	27	19	P1	USS; CT	Abdominal/cornual pregnancy	no	no	Harmonic; Stapling device	Laparoscopic amnioreduction; Hand-assist port through 4cm suprapubic incision
Jihong et al (2009) (10)	27	5	P1	USS	USS at 5, 7 and 8 weeks → missed miscarriage; USS at 12 weeks → right adnexal pregnancy	no	no	Bipolar forceps; endoloop	
Szabo et al (2009) (29)	30	9							
Shahid et al (2010) (11)	33	16	P0	FAST USS	Ruptured ectopic pregnancy	yes (3 lt haemo-peritoneum)	no	Horn excised at later procedure; Harmonic scalpel and bipolar forceps used to extend rupture	Endobag through 3cm suprapubic incision (for fetus and placenta extraction)
Yan (2010) (13)	33	5	P1	USS	Right tubal pregnancy	no	no	Ultrasonic scalpel; bipolar forceps	Posterior colpotomy
Lennox et al (2013) (14)	28	16	P0	USS; MRI	Left RHP	no	KCL	Ligasure; endoloop	Morcellation; Endobag through 2.5cm lateral incision
Present case	29	11	P1	USS	RHP/abdominal pregnancy	no	no	Ligasure; extra-corporeal Roeder's knots	Endobag through 3cm suprapubic incision

The cases in grey shade represent second trimester pregnancies as opposed to the rest which are in the first trimester. Where information is lacking, the respective fields have been left blank. The case of Szabo et al. is published in Hungarian, and we were therefore unable to extract any information from the main text. *RHP* rudimentary horn pregnancy, *MTX* methotrexate, *KCl* potassium chloride, *FAST USS* focused assessment with sonography for trauma, *GnRHa* gonadotrophin-releasing hormone analogue

Extraction of specimens in laparoscopy is often a challenge. In our review, the majority of authors were able to extract their specimens through a small extension of one of the laparoscopic ports (up to 3 cm). Similarly, we extended the suprapubic port to 3 cm and extracted the uterine horn containing the intact pregnancy in a nylon bag. We were thus able to reassure the patient that no destructive techniques (such as morcellation) were applied to remove the fetus. When the size of the pregnancy/fetus was such that morcellation was required, some authors elected to perform feticide with intra-cardiac KCl prior to the laparoscopy [12]. Lennox et al. brought their specimen to the skin (16-week RHP) in an EndoCatch™ bag, then morcellated the tissues and extracted them with Beirer forceps [12]. Contreras et al. performed laparoscopic amnioreduction for a 19-week RHP and used a hand-assist port through a 4-cm suprapubic incision to extract the specimen without morcellation [21]. Kadan and Romano placed their excised horn in an Endo bag, incised it and suctioned its contents laparoscopically; they then extended their right lateral incision slightly for extraction [18]. Alternatively, a posterior colpotomy can be used [13]. Clearly, these methods allow for specimen extraction without the risk of morcellation-associated trophoblast spill and persistent trophoblastic disease, and therefore, laparotomy should not be preferred over laparoscopy on the basis of this argument.

Methotrexate has been used by some authors either with curative intent [22] or as an adjunct to surgery in an attempt to arrest the development of the pregnancy (in combination with intra-cardiac KCl) and reduce the vascularity of the rudimentary horn [5, 23]. Due to the small number of patients, it is not possible to conclude at present whether this method is of any value.

Where available, we attempted to collect data such as operating time, estimated blood loss and hospital stay for the cases shown in Table 1 (excluding the ruptured horn case where excision of the horn was performed at a later procedure). The operating times varied from 45 and 180 min with a mean operating time of 74.6 min. The majority of cases were completed in 50 min, and in one case only, where laparoscopic suturing was required, it took 180 min. Estimated blood loss was reported to range from minimal up to 100 ml, with a mean blood loss of 50 ml. All patients went home either on the first or second post-operative day with a mean hospital stay of 1.25 days.

Conclusion

There exists a growing body of evidence of RHP successfully managed by laparoscopy (20 cases in total). These include second trimester pregnancies as well as a case of a ruptured horn. The surgical technique is now well described. We suggest that when encountered with large dilated vascular pedicles, securing them by extracorporeal Roeder knots is a safe alternative. In advanced gestations, patients must be counselled pre-operatively about the potential need for destructive techniques. In such cases, feticide may need to be performed. Morcellation has been shown to be possible without compromising patient safety from trophoblast spill. The possibility of uncommon presentations such as duplicated or absent ureter should be taken into account pre-operatively, and the ureter must be identified intra-operatively. When the expertise is available, laparoscopy appears to be at least as safe as and potentially superior to laparotomy for the management of RHP.

Statement of informed consent Informed consent was obtained from all patients for which identifying information is included in this article.

This article does not contain any studies with human or animal subjects performed by the any of the authors.

References

1. Nahum GG (2002) Rudimentary uterine horn pregnancy: the 20th-century worldwide experience of 588 cases. J Reprod Med 47:151–163
2. Chopra S, Keepanasseril A, Rohilla M et al (2009) Obstetric morbidity and the diagnostic dilemma in pregnancy in rudimentary horn: retrospective analysis. Arch Gynecol Obstet 280:907–910
3. Sharp HT, Dorsey JH (1997) The 4-S modification of the Roeder knot: how to tie it. Obstet Gynecol 90:1004–1006
4. Fedele L, Bianchi S, Tozzi L et al (1995) Fertility in women with unicornuate uterus. Br J Obstet Gynaecol 102:1007–1009
5. Park JK, Dominguez CE (2007) Combined medical and surgical management of rudimentary uterine horn pregnancy. JSLS 11:119–122
6. Reichman D, Laufer MR, Robinson BK (2009) Pregnancy outcomes in unicornuate uteri: a review. Fertil Steril 91:1886–1894
7. Jurkovic D, Gruboeck K, Tailor A, Nicolaides KH (1997) Ultrasound screening for congenital uterine anomalies. Br J Obstet Gynaecol 104:1320–1321
8. Mavrelos D, Sawyer E, Helmy S et al (2007) Ultrasound diagnosis of ectopic pregnancy in the noncommunicating horn of a unicornuate uterus (cornual pregnancy). Ultrasound Obstet Gynecol 30:765–770
9. van Esch EM, Lashley EE, Berning B, de Kroon CD (2010) The value of hysteroscopy in the diagnostic approach to a rudimentary horn pregnancy. BMJ Case Rep. doi:10.1136/bcr.08.2010.3229
10. Jihong L, Siow A, Chern B (2009) Laparoscopic excision of rudimentary horn pregnancy in a patient with previous caesarean section. Arch Gynecol Obstet 279:403–405
11. Shahid A, Olowu O, Kandasamy G et al (2010) Laparoscopic management of a 16-week ruptured rudimentary horn pregnancy: a case and literature review. Arch Gynecol Obstet 282:121–125
12. Henriet E, Roman H, Zanati J et al (2008) Pregnant noncommunicating rudimentary uterine horn with placenta percreta. JSLS 12:101–103
13. Yan CM (2010) Laparoscopic management of three rare types of ectopic pregnancy. Hong Kong Med J 16:132–136
14. Lennox G, Pantazi S, Keunen J et al (2013) Minimally invasive surgical management of a second trimester pregnancy in a rudimentary uterine horn. J Obstet Gynaecol Can 35:468–472
15. Sharp HT, Dorsey JH, Chovan JD, Holtz PM (1996) The effect of knot geometry on the strength of laparoscopic slip knots. Obstet Gynecol 88:408–411
16. Dickey RP, Hower JF (1995) Ultrasonographic features of uterine blood flow during the first 16 weeks of pregnancy. Hum Reprod 10:2448–2452
17. Dicker D, Nitke S, Shoenfeld A et al (1998) Laparoscopic management of rudimentary horn pregnancy. Hum Reprod 13:2643–2644

18. Kadan Y, Romano S (2008) Rudimentary horn pregnancy diagnosed by ultrasound and treated by laparoscopy—a case report and review of the literature. J Minim Invasive Gynecol 15:527–530

19. Perrotin F, Bertrand J, Body G (1999) Laparoscopic surgery of unicornuate uterus with rudimentary uterine horn. Hum Reprod 14: 931–933

20. Sonmezer M, Taskin S, Atabekoglu C et al (2006) Laparoscopic management of rudimentary uterine horn pregnancy: case report and literature review. JSLS 10:396–399

21. Contreras KR, Rothenberg JM, Kominiarek MA, Raff GJ (2008) Hand-assisted laparoscopic management of a midtrimester rudimentary horn pregnancy with placenta increta: a case report and literature review. J Minim Invasive Gynecol 15:644–648

22. Edelman AB, Jensen JT, Lee DM et al (2003) Successful medical abortion of a pregnancy within a noncommunicating uterine horn. Am J Obstet Gynecol 189:886–887

23. Cutner A, Saridogan E, Hart R et al (2004) Laparoscopic management of pregnancies occurring in a noncommunicating accessory uterine horns. Eur J Obstet Gynecol Reprod Biol 113:106–109

24. Dulemba J, Midgett W, Freeman M (1996) Laparoscopic management of a rudimentary horn pregnancy. J Am Assoc Gynecol Laparosc 3:627–630

25. Yahata T, Kurabayashi T, Ueda H et al (1998) Laparoscopic management of a rudimentary horn pregnancy: a case report. J Reprod Med 43:223–226

26. Yoo EH, Chun SH, Woo BH (1999) Laparoscopic resection of a rudimentary horn pregnancy. Acta Obstet Gynecol Scand 78:167–168

27. Adolph AJ, Gilliland GB (2002) Fertility following laparoscopic removal of rudimentary horn with an ectopic pregnancy. J Obstet Gynaecol Can 24:575–576

28. Chakravati S, Chin K (2003) Rudimentary uterine horn: management of a diagnostic enigma. Acta Obstet Gynecol Scand 82:1153–1154

29. Szabó I, Börzsönyi B, Demendi C, Langmár Z (2009) Successful laparoscopic management of a noncommunicating rudimentary horn pregnancy. Orv Hetil 150:513–515

3

Ultrasound examination before, during, and after office endometrial sampling

Thierry Van den Bosch · Dominique Van Schoubroeck ·
Dirk Timmerman

Abstract Office endometrial sampling is widely used as the first diagnostic test in women with abnormal uterine bleeding. Because office sampling is a blind procedure, the lesion causing the symptoms may be missed. The use of ultrasound before, during, and after office endometrial sampling improves relevant tissue yield. The measurement of the endometrial thickness informs if sampling is indicated. The evaluation of ultrasound features (without or with fluid instillation) may suggest a focal intracavitary lesion necessitating operative hysteroscopy. The knowledge of the uterine cavity length, shape, and flexion may avoid nonrepresentative sampling. The concordance between the tissue yield and the ultrasound findings reflects the reliability of the sampling. If not concordant, further diagnostic steps such as fluid instillation sonography or hysteroscopy are indicated. We conclude that integrating ultrasound in the diagnostic algorithm for uterine intracavitary pathology optimizes office endometrial sampling.

Keywords Ultrasonography · Uterus · Endometrium · Leiomyoma · Metrorrhagia

T. Van den Bosch · D. Van Schoubroeck · D. Timmerman
Department of Development and Regeneration, KU Leuven,
3000 Leuven, Belgium

T. Van den Bosch
Department of Obstetrics and Gynecology, RZTienen, 3300 Tienen,
Belgium

T. Van den Bosch (✉)
KU Leuven Department of Development and Regeneration,
University Hospitals Leuven, Herestraat 49, 3000 Leuven, Belgium
e-mail: thierry.van.den.bosch@skynet.be

Background

Most practitioners favor office endometrial sampling as the first diagnostic test in women with abnormal uterine bleeding. The main reason is that tissue diagnosis is considered pivotal. Depending on the histology of the endometrial sample, further management is planned. The alleged medico legal value of a pathology report is an additional reason in favor of endometrial biopsy. However, because office sampling is a blind procedure, there is no control that the tissue yielded is representative for the patient's problem. If a relevant lesion is missed, management is likely to be inappropriate.

Compared with other office sampling devices such as the Novak or the Vabra curette, the Pipelle® de Cornier [1] has been reported to cause less procedure-related pain while offering a similar diagnostic accuracy [2, 3]. The popularity of the Pipelle® for office endometrial sampling dates from the early 1990s. Stovall et al. [4] reported in 1991 a 97.5 % sensitivity of Pipelle® sampling for endometrial cancer. This study is not very robust since only 40 patients with known endometrial cancer were included. In 1993, Rodrigues et al. [5] measured the endometrial denudation by office sampling in hysterectomy specimens. By Pipelle®, only 4.2 % of the total endometrial surface was sampled and they conclude the method to be unreliable. In 2002, a systematic review by Clark et al. [6], on the accuracy of outpatient endometrial biopsy in the diagnosis of endometrial cancer, reported an excellent positive likelihood ratio of 66.5 (95 % CI, 30.0–147.1) and a good negative likelihood ratio of 0.14 (95 % CI, 0.1–0.3). A possible explanation for the apparent contradiction between Rodrigues' and Clark's conclusions may be the tissue characteristics of endometrial cancer. Malignant endometrial tissue not only tends to protrude into the uterine cavity, it is also more friable because of less intercellular cohesion (Fig. 1). Tumor tissue is thus more prone to be aspirated during Pipelle® sampling.

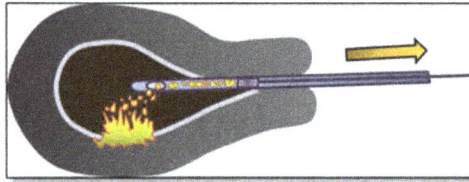

Fig. 1 Pipelle® aspiration biopsie of a focal malignant lesion

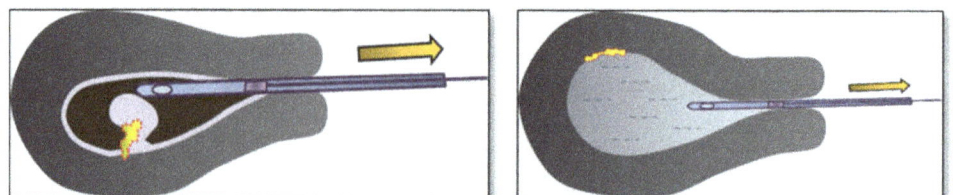

Fig. 3 Ultrasound image of a uniform thin endometrium

Endometrial cancer can be missed by office sampling [7]: small tumors or lesions hidden behind a benign focal lesion may escape the sampler. In the presence of intracavitary fluid or blood, the aspirated material may contain little or no endometrial cells (Fig. 2).

Many benign focal intracavitary lesions, such as endometrial polyps or intracavitary fibroids will not be picked-up by office sampling [8]. Although they are not life threatening, polyps and fibroids cause abnormal bleeding both before and after menopause. It is therefore relevant not to overlook benign focal lesions.

The value of ultrasound before, during, and after office endometrial sampling to improve relevant tissue yield will be discussed in this paper.

Ultrasonography before endometrial sampling

The indication for further testing in case of abnormal bleeding depends on different parameters: in postmenopausal women endometrial investigation may be indicated after a single episode of bleeding, whereas in younger women expectant management may be justified. After menopause, endometrial cancer is to be excluded first, whereas before menopause endometrial malignancy is much less likely. In women of reproductive age presenting with recurrent or persistent abnormal uterine bleeding, endometrial sampling may evidence endometrial hyperplasia, subacute endometritis or luteal dysfunction. However, this issue is beyond the scope of this paper. In this paper, it is assumed that further testing is clinically indicated. In case of (recurrent) abnormal uterine bleeding, the endometrial thickness is measured at transvaginal ultrasonography. If the endometrium is thin and uniform (Fig. 3), endometrial pathology is unlikely [9]. In those cases, endometrial sampling may not be necessary. The proposed threshold

for total endometrial thickness above which further testing is indicated ranges from 3 to 5 mm [10–12].

The evaluation of the endometrium by ultrasound is not limited to an endometrial thickness measurement, but should include a detailed evaluation of the endometrial features at unenhanced ultrasonography, color Doppler imaging, and, if indicated, fluid instillation sonography (FIS), according the International Endometrial Tumor Analysis terms and definitions [13]. If a focal intracavitary lesion is seen, blind sampling is not the diagnostic test of choice because most endometrial polyps and intracavitary fibroids are missed at office sampling [8]. A hysteroscopical resection of these lesions is a more appropriate approach (Fig. 4).

If a diffuse thickening of the endometrium is seen or if endometrial cancer is suspected, office endometrial sampling is indicated. The endometrial thickness at ultrasonography should be correlated with the tissue yield at sampling: the thicker the endometrium, the higher the tissue yield is expected to be [14]. The tissue yield is related to the histology: the highest tissue yield in endometrial cancer, and the lowest tissue yield in endometrial atrophy [14]. To obtain a representative endometrial biopsy, the uterine cavity should be sampled, from the fundus to the endocervical canal. Although the clinician usually feels when the tip of the device touches the fundus, there are some pitfalls. A cesarean section scar defect, extreme uterine retroversion, or an intracavitary fibroid may misleadingly give the impression that the tip of the sampling device touches the fundus (Fig. 5).

The uterine cavity length, the uterine flexion, and the possible presence of an intracavitary fibroid or a cesarean section scar defect assessed by transvaginal ultrasound enable the clinician to ascertain that the sampling device will be introduced deep enough and that the endometrial sample will be representative. One should be aware that sampling disturbs the ultrasound features of the endometrium [15]. The

Fig. 2 Endometrial cancer missed by Pipelle® sampling in case of **a** a small lesion hidden behind a benign focal lesion and **b** in case of intracavitary fluid

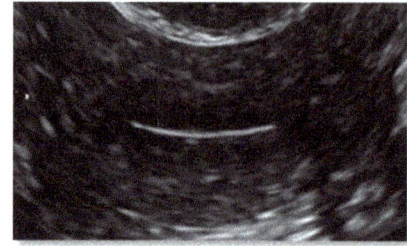

Fig. 4 Diagnostic algorithm

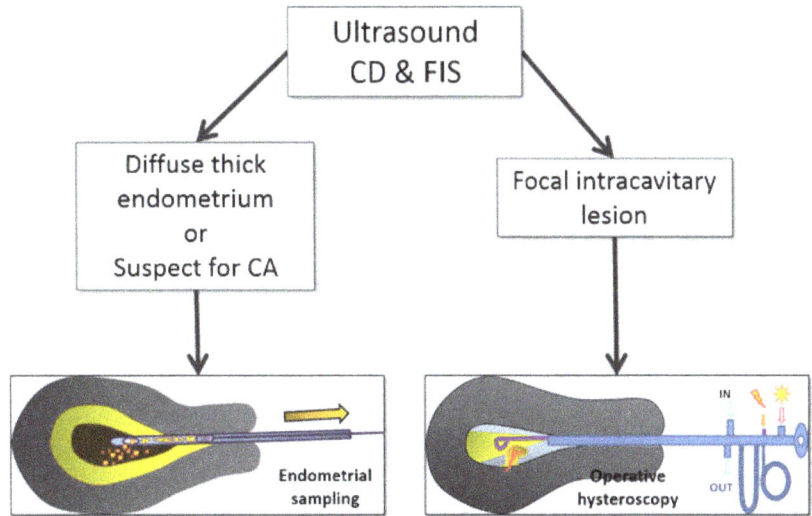

Fig. 5 Incomplete endometrial sampling in case of **a** cesarean scar defect, **b** severe uterine retroflection, **c** proximal benign focal intracavitary lesion

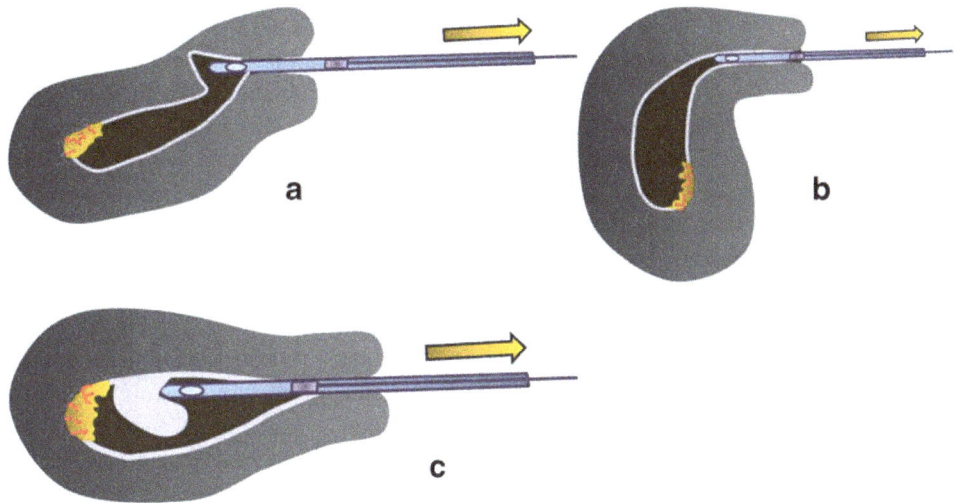

endometrial thickness, as well as other ultrasound characteristics such as the endometrial outline or the echogenicity of the endometrium is altered by the sampling procedure. This is another incentive to perform an ultrasound examination before proceeding with office endometrial biopsy.

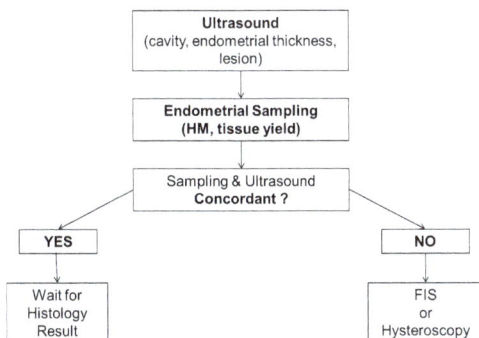

Fig. 6 Diagnostic algorithm based on ultrasound features and findings at endometrial sampling

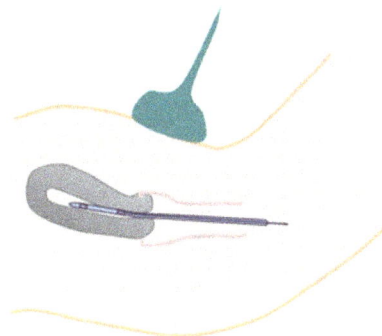

Fig. 7 Endometrial sampling under transabdominal ultrasound guidance

Fig. 8 Pipelle sampling in case
of intracavitary fluid

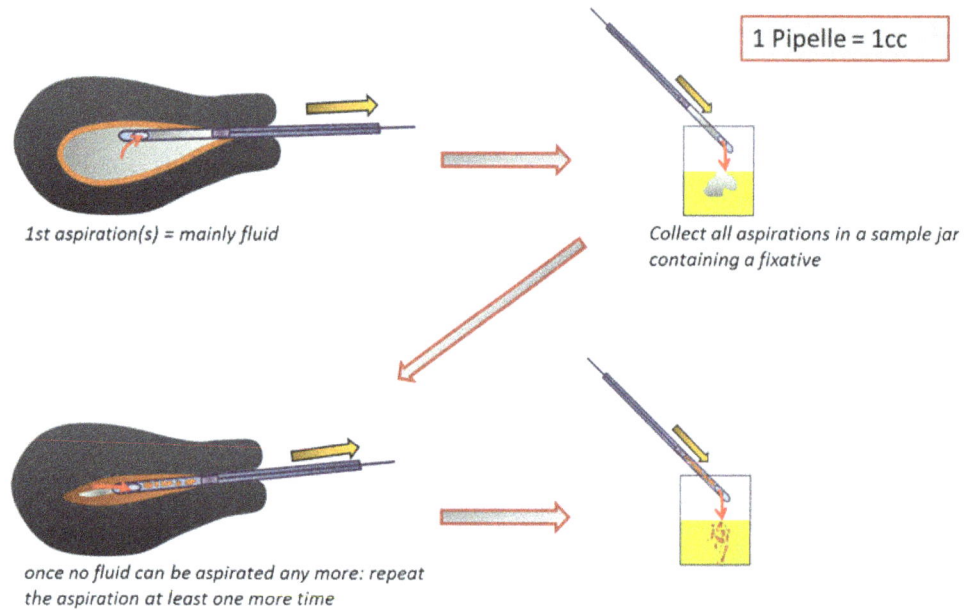

1 Pipelle = 1cc

1st aspiration(s) = mainly fluid

*Collect all aspirations in a sample jar
containing a fixative*

*once no fluid can be aspirated any more: repeat
the aspiration at least one more time*

Ultrasonography during endometrial sampling

After having checked that the hysterometry on the sampling device matches the presampling ultrasound cavity length estimation, the actual tissue aspiration can be started. A Pipelle® sampler is a transparent device, allowing the estimation of the tissue yield during aspiration [14]. Endometrial tissue is visible as small whitish lumps, and can usually easily be differentiated from blood, pus, or mucus within the sampling device. The estimation of the amount of tissue retrieved during sampling correlates well with the tissue yield estimation of the pathologist [14]. Implementing a strict procedure for endometrium biopsy, including presampling ultrasound examination and assessment of the tissue yield during sampling (scored from 1 to 4), in 257 consecutive women with abnormal bleeding, the median endometrial thickness at ultrasound and the median tissue yield score was 18.3 mm and score 4 in the endometrial cancer cases, compared with 11.5 mm and score 2 in endometrial polyp cases, and 3.9 mm and score 1 in endometrial atrophy [14]. If the tissue yield is concordant with

the ultrasound findings (e.g., a thick endometrium and a high tissue yield), the histology result will most probably be reliable. If, on the other hand, the tissue yield is low in a patient with a thickened endometrium at ultrasonography, the lesion could have been missed and one cannot rely upon the histology result. Further testing, such as FIS with saline (SIS) or gel (GIS) [16], or hysteroscopy is needed (Fig. 6).

The insertion of the sampler may be difficult at times. This can be secondary to previous cervical surgery or due to retroversion of the uterus or to a cesarean section scar defect. In order to avoid a "fausse route" and to minimize patient's discomfort, endometrial sampling can be performed under ultrasound guidance. The direction of the sampler's insertion path is guided through transabdominal ultrasound (Fig. 7). This may be easier to do if the woman has some bladder filling.

Ultrasonography after endometrial sampling

Ultrasound examination after sampling should confirm the presampling ultrasound diagnosis: e.g., if the ultrasound image before sampling suggested the presence of blood or clots in the uterine cavity, an ultrasound examination after Pipelle®

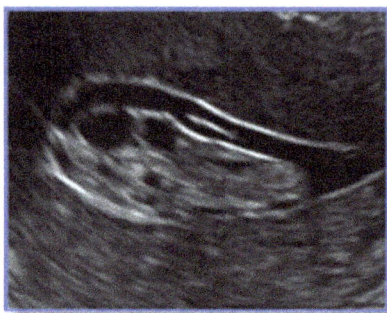

Fig. 9 Endometrial polyp diagnosed at fluid instillation sonography (FIS)

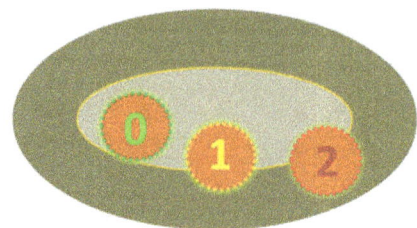

Fig. 10 Grading of intracavitary fibroids [13]

aspiration can confirm that the clots have disappeared and that there are no residual focal lesions. In case of intracavitary fluid, it is important that the sampling is repeated till no fluid can be aspirated any more. Thereafter, at least one additional aspiration is performed for endometrial tissue sampling (Fig. 8).

The woman will hardly experience pain as long as the tip of the sampler is surrounded by fluid and does not touch the cavity wall. When there is no fluid in the cavity anymore, the endometrial mucosa will be sucked against the tip of the sampler, causing patient's discomfort or pain, especially if the endometrium is thin. In case of a thick endometrium at ultrasound and low tissue yield during sampling, a missed focal intracavitary lesion is to be suspected. One can immediately proceed with FIS to detect or exclude a focal lesion (Fig. 9).

Both FIS and hysteroscopy have a similar diagnostic accuracy for the detection of endometrial polyps and intracavitary fibroids [17].

In case of a focal intracavitary lesion, the ultrasound report should also provide additional information to tailor the operation. If one or more polyps are diagnosed, their size and number may determine whether a resection is to be performed as an outpatient's procedure or in theater under general anesthesia or sedation. If one or more fibroids are diagnosed, each lesions' size, grade (Fig. 10), and number should be documented accurately to allow estimation of the technical complexity of the resection procedure [18–25].

A fibroid larger than 2 cm or protruding less than 50 % into the uterine cavity (grade 2) as well as the presence of more than one lesion are known to be technically challenging for the operative hysteroscopist. Ultrasound can give valuable information improving further management planning, such as the need for sedation or anesthesia, the expected operation time, and for informing the patient about the expected procedure's success rate (one or two step procedure).

Conclusion

Transvaginal ultrasound assessment of the uterine cavity informs the clinician if office endometrial sampling is indicated. If the endometrium is very thin and uniform, further testing may not be necessary. If a focal intracavitary lesion is detected, an operative hysteroscopy is warranted—not office sampling. The ultrasound examination also provides valuable information to plan the operative hysteroscopy. If endometrial sampling is to be performed, the ultrasound findings will improve sample quality. Incomplete insertion of the device can be avoided and the tissue yield during sampling can be anticipated by the endometrial thickness measured at ultrasound examination. The added value of ultrasound before,

during, and after endometrial sampling should be validated in future studies.

We conclude that integrating ultrasound in the diagnostic algorithm for uterine intracavitary pathology optimizes endometrial sampling and allows quality control of the sampling procedure.

Declaration of interest The authors report no conflicts in interest. The authors alone are responsible for the content and writing of the paper.

References

1. Cornier E (1984) The Pipelle: a disposable device for endometrial biopsy. Am J Obstet Gynecol 148:109–110
2. Kaunitz AM, Masciello A, Ostrowski M, Rovira EZ (1988) Comparison of endometrial biopsy with the endometrial Pipelle and Vabra aspirator. J Reprod Med 33:427–431
3. Hill GA, Herbert CM 3rd, Parker RA, Wentz AC (1989) Comparison of late luteal phase endometrial biopsies using the Novak curette or PIPELLE endometrial suction curette. Obstet Gynecol 73:443–445
4. Stovall TG, Photopulos GJ, Poston WM, Ling FW, Sandles LG (1991) Pipelle endometrial sampling in patients with known endometrial carcinoma. Obstet Gynecol 77:954–956
5. Rodriguez GC, Yaqub N, King ME (1993) A comparison of the Pipelle device and the Vabra aspirator as measured by endometrial denudation in hysterectomy specimens: the Pipelle device samples significantly less of the endometrial surface than the Vabra aspirator. Am J Obstet Gynecol 168:55–59
6. Clark TJ, Mann CH, Shah HM, Khan KS, Song F, Gupta JK (2002) Accuracy of outpatient endometrial biopsy in the diagnosis of endometrial cancer: a systematic quantitative review. BJOG 109:313–321
7. Van den Bosch T, Cornelis A (1998) Endometrial malignancy missed by office sampling. Aust N Z J Obstet Gynaecol 38:1–2
8. Van den Bosch T, Vandendael A, Van Schoubroeck D, Wranz PAB, Lombard CJ (1995) Combining vaginal ultrasonography and office endometrial sampling in the diagnosis of endometrial disease in postmenopausal women. Obstet Gynecol 85:349–352
9. Van den Bosch T, Van Schoubroeck D, Vergote I, Moerman P, Amant F, Timmerman D (2007) A thin and regular endometrium on ultrasound is very unlikely in patients with endometrial malignancy. Ultrasound Obstet Gynecol 29:674–679
10. Smith-Bindman R, Kerlikowske K, Feldstein VA, Subak L, Scheidler J, Segal M, Brand R, Gracy D (1998) Endovaginal ultrasound to exclude endometrial cancer and other endometrial abnormalities. JAMA 280:1510–1517
11. Tabor A, Watt HC, Wald NJ (2002) Endometrial thickness as a test for endometrial cancer in women with postmenopausal vaginal bleeding. Obstet Gynecol 99:663–670
12. Timmermans A, Opmeer B, Khan K, Bachmann LM, Epstein E, Clark JT, Gupta JK, Bakour SH, Van den Bosch T, van Doorn HC, Cameron ST, Giusa MG, Dessole S, Dijkhuizen FPHLJ, ter Riet G, Mol WJ (2010) Endometrial thickness measurement for detecting endometrial cancer in women with postmenopausal bleeding: a systematic review and meta-analysis. Obstet Gynecol 116:160–167
13. Leone F, Timmerman D, Bourne T, Valentin L, Epstein E, Goldstein SR, Marret H, Parsons AK, Gull B, Istre O, Sepulveda W, Ferrazzi E,

Van den Bosch T (2010) Terms, definitions and measurements to describe the sonographic features of the endometrium and intrauterine lesions: a consensus opinion from the International Endometrial Tumor Analysis (IETA) group. Ultrasound Obstet Gynecol 35:103–112

14. Van den Bosch T, Van Schoubroeck D, Van Calster B, Cornelis A, Timmerman D (2012) Pre-sampling ultrasound evaluation and assessment of the tissue yield during sampling improves the diagnostic reliability of office endometrial biopsy. J Obstet Gynaecol 32:173–176

15. Van den Bosch T, Van Schoubroeck D, Timmerman D (2005) Ultrasound examination of the endometrium before and after Pipelle® endometrial sampling. Ultrasound Obstet Gynecol 26: 283–286

16. Werbrouck E, Veldman J, Luts J, Van Huffel S, Van Schoubroeck D, Timmerman D, Van den Bosch T (2011) Detection of endometrial pathology using saline infusion sonography versus gel instillation sonography: a prospective cohort study. Fertil Steril 95:285–288

17. de Kroon C, De Bock GH, Dieben SWM, Jansen FW (2003) Saline contrast hydrosonography in abnormal uterine bleeding: a systematic review and metaanalysis. BJOG 110:938–947

18. Wamsteker K, Emanuel MH, de Kruif JH (1993) Transcervical hysteroscopic resection of submucous fibroids for abnormal uterine bleeding: results regarding the degree of intramural extension. Obstet Gynecol 82:736–740

19. Emanuel MH, Wamsteker K, Hart AA, Metz G, Lammes FB (1999) Long-term results of hysteroscopic myomectomy for abnormal uterine bleeding. Obstet Gynecol 93:743–748

20. Cravello L, Agostini A, Beerli M, Roger V, Bretelle F, Blanc B (2004) Results of hysteroscopic myomectomy. Gynecol Obstet Fertil 32:825–828, Article in French

21. Marret H, Cottier JP, Alonso AM, Giraudeau B, Body G, Herbreteau D (2005) Predictive factors for fibroids recurrence after uterine artery embolisation. BJOG 112:461–465

22. Di Spiezio SA, Mazzon I, Bramante S, Bettocchi S, Bifulco G, Guida M, Nappi C (2008) Hysteroscopic myomectomy: a comprehensive review of surgical techniques. Hum Reprod Update 14:101–119

23. Rovio PH, Helin R, Heinonen PK (2009) Long-term outcome of hysteroscopic endometrial resection with or without myomectomy in patients with menorrhagia. Arch Gynecol Obstet 279:159–163

24. Camanni M, Bonino L, Delpiano EM, Ferrero B, Migliaretti G, Deltetto F (2010) Hysteroscopic management of large symptomatic submucous uterine myomas. J Minim Invasive Gynecol 17:59–65

25. Lasmar RB, Xinmei Z, Indman PD, Celeste RK, Di Spiezio SA (2011) Feasibility of a new system of classification of submucous myomas: a multicenter study. Fertil Steril 95:2073–2077

4

Pregnancy after transcervical radiofrequency ablation guided by intrauterine sonography

José Gerardo Garza-Leal · Iván Hernández León
David Toub

Abstract Uterine fibroids are a prevalent disorder; with the exception of myomectomy, there are no treatments that are generally accepted as compatible with future fertility and fecundity. Radiofrequency ablation is a minimally invasive treatment modality for uterine fibroids that results in coagulative necrosis and fibroid volume reduction. There have been few reports of pregnancy after laparoscopic and transvaginal radiofrequency ablation of fibroids and no previous reports after a transcervical approach. We report the outcome of the first viable pregnancy after intrauterine sonography-guided radiofrequency ablation of a uterine fibroid.

Keywords Fibroids · Radiofrequency ablation · VizAblate

Uterine fibroids are prevalent and often treated with hysterectomy. While several alternatives to hysterectomy exist, over 200,000 hysterectomies are performed for fibroids each year in the USA [1, 2]. Among alternatives to hysterectomy, only myomectomy is generally considered to be appropriate for women who desire future childbearing. The (ACOG) has advised that uterine artery embolization (UAE) "should be considered investigational or relatively contraindicated in women wishing to retain fertility" [3]. While ACOG has taken note of the reports of successful pregnancies after magnetic resonance imaging-guided focused ultrasound (MRgFUS) therapy [4–8], it maintains that "larger experience is necessary before drawing conclusions" [9].

As with focused ultrasound, radiofrequency energy may be used to thermally ablate fibroid tissue, resulting in coagulative necrosis, fibroid volume reduction, and symptom relief. Few pregnancies have been reported after radiofrequency ablation of uterine fibroids, and none in which the ablation was performed transcervically and under intrauterine sonography guidance. We report the first such viable pregnancy.

Case

A 41-year-old Gravida 4, Para 2 female presented with abnormal uterine bleeding secondary to uterine fibroids and requested treatment. Transvaginal ultrasonography noted the presence of a midline posterofundal type 1 myoma measuring 1.6×1.6 cm. The patient had previously undergone two Cesarean sections and her medical history was otherwise unremarkable. The patient, who desired uterine preservation, was presented with several options, including enrollment in a clinical trial of transcervical radiofrequency ablation (the FAST-EU trial; Clinicaltrials.gov identifier NCT01226290). The FAST-EU trial is a prospective, nonrandomized, single-arm, multisite trial involving ten sites in Mexico (one site), the UK (five sites), and The Netherlands (four sites) and was approved by the Comisión Federal para la Protección contra Riesgos Sanitarios in Mexico along with the ethics committee of the participating hospital, the Hospital Universitario "Dr. José Eleuterio González" de Universidad Autonoma de Nuevo León in Monterrey, Mexico. The FAST-EU trial has

J. G. Garza-Leal · I. H. León
Universidad Autónoma de Nuevo León, Monterrey, Nuevo Leon, Mexico

D. Toub (✉)
Gynesonics, Inc., 604 Fifth Avenue, Suite D, Redwood City, CA 94063, USA
e-mail: dtoub@gynesonics.com

D. Toub
Albert Einstein Medical Center, Philadelphia, PA, USA

been performed in accordance with the ethical standards laid down in the 1964 Declaration of Helsinki and its later amendments.

After a presentation of her care options, the patient elected to be screened for inclusion in the FAST-EU trial. She was using barrier contraception and indicated that she was certain she did not desire future childbearing. The patient met all screening requirements for enrollment and provided her informed consent to participate in the FAST-EU trial and was scheduled for intrauterine sonography-guided, transcervical radiofrequency ablation using the VizAblate® System (Gynesonics, Redwood City, CA, USA).

The VizAblate System uses radiofrequency energy to ablate fibroid tissue and has received CE Marking in the European Union (Fig. 1). The VizAblate treatment device (Fig. 2) is inserted transcervically and includes both an intrauterine sonography probe for visualization and a radiofrequency needle electrode array for treatment. With a single device, the operator identifies each fibroid using the intrauterine sonography probe and ablates a targeted fibroid with the radiofrequency needle electrode array. The VizAblate System features a graphical interface to display the extent of tissue ablation and heat dissipation, so as to optimize the volume of the fibroid ablation while allowing the gynecologist to avoid thermal injury to the uterine serosa and adjacent structures (Fig. 3). The needle electrode array ablates tissue at a constant 105 °C for a specific period of time that is a function of the desired ablation volume. The VizAblate System has been described in further detail elsewhere [10].

The patient's baseline menstrual pictogram score was 330 (the minimum requirement for study entry was 120). Her baseline transformed score on the Uterine Fibroid Symptom and Quality of Life (UFS-QOL) Symptom Severity subscale was 53 % and her transformed health-related quality of life subscale score was 2 %. While there are no well-defined normal limits for the results of the UFS-QOL questionnaire, Spies, and colleagues originally reported transformed symptom severity and health-related quality of life scores for a normal premenopausal female population as 22.5 ± 21.1 and 86.4 ± 17.7, respectively [11]. Screening magnetic resonance imaging (MRI) revealed a 1.3-cm midline posterofundal type 1 myoma; there was no suggestion of adenomyosis.

In July, 2012, after a negative pregnancy test, the patient underwent treatment with the VizAblate System under conscious sedation with midazolam and fentanyl. After mechanical cervical dilatation to 25 Fr in the usual fashion, the VizAblate treatment device was introduced into the endometrial cavity. Intrauterine sonography was used to survey the uterus and revealed the type 1 myoma. Using the graphical interface, the ablation location and size were planned by the operating gynecologist so as to maximize the ablation volume of the fibroid while avoiding thermal injury to the uterine serosa. This was accomplished prior to introduction of any device elements within the fibroid. Once the operator was satisfied that the planned ablation was optimal and safe, the distal tip of the VizAblate treatment device was articulated to 45° and the fibroid was penetrated with a trocar that permitted the needle electrode array to be deployed within the myoma. This was entirely performed under intrauterine sonographic guidance. Rotation of the VizAblate treatment device with concomitant intrauterine sonography in multiple planes confirmed that the uterine serosa was out of harm's way; the planned ablation and its dissipated heat were contained within the uterine serosal margin. A 1.5-cm wide ablation of the targeted fibroid was created with the VizAblate System. This required an ablation duration of 4 min at a temperature of 105 °C; total procedure time was 16 min. The patient tolerated the procedure well and was discharged that same day. There were no complications reported during or after radiofrequency ablation.

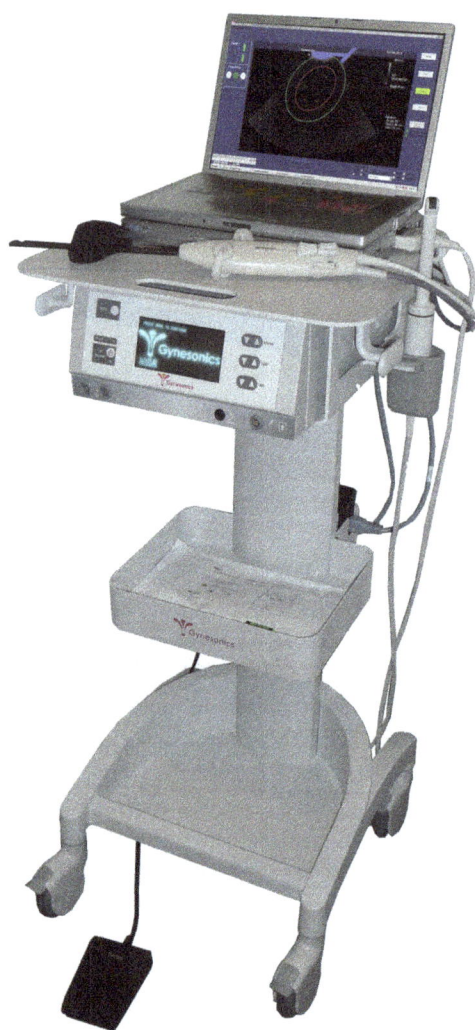

Fig. 1 The VizAblate System. The ultrasound display is provided by the laptop, while the RF generator resides on the second shelf from the bottom

Fig. 2 The VizAblate Treatment
Device

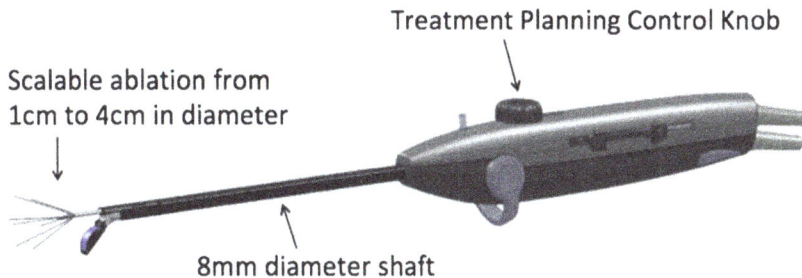

Treatment Planning Control Knob

Scalable ablation from
1cm to 4cm in diameter

8mm diameter shaft

Contrast-enhanced MRI at baseline demonstrated that the total and perfused fibroid volumes were each 1.2 cc, indicating 100 % perfusion of the fibroid. At 3 months, both were reduced to 0.1 cc, so that both total and perfused fibroid volumes were diminished by 91.7 % from baseline (Fig. 4). The maximum fibroid diameter was reduced from 1.3 to 0.7 cm, a 46.2 % reduction. In terms of symptom relief, the patient's menstrual blood loss was reduced by 45 %, as reflected by her 3-month menstrual pictogram score; it fell to 181 from her baseline of 330. The Symptom Severity Score subscale of the UFS-QOL questionnaire fell by 64 %, from 53 to 19 %. There was similarly improvement in the health-related quality of life sub-scale, rising from 2 to 97 %, an increase of 4750 %.

On January 30, 2013, the patient returned for 6-month follow-up and noted that she did not complete her 6-month menstrual pictogram or UFS-QOL questionnaire, as she had not had a period since November 5, 2012. A transvaginal sonogram that day revealed a crown-rump length of 6.1 cm, corresponding to a 12 4/7-week intrauterine pregnancy. This was consistent with her dates by last menstrual period, with an estimated date of confinement of August 12, 2013. The patient desired to continue her pregnancy and was provided with routine prenatal care. Her pregnancy was unremarkable except for the development of gestational diabetes that was controlled with diet.

On July 30, 2013 at 38 1/7 weeks' gestation, because of her two prior Cesarean deliveries, the patient underwent an elective repeat Cesarean section with intrapartum tubal ligation. This resulted in the birth of a live-born male infant weighing 3,150 g who received Apgar scores of 9 at 1 min and 10 at 5 min. Both the infant and mother did well, and there were no complications. The operative report did not note any findings related to fibroids or the prior ablation; there was no indication of a preexisting uterine defect.

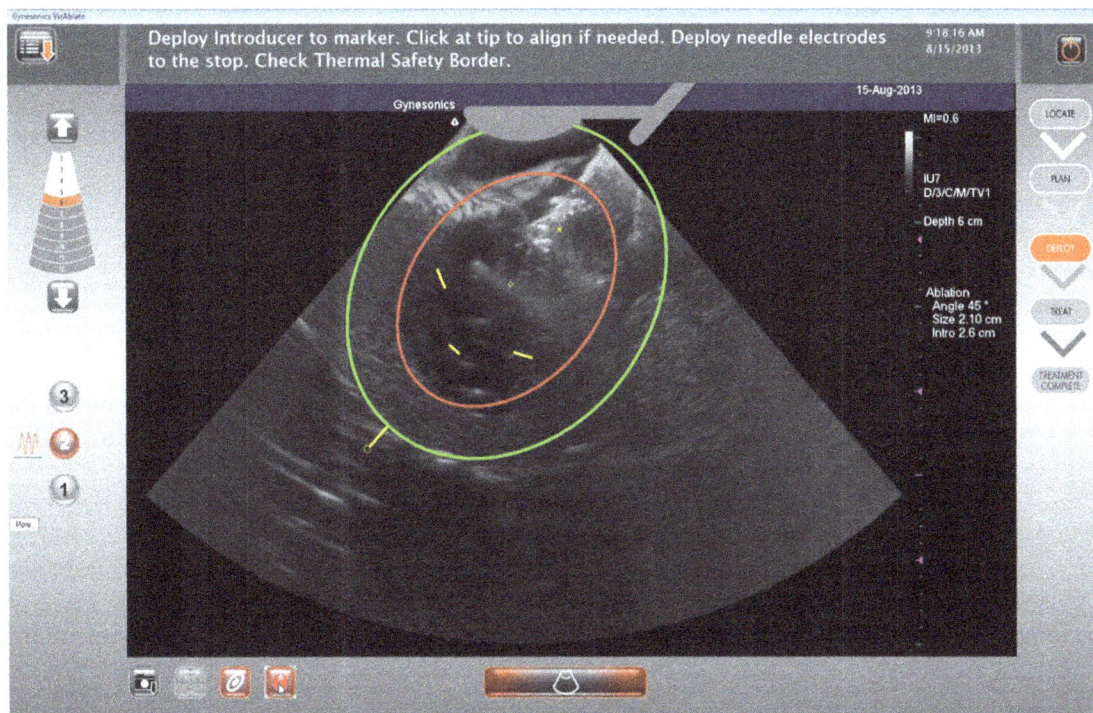

Fig. 3 Intrauterine sonogram of a submucosal fibroid with the VizAblate treatment guides visible (Mean Treatment Region in *red* and Thermal Safety Border in *green*). The mean treatment region delineates where the ablation will occur and the thermal safety border demarcates the extent of thermal spread beyond the ablation. The serosa is visible as an echogenic border around the uterus

Fig. 4 Reduction in total and perfused uterine fibroid volume; baseline, 24 h and 3-month contrast-enhanced MRI images. *Green arrow* tip designates the fibroid

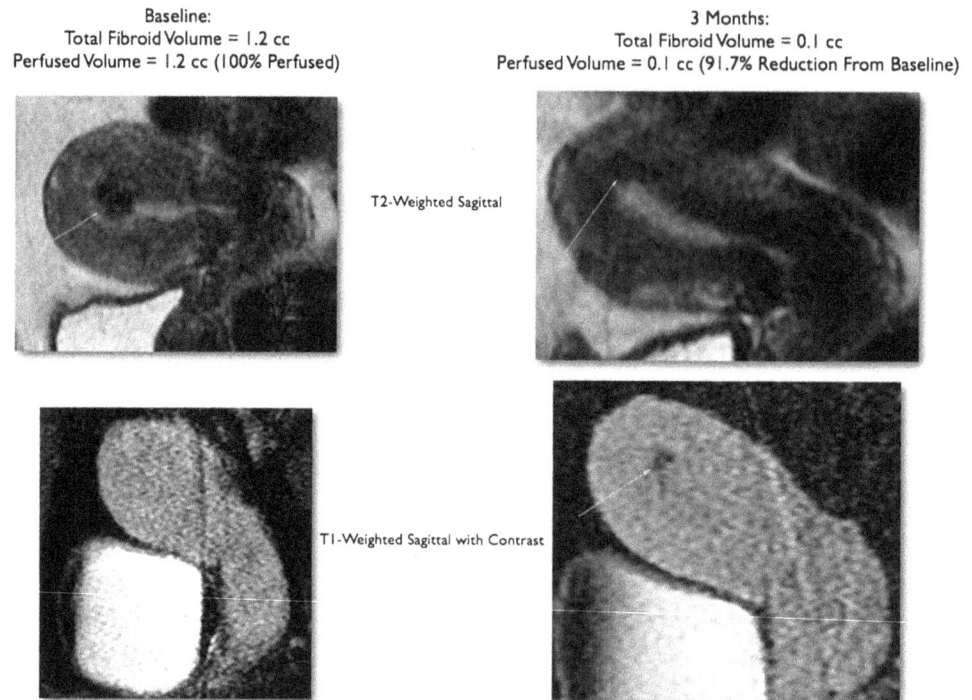

Baseline:
Total Fibroid Volume = 1.2 cc
Perfused Volume = 1.2 cc (100% Perfused)

3 Months:
Total Fibroid Volume = 0.1 cc
Perfused Volume = 0.1 cc (91.7% Reduction From Baseline)

T2-Weighted Sagittal

T1-Weighted Sagittal with Contrast

Discussion

There is interest in a fibroid treatment that is minimally invasive, does not require general anesthesia, and preserves fertility. Hysteroscopic myomectomy is generally considered to preserve fertility, but may be technically challenging and is limited in its ability to treat larger and/or deeper type 1 and type 2 myomata; it is not generally feasible for resection of FIGO types 3, 4, or 2–5 fibroids. Radiofrequency ablation is an established technology that has been used to effectively treat uterine fibroids [12–20]. Most studies have involved a laparoscopic, percutaneous or transvaginal approach for ablation under laparoscopic, transabdominal or transvaginal sonography. Because the imaging modality is not typically coupled with the radiofrequency treatment device, it can be unwieldy and challenging to perform adequate radiofrequency ablation of fibroids through such approaches. Transcervical radiofrequency ablation, using an intrauterine sonography probe intimately coupled to the treatment device, provides an incisionless approach to treating fibroids. It does not require general anesthesia or uterine distension and can ablate fibroids that include those that are not amenable to hysteroscopic myomectomy. This represents another method by which uterine fibroids may be managed, blending intrauterine sonography for imaging with radiofrequency ablation for treatment.

At present, myomectomy is the only surgical fibroid treatment that is generally considered to be compatible with future pregnancy. Nonetheless, there have been reports describing successful pregnancies after ablative therapies such as MRgFUS and radiofrequency ablation.

In the MRgFUS literature, there have been several reports of successful pregnancies after treatment. Rabinovici and colleagues provided a case report of a 36-year-old woman who underwent MRgFUS for focal adenomyosis [7]. She conceived spontaneously and had an uneventful pregnancy, undergoing a normal spontaneous vaginal delivery at term. There was no evidence of any uterine abnormalities postpartum. In 2008, Rabinovici and his associates also reported the experience with pregnancy after MRgFUS from a prospective registry involving 13 treatment sites in seven nations [6]. There were 54 pregnancies occurring in 51 women, with a mean time to conception of 8 months after MRgFUS. The live birth rate was 41 %, with a 28 % spontaneous abortion rate, an 11 % rate of elective abortion, and a 20 % rate of ongoing pregnancies beyond 20 gestational weeks. The mean birth weight was 3.3 kg, and the vaginal delivery rate was 64 %. No uterine ruptures were noted. Zaher has also published two separate cases of successful pregnancies after MRgFUS, including one patient who underwent assisted reproduction after her fibroid treatment [8, 21].

With regard to pregnancy after contemporary radiofrequency ablation technology, Kim and colleagues treated 69 women with symptomatic fibroids, 13 of whom desired future fertility, using a single-needle radiofrequency electrode connected to a transvaginal sonography probe [20]. Three patients (4.3 %) conceived and had uncomplicated pregnancies and deliveries (one Cesarean section and two normal spontaneous vaginal deliveries). Again, no uterine ruptures were noted. Berman and colleagues reported their experience in treating a patient with seven fibroids ranging up to 6.1 cm in diameter via laparoscopic radiofrequency ablation with a separate laparoscopic sonography probe for imaging [22]. The patient conceived approximately 3.5 months after treatment and underwent a normal spontaneous vaginal delivery of a 3,487-g infant with Apgar scores of 9 at 1 min and 9 at 5 min. Post-ablation and post-delivery MRI images indicated a myometrial thickness of 9.6 mm, including beneath the ablation site, suggesting the absence of any myometrial defect.

The experience of our patient adds to this growing literature base relating to thermal ablation of uterine fibroids, particularly via radiofrequency energy. The patient had evidence of symptomatic relief and reductions in both total and perfused fibroid volumes at 3 months, but a longer term assessment was interrupted by her pregnancy. Her pregnancy resulted in a normal outcome via elective repeat Cesarean section.

Many treatment options exist for uterine fibroids, and radiofrequency ablation represents another component in this armamentarium. Additional study must be done to establish the appropriate role of radiofrequency ablation in women who desire future pregnancy. It is not yet established if focal ablation of myomata would typically result in endometrial and/or myometrial injury that would have a negative impact on fertility or fecundity, for example.

Note: Informed consent was obtained from all patients in order to be included in the FAST-EU trial, and this applied to the patient described in this case report.

References

1. Day Baird D, Dunson DB, Hill MC et al (2003) High cumulative incidence of uterine leiomyoma in black and white women: ultrasound evidence. Am J Obstet Gynecol 188(1):100–107
2. Dembek CJ, Pelletier EM, Isaacson KB et al (2007) Payer costs in patients undergoing uterine artery embolization, hysterectomy, or myomectomy for treatment of uterine fibroids. J Vasc Interv Radiol 18(10):1207–1213
3. Committee ACOG (2004) Opinion. Uterine artery embolization. Obstet Gynecol 103(2):403–404
4. Gavrilova-Jordan LP, Rose CH, Traynor KD et al (2007) Successful term pregnancy following MR-guided focused ultrasound treatment of uterine leiomyoma. J Perinatol 27(1):59–61
5. Qin J, Chen JY, Zhao WP et al (2012) Outcome of unintended pregnancy after ultrasound-guided high-intensity focused ultrasound ablation of uterine fibroids. Int J Gynaecol Obstet 117(3):273–277
6. Rabinovici J, David M, Fukunishi H et al (2010) Pregnancy outcome after magnetic resonance-guided focused ultrasound surgery (MRgFUS) for conservative treatment of uterine fibroids. Fertil Steril 93(1):199–209
7. Rabinovici J, Inbar Y, Eylon SC et al (2006) Pregnancy and live birth after focused ultrasound surgery for symptomatic focal adenomyosis: a case report. Hum Reprod 21(5):1255–1259
8. Zaher S, Lyons D, Regan L (2011) Successful in vitro fertilization pregnancy following magnetic resonance-guided focused ultrasound surgery for uterine fibroids. J Obstet Gynaecol Res 37(4): 370–373
9. ACOG practice bulletin. Alternatives to hysterectomy in the management of leiomyomas. Obstet Gynecol 2008;112(2 Pt 1): 387–400
10. Garza-Leal J, Toub D, León I et al (2011) Transcervical, intrauterine ultrasound-guided radiofrequency ablation of uterine fibroids with the VizAblate System: safety, tolerability, and ablation results in a closed abdomen setting. Gynecol Surg 8(3):327–334
11. Spies JB, Coyne K, Guaou Guaou N et al (2002) The UFS-QOL, a new disease-specific symptom and health-related quality of life questionnaire for leiomyomata. Obstet Gynecol 99(2):290–300
12. Banks E, Harris M, Garza-Leal J et al (2012) Prospective 12-month follow-up of menstrual blood loss reduction following 135 consecutive cases of radiofrequency volumetric thermal ablation of symptomatic fibroids. J Minim Invasive Gynecol 19(6):S1
13. Bergamini V, Ghezzi F, Cromi A et al (2005) Laparoscopic radiofrequency thermal ablation: a new approach to symptomatic uterine myomas. Am J Obstet Gynecol 192(3):768–773
14. Carrafiello G, Recaldini C, Fontana F et al (2010) Ultrasound-guided radiofrequency thermal ablation of uterine fibroids: medium-term follow-up. Cardiovasc Intervent Radiol 33(1):113–119
15. Cho HH, Kim JH, Kim MR (2008) Transvaginal radiofrequency thermal ablation: a day-care approach to symptomatic uterine myomas. Aust N Z J Obstet Gynaecol 48(3):296–301
16. Chudnoff SG, Levine DJ, Galen DI et al (2012) Prospective 12-month follow-up of quality-of-life improvement following 135 consecutive cases of laparoscopic and ultrasound-guided radiofrequency ablation of fibroids. J Minim Invasive Gynecol 19(6):S45
17. Ghezzi F, Cromi A, Bergamini V et al (2007) Midterm outcome of radiofrequency thermal ablation for symptomatic uterine myomas. Surg Endosc 21(11):2081–2085
18. Guido RS, Macer JA, Abbott K et al (2013) Radiofrequency volumetric thermal ablation of fibroids: a prospective, clinical analysis of two years' outcome from the Halt trial. Health Qual Life Outcomes 11(1):139
19. Iversen H, Lenz S, Dueholm M (2012) Ultrasound-guided radiofrequency ablation of symptomatic uterine fibroids: short-term evaluation of effect of treatment on quality of life and symptom severity. Ultrasound Obstet Gynecol 40(4):445–451
20. Kim CH, Kim SR, Lee HA et al (2011) Transvaginal ultrasound-guided radiofrequency myolysis for uterine myomas. Hum Reprod 26(3):559–563
21. Zaher S, Lyons D, Regan L (2010) Uncomplicated term vaginal delivery following magnetic resonance-guided focused ultrasound surgery for uterine fibroids. Biomed Imaging Interv J 6(2):e28
22. Berman JM, Puscheck EE, Diamond MP (2012) Full-term vaginal live birth after laparoscopic radiofrequency ablation of a large, symptomatic intramural fibroid: a case report. J Reprod Med 57(3–4):159–163

5

Hysteroscopy training and learning curve of 30° camera navigation on a new box trainer: the HYSTT

J. A. Janse · C. J. Tolman · S. Veersema
F. J. M. Broekmans · H. W. R. Schreuder

Abstract Despite the upcoming use of hysteroscopy and increased applicability during the last decades, little work has been done regarding the development of hysteroscopic training models in comparison to laparoscopy. Camera navigation is often perceived to be an easy task, but it is far from an innate ability, especially when an angled optic is used. This study investigated the learning curve of hysteroscopic 30° camera navigation on a new box trainer: Hysteroscopic Skills Training and Testing (HYSTT). This prospective study (Canadian Task Force II-2) enrolled 30 novices (medical students) and ten experts (gynecologists who had performed >100 diagnostic 30° hysteroscopies). All participants performed nine repetitions of a 30° camera exercise on the HYSTT. Novices returned after 2 weeks and performed a second series of five repetitions to assess retention of skills. The parameter procedure time and structured observations on performance using the Global Rating Scale provided measurements for analysis. The learning curve is represented by improvement per procedure. Two-way repeated-measures analysis of variance was used to analyze learning curves. Effect size (ES) was calculated to express the practical significance of the results (ES $\geq$0.50 indicates a large learning effect). For both parameters, significant improvements were found in novice performance within nine repetitions. Moderate to large learning effects were established ($p < 0.05$; ES 0.44–0.71). Retention of skills and prolonged learning curves were observed. The learning curve, established in this study, of hysteroscopic 30° camera navigation skills on the HYSTT box trainer, indicates a good training capacity and provides the first step towards recommended implementation into a training curriculum.

Keywords Hysteroscopy · Training · Camera navigation · Box trainer · Simulation

Background

The exponential growth of minimally invasive surgery and the limited resident availability for educational endeavors by work hour restrictions are recent changes in modern medicine that have led to the increasing demand of valid simulation training models [1]. For developing endoscopic skills, simulators offer a safe, effective and attractive way of repeatedly training these skills without causing discomfort or harming patients [2, 3]. Thus far, the beneficial results of simulator training are mainly derived from studies on laparoscopy [4, 5].

Hysteroscopy is generally considered as a safe procedure with a low complication rate [6, 7]. Its practice ranges from diagnostics in an outpatient setting to a surgical alternative in the operation room for many gynecological problems. Despite the upcoming use of hysteroscopy and increased applicability during the last decades, little work has been done regarding the development of hysteroscopic training models in comparison to laparoscopy.

Recently, the Hysteroscopic Skills Training and Testing (HYSTT) method has been developed under auspices of the European Academy of Gynaecological Surgery (Leuven, Belgium). This box trainer aims at practicing camera navigation skills with a 30° angled hysteroscope. Camera navigation is often perceived to be an easy task, but it is far from an innate

J. A. Janse (✉) · S. Veersema
Department of Gynaecology and Obstetrics, St. Antonius Hospital,
Koekoekslaan 1, 3430 EM Nieuwegein, the Netherlands
e-mail: julienne.janse@gmail.com

C. J. Tolman · F. J. M. Broekmans · H. W. R. Schreuder
Division of Woman and Baby, Department of Reproductive
Medicine and Gynaecology, University Medical Center Utrecht,
Utrecht, the Netherlands

ability. Psychomotor skills need to be learned to overcome the barriers that are known for endoscopic skills in general, namely the fulcrum effect, a two-dimensional environment, a fixed access point, and decreased range of motion [8]. In addition, skills unique to camera navigation include maintaining a correct horizontal axis while centering the operative field and holding a steady image. Further dexterity and knowledge is required for correct use of the additional degrees of freedom afforded by an angled scope [8–10], which is used routinely in many hysteroscopic procedures [9, 11]. In a national UK survey among gynecologists, a disappointing percentage of 25.8% of all responders that use a 30° hysteroscope showed understanding of the principles of 30° angled view [9].

Camera navigation is a basic and essential skill for performing hysteroscopic procedures, especially when an angled scope is used. The HYSTT box trainer might provide a simple, effective and feasible answer to the need for training this skill.

The objective of the present study was to investigate the effectiveness of repetitive training on the HYSTT. This was sought to be achieved by determining the learning curve of novice participants and by investigating whether novices can improve and retain their skills, and whether they can approximate the expert level.

Methods

Participants

From April to June 2012, 30 novices and ten experts voluntarily conducted a series of repetitions on the HYSTT. Medical students of the University of Utrecht participated as novices, during or after their gynecology internship. The novices had a basic understanding of hysteroscopy but had never previously performed nor assisted in a hysteroscopic procedure. All novices were invited to participate via oral and written means, and all agreed. Ten gynecologists served as experts to set a reference for novice performance. For the present study, a gynecologist was considered a hysteroscopy expert after performing >100 diagnostic hysteroscopies with a 30° scope and still practicing diagnostic hysteroscopy on a weekly base. All gynecologists were personally invited and all agreed to participate. None had any experience of performing hysteroscopy on this box trainer.

The study was exempt from Institutional Review Board approval, since no potential harm could be done to humans or nonhumans. All participants gave oral consent prior to the start of the study.

Box trainer

The HYSTT has been developed under auspices of the European Academy of Gynaecological Surgery (Leuven, Belgium) and consists of a plastic uterus model in which 14 numbers

and characters are placed at 14 anatomical locations, known as: isthmus anterior/posterior/left/right, mid anterior/posterior/left/right, fundus anterior/posterior, cornua left/right and tubal ostium left/right. Six models are available in which each location contains a different number or character (model A–F). This plastic uterus is placed in a silicone model of a vulva, which in turn is situated in a plastic model of a female pelvis (Fig. 1). A 30° hysteroscope (Karl Storz diagnostic continuous-flow) connected to a video-camera, light source and monitor (Telepack, Karl Storz) were used.

Exercises

Beforehand, a survey was administered to obtain baseline characteristics. The novices received a short standardized oral introduction on hysteroscopy, the box trainer and study protocol. The experts received a standardized oral introduction on the box trainer and study protocol. Figure 2 displays the scheme of exercises per group. One-minute practice time was given to each participant to obtain familiarization with the HYSTT model. One investigator (C.J.T.) supervised all tests to limit intersupervisor bias. Both groups conducted a series of nine exercises. In detail, the exercise was as follows: the supervisor read out an anatomical location (e.g., fundus posterior), after which the participant had to navigate to that specific location and visualize the associated number or character within a black circle with a diameter of 2.5 cm. Once this was correctly and readably visualized and named, the next command was read out. Video 1 (Supplemental Material) shows a short display of the model and exercise. During each repetition, the participants had to identify as many targets in a correct manner with a maximum of 14. Each repetition ended after 3 min, after which the total number of correctly visualized objects was noted. We chose to end each repetition after 3 min, as specified by the European Academy and because we wanted to limit the training duration per

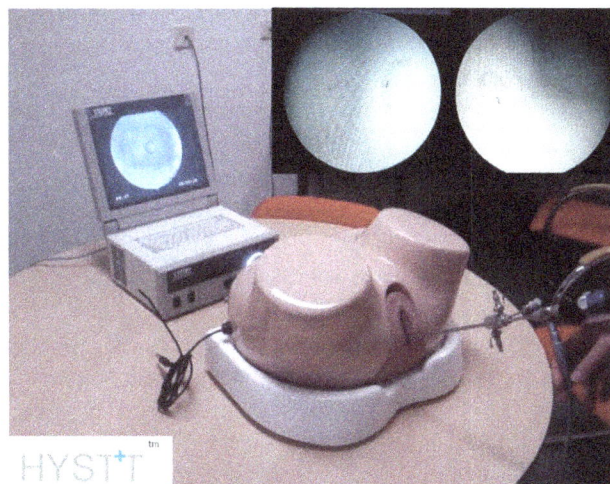

Fig. 1 Set-up Hysteroscopic Skills Training and Testing (*HYSTT*) box trainer

Fig. 2 Scheme of exercises. Note: of all repetitions, the even-numbered repetitions were meant for training by the supervisor; during the odd-numbered repetitions no training was provided because these performances were used solely for data analysis

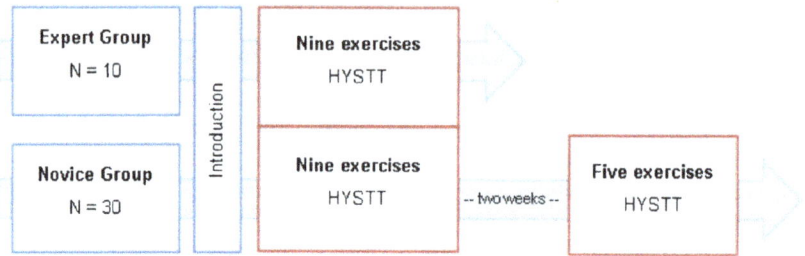

participant to 30 min per session, to optimize the concentration of the subjects. If a participant identified all 14 objects within 3 min, the time to finish the exercise was marked. Each repetition contained a completely different sequence of commands and uterus model A was switched to model B after five repetitions for every participant. This switch was performed since five different command sequences were available per model.

Of all nine repetitions, the first, third, fifth, seventh and ninth repetitions were used for data analysis. The other repetitions were meant for training by the supervisor and consisted of answering questions of the participants and giving tips and tricks on the procedure. For this reason, the even-numbered repetitions had a different duration and goal and were consequently excluded from further analysis. During the odd-numbered repetitions, no questions could be asked nor were any tips given because these performances were used solely for data analysis. To assess retention of skills, after 2 weeks, novices returned for a second series of five repetitions (model C). The first, third and fifth repetitions were used for data analysis. The other repetitions were meant for training by the supervisor and were excluded from further analysis.

Outcome measures

The main outcome parameter was procedure time, measured as time needed to finish a repetition, by identifying all 14 signs with a limit of 3 min. If less than 14 signs were identified in 3 min, the total number of correctly visualized signs (n) in 3 min was recorded by the investigator. This score was then converted to the parameter time using the following formula: $180 \text{ s} \times (14/n) = \text{score}$ (in seconds). Participants were not assessed only by procedure time because performing a procedure very fast does not necessarily mean it is performed properly and/or with good results. For that reason, a 5-point Global Rating Scale (GRS) was used to assess competence from another (clinical) perspective. The GRS was adjusted for hysteroscopic 30° camera navigation training (Fig. 3) and has not yet been validated [12]. Aspects that were rated included respect for tissue, handling of the hysteroscope, time and motion, flow and forward planning and procedure knowledge. Blinding was not possible due to the clear differences between age and status of the groups and the necessity to score both the simulator screen and the participant behavior.

Expert opinion

To investigate the expert opinion on this new box trainer, the experts completed a questionnaire at the end of the training session. The experts rated six statements on a 5-point Likert scale, concerning the applicability of the HYSTT for testing and training camera navigation, for training residents and/or medical students and for learning anatomy. The experts also valued the realism of the HYSTT in simulating a diagnostic hysteroscopy.

Statistical analysis

Data were analyzed using commercially available software (SPSS version 20.0; SPSS, Inc., Chicago, IL, USA). No power analysis was performed prior to the study. To analyze the improvement within the novice group, a sample size of 30 was considered sufficient.

The independent t-test and chi-square test were used to compare general demographic data of the experts and novices. Two-way repeated measures analysis of variance was used to analyze learning curves. The between-subject factor group was added to investigate novice and expert performance separately. Retention of skills was investigated by within-subject contrasts and was assessed by comparing the last repetition of both series; a significant improvement by repetitive training was defined as a prolonged learning curve [13]. A p value of <0.05 was considered as statistically significant for all tests.

GRS 1 Respect for tissue	Scope frequently pushed into wall of uterus.		Scope occasionally pushed into wall of uterus.	No trauma to uterus with scope.	
	1	2	3	4	5
GRS 2 Time and motion	Many unnecessary moves.		Made some unnecessary moves, but time more efficient.	No unnecessary moves and time is maximized.	
	1	2	3	4	5
GRS 3 Handling of hysteroscope	Scope poorly aligned during procedure.		Moderate use of scope angle during procedure.	Scope always set in good angle throughout the procedure.	
	1	2	3	4	5
GRS 4 Flow of procedure and forward planning	Frequently stopped or needed advice or assistance from examiner.		Demonstrated ability to think forward with relatively steady progression of procedure.	Obviously planned procedure from beginning to end with fluid motion.	
	1	2	3	4	5
GRS 5 Knowledge of procedure	Deficient knowledge. Needed specific instruction at most procedural steps.		Knew all important aspects of procedure.	Demonstrated familiarity with all aspects of procedure.	
	1	2	3	4	5

Fig. 3 Global Rating Scale, adjusted for hysteroscopic 30° camera navigation training

Means and 95% confidence intervals (CI) were used to compare data for the learning curves because these are applicable to the analysis of variance.

While statistical significance provides information on evidence of any effect at all, the practical significance of the results was quantified by the effect size (ES), which indicates whether a learning effect is meaningful or important [14]. The ES is independent of sample size and a scale-free index. The ES was extracted from the analysis of variance output in SPSS. ES of 0.10, 0.30 and 0.50 were considered to indicate small (negligible), medium (moderate) and large (crucial) effects, respectively. ES was considered relevant only if a significant ($p < 0.05$) result was found.

Findings

Demographic data

General demographic data of novices and experts are given in Table 1. As expected, there is a significant difference between gender ($p < 0.001$), age ($p < 0.001$) and prior hysteroscopy experience ($p < 0.001$). To assess retention of skills, novices returned after a median of 14 days (range, 11–19 days) for a second series of repetitions. None of the experts had previous experience of performing exercises on HYSTT.

Learning curve

The main outcome measure was procedure time. The secondary outcome parameter was clinical performance, which was assessed by the mean GRS score. Results of novice performance in both series of repetitions are given in Table 2 (original measurements). A graphic presentation of the novice learning curve with the expert performance as a reference curve is shown in Fig. 4.

Novices showed a significant and moderate learning effect for the time needed to complete a repetition ($p < 0.05$, ES=0.44). A large difference was observed between experts and novices in procedure time, in favour of the experts (experts, mean 215.8 s, 95% CI 154.9 – 276.7 s; novices, 869.4 s, 95% CI 570.1–1,168.6 s). As recognized in the graph, novices progressed towards expert level in time and reached a plateau phase at the seventh repetition, while experts performed stable after their first exercise. Both plateau phases did not coincide (experts, mean 108.3 s, 95% CI 87.8–128.8 s; novices, mean 154.3 s, 95% CI 130.3–178.3 s).

For mean GRS score, the novice group demonstrated a significant and large learning effect ($p < 0.05$, ES=0.71). The expert group received higher GRS scores from the start (experts, mean 3.4, 95% CI 3.0 – 3.8; novices, mean 1.8, 95% CI 1.6 – 2.1) and the difference between both groups only moderately decreased. No plateau phase was recognized in the novice learning curve.

Table 1 Baseline characteristics of all participants

		Novices (N=30)	Experts (N=10)	
Demographic data				
Sex, male/female, No. (%)		6:24 (20:80)	8:2 (80:20)	
Age, median in years (range)		24.0 (21 – 27)	51.5 (42 – 56)	
Handedness, right/left, No. (%)		27:3 (90:10)	10:0 (100:0)	
Days between series, median (range)		14 (11–19)	NA	
Training experience in hysteroscopy, No. (%)			Animal Box VR	
0 h		30 (100)	5 (50) 7 (70) 7 (70)	
1–10 h		0	5 (50) 3 (30) 3 (30)	
>10 h		0	0 0 0	
Novice experience				
Hysteroscopies seen, No. (%)				
0		17 (56.7)		
1–10		12 (40.0)		
> 10		1 (3.3)		
Hysteroscopies performed, No. (%)		0 (100)		
Expert experience				
Hysteroscopies performed,[a] No. (%)			Level 1 Level 2 Level 3	
0			0 0 0	
1–30			0 0 2 (20)	
31–50			0 0 3 (30)	
>50			10 (100) 10 (100) 5 (50)	

NA not applicable, *Animal* animal cadaver model, *Box* box trainer, *VR* virtual reality simulator

[a] According to European Society for Gynaecological Endoscopy (ESGE) classification of hysteroscopic complexity [15]

Table 2 Results of novice performance in both series

Parameter	First series: learning curve			Second series: retention of skills	
	First repetition	Last repetition	Significance[a]	Last repetition	Significance[b]
Time (s)	869.4 (95% CI, 570.1–1168.6)	154.3 (95% CI, 130.3–178.3)	$p < 0.05$, ES=0.44	121.0 (95% CI, 103.3–138.8)	$p < 0.05$[c], ES=0.35
Mean GRS (5-point scale)	1.83 (95% CI, 1.59–2.08)	3.78 (95% CI, 3.50–4.06)	$p < 0.05$, ES=0.71	4.13 (95% CI, 3.95–4.32)	$p < 0.05$[c], ES=0.65

CI confidence interval, *ES* effect size (only applicable if result is significant), *GRS* Global Rating Scale

[a] Implicates significance of comparison between first and last repetition of first series (analysis of variance)

[b] Implicates significance of comparison between last repetition of first and second series (analysis of variance)

[c] Indicates prolonged learning curve

Retention of skills

For both procedure time and GRS, analysis of novice performance after 2 weeks showed retention of skills. Comparing the last repetitions of both series, no significant decrease in performance was found. Instead, a significant improvement of performance parameters was observed by repetitive training ($p < 0.05$, ES=0.35–0.65), indicating a prolonged learning curve (Table 2).

Expert opinion

All experts completed the questionnaire concerning the realism and training capacity of the HYSTT. Table 3 summarizes the scores awarded by the experts. The ability to test and train camera navigation skills was scored with a median of 5.00 points on a 5-point Likert scale. The experts indicated the HYSTT to be very applicable in training residents (median 4.90). The box trainer was considered less applicable for training medical students (median 3.50) and for learning anatomy (median 3.00). The realism of the HYSTT in simulating a diagnostic hysteroscopy was awarded a median of 3.00 points.

Discussion

The present study assessed the learning curve for performance of hysteroscopic 30° camera navigation skills using the HYSTT, a new box trainer for diagnostic hysteroscopy. For all parameters, significant improvements were found in novice performance within nine repetitions. Retention of skills was demonstrated and a prolonged learning curve was established. These results indicate an adequate training capacity of the HYSTT and the effectiveness of repetitive training. One or more training sessions substantially improve the acquisition of 30° camera navigation skills on the HYSTT.

Strong points of this study are its realistic study design, additional assessment of retention of skills, and that one investigator supervised all tests in both groups. Furthermore, the use of ES adds information as to whether significant learning curves can be translated into meaningful and important learning effects. Besides procedure time, a clinical parameter (GRS) was used to assess competence from another perspective. Performing a procedure very fast does not necessarily mean it is performed properly and/or with good results.

Differences between the performance levels of both groups give an indication of construct validity, which is an important

Fig. 4 Learning curve for novices (*blue*) and experts (*green*) in the first series of exercises and for novices in the second series

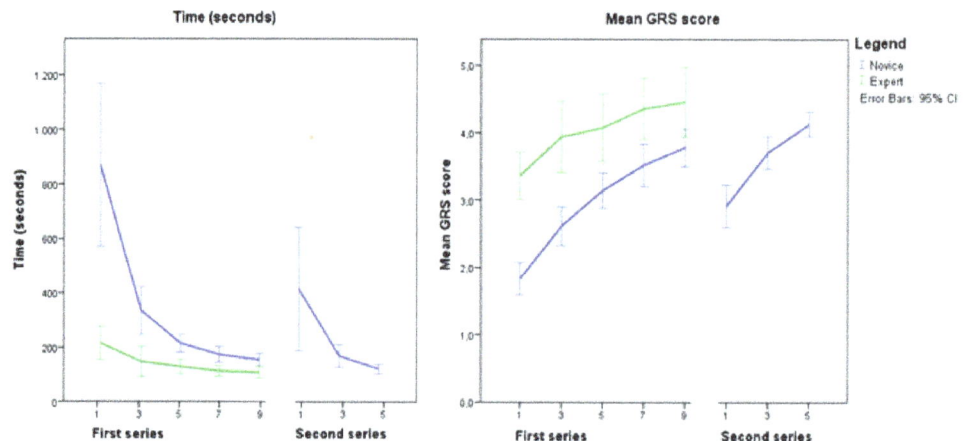

Table 3 Results of expert opinion

The HYSTT…	Experts ($N=10$)
1. … is able to *train* 30° hysteroscopic camera navigation skills	5.00 (4.75–5.00)
2. … is able to *test* 30° hysteroscopic camera navigation skills	5.00 (4.00–5.00)
3. … is applicable for training OBGYN residents	5.00 (5.00–5.00)
4. … is applicable for training medical students	3.50 (2.75–5.00)
5. … is applicable for learning uterine anatomy	3.00 (1.75–4.00)
6. … simulates a diagnostic hysteroscopy realistically	3.00 (2.00–4.00)

Median scores (with interquartile ranges) are given on a 5-point Likert scale

investigation before implementation of a model into a training curriculum [16]. The results imply that the HYSTT is indeed able to teach and evaluate those skills that are intended to be taught and measured, by differentiating between levels of expertise. However, the present study was not designed to investigate construct validity or powered to differentiate. Therefore, the indication of construct validity should be interpreted with caution.

The GRS was adjusted for hysteroscopic 30° camera navigation training and has not yet been validated, though similar rating scales have been implemented and validated for use in a general hysteroscopic training program and diagnostic cystoscopy in urology [17, 18].

It can be argued whether the first repetition(s) should be used for data analysis in a study assessing the learning curve, considering the improvement in performance parameters for both groups. The time needed to become familiar with a simulation model could influence results. The chosen study design reflects reality and integrates the possibility of feedback and training in the process [19]. The expert curve functions as a reference, and possible improvement during the first cases is likely to represent reality. Experts also must become accustomed to the new environment because this is by definition a deduction of reality.

The learning curve for GRS shows that the experts continue to improve their score until the seventh repetition, which might be a later plateau phase than one expects. A possible explanation could be that the white plastic HYSTT model does not resemble the uterus in a very close matter, as indicated by the expert opinion. The anatomical terms were considered confusing for several uterine locations. For example, "cornua" implies the *region* where a fallopian tube enters the uterine cavity. The HYSTT model contains specific *spots* for both "cornua" and "tubal ostium", which are located very close to each other and without any further clues concerning the differentiation between these anatomical terms. These locations were frequently mixed up by several experts throughout the repetitions, which led to lower GRS scores. Also, in the HYSTT model, the cervical canal is absent and

therefore the hysteroscope can slip out of the uterus without visual warning.

To improve the use and applicability of the HYSTT, the realism of the model might be enhanced by improving the visual aspects of the uterine cavity, e.g., silicone material with realistic colour effects, augmented uterine shape with real tubal ostia and a cervical canal. A different possibility might be to remove the cornual locations and change the anatomical terms into more general terms, e.g., front/mid/rear, combined with anterior/posterior/left/right.

A recent study by the current authors investigated the learning curve of hysteroscopic sterilization on a virtual reality (VR) simulator [20]. The curves of both training models show similar shapes, indicating an adequate training capacity of repetitive training for both exercises and models. Concerning procedure time, the novices learned somewhat faster and reached a plateau phase within nine repetitions on the camera navigation box trainer in comparison to the VR sterilization simulator. Regarding GRS score, the novice group showed a slightly greater improvement of clinical skills on the VR sterilization simulator; a prolonged learning curve was observed for both training models.

Enabling a good training model to be successful in daily practice, it should be implemented into a well-thought-out training curriculum [21, 22]. This curriculum preferably contains training sessions taking place on an interval basis rather than massed into a short period of extensive practice. In addition, expert performance should be used to provide a proficiency criterion [21]. This gives trainees an objectively established goal they would have to reach before progressing to a next level or the operating room. Furthermore, feasibility is important to consider, for easy employment of the training model in a curriculum. The present box trainer showed promising results for interval training and the expert level was determined to provide an indication of the proficiency criterion. Also, the HYSTT is portable and reusable and the instruments are available at any institution providing hysteroscopic procedures.

Assessment of predictive validity is a further important step in determining the applicability of a simulator in a training curriculum. The predictive validity indicates the extent to which the training model predicts future performance and there remains a paucity of predictive validity testing of gynecologic simulators at this time, especially for hysteroscopy.

Conclusions

In conclusion, the learning curve of the present box trainer for hysteroscopic 30° camera navigation skills indicate a good training capacity because large improvements were made for novice training on this box trainer. Furthermore, retention of skills and prolonged learning curves were observed for both parameters procedure time and GRS. In addition, experts awarded the HYSTT the highest scores for training camera skills and applicability in residency training. Improvements can be made on the realism and anatomy of the uterus model.

Acknowledgements We thank all the participants who voluntarily participated in this study. We also thank M.J.C. Eijkemans, associate professor in BioStatistics from the Julius Center for Health Sciences and Primary care, University of Utrecht, the Netherlands, for his help with the statistical analysis.

Contribution to authorship All authors meet the criteria to qualify for authorship, in detail: JJ designed and planned the study, analyzed the data and wrote the manuscript. CT collected and analyzed the data and wrote the manuscript. SV helped with the study design and revised the manuscript. FB helped with the study design and revised the manuscript. HS designed the study, assisted in analyses and revised the manuscript. All authors accept the responsibility for the paper as published.

References

1. Diesen DL, Erhunmwunsee L, Bennett KM, Ben-David K, Yurcisin B, Cepaa EP, Omotosho PA, Perez A, Pryor A (2011) Effectiveness of laparoscopic computer simulator versus usage of box trainer for endoscopic surgery training of novices. J Surg Educ 68:282–289

2. Gallagher AG, Cates CU (2004) Virtual reality training for the operating room and cardiac catheterization laboratory. Lancet 364:1538–1540

3. Larsen CR, Soerensen JL, Grantcharov TP, Dalsgaard T, Schouenborg L, Ottosen C, Schroeder TV, Ottesen BS (2009) Effect of virtual reality training on laparoscopic surgery: randomised controlled trial. BMJ 338:b1802

4. Schreuder HW, van den Berg CB, Hazebroek EJ, Verheijen RH, Schijven MP (2011) Laparoscopic skills training using inexpensive box trainers: which exercises to choose when constructing a validated training course. BJOG 118:1576–1584

5. Larsen CR, Oestergaard J, Ottesen BS, Soerensen JL (2012) The efficacy of virtual reality simulation training in laparoscopy: a systematic review of randomized trials. Acta Obstet Gynecol Scand 91:1015–1028

6. Jansen FW, Vredevoogd CB, van Ulzen K, Hermans J, Trimbos JB, Trimbos-Kemper TC (2000) Complications of hysteroscopy: a prospective, multicenter study. Obstet Gynecol 96:266–270

7. Aydeniz B, Gruber IV, Schauf B, Kurek R, Meyer A, Wallwiener D (2002) A multicenter survey of complications associated with 21,676 operative hysteroscopies. Eur J Obstet Gynecol Reprod Biol 104:160–164

8. Korndorffer JR Jr, Hayes DJ, Dunne JB, Sierra R, Touchard CL, Markert RJ, Scott DJ (2005) Development and transferability of a cost-effective laparoscopic camera navigation simulator. Surg Endosc 19:161–167

9. Tawfeek S, Scott P (2010) National inpatient diagnostic hysteroscopy survey. Gynecol Surg 7:53–59

10. Yee KA, Karmali S, Sherman V (2009) Validation of a simple camera navigation trainer. J Am Coll Surg 209:753–757

11. Di Spiezio SA, Taylor A, Tsirkas P, Mastrogamvrakis G, Sharma M, Magos A (2008) Hysteroscopy: a technique for all? Analysis of 5,000 outpatient hysteroscopies. Fertil Steril 89:438–443

12. Martin JA, Regehr G, Reznick R, MacRae H, Murnaghan J, Hutchison C, Brown M (1997) Objective structured assessment of technical skill (OSATS) for surgical residents. Br J Surg 84:273–278

13. Maagaard M, Sorensen JL, Oestergaard J, Dalsgaard T, Grantcharov TP, Ottesen BS, Larsen CR (2011) Retention of laparoscopic procedural skills acquired on a virtual-reality surgical trainer. Surg Endosc 25:722–727

14. Hojat M, Xu G (2004) A visitor's guide to effect sizes: statistical significance versus practical (clinical) importance of research findings. Adv Health Sci Educ Theory Pract 9:241–249

15. European Society for Gynaecological Endoscopy (2013) Classification hysteroscopy. http://www.esge.org/media/files/hystt%20identification%20form.pdf. Accessed 29 May 2013

16. McDougall EM (2007) Validation of surgical simulators. J Endourol 21:244–7

17. VanBlaricom AL, Goff BA, Chinn M, Icasiano MM, Nielsen P, Mandel L (2005) A new curriculum for hysteroscopy training as demonstrated by an objective structured assessment of technical skills (OSATS). Am J Obstet Gynecol 193:1856–1865

18. Matsumoto ED, Hamstra SJ, Radomski SB, Cusimano MD (2001) A novel approach to endourological training: training at the Surgical Skills Center. J Urol 166:1261–1266

19. Verdaasdonk EGG, Stassen LPS, Schijven MP, Dankelman J (2007) Construct validity and assessment of the learning curve for the SIMENDO endoscopic simulator. Surg Endosc 21:1406–12

20. Janse JA, Goedegebuure RSA, Veersema S, Broekmans FJM, Schreuder HWR (2013) Hysteroscopic sterilization using a virtual reality simulator: assessment of learning curve. JMIG 20:775–782

21. Gallagher AG, Ritter EM, Champion H, Higgins G, Fried MP, Moses G, Smith CD, Satava RM (2005) Virtual reality simulation for the operating room: proficiency-based training as a paradigm shift in surgical skills training. Ann Surg 241:364–372

22. Zevin B, Levy JS, Satava RM, Grantcharov TP (2012) A consensus-based framework for design, validation, and implementation of simulation-based training curricula in surgery. J Am Coll Surg 215:580v586

6

Systematic review of the outcome associated with the different surgical treatment of bowel and rectovaginal endometriosis

Magdy Mohammed Moustafa ·
Mohamed Abdel Aleem Elnasharty

Abstract Background: Treatment of deep endometriosis involving the bowel is controversial. There is limitation of medical treatment. Several surgical techniques are used. All of them are associated with potential intraoperative complications and long-term hazards for the bladder, bowel and sexual function. Objectives: This study seeks to review systematically different types of surgical treatment of bowel endometriosis which include mucosal skinning (shaving), disc excision, and segmental resection. The review includes the number of participants, histology, symptomatology, preoperative assessment, types and access of surgery, complications, hospital stay, length and way of follow up, symptom improvement, recurrence, and effects on fertility. Study strategy: All published articles on surgical treatment of endometriosis (shaving, rectovaginal endometriosis, disc excision, and segmental resection), identified through MEDLINE, EMBASE, CINAHL, and Cochran library during 1970–2011. Grey literatures were searched as well. Selection criteria: The terms 'endometriosis', 'bowel', surgical, and complications were used. Articles describing 50 patients or more who had bowel surgery for endometriosis were only included. Data collection and analysis: Data did not permit a meaningful meta-analysis. Main results: We analyzed 36 articles after thorough literature search. It described 2,414 of mucosal skinning/rectovaginal endometriosis, 381 of disc excision, and 2,728 of bowel resection for deep endometriosis involving the bowel. The indication for surgery was stated in most of the studies. Histology was confirmed in the majority; however, completeness of the excision was stated in few articles. There is significant improvement of symptoms with all

types of surgery. Complications were higher in segmental resection than conservative surgery (shaving and disc excision) especially leakage and fistula formation. The duration of surgery and hospital stay was shorter in conservative surgery unless there were complications or if associated with other surgeries. Fertility outcome was favourable in all. The recurrence and reoperation rate was higher in one study only in the shaving group, but otherwise was comparable to the resection group. Conclusion: There was no difference in the outcome between different types of surgery which indicates that we should adopt the conservative surgery if possible. The heterogeneity of the studies makes it difficult to do any valuable statistical analysis. There should be standardization in clinical trials evaluating bowel surgery for endometriosis.

Keywords Deep endometriosis · Rectovaginal endometriosis · Shaving techniques · Bowel resection

Introduction

Endometriosis is a gynaecological disease defined by histological presence of endometrial glands and stroma outside the uterine cavity, most commonly implanted over visceral and peritoneal surfaces within the female pelvis [1].

Deep endometriosis is defined as adenomyosis externa, mostly presents as a single nodule larger than 1 cm in diameter, in the vesicouterine fold or close to the lower 20 cm of the bowel [2]. It is surgically challenging when involving organs, such as the bowel, bladder, or ureter [3, 4].

Sites of endometriosis affecting the bowel

The term 'bowel endometriosis' should be used when endometrial-like glands and stroma infiltrate the bowel wall reaching at least the subserous fat tissue or adjacent to the

M. M. Moustafa (✉)
Frimley Park Hospital, Surrey, UK
e-mail: magdy_moustafa@live.co.uk

M. A. A. Elnasharty
Cairo University Hospital, Cairo, Egypt

neurovascular branches (subserous plexus). As initially suggested by Chapron et al. [5], endometriotic foci located on the bowel serosa should be considered peritoneal and not bowel endometriosis. The most frequent location of bowel involvement with endometriosis is the sigmoid colon (over 65 % of the cases), followed by the rectum, the ileum, the appendix, and the caecum [6]. Gastric and transverse colonic diseases are also reported by Remorgida et al. [7].

Why it is important to do this review

Endometriosis generally affects otherwise healthy young women with high expectations of well-being and quality of life. In this population, complications and side effects of surgery are not easily tolerated, and the recurrence of symptoms can be especially frustrating. It is doubtful that the primary surgery, however beautifully and skilfully performed, would remove all viable endometriotic 'cells' or microscopic endometriotic lesions invisible to the naked eyes under the laparoscopy and eliminate recurrence altogether. Theoretically, just one single viable cell can, under suitable milieu and conditions, propagate and grow into a colony [8]. Conceivably, recurrence after surgery occurs because of in situ regrowth of residual endometriotic lesions or cells not completely removed in the surgery, growth of microscopic endometriosis undetected at surgery, or the development of de novo lesions, or a combination of these.

Obviously, the recurrence rate varies with the definition of recurrence (subjective feeling of pain or more objective clinical/instrumental measurements), type of endometriosis, methods of surgery or post-operation intervention, if any, disease severity, type of hospital where the surgery is performed, and the skills of the surgeons who performed the surgery, among many known or potential factors that may influence the recurrence risk. Although it is self-evident that the recurrence rate increases as the length of follow-up, occasionally some studies, which involve patients recruited consecutively during a certain time window, only report an 'overall recurrence rate', giving few clues to the duration of follow-up. This kind of 'recurrence rate' is next to useless when making comparison among studies since it simply means little if anything without specifying the time elapsed since surgery [8].

In the experience of Anaf et al. [9], as well as in the available literature, the presence of a rectovaginal endometriotic nodule is always associated with pelvic pain, dysmenorrhoea, and/or deep dyspareunia [8, 10–13]. However, Fedele et al. [14] followed 88 patients with untreated asymptomatic rectovaginal endometriosis for 1 to 9 years. Pain symptoms and clinical and transrectal ultrasonographic findings were evaluated before and every 6 months after diagnosis. Progression of the disease and appearance of specific symptoms rarely occurred in patients with asymptomatic rectovaginal endometriosis.

Medical management of deep endometriosis (DIE) with colorectal extension (with non-steroidal anti-inflammatory drugs, oral contraceptives, gestogens, antigestogens, or GnRH agonists) is based on suppression of the symptoms, is not curative, and is often associated with significant side effects [15–17]. It is not clear if the medical management approach prevents disease progression, especially in more severe cases of endometriosis with colorectal extension. In addition, discontinuation of this therapy commonly results in recurrence [18].

De Cicco et al. [4] struggled to find good quality studies with accurate reports of the essential information needed to fully appreciate the risks associated with segmental resection for endometriosis. In the studies they reviewed, the majority was retrospective case series, with only four of the 30 studies presented containing more than 100 participants. Indeed, 77 % of the studies included contained fewer than 50 participants. What they do not know from these smaller studies is whether the reported cases reflect the complication rate during the surgeons learning curve. As the major complications rate vary considerably (from 0 % to 48 %), it is likely that the results are heavily influenced by the current experience of the surgeons. It may be the higher morbidity reported in the smaller studies reflects the true situation in units only performing few cases a year. Importantly, there are no reports on fertility rates in women who experienced severe complications, such as faecal peritonitis, which is likely to have resulted in significant adhesive disease.

Paya et al. [19] in their review of surgical treatment of rectovaginal endometriosis concluded that although the studies published to assess the effect of different surgical techniques on the treatment of rectovaginal endometriosis showed a great heterogeneity in their characteristics and methodology, we can say that whenever technically possible, the more conservative techniques, shaving, and discoid intestinal resection would be recommended since they present a lower rate of complications with similar recurrence and greater rates of gestation. In relation to the surgical approach, two main groups can be observed: those who propose a more aggressive approach and tend to defend the systematic intestinal resection under the premise that a more radical approach would be more effective (segmental resection of the rectum and/or sigmoid colon) and those that argue for a more conservative approach basing their argument on the lack of scientific evidence of better results with more radical techniques and the association of these techniques with higher-long-term morbidity and a lower quality of life for patients(shaving of the rectal, disc excision of the anterior rectal wall).

So what advice could we sensibly give women who need to decide on whether they opt for surgical treatment of lower bowel endometriosis? Until we have robust data, it is difficult to provide women with accurate information about the surgical risk. Based on the larger studies in the review by De Cicco et al. [4], we can advise that the chances of having a major surgical complication are probably around 10 % in the bowel resection.

Wright and Ballard [18], continue to remain unclear about the efficacy of rectal surgery for endometriosis.

Yet, in order for women to be able to make an informed choice about whether to have bowel surgery for endometriosis, it is essential that they have accurate information about both the benefits and risks associated with the procedure. We will try in this review to explore the surgical option by looking at large studies.

Methods

We included only the randomized, retrospective or prospective studies with 50 patients or more of bowel surgery for endometriosis which include excision of rectovaginal septum, mucosal skinning, disc excision, and bowel resection. The route of surgery could be laparotomy, laparoscopy, with or without the help of vaginal or transanal approach. The outcome measures include:

1. Significant complications (anastomotic leaks, stenosis of anastomosis, rectovaginal fistula, vesicovaginal fistula, bowel dysfunction, bladder dysfunction, ureteric injury, haemorrhage necessitating blood transfusion, colostomy, or ileostomy and reoperation).
2. Improvement of symptoms related to endometriosis (pelvic pain, dyspareunia, dyschezia, and dysmenorrhoea). Assessment of improvements can be either clinically, questionnaire, or visual analogue scale. Quality of life after surgery will be looked at as well.
3. Fertility outcome.

We searched the electronic database such as MEDLINE (from 1970 to the end of 2011), CINAHL (from 1981 to the end of 2011), EMBASE (from 1980 to end of 2011), and Cochrane library for relevant studies. The following keywords: endometriosis, bowel, surgical, and complications were searched. The Biotechnology Research Abstracts and all registers included in the meta Register of Controlled Trials (mRCT) were also searched.

Grey literature search was performed using the SIGLE system (System for Information on Grey Literature in Europe). The references of retrieved key articles, together with the proceedings of relevant conferences, were hand-searched to identify other potentially eligible studies for inclusion in the analysis missed by the initial search or any unpublished studies. We also searched the index to thesis. The review will include only the studies published in English.

Study characteristics

- Setting:
  - Single or multicentre
  - Location
  - Timing and duration
- Size:
  - Number of included women
  - Number of women lost in follow-up
  - Number of women analyzed
- Duration and way of follow-up
- Type of surgery
- Duration of surgery
- Hospital stay
- Complications
- Fertility issues

  Figure 1 shows the research pathway.

Results

From 1987 to December 2011, 36 articles (5539 patients) were analysed describing 2,414 of mucosal skinning/rectovaginal septum, 381 of disc excision, and 2,728 of bowel resection for deep endometriosis involving the bowel [20–55] (Table 1). There is progressive shift from laparotomy to laparoscopy. Around half of the studies in this review (19 studies) were between 2007 and 2011.

We will use the reference's number for description rather than the authors' names if required. The case series which deal with shaving only [27, 28, 34, 47], will be named as 'the shaving group', and those which discuss the bowel resection only [22, 25, 26, 30, 36, 37, 40, 42, 49, 51] will be named as 'the resection group'. The rest of the studies will be called 'the mixed group'. There were no clear subdivisions between different types of surgery in the latter group except in these studies [23, 31, 35, 38, 39, 43, 45]. Cases with disc excision in the previous studies within the mixed group were analyzed separately (Fig. 2). Complications rate in this group varied from 0 % to 23 %. Recurrence was only discussed in [23] (3 rectal endometriosis and 7 pelvic endometriosis). Fertility after disc excision was 11 % which was mentioned only in one case series [43].

Types of the studies

There were 15 retrospective and 20 prospective studies in this review. The only randomized study in this systematic review was in study [26]. It was a comparison between laparoscopic assisted and open colorectal resection.

Fig. 1 Flow chart of the research pathway

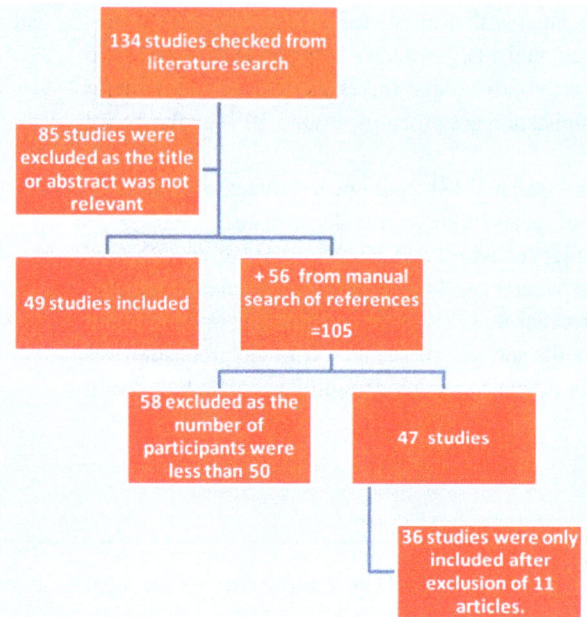

Route of surgery

Laparotomy was the only access of surgery in these studies [21]: (130) [24], (77) [29], (100) [54], and (163). A combination of laparoscopy and laparotomy was the route of surgery in these studies [23, 26, 27, 32, 33, 35, 52, 53, 55]. In the rest of the studies, laparoscopy was the primary access of surgery (23

studies). There were conversions to laparatomy in 103 cases out of 4,946(2.1 %). In the shaving group, all the procedures were laparoscopic. There were 3 conversions out of 1,181 laparoscopies (0.25 %). All the studies in the resection group except [26, 29] (50 % had laparotomy), laparoscopy was the only surgical route. Conversions were done in 35 out of 1,608 laparoscopies (2.2 %) [Table 2].

Table 1 The studies and the number of patients in the systematic review

References	No. of patients	References	No. of patients
Alvez Pereira et al. [20]/Brazil	168	Kondo et al. [38]/France	225
Bailey et al. [21]/USA	130	Maytham et al. [39]/UK	54
Bassi et al. [22]/Brazil	151	Mereu et al. [40]/Italy	192
Brouwer and Woods [23]/Australia	213	Meuleman et al. [41]/Belgium	56
Coronado et al. [24]/USA	77	Minelli et al. [42]/Italy	357
Darai et al. [25]/France	71	Mohr et al. [43]/USA	187
Darai et al. [26]/France	52	Nezhat et al. [44]/USA	185
Donnez et al. [27]/Belgium	500	Pandis et al. [45]/UK	134
Donnez and Squifflet [28]/Belgium	500	Redwine and Wright [46]/USA	84
Dousset et al. [29]/France	100	Reich et al. [47]/USA	100
Dubernard et al. [30]/France	58	Ribeiro et al. [48]/Brazil	125
Duepree et al. [31]/USA	51	Ruffo et al. [49]/Italy	436
Fedele et al. [32]/Italy	83	Slack et al. [50]/UK	128
Ford et al. [33]/UK	60	Stepniewska et al. [51]/Italy	60
Hollett-Caines et al. [34]/Canada	81	Tarjanne et al. [52]/Finland	60
Jatan et al. [35]/Australia	95	Varol et al. [53]/Australia	169
Kavallaris et al. [36]/Germany	55	Weed and Ray [54]/USA	163
Keckstein and Wiesinger [37]/Austria	202	Wills et al. [55]/Australia	177

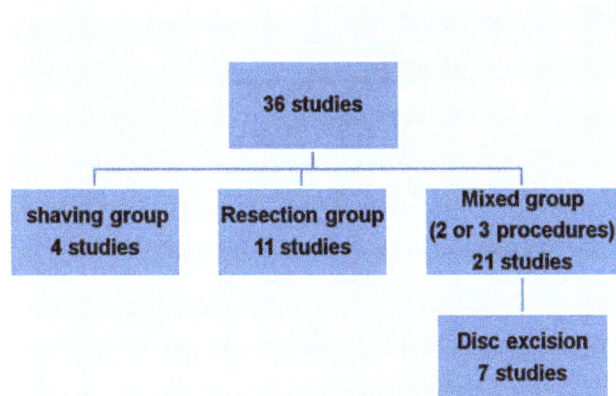

Fig. 2 Subdivision of the study group

Site of the lesion

The rectum (or the rectovaginal septum) was involved in all the studies. The colon (mainly the sigmoid), appendix, and the terminal ileum were also involved in addition to the rectum in some studies to a variable degree.

Symptomatology

Pelvic pain, dysmenorrhoea, dyspareunia, infertility, dyschezia, rectal bleeding, and change of bowel habits are the most common symptoms of endometriosis and the cause of referral. Studies [38, 48, 55] did not mention what the symptoms that the patients were referred with.

Histology examination

It was not clearly stated that the specimen removed was sent for histology, in 13 case series [22, 23, 26, 31, 34, 35, 37, 40, 44, 47, 49, 52, 53] out of 36 studies(36 %) [Table 3].

The completeness of the excision was discussed only in 4 articles [25, 29, 36, 53]. It was reported as complete in the last three case series. Darai et al. [25] stated that the completeness of excision was confirmed in 69/ 70 patients.

Preoperative assessment

It was not mentioned in 3 studies [21, 31, 52] (Table 4). Laparoscopy was used as an initial assessment in these studies [23, 33, 36, 39, 43, 47, 50, 53–55]. Visual analogue was used in four studies as part of the preoperative assessment [40, 41, 46, 51]. Other methods of preoperative assessment included in the study include transvaginal/endorectal ultrasound, colonoscopy/sigmoidoscopy, double contrast barium enema, MRI, and CT scan. CA125 was requested in only one study [42].

Table 2 Route of surgery

References	A Laparosopy/B Laparotomy/C Conversion	References	Laparosopy/ laparotomy
Alvez Pereira et al. [20]	A 168, C 1	Kondo et al. [38]	A 220, B 5, C 9
Bailey et al. [21]	B 130	Maytham et al. [39]	A 54, C 2
Bassi et al. [22]	A 151	Mereu et al. [40]	A 192, C 5
Brouwer and Woods [23]	A 152, B 61, C 2	Meuleman et al. [41]	A 56
Coronado et al. [24]	B 77	Minelli et al. [42]	A 357, C14
Darai et al. [25]	A 71, C 7	Mohr et al. [43]	A 187, C 2
Darai et al. [26]	A 26, B 26, C 2	Nezhat et al. [44]	A 184, B 1
Donnez et al. [27]	A 497, B 3	Pandis et al. [45]	A 134, C 1
Donnez and Squifflet [28]	A 500	Redwine and Wright [46]	A 84
Dousset et al. [29]	B 100	Reich et al. [47]	A 100
Dubernard et al. [30]	A 58, C 7	Ribeiro et al. [48]	A 125
Duepree et al. [31]	A 51, C 4	Ruffo et al. [49]	A 436, C 14
Fedele et al. [32]	A 21, B 62	Slack et al. [50]	A 128
Ford et al. [33]	A 48, B 12, C 2	Stepniewska et al. [51]	A 60
Hollett-Caines et al. [34]	A 81	Tarjanne et al. [52]	A 23, B 37
Jatan et al. [35]	A 91, B 4, C 13	Varol et al. [53]	A 145, B 24
Kavallaris et al. [36]	A 55	Weed and Ray [54]	B 163
Keckstein and Wiesinger [37]	A 202	Wills et al. [55]	A 158, B 19, C 14

Table 3 Histology

References	No.	Histology
Alvez Pereira et al. [20]	168	Confirmed in 155
Bailey et al. [21]	130	Confirmed
Bassi et al. [22]	151	NA
Brouwer and Woods [23]	213	NA
Coronado et al. [24]	77	Confirmed
Darai et al. [25]	71	Confirmed in 70
Darai et al. [26]	52	NA
Donnez et al. [27]	500	Confirmed
Donnez and Squifflet [28]	500	Confirmed
Dousset et al. [29]	100	Confirmed
Dubernard et al. [30]	58	Confirmed in 57
Duepree et al. [31]	51	NA
Fedele et al. [32]	83	Confirmed
Ford et al. [33]	60	Confirmed in 55
Hollett-Caines et al. [34]	81	NA
Jatan [35]	95	NA
Kavallaris et al. [36]	55	Confirmed
Keckstein and Wiesinger [37]	202	NA
Kondo et al. [38]	225	Confirmed
Maytham et al. [39]	54	Confirmed
Mereu et al. [40]	192	NA
Meuleman et al. [41]	56	Confirmed in 42
Minelli et al. [42]	357	Confirmed
Mohr et al. [43]	187	Confirmed 183
Nezhat et al. [44]	185	NA
Pandis et al. [45]	134	Confirmed in 132
Redwine and Wright [46]	84	Confirmed in 73
Reich et al. [47]	100	NA
Ribeiro et al. [48]	125	Confirmed
Ruffo et al. [49]	436	NA
Slack et al. [50]	128	Confirmed
Stepniewska et al. [51]	60	Confirmed
Tarjanne et al. [52]	60	NA
Varol et al. [53]	169	NA
Weed and Ray [54]	163	Confirmed in 158
Wills et al. [55]	177	Confirmed n 174

Operation time and hospital stay

The shaving group got less operating time (69–178 min) and hospital stay (1.5- 2.8 days), than the resection group (181–390 min) and (3.1–9 days), respectively (Tables 5, 6, and 7).

Effect of surgery on symptoms

Pelvic pain

The effect of surgery was not mentioned in these studies [35, 38, 40, 42, 45, 48, 49, 51, 54, 55]. The improvement of pain,

Table 4 Preoperative assessment

Preoperative assessment
Clinical examination and TV scan [20]
Not described [21]
Clinical examination and TV scan [22]
Laparoscopy 60 %, EUA 70 %, colonoscopy 13 % [barium enema, TV scan, and endorectal ultrasound], rarely used [23]
Clinical examination, proctosigmoidoscopy [24]
All women underwent both MRI and endorectal ultrasound [25]
Clinical examination, TV scan, rectal endoscopy [26]
Clinical examination, barium enema [27]
Clinical examination, TVS, TRUS, barium enema, and MRI [28]
Clinical examination, MRI, rectal US, CT scan (if indicated) [29]
MRI, endorectal ultrasound [30]
Not mentioned [31]
Clinical examination and endorectal ultrasound [32]
Staging laparoscopy and rectal examination [33]
Not mentioned [34]
Clinical examination, TV scans [35]
Ultrasound and laparoscopy and then referred if bowel endometriosis has been diagnosed [36]
Clinical examination, TV scan and endorectal ultrasound, MRI, and colonoscopy [37]
Clinical examination, TV scans, MRI, endorectal ultrasound [38]
Initial diagnostic laparoscopy, MRI, TV scan [39]
Clinical examination, TV scan, endorectal ultrasound, double contrast barium enema [40]
Clinical examination, TV scan, barium enema with double contrast, IVP [41]
Clinical examination, CA125, TV scan, endorectal ultrasound, MRI, and double contrast barium meal [42]
All patients were referred with a diagnosis of bowel endometriosis by previous laparoscopy [43]
Clinical examination, barium enema, and sigmoidoscopy [44]
Clinical examination, TV scan+/−MRI, colonoscopy [45]
Clinical examination, barium studies, MRI, CT or endoscopic evaluation. A questionnaire (visual analogue) used before or after surgery [46]
Laparoscopy in all the cases [47]
Clinical examination, TV scan, MRI [detect 80.8 %], colonoscopy [detect 43.2 %], and endorectal ultrasound [48]
Clinical examination, TV scan and endorectal ultrasound, MRI, and double contrast barium enema [49]
Clinical examination, selective MRI, and barium enema. Some referred after initial laparoscopy [50]
Clinical examination, TV scan, double contrast barium enema, visual analogue [51]
Not described [52]
Clinical examination, all of them had at least one laparoscopy before [53]
Clinical examination, radiological (not specified), laparoscopy [54]
Preoperative laparoscopy in the majority, colonoscopy performed on an individual basis [55]

MRI magnetic resonance imaging, *TV* transvaginal, *EUA* examination under anaethesia, *TRUS* transrectal ultrasound, *US* ultrasound

Table 5 Operation time and hospital stay in the shaving group

References	Mean operating time	Mean hospital stay
Donnez et al. [27]	69 (40–132) min	2.8 (2–5) days
Donnez and Squifflet [28]	78 (50–218) min	1.5 (1–7) days
Hollett-Caines et al. [34]	NA	NA
Reich et al. [47]	178 (40–475) min	NA

NA not available

either partial or complete varied between 64 % [53] to 97 % [43]. In the shaving group, the improvement was between 88 % and 96 %. In the resection group, there is no comment in these case series [40, 41, 49, 51], while the others [28, 29, 37] showed improvement between 90 % and 96 % or significant improvement [22, 25, 26, 30].

Dysmenorrhea improvement

The effect was not mentioned in these studies [21, 24, 34, 35, 37, 38, 40, 43–45, 47, 49–51, 53–55]. In the other series, the improvement varies between 28 % and 100 %. In the shaving group, it was mentioned in two studies only [27, 28] and the improvement was between 91 % and 100 %.

Rectal bleeding

This was only mentioned in 4 studies [20, 21, 30, 36]. Rectal bleeding disappeared after surgery in 3 studies [20, 21, 36] and remained the same in the fourth [30]. It was not an issue in the shaving group.

Dyspareunia

There was no direct comment on dyspareunia in these studies [24, 34, 35, 38, 40, 45, 47–49, 51–55]. In the other studies, all

the patients showed improvement, which was expressed either as percentage (70–100 %), using the score of 10 to compare between the preoperative and postoperative condition, or using the expression of significant improvement. In the shaving group the improvement varies between 91 % and 100 % [28, 29].

Dyschezia

There was no direct comment on dyschezia in these studies [21, 24, 27, 33–35, 37, 38, 40, 41, 43–45, 47–49, 51–55]. Improvement varied between 59 % and 100 %. In the shaving group, the improvement was 91.2 % [28].

Quality of life and way of follow-up

Quality of life score was carried out in these studies [22, 26, 30, 33, 39, 41]. SF-36 health status questionnaire was used in [22, 26, 30]. EQ-5D quality of life score was used in [33]. All these assessments showed significant improvement.

In the shaving group, QOL was not assessed in any study. In the resection group, QOL was assessed in 3 case series [22, 26, 30].

Recurrence of endometriosis and reoperation

Fifteen case series reported recurrence of endometriosis [20]: (4 %) [23], (4.7 %) [26], (5 %) [29], (7.8 %) [32], (30 %) [35], (5 %) [36], (6.6 %) [41], (2–7 %) [42], (8.4 %) [43], (8.4 %) [44], (4.3 %) [47], (50 % in 2nd laparoscopy–67 % in 3rd laparoscopy) [52], (48 %) [53], (15 %), and [54](4.9 %).

Reoperation reported in these series [20]: (2.4 %) [27], (1.2 %) [28], (2.4 %) [32], (25 %) [33], (6 %) [35], (5 %) [20], (4 %) [40], (10.4 %) [41], (9 %) [42], (3.8 %) [43],

Table 6 Operation time and hospital stay in the resection group

Reference	Mean operating time	Mean hospital stay
Bassi et al. [22]	NA	NA
Darai et al. [25]	(6.5±2.1) h 1st half of the study/5.9±1.8 h 2nd half of the study	NA
Darai et al. [26]	260 (150–510) min [lap], 221 (95–480) min [open]	8.3 (5–19) days [lap], 9.4 (4–20) days [open]
Dousset et al. [29]	NA	NA
Dubernard et al. [30]	NA	NA
Kavallaris et al. [36]	190 (165–230) min	8.3 (7–11) days
Keckstein and Wiesinger [37]	181 (45–260) min	NA
Mereu et al. [40]	326.7 (97.7) min	3.1 (2–17) days
Minelli et al. [42]	300 (85–720) min	8 (3–36) days
Ruffo et al. [49]	312 (60–720) min	9 (3–44) days
Stepniewska et al. [51]	NA	NA

NA not available, *lap* laparoscopic

Table 7 Operation time and hospital stay in the mixed group

References	Mean operating time	Mean hospital stay
Alvez Pereira et al. [20]	6.5 (5.8–7.2)h	NA
Bailey et al. [21]	NA	NA
Brouwer and Woods [23]	NA	NA
Coronado et al. [24]	NA	7.4 days
Duepree et al. [31]	187 (145–277)min	2 (1–4)days/33 % of excisions were as an outpatients
Fedele et al. [32]	NA	NA
Ford et al. [33]	146 (36–420)min	4.6 (1–10)days
Jatan [35]	NA	3.1 days (0–17) varies according to type of surgery
Kondo et al. [38]	155 (110–371)min	3.2 (1–25)days
Maytham et al. [39]	NA	3 (1–13)days
Meuleman et al. [41]	436 (180–780)min	NA
Mohr et al. [43]	NA	2 (0–180)days
Nezhat et al. [44]	(55–245)min	175 discharged within 24 h; 9 discharged in 2–4 days
Pandis et al. [45]	95 (30–270)min	2 (1–7)days
Redwine and Wright [46]	NA	NA
Ribeiro et al. [48]	110 (40–420)min	7 (6–20)days
Slack et al. [50]	106 (35–240)min	NA
Tarjanne et al. [52]	NA	NA
Varol et al. [53]	NA	Average of 2 days in laparoscopy, 7 days in the case of laparotomy
Weed and Ray [54]	NA	NA
Wills et al. [55]	NA	NA

NA not available

(21 %) [44], (16 %) [46], (19.4 %) [47], (36 %) [50], (2.3 %) [52], (10 %) [53], (36 %), and (20 %) [54].

The recurrence in the shaving group was 5 % [27], 7.8 % [28], 50–67 % [47], while reoperation rate was 1.2 % [27], 2.4 % [28], and 36 % [47]. In the resection group, the recurrence rate varied between 6.6 % and 8.4 %. The reoperation rate was 3.8 % and 10.4 %.

Follow-up

There were no data on the follow up in 4 studies [38, 48, 54, 55]. In the rest of the studies, there was wide range of duration of follow up which varied between 1 month and 11 years. The follow-up duration in the shaving group [27, 28, 34, 47] varied between 1 year and 11 years. All the patients were followed up in these studies [20–22, 24–26, 28, 29, 31, 34, 37, 40, 41, 45, 49, 51, 53]. In the rest of the studies, the number of patients who were followed up varied between 27 % and 98 %.

Fertility outcome

There were data of the effect of surgery on the fertility in 16 studies (44 %) [21, 24, 25, 28, 32, 34, 36, 37, 41–43,

46, 47, 51, 54] (Table 8). The pregnancy rate was between 11.5 % and 84 %. The success rate includes both cases of spontaneous pregnancy and assisted conception. There were 640 pregnancies in 1,232 women (52 %). In the shaving group [28, 34, 47], the pregnancy rate was 84 %, 57 %, and 74 %, respectively. In the resection group, it was recorded in 5/11 (45 %). The success rate was between 11.5 % and 65 %.

Complications

The intraoperative and postoperative complications of surgery were reported in 34 articles (Table 9). The overall complication rate after surgery was 13.9 % (744/5349). It varied from 1.2 % to 40 %. Leakage occurred in 38/744 cases (5.1 %), fistula 93/744 (12.5 %), bowel obstruction/stricture 55/744 (7.3 %), bladder dysfunction 171/744 (23 %), and bowel dysfunction 55/744 (7.4 %). In the shaving group, the complications rate was 2.8 %. In studies in which segmental resection was the only surgical route [22, 25, 26, 29, 30, 36, 40, 42, 49, 51], the complications rate was 447/1,512 (29.6 %). Keckstein and Weisinger [37] and Tarjanne et al. [52] were excluded as the complications were not discussed (190 patients). The complications include the minors and majors.

Table 8 Effect of surgery on fertility

References	Fertility
Alvez Pereira et al. [20]	NA
Bailey et al. [21]	57 % (24/49 spontaneous pregnancy+4/49 assisted conception=28/49)
Bassi et al. [22]	NA
Brouwer and Woods [32]	NA
Coronado et al. [24]	39.4 % (13/33, no details if it is spontaneous or assisted)
Darai et al. [25]	NA
Darai et al. [26]	11.5 % (6[spontaneous]/26 laparoscopy group+0/26 open surgery=6/52)
Donnez et al. [27]	NA
Donnez and Squifflet [28]	84 % [221 spontaneous+107 assisted/388]
Dousset et al. [29]	NA
Dubernard et al. [30]	NA
Duepree et al. [31]	NA
Fedele et al. [32]	34 % (17/50, no details if it is spontaneous or assisted)
Ford et al. [33]	NA
Hollett-Caines et al. [34]	57 % (26/46, 14 spontaneous, 5 clomid tablets, 7 IVF)
Jatan [35]	NA
Kavallaris et al. [36]	65 % (11/17, 7 with spontaneous pregnancy and 4 after assisted conception)
Keckstein and Wiesinger [37]	50 % (18/36, no details if it is spontaneous or assisted)
Kondo et al. [38]	NA
Maytham et al. [39]	NA
Mereu et al. [40]	NA
Meuleman et al. [41]	48 % [16/33, 7/16(44 %) spontaneously, 9/16(56 %) assisted]. Cumulative pregnancy rate 31 %, 49 %, 55 %, and 70 % after1, 2, 3, and 4 years.
Minelli et al. 2009 [42]	41.6 %(47/113, Spontaneous 13(20 %) & assisted 51(80 %).64 pregnancies/47).
Mohr et al. [43]	23/178=13 % [16/93 shaving group=17 %, 4/38 disc excision group=11 %, 3/47 segmental resection group=6 %]
Nezhat et al. [44]	41 % (25/61)
Pandis et al. [45]	NA
Redwine and Wright [46]	43 % (12/28) 5 of these requiring assisted conception.
Reich et al. [47]	74 % (34/46), viable intrauterine pregnancy (32/46)
Ribeiro et al. [48]	NA
Ruffo et al. [49]	NA
Slack et al. [50]	NA
Stepniewska et al. [51]	35 % (17/48), the monthly fecundity rate (2.3)
Tarjanne et al. [52]	NA
Varol et al. [53]	NA
Weed and Ray [54]	42.6 % (23/54; no details if it is spontaneous or assisted)
Wills et al. [55]	NA

NA not available

Stoma formation

Colostomy or ileostomy can be done prophylactically before bowel resection (Table 10). In some studies, it was done as part of the treatment of complications of bowel surgery. In the shaving group, there was no colostomy or ileostomy in 3 studies [27, 28, 34] and there was no comment in the fourth [47]. In the resection group, there were no data in 2 studies [26, 37] and no stoma in another 2 studies [22, 51]. There were stoma formations in the rest of the studies in the same group [25, 29, 30, 36, 40, 42, 49]. In the disc excision subgroup, there was stoma formation in all of them [23, 31, 35, 38, 39, 44, 45].

Discussion

There is a need for strong and energetic debate to weigh up the benefits and risks of debulking surgery (shaving and disc excision) and radical surgery (bowel resection).

Unfortunately, we have only one randomized trial [26] in this study, comparing laparoscopic versus open colorectal resection for endometriosis. Ideally other randomized studies, one to compare medical and surgical treatment, and the other, to evaluate different types of surgical treatment, are required. To avoid losing large case series, e.g [27, 38], we included 15 retrospective studies (42 %), in spite of the limitations of this type of research.

As we have different types of studies describing varieties of surgeries, with different techniques, done by gynaecologists, surgeons or both, with different ways and time of follow-up, we should interpret the results with caution. De Cicco et al. [4] stated that it would greatly facilitate and permit meta-analysis if journals agreed on the format of reporting and when individual data could be submitted.

All the symptoms significantly improved after surgery. The follow-up in some studies was up to 11 years, and on the other hand, it was just a month in some. It does not look that there is difference between different types of surgery.

Type of surgery

Laparoscopy is taking over from open surgery. It allows accurate diagnosis due to improved visualization of pelvic structures as well as better access to the deep pelvis in cases of rectovaginal septum involvement [53]. Laparoscopy was the only route in the shaving group. The conversion rate in all laparoscopies was quiet low (2.1 %). It is lower in the shaving group (0.25 %) rather than the resection group (2.2 %). This is to add to the advantages of conservative surgery over resection.

Table 9 Complications

Ref.	No.	Number of complications	Leak	Fistula	He	Infection	Obstruction/ stricture	Other major	Bladder dysfunction	Bowel dysfunction	Other minim
Alvez Pereira et al. [20]	168.	13 (7.6 %).	1	3		2	3			4	
Bailey et al. [21]	130	6 (4.6 %)				1	4		1		
Bassi et al. [22]	151	11 (7.3 %)				1	2		1	1	6
Brouwer and Woods [23]	213	15 (7 %)	1		1	2	3	6	2		
Coronado et al. [24]	77	9 (11.6 %)						2			7
Darai et al. [25]	71	9 (12.7 %)		6		3					
Darai et al. [26]	52	2 (7.6 %) laparoscopy; 10 (40 %); open surgery	?	?	?	?	?	?	?	?	?
Donnez et al. [27]	500	8 (1.6 %)				2		4	4		
Donnez and Squifflet [28]	500	15 (3 %)						11	4		
Dousset et al. [29]	100	32 (32 %)	2	4	2				16		6
Dubernard et al. [30]	58	9 (15.5 %)		6		1		2			
Duepree et al. [31]	51	10 (19.6 %)	1			2		5	1		1
Fedele et al. [32]	83	1 (1.2 %)					1				
Ford et al. [33]	60	7 (11.7 %)				3		4			
Hollett-Caines et al. [34]	81	1 (1.2 %).				1					
Jatan [35]	95	8 (8 %)				2	2	1	1		2
Kavallaris et al. [36]	55	18 (32.7 %)	2			1		1	14		
Keckstein and Wiesinger [37]	130	NA									
Kondo et al. [38]	225	26 (4.6 %)	1	15	3	3	4				
Maytham et al. [39]	54	9 (16.6 %)	3			1	5				
Mereu et al. [40]	192	61 (31.8 %)	9	12		2	1	20	9	5	3
Meuleman et al. [41]	56	3 (5 %)	1	1		1					
Minelli et al. [42]	357	44 (12.3 %) author's figure; 125 (35 %)	4	19	3	9		9	30	15	36
Mohr et al. [43]	187	33 (17.6 %)	1	2		2	1	3	1		23
Nezhat et al. [44]	185	20 (10.8 %)						20			
Pandis et al. [45]	134	18 (10.2 %; 25 in 18 patients				1		17	7		
Redwine and Wright [46]	84	2 (2.4 %)									2
Reich et al. [47]	100	1/100 (1 %)				1					
Ribeiro et al. [48]	125	12 (9.6 %)		2		1		1	3		5
Ruffo G et al. [49]	436	146/436 (33.4 %)	9	14	9	3	16	6	71	15	3
Slack et al. [50]	128	10 (7.8 %)		4				1	5		
Stepniewska et al. [51]	60	24 (40 %)		2	2	0	1	2	1	15	1
Tarjanne et al. [52]	60	NA		NA	NA				NA	NA	NA
Varol et al. [53]	169	21 (12.4 %)		1	3			5			12
Weed and Ray [54]	163	33 (20 %)					7	26			
Wills et al. [55]	177	16 (9 %)	3	2		2		9			

No number of the patients in each study, *Hge* haemorrhage, *?* no details of the postoperative complications, *NA* not available, *Ref* reference

Histology confirmation

Histological examination is essential to confirm the diagnosis and to exclude other pathology. Excision should be complete in order to achieve maximal pain relief and minimal recurrence. However, De Cicco [4] stated that there is no data to substantiate this. Histology was reported in 23 studies (64 %) and confirmed in 41–100 % of the specimen. However, there were no data about the completeness of the excision. Absence of clear documentation on the histology is considered as a weakness of the study. Kavallaris et al. [56] noted that a distance of 2 cm between the margin and the main lesion

Table 10 Stoma required before, during, and after surgery

References	Stoma
Alvez Pereira et al. [20]	0
Bailey et al. [21]	0
Bassi et al. [22]	0
Brouwer and Woods [23]	X7, loop ileostomy was required (5 %).
Coronado et al. [24]	0
Darai et al. [25]	X5 colostomy and a Hartmann procedure in one (6.9 %).
Darai et al. [26]	NA
Donnez et al. [27]	0
Donnez and Squifflet [28]	0
Dousset et al. [29]	X96 defunctioning ileostomy was done.
Dubernard et al. [30]	X6 (5 of rectovaginal fistula colostomy and the last had Hartmann procedure)
Dupree et al. [31]	X1, due to combined ileal and rectal injury
Fedele et al. [32]	0
Ford et al. [33]	X2 temporary (one intraoperative) and the second postoperatively (rectal perforation)
Hollett-Caines et al. [34]	0
Jatan [35]	X2
Kavallaris et al. [36]	X2, Ileostomy (left for 4 months)
Keckstein and Wiesinger [37]	NA
Kondo et al. [38]	X1, protective ileostomy
Maytham et al. [39]	X1, temporary defunctioning loop colostomy
Mereu et al. [40]	X3 ,temporary ileostomy,2 temporary colostomy
Meuleman et al. [41]	0
Minelli et al. [42]	X41, temporary ileostomy X41 (11.5 %)
Mohr et al. [43]	X2, ileostomy done preoperatively
Nezhat et al. [44]	0
Pandis et al. [45]	X2, Ileostomy
Redwine and Wright [46]	0
Reich et al. [47]	No data
Ribeiro et al. [48]	0
Ruffo et al. [49]	X61 primary ileostomy, 8 required permanent ileostomy, colostomy X2, Hartmannx1
Slack et al. [50]	X3 temporary
Stepniewska et al. [51]	0
Tarjanne et al. [52]	NA
Varol et al. [53]	X1, closed after 10 weeks after healing of rectovaginal fistula
Weed and Ray [54]	X3 temporary, one permanent
Wills et al. [55]	X3 ileostomies, one elective and 2 due to anastomotic leak

was not sufficient to obtain endometriosis free margins in more than one-third of the patients. Furthermore, margins of the resected bowel specimen were still positive for endometriosis in 6 patients (19 %) after bowel resection was performed in an area with a distance of at least 3 cm from the edges of the palpated lesions, free of any indurations at manual palpation, and free of any serosal or muscular visible endometriosis implant [56]. The same was discussed by Anaf et al. [57, 58] and Roman et al. [59] with a positive margin around 10 %. Neural metastasis hypothesis provides an explanation. This might explains the recurrence of symptoms and endometriosis in segmental resection.

Complications

The overall complication rate after surgery was 13.9 %. In the shaving group, the complications rate was 2.8 % while it was 29.6 % in the resection group. It is obvious that conservative surgery carries low risk. Although most of it was related to bowel surgery, additional surgery, such as ureterolysis, uterosacral ligament resection, and hysterectomy, might contribute as well. Opening of the vagina contributes to the complication, in spite being not always reported. This pleads for the introduction of a systematic protective colostomy in case of concomitant vaginal and rectal resection as already applied in some studies [39]. Additionally, extensive electro coagulation can lead to necrosis of the posterior vaginal cuff with a higher risk for rectovaginal fistulae and abscesses [30].

Pelvic denervation can lead to urine retention, de novo dysuria, and sexual dysfunction. Nerve sparing technique is required, in spite that it is not always possible if there are large nodules with bilateral extension. Care must always be taken to preserve the pelvic autonomic nerves, as they are the pathway for the neurogenic control of rectal, bladder, and sexual arousal function. The identification of the inferior hypogastric nerve and plexus was feasible and performed in acceptable operative time [60]. They believe that a trained laparoscopic surgeon should have a good knowledge not only of the retroperitoneal anatomy, but also of the pelvic neuro-anatomy as this qualification could prohibit long-term bladder and voiding dysfunction.

The shaving technique allows preservation of the nerves by avoiding deep lateral rectal dissection (necessary for recto sigmoid resection). Indeed, lateral dissection is mandatory only in the case of lateral extension of the disease with ureteral involvement and, even in this case, rarely involves dissection of the postero-lateral compartment of the rectum [61]. The case series of Kondo et al. [20] suggests that the major complication rate is likely to be lower in women undergoing a mucosal skinning procedure relative to those having a segmental resection. Women also need to be advised that the complication rate may be higher in units that have relatively little experience of this surgery and, as recommended by the RCOG, the surgeon should quote his/her own complication rate.

Bladder dysfunction constitutes 23 % of the whole complications followed by fistula formation (12.5 %). Anastomotic leakage is a feared complication of colorectal surgery and if unrecognized may be associated with a mortality as high as 39 %. Minor cases may also cause late functional problems [50]. The functional problems are less frequent after a sigmoid than after a rectum resection. As the discoid resection is easier at the level of the rectum, Ret Davalos et al. [62] would suggest an avoidance of resection for lower lesion, if possible. Surgeons should work hard to minimize these serious complications.

Follow-up

The wide variation in the follow-up and the high proportion of the patients who lost in the follow-up are considered to be weakness in this study. There were no follow-up in four studies [38, 48, 54, 55] and very short follow-up (between 1–3 months) in another four studies [31, 40, 45, 49]. All the participants were followed-up in 18 studies only. Study [53] reported at 35 months follow-up that 61 women (36 %) required further surgery for pain. The average time between primary and repeat surgery was 16 months. This explains the value of long-term follow-up. The value of surgery could be overestimated by short follow-up.

Recurrence

It is difficult to distinguish between residual and recurrent disease [63]. Excluding Reich et al. [47], the improvement, recurrence, and reoperation rate are comparable between the two groups, but with higher rate of complications in the resection group.

It is difficult to gauge the proportion of women suffering from pelvic pain due to genuine recurrence of endometriosis and those with postoperative adhesions related to severe complications, such as pelvic abscesses or peritonitis [61]. Resection of deep nodular endometriosis, which is innervated abundantly by sensory C cholinergic and adrenergic nerve fibres, as recently demonstrated [64].

Investigations confirmed high nerve fibre density in deep infiltrating lesions, mainly observed near the intestinal lining. Considering that in bowel resection, the margin are not free in around 10 % [57, 58], it should not be undertaken as first line therapy ,but as secondary-line approach in the case of recurrence with stenosis >80 % after shaving [61].

Paya et al. [19] did a comparative study between different surgeries for rectovaginal endometriosis in four case series (see the table below). All of them are observational studies in which the treatment option was not decided randomly; rather, it was made in terms of clinical criteria or in consensus with the patients. Two studies were part of our systematic analysis [23, 43]. Although some of the outcomes and the way they

were assessed are not directly comparable between papers, one can see a tendency that points to a similar symptomatic improvement among the different techniques and a greater rate of surgical complications among the most radical approaches.

The results of the discoid resection analyzed in comparative studies show that the rate of severe complications remains low; the symptomatic improvement stands around 90 %, and the rate of relapse between 5 % and 14 % (Table 11).

More prospective follow-up studies with large sample sizes and clear definitions of endometriosis recurrence (using life table analysis to calculate the cumulative endometriosis recurrence rate) are needed to compare endometriosis recurrence between patient groups receiving different surgical techniques for the treatment of endometriosis with colorectal lesions.

Fertility

The association between endometriosis and infertility is still undefined and there is no consensus on the best treatment options for various clinical conditions [67]. On the basis of three studies [68–70], there seems to be a negative correlation between the stage of endometriosis and the spontaneous cumulative pregnancy rate after surgical removal of endometriosis, but statistical significance was reached only in one study [70].

In our study, we looked at the fertility for women wished to conceive after surgery, either with a documented infertility or not. It was difficult to do a separate analysis of the effect of surgery on infertile women because of the absence of clear documentation or definition of infertility in some studies. Fertility was discussed in 44 % of the studies with a pregnancy rate between 11.5 % and 84 %. The highest was in the shaving group [38].

Rectovaginal endometriosis is a benign condition with limited tendency to progress [32]. In a comparative non randomized study, between resection of rectovaginal endometriosis and expectant treatment, the results did not suggest that excision of rectovaginal plaques improves the incidence of pregnancy and reduces time to conception in women with endometriosis associated infertility [67]. There is no randomized controlled study or met analysis available to answer the question of whether surgical excision of moderate to severe endometriosis enhances pregnancy rate. However, other studies suggest that complete removal of deep infiltrating endometriosis potentially improve fertility [40]. Even in the subfertile population, a good spontaneous pregnancy rate can be achieved after conservative surgery. The spontaneous pregnancy rate in Gordts 2013 study [71] was 50 % in his fertility unit.

If infertility is of primary concern, the lower complication rates and better chance for fertility offered by the less invasive shaving approach justifies initially using this technique [43].

Table 11 Comparison of different types of surgery

		Moher et al. [43] 24 months	Brouwer and Woods [23] 68 months	Fanfani et al. [65] 32 months	Roman et al. [66] 26 months
Shaving	Number	100	18		
	Complications	Total 6 %	Total 17 %, PA 5.6 %		
	Improvement	80 %			
	Relapse		22.2 %		
	Fertility	17 %			
Discoid excision	Number	39	58	48	16
	Complications	Total 23 %, RVF 3 %, PA 5 %	Total 2 %, CA 2 %	Total 59.7 %, RVF 2.1 %, PA 2.1 %, ID 2.1 %	ID 19 %
	Improvement	92 %		88 %	86 %
	Relapse		5.17 %	13.8 %	
	Fertility	11 %			13 %
Segmental intestinal resection	Number	48	137	88	25
	Complications	Total 38 %, BD 2 %, CA 6 %	Total 8 %, PA 1.4 %, CA:2.2 %+, BD 1.4 %, ID 9 %	Total 59.7 %, RVF 3.4 %, PA 2.2 %, BD 14.7 %, CA 1.1 %, ID 4.5 %	BD 8 %, ID 64 %
	Improvement	92 %		93 %	83 %
	Relapse		2.19 %	11.5 %	
	Fertility	3 %			12 %

RVF rectovaginal fistula, *CA* complications of anastomosis, *PA* pelvic abscess, *BD* bladder dysfunction, *ID* intestinal dysfunction

The highest pregnancy rate (84 %) in our study was in study No [28], in which shaving technique was only used. The pregnancy rate in the shaving group (57–84 %) is comparable to that of the resection group (11.5–65 %) [Table 8].

Donnez and Squifflet [28] explained the high pregnancy rate to the following:

- Lesions are resected without extension or lateral dissection, frequently associated with subsequent adhesions in case of bowel resection.
- Nodules are not associated with severe peritoneal endometriosis or ovarian endometriomas.
- Use of the combined technique, when ovarian endometrioma are present, as demonstrated by Donnez et al. [72].

Meuleman et al. [73] stated that the fertility wish of patients with advanced endometriosis with colorectal extension is underestimated in the papers reviewed. The indication of infertility with or without pain is only 22–36 % of all patients included in these papers. Most patients have a combined problem of pain and unfulfilled or uncompleted child wish, which may be formulated by the patient passively (wish for preservation/restoration of fertility during surgery, without well-defined child wish in the near or distant future). Furthermore, it is important to realize that many women with pelvic endometriosis and colorectal extension have been told for many years that they will never become pregnant as a result of their disease. Additionally, before surgery these women are in pain, implying that their first concern is how

to stop the pain, rather than a child wish. In these women, child wish may only emerge after a successful removal of the endometriosis and pain reduction.

Life table analysis was used to calculate the cumulative pregnancy rate in only 4 out of 16 (25 %) studies reporting fertility outcome [24, 34, 41, 51]. This is surprising in view of the fact that it has been generally accepted that life table analysis is the best way to calculate fertility outcome while controlling for the duration of follow-up and dropout rate for each patient. Overall, this observation supports the need for prospective follow-up studies with sufficient duration of follow-up and complete follow-up of all operated patients.

Quality of life (QOL)

As we have shown before, there was wide range of methods of follow up to assess the outcome including QOL. SF-36 and EQ-5D were used to measure QOL. The EQ-5D is a short-generic patient-rated questionnaire for subjectively describing and valuing health-related quality of life; it is often used as an outcome measure in both clinical and health care services research. The EQ-5D questionnaire comprises five questions (items) relating to current problems in the dimensions mobility', 'self-care', 'usual activities', 'pain/discomfort', and 'anxiety/depression. Responses in each dimension are divided into three ordinal levels coded (a) no problems, (b) moderate problems, and (c) extreme problems. The SF-36 is composed of 36 questions that estimates a total of 8 domains of physical health (physical functioning, role physical, bodily pain, general health) and mental health (vitality, social functioning, role-emotional, and mental health). It may be applied to individuals 18 years of age up to advanced ages, with different medical conditions, and undergoing different types of treatment.

There were improvement in QOL in the four studies using SF-36 and EQ-5D. Three of them were from the resection group and the other one from the mixed group. The SF-36 questionnaire was applied before and after surgery in Dubernard et al. [30]. These scores were lower after surgery in 11 cases (7.3 %). In two patients, the poorer scores after surgery were a result of the persistence of abdominal pain after treatment, whereas the other patients went on to have some form of clinical complication that did not appear to be directly associated with the laparoscopic intervention alone. Bassi et al. [22] stated that patients reported deterioration both in bowel symptoms and in pain after surgery is attributed to post operative fibrosis. More and large studies with a long-term follow-up using the same validated QOL questionnaire are required to allow comparison between the different surgical techniques used and to confirm the positive impact of each type of surgery on the QOL.

Stoma formation

Obviously, having stoma is very embarrassing to any woman. She should feel that the gain is going to have from surgery is worthwhile, so she can cope with having stoma for some time. No recorded cases of stoma formation were in the shaving group but there were in all the disc excision subgroup and in 7 case series in the resection group. This again emphasizes the value of doing the minimum surgery needed, to get the best outcome at a cheap price.

Conclusion

Implications for practice

Most of the studies documented the clinical outcome for bowel surgery in deep endometriosis regarding postoperative complication rate and relief of symptoms. However, less than 50 % of the studies included data with respect to the recurrence rate, fertility outcome, and quality of life. It is difficult to estimate the actual pregnancy and recurrence rates in some studies because of the short-term follow-up. A patient who has been lost or not included in the follow-up is not necessarily cured, but has possibly moved to another area or turned to another gynaecologist because of the lack of satisfaction or complications.

There was no difference in the outcome between conservative surgery and bowel resection. It is important to make every effort to get the best result from the minimum number of surgical interventions. Precise preoperative diagnosis, advanced laparoscopic surgical skills, and multidisciplinary approaches are considered to be the baseline for successful treatment.

Further studies

We need to have standardization in the clinical trial regarding the methodology, outcome variables, and long-term follow-up. A definition should be used to record postoperative complications, document pelvic pain (dysmenorrheal, dyspareunia, chronic non-menstrual pelvic pain) and assess quality of life, fertility (pregnancy rate), and recurrence rate after surgery for endometriosis. Health professionals are encouraged to report unequivocally and completely in much needed prospective studies with large sample sizes and complete follow up of all patients for a reasonable period of time after surgery [4]. This enables meta-analysis to be done with a reliable conclusion and recommendation.

Disclosure of interest The author had no financial interest.

Funding None.

References

1. Giudice LC, Kao LC (2004) Endometriosis. Lancet 364:1789–1799
2. Koninckx PR, Martin DC (2012) Deep endometriosis: a consequence of infiltration or retraction or possibly adenomyosis externa. Fertil Steril 58:924–928
3. Koninckx PR, Martin D (1994) Treatment of deeply infiltrating endometriosis. Curr Opin Obstet Gynecol 6:231–234
4. De Cicco C, Corona R, Schonman R, Mailova K, Ussia A, Koninckx PR (2010) Bowel resection for deep endometriosis : a systematic review. BJOG 118:285–291
5. Chapron C, Fauconnier A, Viera M, Barakat H, Dousset B, Pansini V, Vacher-Lavenu MC, Dubuisson JB (2003) Anatomical distribution of deeply infiltrating endometriosis: surgical implications and proposition for classification. Hum Reprod 18:157–161
6. Redwine DB (2004) Intestinal endometriosis. In: Redwine DB (ed) Surgical Management of Endometriosis. Taylor & Francis, London, pp 157–173
7. Remorgida V, Ferrero S, Fulcher E, Ragni N, Martin DC (2007) Bowel endometriosis: presentation, diagnosis, and treatment. Obstet Gynecol Surv 62(7):461–469
8. Sun-Wei G (2009) Recurrence of endometriosis and its control. Hum Reprod Update 15(4):441–461
9. Anaf V, Simon PH, El Nakadi L, Fayt I, Buxant F, Simonart T, Peny MO, Noel JC (2000) Relationship between endometriotic foci and nerves in rectovaginal endometriotic nodules. Hum Reprod 15:1744–1750
10. Cornillie FJ, Oosterlynck J, Lauweryns M, Koninckx PR (1991) Suggestive evidence that endometriosis is a progressive disease,

whereas deeply infiltrating endometriosis is associated with pelvic pain. Fertil Steril 55:759–765

11. Donnez J, Nisolle M, Casanas-Roux F, Bassil S, Anaf V (1995) Rectovaginal septum, endometriosis or adenomyosis: laparoscopic management in a series of 231 patients. Hum Reprod 10:630–635

12. Clayton RD, Hawe JA, Love JC, Wilkinson N, Garry R (1999) Recurrent pain after hysterectomy and bilateral salpingo-oophorectomy for endometriosis: evaluation of laparoscopic excision of residual excision. Br J Obstet Gynaecol 106(7):740–744

13. Porpora MG, Koninckx PR, Piazze J, Natili M, Colagrande S, Cosmi EV (1999) Correlation between endometriosis and pelvic pain. J Am Assoc Gynecol Laparosc 6:429–434

14. Fedele L, Bianchi S, Zanconato G, Raffaelli R, Berlanda N (2004) Is rectovaginal endometriosis a progressive disease? Am J Obstet Gynecol 191:1539–1542

15. Telimaa S (1988) Danazol and medroxyprogesterone acetate inefficient in the treatment of infertility in endometriosis. Fertil Steril 50:872–875

16. Marana R, Paielli F, Muzil L, Dell'Acqua S, Mancuso S (1994) GnRH analogs versus expectant management in minimal –mild endometriosis-associated infertility. Acta Eur Fertil 25:37–41

17. Vercellini P, Crosignani PG, Somigliana E, Berlanda N, Barbara G, Fedele L (2009) Medical treatment for rectovaginal endometriosis : what is the evidence ? Hum Reprod 24:2504–2514

18. Wright J, Ballard K (2011) The surgical management of rectovaginal endometriosis: plus ca change? BJOG 118(3):274–277

19. Paya V, Hidalgo-Mora JJ, Diaz-Garcia C, Pellicer A (2011) Surgical treatment of rectovaginal endometriosis with rectal endometriosis. Gynecol Surg 8:269–277

20. Alvez Pereira RM, Zanatta A, Lima Preti CD, Felipe de Paula FJ, Alvez da Motta EL, Serafini PC (2009) Should the gynaecologist perform laparoscopic bowel resection to treat endometriosis? Results over 7 years in 168 patients. J Minim Invasive Gynecol 16(4):427–429

21. Bailey HR, Ott MT, Hartendorp P (1994) Aggressive surgical management for advanced colorectal endometriosis. Dis Colon Rectum 37:747–753

22. Bassi MA, Podgaec S, Antonio D, D'Amico Filho N, Alberto Petta C, Abrao MS (2011) Quality of life after segmental resection of the rectosigmoid by laparoscopy in patients with deep infiltrating endometriosis with bowel involvement. Minim Invasive Gynecol 18:730–733

23. Brouwer R, Woods RJ (2007) Rectal endometriosis: results of radical excision and review of published work. Aust N Z J Surg 77:562–571

24. Coronado C, Randolph B, Franklin RR, Valdes CT, Lotez EC (1990) Surgical treatment of symptomatic colorectal endometriosis. Fertil Steril 53(3):411–416

25. Darai E, Ackerman G, Bazot M, Rouzier R, Dubernard G (2007) Laparoscopic segmental colorectal resection for endometriosis: limits and complications. Surg Endosc 21:1572–1577

26. Darai E, Dubernard G, Coutant C, Coutan C, Frey C, Rouzier R, Ballester M (2010) Randomized trial of laparoscopically assisted versus open colorectal resection for endometriosis: morbidity, symptoms, quality of life and fertility. Ann Surg 251:1018–1023

27. Donnez J, Nisolle M, Gillerot S, Smets M, Basil S, Casanas- Roux F (1997) Rectovaginal septum adenomyotic nodules: a series of 500 cases. Br J Obstet Gynaecol 104:1014–1018

28. Donnez J, Squifflet J (2010) Complications, pregnancy and recurrence in a prospective series of 500 patients operated on by the shaving technique for deep rectovaginal endometriotic nodules. Hum Reprod 25(8):1949–1958

29. Dousset B, Leconte M, Borghese B, Millischer AE, Roseau G, Akwright S, Chapron C (2010) Complete surgery for low rectal endometriosis. Long term results of a 100- case prospective study. Ann Surg 251:887–895

30. Dubernard G, Piketty M, Rouzier R, Houry S, Bazot M, Darai E (2006) Quality of life after laparoscopic colorectal resection for endometriosis. Hum Reprod 21(5):1243–1247

31. Duepree HJ, Senagore AJ, Delaney CP, Marcello P, Brady KM, Falcone T (2002) Laparoscopic resection of deep pelvic endometriosis with rectosigmoid involvement. J Am Coll Surg 195:754–758

32. Fedele L, Bianchi S, Zanconato G, Bettoni G, Gotsch F (2004) Long-term follow-up after conservative surgery for rectovaginal endometriosis. Am J Obstet Gynecol 190:1020–1024

33. Ford J, English J, Miles WA, Giannopoulos T (2004) Pain, quality of life and complications following the radical resection of rectovaginal endometriosis. BJOG 111:353–356

34. Hollett-Caines J, Vilos GA, Penava DA (2003) laparoscopic mobilization of the rectosigmoid and excision of the obliterated cul-de-sac. J Am Assoc Gynecol Laparosc 10(2):190–194

35. Jatan AK, Solomon MJ, Young J, Cooper M, Pathma-Nathan N (2006) Laparoscopic management of rectal endometriosis. Dis Colon Rectum 49(2):169–174

36. Kavallaris A, Chalvatzas N, Hornemann A, Banz C, Diedrich K, Agic A (2011) 94 months follow up after laparoscopic assisted vaginal resection of septum rectovaginale and rectosigmoid in women with deep infiltrating endometriosis. Arch Gynecol Obstet 283:1059–1064

37. Keckstein J, Wiesinger H (2005) Deep endometriosis, including intestinal involvement –the interdisciplinary approach. Minim Invasive Ther Allied Technol 14:160–166

38. Kondo W, Bourdel N, Tamburro S, Cavoli D, Jardon K, Rabischong B, Botchorishvili R, Pouly JL, Mage G, Canis M (2011) Complications after surgery for deeply infiltrating pelvic endometriosis. BJOG 118:292–298

39. Maytham G, Dowson H, Levy B, Kent A, Rockall TA (2010) Laparoscopic excision of rectovaginal endometriosis : report of a prospective study and review of the literature. Color Dis 12:1105–1112

40. Mereu L, Giacomo R, Stefano L, Barbieri F, Zaccoletti R, Fiaccavento A, Stepniewska A, Pontrelli G, Minelli L (2007) Laparoscopic treatment of deep endometriosis with segmental colorectal resection:short term morbidity. Minim Invasive Gynecol 14:463–469

41. Meuleman C, D'Hoore A, Van Cleynenbreugel B, Berks N, D'Hooghe T (2009) Outcome after mutidisciplinary CO2 laser laparoscopic excision of deep infiltrating colorectal endometriosis. Reprod Biomed Online 18:282–289

42. Minelli L, Fanfani F, Fagotti A, Rffo G, Ceccaroni M, Mereu L, Landi S, Pomini P, Scambia G (2009) Laparoscopic colorectal resection for bowel endometriosis; feasibility, complications, and clinical outcome. Arch Surg 144(3):234–239

43. Mohr C, Nezhat FR, Nezhat CH, Seidman DS, Nezhat CR (2005) Fertility consideration in laparoscopic treatment of infiltrative bowel endometriosis. JSLS 9:16–24

44. Nezhat F, Nezhat C, Pennington E (1992) Laparoscopic treatment of infiltrative rectosigmoid colon and rectovaginal septum by the technique of videolaparoscopy and the CO2 laser. Br J Obstet Gynaecol 99:664–667

45. Pandis GK, Saridogan E, Windsor AC, Gulumser C, Cohen RG, Cutner AS (2010) Short term outcome of fertility –sparing laparoscopic excision of deeply infiltrating pelvic endometriosis performed in a tertiary centre. Fertil Steril 93:39–45

46. Redwine DB, Wright JT (2001) Laparoscopic treatment of complete obliteration of the cul-de-sac associated with endometriosis; long term follow up of en bloc resection. Fertil Steril 76:358–365

47. Reich H, Mc Glynn F, Salvat J (1991) Laparoscopic treatment of Cul-de-sac Obliteration secondary to retrocervical deep fibrotic endometriosis. J Reprod Med 36(7):516–522

48. Riberiro PA, Rodrigues FC, Kehdi IP, Rossini L, Abdalla HS, Donadio N, Aoki T et al (2006) Laparoscopic resection of intestinal

endometriosis : a 5-year experience. J Minim Invasive Gynecol 13: 442–446

49. Ruffo G, Scopelliti M, Scioscia M, Ceccaroni M, Mainardi P, Minelli L (2010) Laparoscopic colorectal resection for deep infiltrating endometriosis:analysis of 436 cases. Surg Endosc 24:63–67

50. Slack A, Child T, Lindsey I, Kennedy S, Cunningham C, Mortensen N, Koninckx P, Mc Veigh E (2007) Urological and colorectal complications following surgery for rectovaginal endometriosis. BJOG 114:1278–1282

51. Stepniewska A, Pomini P, Bruni F, Mereu L, Ruffo G, Ceccaroni M, Scioscia M, Guerriero M, Minelli L (2009) Laparoscopic treatment of bowel endometriosis in infertile women. Hum Reprod 24(7):1619–1625

52. Tarjanne S, Sjoberg J, Heikinheimo O (2010) Radical excision of rectovaginal endometriosis results in high rate of pain relief –results of a long term follow up study. Acta Obstet Gynecol Scand 89:71–77

53. Varol N, Maher P, Healey M, Woods R, Wood C, Hill D, Lolatgis TJ (2003) Rectal surgery for endometriosis- should we be aggressive? Am Assoc Gynecol Laparosc 10:182–189

54. Weed JC, Ray JE (1987) Endometriosis of the bowel. Obstet Gynecol 69(5):727–730

55. Wills H, Reid GD, Cooper MJW, Tsalitas J, Morgan M, Woods RJ (2008) Bowel resection for severe endometriosis: an Australian series of 177 cases. Aust N Z J Obstet Gyaecol 49:415–418

56. Kavallaris A, Kohler C, Kuhne-Heid SA (2003) Histological extent of rectal invasion by rectovaginal endometriosis. Hum Reprod 18(6): 1323–1327

57. Anaf V, El Nakadi I, Simon P, Van de Stadt J, Fayt L, Simonart T, Noel JC (2004) Preferential infiltration of large bowel endometriosis along the nerves of the colon. Hum Reprod 19(4):996–1002

58. Anaf V, El Nakadi I, De Moore V, Coppens E, Zalcman M, Noel JC (2009) Anatomic signifcance of a positive barium enema in deep infitrating endometriosisof the large bowel. World J Surg 33:822–827

59. Roman H, Puscasiu L, Kouteich K, Gromez A, Resch B, Marouteau-Pasquier N, Hochain P, Tuech JJ, Scotte M, Marpeau L (2007) Laparoscopic management of deep endometriosis with rectal affect. Chirurgia 102:421–428

60. Kavallaris A, Banz C, Chalvatzas N, Hornemann A, Luedders DK, Bohmann M (2011) Laparoscopic nerve-sparing surgery of deep infiltrating endometriosis :description of the technique and patients' outcome. Arch Gynecol Obstet 284:1642–1649

61. Donnez J, Jadoul P, Colette S, Luyckx M, Squifflet J, Donnez O (2013) Deep rectovaginal endometriotic nodules:perioperative complications from a series of 3298 patients operated on the shaving technique. Gynecol Surg 10(1):31–40

62. Ret Davalos ML, De Cicco C, D'Hoore A, De Decker B, Koninckx PR (2007) Outcome after rectum or sigmoid resection. A review for gynaecologists. Minim Invasive Gynecol 14(1):33–38

63. McDonough PG (2001) Are basic assumptions correct-is endometriosis a progressive self destructive disease? Fertil Steril 75:230

64. Wang G (2009) Rich innervation of deep infiltrating endometriosis. Hum Reprod 24:827–834

65. Fanfani F, Fagotti A, Gagliardi ML, Ruffo G, Ceccaroni M, Scambia G, Minelli L (2010) Discoid or segmental rectosigmoid resection for deep infiltrating endometriosis : a case–control study. Fertil Steril 94: 444–449

66. Roman H, Loise C, Resch B, Tuech JJ, Hochain P, Leroi AM, Marpeau L (2010) Delayed functional outcomes associated with surgical management of deep rectovaginal endometriosis with rectal involvement :giving patients an informed choice. Hum Reprod 25: 890–899

67. Vercellini P, Pietropaolo G, Giorgi OD, Daguati R, Pasin R, Crosignani PG (2006) Reproductive performance in infertile women with rectovaginal endometriosis: Is surgery worthwhile? Am J Obstet Gynecol 195(5):1303–1310

68. Adamson GD, Hurd SJ, Pasta DJ, Rodriguez BD (1993) Laparoscopic endometriosis treatment :is it better? Fertil Steril 59: 35–44

69. Guzick DS, Silliman NP, Adamson GD, Buttram VC Jr, Canis M, Malinak LR (1997) Prediction of pregnancy in infertile women based on the American Society for Reproductive Medicine's revised classification of endometriosis. Fertil Steril 67:822–829

70. Osuga Y, Koga K, Tsutsumi O, Yano T, Maruyama M, Kugu K (2002) Role of laparoscopy in the treatment of endometriosis associated infertility. Gynecol Obstet Invest 53(Suppl 1):33–39

71. Gordts S, Puttemans P, Campo R, Valkenburg M, Gordts S (2013) Outcome of conservative surgical treatment of deep infiltrating endometriosis. Gynecol Surg 10:137–141

72. Donnez J, Lousse JC, Jadoul P, Squifflet J (2010) Laparoscopic management of endometriomas using a combined technique of excisional (cystectomy) and ablative surgery. Fertil Steril 94(1):28–32

73. Meuleman C, Tomassetti C, D'Hoore A, Van Cleynenbreuguel B, Penninckx F, Vergote I, D'Hooghe T (2011) Surgical treatment of deeply infiltrating endometriosis with colorectal involvement. Hum Reprod Update 17:311–326

7

Septate uterus: nosographic overview and endoscopic treatment

Antonio Perino · Francesco Forlani · Antonio Lo Casto · Giuseppe Calì · Gloria Calagna · Stefano Rotolo · Gaspare Cucinella

Abstract To comment on the prevalence, diagnosis, and treatment of the septate uterus, with special reference to hysteroscopic metroplasty and its effect on reproductive outcome, we searched publications in PubMed and Embase. Original articles, meta-analysis, reviews, and opinion articles were selected. The studies suggest that the prevalence of the septate uterus is increased in women with repeated pregnancy loss and infertility. Reliable diagnosis depends on accurate assessment of the uterine fundal contour and uterine cavity by means of magnetic resonance and three-dimensional ultrasound. Pertinent published data comparing pregnancy outcome before and after hysteroscopic metroplasty indicated a marked improvement after surgery. Magnetic resonance and three-dimensional ultrasound represent the gold standard for diagnosis of septate uterus. Hysteroscopic metroplasty with its simplicity, minimal postoperative sequelae, and improved reproductive outcome is the gold standard for treatment, not only in patients with recurrent pregnancy loss and premature labor but also in patients with infertility, especially if in vitro fertilization is being contemplated.

Keywords Septate uterus · Miscarriage · Infertility · Hysteroscopy · Metroplasty

A. Perino · F. Forlani (✉) · G. Calagna · S. Rotolo · G. Cucinella
Department of Obstetrics and Gynecology, University Hospital "P. Giaccone", Palermo, Italy
e-mail: forlani81@gmail.com

A. Lo Casto
Department of Radiological Sciences, DIBIMEF, University Hospital "P. Giaccone", Palermo, Italy

G. Calì
Department of Obstetrics and Gynecology, ARNAS Civico, Di Cristina e Benfratelli, Palermo, Italy

Introduction

Septate uterus results from the incomplete or completely failed fusion of Müllerian ducts and is the most common type among congenital uterine anomalies [1, 2]. Two types of septate uterus are described: the *complete septate uterus*, in which the septum divides the whole uterine cavity, and the *subseptate uterus*, in which a partial separation of uterine cavity does not reach the cervix (Fig. 1a, b). Failure of fusion may even occur at a lower level, so that two cervices and even a vaginal septum may be present [3–6] (Fig. 1, d). The European Society of Human Reproduction and Embryology (ESHRE) and the European Society for Gynecological Endoscopy (ESGE) developed a new updated classification system of congenital uterine anomalies [7]. The uterus septum (category U2) was defined as the uterus with normal outline and an internal indentation at the fundal midline exceeding 50 % of the uterine wall thickness. This indentation is characterized as septum and could divide partly or completely the uterine cavity, including in some cases cervix and/or vagina (cervical and vaginal coexistent anomalies). The true prevalence of Müllerian anomalies in the general population remains unknown. Mainly based on clinical exam, early investigations on congenital uterine anomalies were limited by the lack of diagnostic tools. A meta-analysis of 94 observational studies comprising nearly 90,000 women indicated a prevalence of 5.5 % in the unselected population, 8.0 % in infertile women, 13.3 % in those with a history of miscarriage, and 24.5 % in those with miscarriage and infertility [8]. Furthermore, canalization defects (subseptate or septate uteri) had a prevalence of 2.3 % in the unselected population but were encountered significantly more frequently in women with previous miscarriage (5.3 %) [8]. In addiiton, septate uterus is associated with higher first and second trimester abortion rates, preterm labor, abnormal labor, intrauterine growth restriction, and infertility. These conditions may be attributed to

Fig. 1 Sepatate uterus: partial (**a**) and complete (**b**). Uterine septum involving the cervix (**c**) and vagina (**d**)

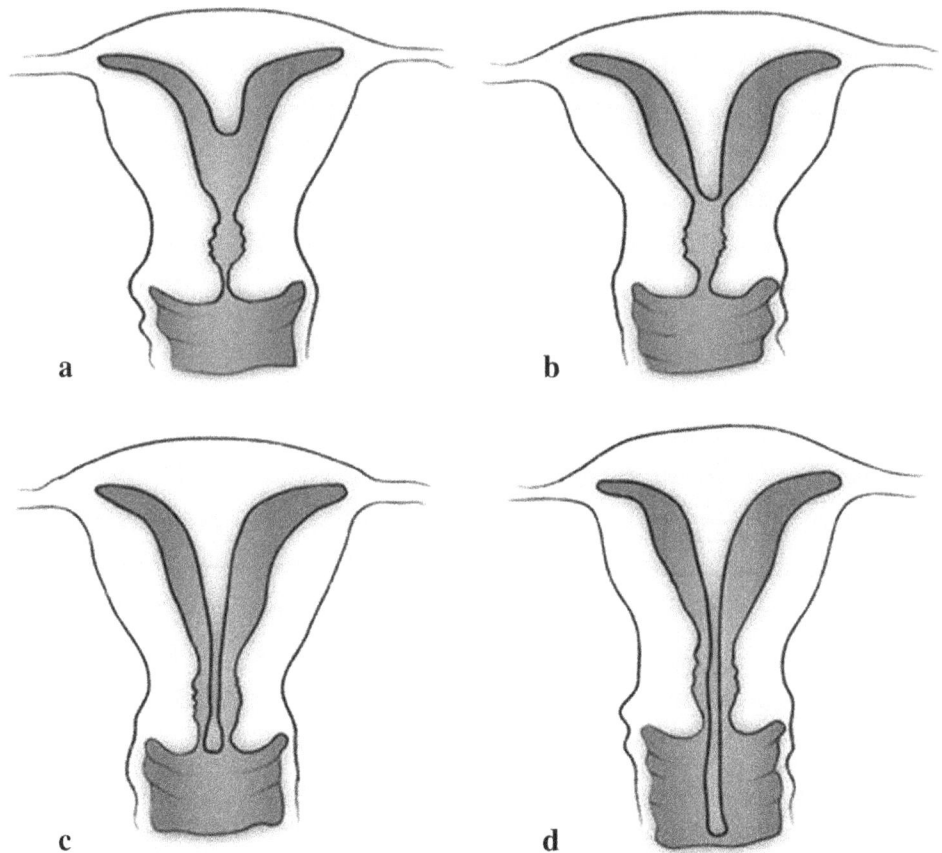

several factors, as diminished blood supply [9], distortion of the uterine cavity, increased intrauterine pressure with resultant cervical incompetence [10], and altered estrogen and progesterone receptor expression [11]. Thus, surgical correction of septate uterus should be considered a first-line treatment whenever indications are present.

Currently, surgical treatment of septate uterus has been significantly simplified by the introduction of hysteroscopic metroplasty, which has almost completely replaced the abdominal approach. Although the reproductive outcome of abdominal and hysteroscopic procedures is similar [12, 13], the latter is associated with a reduced complication rate and shorter hospital stay. Therefore, hysteroscopic metroplasty is currently considered the gold standard of these uterine anomalies, as it increases the reproductive outcome with less cost in terms of risk of complications and outflow of resources. Nonetheless, currently available data come mainly from uncontrolled retrospective studies, and to date no randomized trials have been conducted. Considering the resulting lack of evidence, analysis regarding the efficacy of hysteroscopic metroplasty cannot be considered conclusive. Herein, we want to focus on the most relevant literature findings about diagnosis and management of the uterine septum; we also want to analyze the impact of this disease on reproductive outcome.

Methods

The authors performed a comprehensive search on the PubMed and EMBASE database for published studies with the following keywords: "septate uterus," "hysteroscopic metroplasty," "uterine anomalies," "infertility," and "recurrent miscarriage." We selected studies evaluating diagnosis, impact on fertility, hysteroscopic treatment of septate uterus including original articles, meta-analysis, reviews, and opinion articles published up to August 2013. The authors analyzed embryology, diagnosis, and role of surgical correction on reproductive outcome.

Findings

Embryology and genetics

In the embryo of 5 to 6 weeks of gestational age, the Müllerian ducts become apparent. They stem from the urogenital ridge as a groove of the coelomic epithelium, growing caudally their medial walls fuse in the midline around 9 weeks and finally join the endodermal evaginations of the urogenital sinus. The process concludes at the end of the first trimester with the resorption of the septum, around 19–20 weeks of gestation [14].

Studies conducted on women affected by genetic syndromes, including Müllerian anomalies and knockout mouse models, have allowed the identification of several genes, which play a significant role in the development of the female reproductive system and in the pathogenesis of uterine malformations [15]. An altered expression of the *Bcl-2* gene in uterine septum may prevent apoptosis and uterine septum regression [16]. Mikkilä et al. described an X-linked laterality sequence, in which obligate carrier females had uterine septum and hypertelorism [17]. Ergün et al. reported a rare familial aggregation in three sisters with different degrees of septate uterus [18].

Despite advances in molecular biology and genetics, the precise pathophysiology of septate uterus remains unveiled. The majority of the authors agree that the origin of nearly all uterine malformations is consistent with a polygenic/multifactorial etiology [18, 19].

Diagnosis

Congenital uterine anomalies are usually asymptomatic and may present with delayed menarche, primary infertility, or recurrent pregnancy loss. Although diagnosis of reproductive malformations can be made during gynecological examination if obvious anomalies of the vagina and cervix are present, the identification of uterine malformations mainly depends on imaging findings. Furthermore, surgical treatment produces clear benefits in terms of reproductive outcome only in the case of a septate uterus; therefore, it is crucial to differentiate this condition from other uterine anomalies [1–8, 20]. An ideal diagnostic tool should assess two main key points: the shape of the uterine cavity (with the position of tubal ostium) and the external uterine outline. Gubbini et al. proposed a simple, systematic, and reproducible subclassification system for uterine anomalies previously classified by the American Ferility Society as classes V and VI, to achieve a precise definition of each uterine anomaly and determine the specific surgical management [21].

Hysterosalpingography has been the primary diagnostic tool used to detect uterine cavity malformations and is still currently indicated in the early stages of evaluation of the infertile couple. Despite being able to supply important information regarding tubal patency, it does not provide any information on uterine wall or external uterine contour. Moreover, this technique is not reproducible and is not free from risks arising from radiating exposure and/or upper reproductive tract infection [22].

Two-dimensional ultrasound (2D US) mainly performed through an endovaginal approach, offers clear information about the uterine cavity, internal uterine walls, and external uterine outline. Being economic and reproducible, its use is widespread but accuracy chiefly depends on the clinician's experience [23–25]. Sensitivity of 2D US ranges from 88 to 93 % and specificity from 94 to 99 %, with a positive predictive value around 50–55 % and a negative predictive value ranging between 88 and 100 % [26–30]. In addition, sonohysterography in which a transonic means expands the uterine cavity enhances ultrasound accuracy in the identification of uterine anomalies providing more detailed information about uterine cavity contour [31–37].

Hysteroscopy offers a direct visual inspection of the cervical canal and uterine cavity. Modern mini-hysteroscopy, combining miniaturization with adequate image quality, has been widely used as a screening tool [38, 39]. However, it cannot provide any information about uterine wall or external uterine outline. The combined hysteroscopic–laparoscopic approach is considered the best approach in the assessment of women with congenital reproductive malformations, as both internal and external aspect of the uterus can be explored [40]. In addition, coexistent tubal and ovarian anomalies, peritoneal adhesion, or endometriosis can be identified and treated. Nonetheless, like diagnostic tools, this combined approach cannot provide objective measurable data as diagnosis relies on the subjective impression of the examiner. Furthermore, because of the invasive nature, it should not be used as a primary diagnostic tool. The techniques so far described are widely used in the study of Müllerian anomalies, but, if they are considered separately, none is able to provide adequate data on both the uterine cavity and external contour of the uterus. Currently, magnetic resonance imaging (MRI) and three-dimensional ultrasound (3D US) are the only techniques that can assess both aspects contemporarily.

As MRI accuracy in diagnosis of uterine malformations has been demonstrated by several studies [41–44], 3D US represents a good, emerging alternative as it provides image quality similar to that of MRI, being better tolerated by patients and cheaper. A recently introduced MR technique, 3D fastrecovery fast spin-echo (FRFSE) cube can be used to produce high-resolution volumetric image sets. The image data can be reformatted in any plane eliminating the possibility of suboptimal plane prescription using 2D FRFSE technique, regardless of the prescribed plane during the image acquisition (Fig. 2). This is advantageous because variable uterine anatomy in case of Müllerian anomaly may obstacle a correct choice of cross sectional planes in 2D imaging. Furthermore, acquiring just one image volumetric sequence instead of multiple sequences on different planes decreases the MR exam acquisition time with a positive impact on patient comfort [45].

Ghi et al. [46] demonstrated the efficacy of 3D US in differentiating arcuate, subseptate, septate, and bicornuate uterus by analysis of the outer profile of the uterus in coronal plane scans. A bicornuate uterus is diagnosed if a fundal

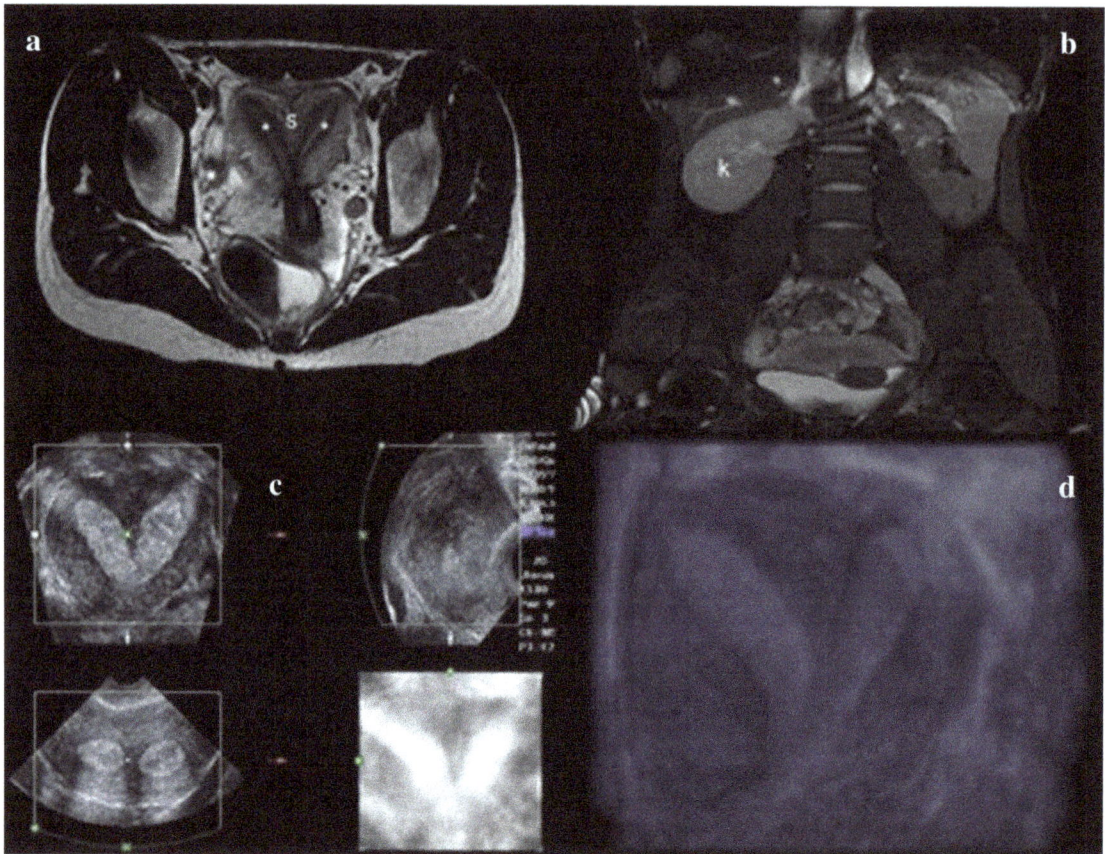

Fig. 2 A case of septate uterus. Axial reformatted 3D FRFSE cube T2 image (**a**): two distinguished uterine horns (*asterisk*) with an interposed, complete septum (*s*) reaching the internal os are depicted. Coronal GE T2 fat-saturated image (**b**). Agenesia of the left kidney with hypertrophy of the right kidney (*k*). 3D ultrasonography image of septate uterus (**c, d**)

external indentation higher than or equal to 10 mm divides two separated uterine cornua; conversely, septate, subseptate, and arcuate uteri present a convex fundal outline or a fundal indentation inferior than 10 mm. While in the septate uterus the septum completely divides the cavity from fundus to cervix, in the subseptate and arcuate uteri the septum is bulging inside the uterine cavity drawing an acute or obtuse angle at its central point, respectively.

Bermejo et al. [44] found a high degree of concordance between 3D US and MRI in the diagnosis and classification of uterine malformations [47]. To differentiate bicornuate from septate uteri using 3D US, they used a formula to analyze coronal plane scans, proposed by Troiano and McCarthy [48]: if a line passing through tubal ostia crosses the fundus or its distance from the fundus is less than or equal to 5 mm, it is a bicornuate uterus; if distance is more than 5 mm, it is considered septate uterus, regardless of fundus shape (Fig. 3). Faivre et al. [49] following the diagnostic criteria proposed by the American Fertility Society (AFS) [50] and previously used by Woefler et al. [51] experienced higher diagnostic accuracy of 3D US in detecting septate uterus and differentiating septate from bicornuate uterus, compared with hysteroscopy and MRI. Moreover, the same authors have proposed the use of

3D sonohysterography when endometrium appears thin or irregular or if other uterine pathologies coexist.

Thus, clinical assessment of women with suspected Müllerian anomalies should be addressed with 3D US, especially before the surgery. With regard to MRI, its high costs

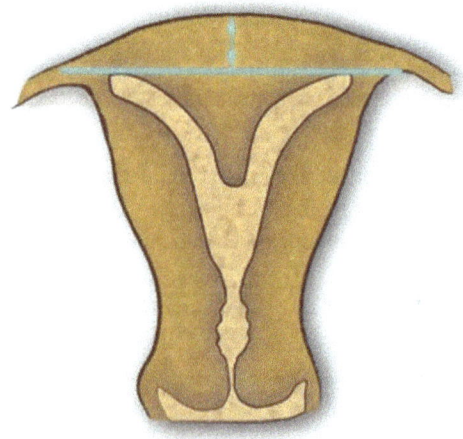

Fig. 3 Septate uterus: the fundus is more than 5 mm (*arrow*) above the line passing through tubal ostia

together with the need of uterine malformation experienced clinicians, limit its use to doubtful or complex cases.

Surgical technique

Historically, metroplasty for septate uterus has been approached by laparotomic hysterotomy and only in the case of recurrent pregnancy loss. Although both Tompkins and Jones' procedure provided quite good results [52, 53], these were highly morbid procedures, resulting in a long time before conception and a subsequent cesarean delivery [54].

In 1974, Edstrom first described the hysteroscopic resection of the uterine septum [55]. Since then, the hysteroscopic surgical technique have been refined and so have been significant diffusion, technical developments have led to miniaturization and improvement of endoscopes resulting in a safer, less-invasive diagnostic and therapeutic tool [56]. Currently, two types of instrument are available for the procedure, namely resectoscope and mini-hysteroscopy, both supporting bipolar and monopolar cautery (Fig. 4). It is best to perform metroplasty in the follicular phase when the endometrium is thin; otherwise, it is possible to administer hormonal therapy

as gonadotropin-releasing hormone analog (GnRH-a) prior to surgery. The surgical technique consists briefly in the incision of the septum, beginning from its inferior apex and proceeding slowly toward the fundus; after, the septum is thinned from both sides under vision while continuously monitoring the position of the ostia, it is then incised in the midsection. As the septum is cut transversely, both edges will retract anteriorly and posteriorly.

The most critical step of this procedure is determining the end point of the resection: if keeping the incision too superficial, it may result in a residual septum and eventually will require an additional operation, whereas, carrying the resection too deep into the fundus, it can lead to intraoperative uterine perforation or uterine rupture during labor or, worse, during subsequent pregnancies.

The procedure usually ends when both ostia are clearly visible from a panoramic view of the uterine cavity and the tip of the instrument can be moved freely from one side to the other, otherwise, when the septum has been adequately resected and minimal bleeding coming from myometrial vessels appears from the bottom of the incision. A few months after surgery, a hysteroscopic evaluation of the uterine cavity may be performed to reveal potential postoperative adhesions

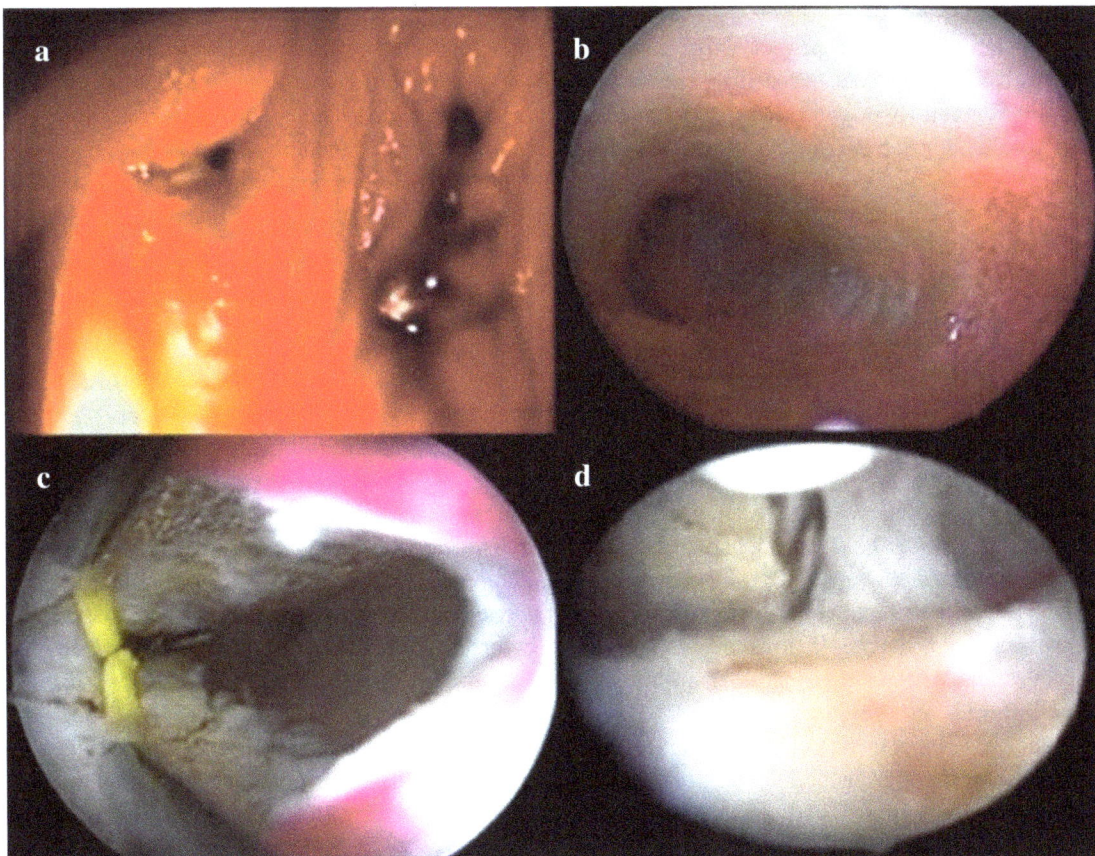

Fig. 4 Septate uterus with double cervix (**a**, **b**). Resettoscopic metroplasty with monopolar electrode (**c**). Small-diameter hysteroscopy with VersaPoint bipolar system (**d**)

or a residual septum thicker than 1 cm. The majority of the authors agree that a residual septum inferior to 1 cm does not worsen the reproductive outcome [57].

The use of laparoscopy, once considered mandatory both during diagnosis (mainly to differentiate the septate from bicornuate uterus) and during surgery (to reveal the relative thickness of the remaining myometrium, through transillumination) has now become quite uncommon. Laparoscopy is occasionally used to conclude a diagnostic work-up in infertile women and is mainly reserved to treat coexisting pathologies.

Traditional resectoscopic techniques make use of 22 or 26 Fr endoscope equipped with a monopolar or bipolar 90° loop. The procedure is usually performed in the operating theater under general or locoregional anesthesia and is preceded by the dilatation of the cervical canal and distension of the uterine cavity with a non-electrolytic medium if monopolar cautery is used, or with saline solution if bipolar loop is used. It is well known that bipolar energy reduces thermal injury to adjacent tissue compared with monopolar cautery, allowing the use of saline solution as distension media at the same time, which may provide a greater margin in fluid intravasation.

A further advance in the hysteroscopic approach to septate uterus has been achieved in the last decade thanks to the miniaturization of hysteroscopes that allows diagnosis and treatment in the same operative session, with the so-called "see-and-treat" hysteroscopy.

Currently, operative hysteroscopes of small diameter with continuous flow features and operative sheaths are available. Such hysteroscopes allow the use of microscissors or 5 Fr bipolar electrodes. No cervical dilatation is needed, thus reducing cervical trauma, operating time, risk of uterine perforation, and subsequent cervical incompetence, especially in nulliparous infertile women [58]. In addition, numerous studies indicate the possibility to perform the "office" procedure with a short intravenous sedation or no analgesia [53–55]. The efficacy and safety of office hysteroscopy with a VersaPoint device were assessed by two major studies that compared this technique with traditional monopolar [54–57]. Although reproductive outcomes (pregnancy rate, live births rate, and miscarriages rate) were similar in both techniques, hysteroscopy performed with VersaPoint was found to be safer and easier (as no dilatation was needed). Furthermore, it granted better haemostasis and could be used both in nulligravide and in women with stenosis of the cervical canal. Colacurci et al. [54] in a randomized, multicentre trial found no difference in reproductive outcomes between women treated by a bipolar microelectrode and those treated by resectoscope with monopolar knife, whereas operative time, fluid absorption, and complication rates were higher with resectoscopy.

Although, "office" hysteroscopic metroplasty with bipolar electrodes is fully equivalent to monopolar resectoscope in terms of reproductive outcome, the choice of either depends on the costs of the instrumentation, the availability of the operating room, operative time and complication rate.

The advantages of classic resectoscopy include availability and low cost instruments. Conversely, considering the advantages in terms of operative time, increased safety and higher feasibility, mini-hysteroscopy is a viable alternative to traditional resectoscopy and therefore should be preferred in case of subseptate uterus (class Vb).

Only in the case of septate uterus (septum extends up to the cervix) should the use of the classic resectoscope be preferred, as a continuous loss of distension medium through a widely patent cervical canal may occur; this can lead to insufficient expansion of the uterine cavity and hence a suboptimal view of the surgical field.

Septate uterus and reproductive outcome

Obstetric complications Approximately 20–25 % women with septate uterus experience obstetric complications and, among these, recurrent miscarriage and preterm labor are the most common [59].

A retrospective review conducted in 2001 on 198 women with septate uterus and a total of 499 pregnancies, indicated a prevalence of 44.1 % of miscarriage, 22.3 % of preterm labor, and 32.9 % for term delivery [60]. Similar results have been reported by other authors during the last years, confirming poor pregnancy outcome related to the presence of uterine septum. Therefore, reproductive outcome in women with septate uterus is the reference parameter used to assess the efficacy of hysteroscopic metroplasty. Numerous studies have already demonstrated a significant decrease of abortion and preterm labor rate in women treated with hysteroscopic metroplasty [61–69]. In a series of 366 pregnancies following hysteroscopic septum resection, just 60 cases of recurrent abortion (16.4 %) and 25 cases of preterm labor (6.8 %) were observed. These results were significantly improved when compared with preoperative rates, 86.4 % for miscarriage and 9.8 % for preterm labor [60].

The prophylactic role of metroplasty in asymptomatic or nulliparous women is still debated. The increased risk of uterine rupture in subsequent pregnancies and the need for a cesarean section would limit the surgical removal of the septum only to symptomatic women [59, 70]. Conversely, scientific evidence indicates a clear association between septate uterus and poor pregnancy outcome and a significant improvement of the reproductive outcome after resection. Considering the safety and feasibility of hysteroscopic metroplasty in the hands of an experienced surgeon, several authors have taken into account the possibility of using it as a prophylactic tool [71].

Infertility During the last two decades, contradictory results about the role of uterine malformations in fertility have been reported [23, 60, 72, 73]. Although uterine malformations may interfere with embryonic implantation and placentation [67], a review by Grimbizis et al. [60] found a similar prevalence of uterine malformations in infertile women and in the general population. These findings were confirmed by other authors [20, 66]. Thus, a direct correlation between uterine malformations and infertility should be excluded. Conversely, arcuate uterus is the most common uterine malformation in the fertile population and, in addition, the prevalence of septate uterus among infertile women is twice as high as that observed in the general population. These data support a relation between septate uterus and female infertility [74], especially in secondary infertility [66].

The discrepancy of data available in literature is reflected in clinical practice when metroplasty is used in cases of unexplained female infertility, to improve pregnancy rates. Still, data available are not conclusive, coming mostly from retrospective studies, conducted over small numbers of patients, often selected by different criteria.

A systematic review conducted by Homer et al. found a pregnancy rate of 48 % after resection in women with primary sterility and thereby supporting the use of hysteroscopic metroplasty in these cases [69]. The first prospective study on the use of metroplasty in infertile women was published in 2004 by Pabuccu et al. [73], reporting a postoperative spontaneous pregnancy rate of 41 % in women with infertility of unknown cause. These results were confirmed by prospective controlled trial by Mollo et al. on 44 women affected by septate uterus and otherwise unexplained infertility and 132 women with unexplained infertility as control [71]; the authors found a significantly higher pregnancy rate (38.6 vs 20.4 %) and live birth rate (34.1 vs 18.9 %) in the metroplasty group than in the control group. Similar outcome is achieved from a study by Shokeir et al. in 2011 [34], highlighting a postoperative pregnancy rate of 40.7 % with 80 % spontaneous conceptions. Although there are no randomized controlled trials, published data from 1986 to 2011 of hysteroscopic metroplasty in patients with primary infertility showed a pregnancy rate of about 40 % (16–74 %) (Table 1).

With regard to the need for metroplasty prior to a program for assisted reproduction (hence consisting of an infertile female population), most authors agree with the benefits of hysteroscopic resection of endometrial polyps, submucous fibroids, and uterine septum in terms of reproductive outcome. Tomazevic et al. studied approximately 2,500 patients affected by septate uterus (complete, subseptate uterus, and arcuate uterus) and undergoing an assisted reproduction program. They found that hysteroscopic metroplasty prior to in vitro

Table 1 Pregnancy rate after hysteroscopic metroplasty for the septate uterus in women with primary infertility

Author	No. of patients who underwent hysteroscopic metroplasty for septate uterus	No. of patients with primary infertility	Pregnancy rate (%)
Fayez [11]	19	7	36
Perino [54]	24	8	33
Daly [55]	70	15	21
Marabini [74]	40	14	35
Pabuccu [75]	59	10	16
Colacurci [76]	69	21	30
Venturoli [77]	69	36	52
Pabuccu [71]	61	25	40
Colacurci [52]	35	26	74
Mollo[69]	44	17	38
Wang [78]	6	2	33
Pai [79]	64	33	51
Tongue [80]	102	44	43
Total	662	258	39

fertilization (IVF) or intracytoplasmic sperm injection, significantly increased pregnancy rates and live birth rates [75]. Therefore, in accordance with Homer [69], they conclude that hysteroscopic correction of uterine abnormalities is a feasible, safe technique that improves reproductive outcome not only in women with recurrent pregnancy loss and preterm labor but also in infertile women, especially if IVF is being contemplated.

Conclusions

Septate uterus results from the incomplete or completely failed fusion of Müllerian ducts. Approximately 20–25 % of women with septate uterus experience obstetric complications that required a hysteroscopic surgery. Although obstetric complications represent the main indications for metroplasty, a possible negative role of uterine septum in case of otherwise unexplained infertility cannot be excluded. The scientific evidence does not show a direct etiological nexus but are not conclusive and require further study. According to the latest data, considering the simplicity and safety of hysteroscopic metroplasty, it seems safe to indicate the use in infertile women, especially if nulliparous over 35 years of age [23] or who intend to undergo a program of PMA [59].

References

1. Raga F, Bauset C, Remohi J, Bonilla-Musoles F, Simon C, Pellicer A (1997) Reproductive impact of congenital Mullerian anomalies. Hum Reprod 12:2277–2281
2. Taylor E, Gomel V (2008) The uterus and fertility. Fertil Steril 89:1–16
3. Giraldo JL, Habana A, Duleba AJ, Dokras A (2000) Septate uterus associated with cervical duplication and vaginal septum. J Am Assoc Gynecol Laparosc 7(2):277–279
4. Hundley AF, Fielding JR, Hoyte L (2001) Double cervix and vagina with septate uterus: an uncommon müllerian malformation. Obstet Gynecol 98(5 Pt 2):982–985
5. Wai CY, Zekam N, Sanz LE (2001) Septate uterus with double cervix and longitudinal vaginal septum. A case report. J Reprod Med 46(6):613–617
6. Saygili-Yilmaz ES, Erman-Akar M, Bayar D, Yuksel B, Yilmaz Z (2004) Septate uterus with a double cervix and longitudinal vaginal septum. J Reprod Med 49(10):833–836
7. Grimbizis GF, Gordts S, Di Spiezio Sardo A, Brucker S, De Angelis C, Gergolet M et al (2013) The ESHRE-ESGE consensus on the classification of female genital tract congenital anomalies. Gynecol Surg 10(3):199–212
8. Chan YY, Jayaprakasan K, Zamora J, Thornton JG, Raine-Fenning N, Coomarasamy A (2011) The prevalence of congenital uterine anomalies in unselected and high-risk populations: a systematic review. Hum Reprod Update 17(6):761–771
9. Burchell RC, Creed F, Rasoulpour M, Whitcomb M (1978) Vascular anatomy of the human uterus and pregnancy wastage. Br J Obstet Gynaecol 85:698–706
10. Candiani GB, Fedele L, Zamberletti D, De Virgiliis D, Carinelli S (1983) Endometrial patterns in malformed uteri. Acta Eur Fertil 14:35–42
11. Rock JA, Murphy AA (1986) Anatomic abnormalities. Clin Obstet Gynecol 29:886–911
12. Fayez JA (1986) Comparison between abdominal and hysteroscopic metroplasty. Obstet Gynecol 68:399–403
13. Heinonen PK (1997) Reproductive performance of women with uterine anomalies after abdominal or hysteroscopic metroplasty or no surgical treatment. J Am Assoc Gynecol Laparosc 4:311–317
14. Valle RF, Ekpo GE (2013) Hysteroscopic metroplasty for the septate uterus: review and metanalysis. J Minim Invasive Gynecol 20(1):22–42
15. Connell MT, Owen CM, Segars JH (2013) Genetic syndromes and genes involved in the development of the female reproductive tract: a possible role for gene therapy. J Genet Syndr Gene Ther 4:2
16. Lee DM, Osathanondh R, Yeh J (1998) Localization of Bcl-2 in the human fetal müllerian tract. Fertil Steril 70:135–140
17. Mikkila SP, Janas M, Karikoski R, Tarkkila T, Simola KO (1994) X-linked laterality sequence in a family with carrier manifestations. Am J Med Genet 49:435–438
18. Ergun A, Pabuccu R, Atay V, Kucuk T, Duru NK, Gungor S (1997) Three sisters with septate uteri: another reference to bidirectional theory. Hum Reprod 12:140–142, 9
19. Wu MH, Hsu CC et al (1997) Detection of congenital Mullerian duct anomalies using three-dimensional ultrasound. J Clin Ultrasound 25(9):487–492
20. Saravelos SH, Cocksedge KA, Li TC (2008) Prevalence and diagnosis of congenital uterine anomalies in women with reproductive failure: a critical appraisal. Hum Reprod Update 14(5):415–429
21. Gubbini G, Di Spiezio Sardo A, Nascetti D, Marra E, Spinelli M, Greco E, Casadio P, Nappi C (2009) New outpatient subclassification system for American Fertility Society classes V and VI uterine anomalies. J Minim Invasive Gynecol 16(5):554–561
22. Reuter K, Daly DC, Cohen SM (1989) Septate versus bicornuate uteri: errors in imaging diagnosis. Radiology 172:749–752
23. Kupesic S (2001) Clinical implications of sonographic detection of uterine anomalies for reproductive outcome. Ultrasound Obstet Gynecol 18:387–400
24. Mazouni C, Girard G, Deter R, Haumonte J-B, Blanc B, Bretelle F (2008) Diagnosis of Mullerian anomalies in adults: evaluation of practice. Fertil Steril 89:219–222
25. Ludwin A, Pityński K, Ludwin I, Banas T, Knafel A (2013) Two- and three-dimensional ultrasonography and sonohysterography versus hysteroscopy with laparoscopy in the differential diagnosis of septate, bicornuate, and arcuate uteri. J Minim Invasive Gynecol 20(1):90–99
26. Nicolini U, Bellotti M, Bonazzi B, Zamberletti D, Candiani GB (1987) Can ultrasound be used to screen uterine malformations? Fertil Steril 47:89–93
27. Fedele L, Ferrazzi E, Dorta M, Vercellini P, Candiani GB (1988) Ultrasonography in the differential diagnosis of "double" uteri. Fertil Steril 50:361–364
28. Salle B, Sergeant P, Gaucherand P, Guimont I, de Saint Hillaire P, Rudigoz RC (1996) Transvaginal hysterosonographic evaluation of septate uteri: a preliminary report. Hum Reprod 11:1004–1007
29. Storment JM, Kaiser JR, Sites CK (1998) Transvaginal ultrasonographic diagnosis of uterine septa. J Reprod Med 43:823–826
30. Perino A, Catinella E, Comparetto G, Venezia R, Candela P, Cimino C, Zangara C, Mencaglia L (1987) Hysteroscopic metroplasty: the role of ultrasound in the diagnosis and monitoring of patients with uterine septa. Acta Eur Fertil 18(5):349–352
31. Grimbizis GF, Tsolakidis D, Mikos T, Anagnostou E, Asimakopoulos E, Stamatopoulos P, Tarlatzis BC (2010) A prospective comparison of transvaginal ultrasound, saline infusion sonohysterography, and diagnostic hysteroscopy in the evaluation of endometrial pathology. Fertil Steril 94:2720–2795
32. Guimarães Filho HA, Mattar R, Pires CR, Araujo Junior E, Moron AF, Nardozza LMM (2006) Comparison of hysterosalpingography, hysterosonography and hysteroscopy in evaluation of the uterine cavity in patients with recurrent pregnancy losses. Arch Gynecol Obstet 274:284–288
33. Guven MA, Bese T, Demirkiran F, Idil M, Mgoyi L (2004) Hydrosonography in screening for intracavitary pathology in infertile women. Int J Gynecol Obstet 86:377–383
34. Shokeir T, Abdelshaheed M, El-Shafie M, Sherif L, Badawy A (2011) Determinants of fertility and reproductive success after hysteroscopic septoplasty for women with unexplained primary infertility: a prospective analysis of 88 cases. Eur J Obstet Gynecol Reprod Biol 155(1):54–57
35. Shokeir S, Abdelshaheed M (2009) Sonohysterography as a first-line evaluation for uterine abnormalities in women with recurrent failed in vitro fertilization-embryo transfer. Fertil Steril 91(suppl 4):1321–1322
36. Tur-Kaspa I, Gal M, Hartman M, Hartman J, Hartman A (2006) A prospective evaluation of uterine abnormalities by saline infusion sonohysterography in 1009 women with infertility or abnormal uterine bleeding. Fertil Steril 86:1731–1735
37. Valenzano MM, Mistrangelo E, Lijoi D, Fortunato T, Lantieri PB, Risso D, Costantini S, Ragni N (2006) Transvaginal sonohysterographic evaluation of uterine malformations. Eur J Obstet Gynecol Reprod Biol 124:246–249
38. Campo R, Van Belle Y, Rombauts L, Brosens I, Gordts S (1999) Office mini-hysteroscopy. Hum Reprod Update 5:73–81
39. Gordts S, Campo R, Puttemans P, Verhoven H, Gianaroli L, Brosens J, Brosens I (2002) Investigation of the infertile

couple: a one stop outpatient endoscopy-based approach. Hum Reprod 17:1684–1687

40. Philbois O, Guye E, Richard O, Tardieu D, Seffert P, Chavrier Y, Varlet F (2004) Role of laparoscopy in vaginal malformation. An experience in 22 children. Surg Endosc 18:87–91

41. Fedele L, Dorta M, Brioschi D, Massari C, Candiani GB (1989) Magnetic resonance evaluation of double uteri. Obstet Gynecol 74:844–847, 11

42. Carrington BM, Hricak H, Nuruddin RN, Secaf E, Laros RK Jr, Hill EC (1990) Mullerian duct anomalies: MR imaging evaluation. Radiology 176:715–720

43. Pellerito JS, McCarthy SM, Doyle MB, Glickman MG, DeCherney AH (1992) Diagnosis of uterine anomalies: relative accuracy of MR imaging, endovaginal sonography and hysterosalpingography. Radiology 183:795–800

44. Fischetti SG, Politi G, Lomeo E, Garozzo G (1995) Magnetic resonance in the evaluation of Mullerian duct anomalies. Radiol Med 89:105–111

45. Agrawal G, Riherd JM, Busse RF, Hinshaw JL, Sadowski EA (2009) Evaluation of uterine anomalies: 3D FRFSE cube versus standard 2D FRFSE. AJR 193:558–562

46. Ghi T, Casadio P, Kuleva M, Perrone AM, Savelli L, Giunchi S et al (2009) Accuracy of three-dimensional ultrasound in diagnosis and classification of congenital uterine anomalies. Fertil Steril 92(2):808–813

47. Bermejo C, Ten Martínez P, Cantarero R, Diaz D, Pérez Pedregosa J, Barrón E, Labrador E et al (2010) Three-dimensional ultrasound in the diagnosis of Müllerian duct anomalies and concordance with magnetic resonance imaging. Ultrasound Obstet Gynecol 35:593–601

48. Troiano R, Mc Carthy S (2004) Mülleriane duct anomalies: imaging and clinical issues. Radiology 233:19–34

49. Faivre E, Fernandez H, Deffieux X, Gervaise A, Frydman R, Levaillant JM (2012) Accuracy of three-dimensional ultrasonography in differential diagnosis of septate and bicornuate uterus compared with office hysteroscopy and pelvic magnetic resonance imaging. J Minim Invasive Gynecol 19(1):101–106

50. The American Fertility Society (1988) The American Fertility Society classi- fication of adnexal adhesions, distal tubal occlusion, tubal occlusion secondary to tubal ligation, tubal pregnancies, Mullerian anomalies and intrauterine adhesions. Fertil Steril 49:944–955

51. Woelfer B, Salim R, Banerjee S, Elson J, Regan L, Jurkovic D (2001) Reproductive outcomes in women with congenital anomalies detected by three-dimensional ultrasound screening. Obstet Gynecol 98:1099–1103

52. Manuale per un'isteroscopia moderna. Gruppo Isteroscopisti della Scuola Italiana di Chirurgia Mini Invasiva Ginecologica. Cap 19.

53. Bettocchi S, Ceci O, Nappi L, Pontrelli G, Pinto L, Vicino M (2007) Office hysteroscopic metroplasty: three "diagnostic criteria" to differentiate between septate and bicornuate uteri. J Minim Invasive Gynecol 14(3):324–328

54. Colacurci N, De Franciscis P, Mollo A, Litta P, Perino A, Cobellis L, De Placido G (2007) Small-diameter hysteroscopy with VersaPoint versus resectoscopy with a unipolar knife for the treatment of septate uterus: a prospective randomized study. J Minim Invasive Gynecol 14(5):622–627

55. Edstrom K (1974) Intrauterine surgical procedures during hysteroscopy. Endoscopy 6:175–181

56. Perino A, Castelli A, Cucinella G, Biondo A, Pane A, Venezia R (2004) A randomized comparison of endometrial laser intrauterine thermotherapy and hysteroscopic endometrial resection. Fertil Steril 82(3):731–734

57. Litta P, Spiller E, Saccardi C, Ambrosini G, Caserta D, Cosmi E (2008) Resectoscope or VersaPoint for hysteroscopic metroplasty. Int J Gynaecol Obstet 101(1):39–42

58. Lavergne N, Aristizabal J, Zarka V, Erny R, Hedon B (1996) Uterine anomalies and in vitro fertilization: what are the results? Eur J Obstet Gynecol Reprod Biol 68:29–34

59. Lourdel E, Cabry-Goubet R, Merviel P, Grenier N, Oliéric M-F, Gondry J (2007) Septate uterus: role of hysteroscopic metroplasty. Gynécol ObstétFertil 35:811–818

60. Grimbizis GF, Camus M, Tarlatzis BC, Bontis JN, Devroey P (2001) Clinical implications of uterine malformations and hysteroscopic treatment results. Hum Reprod Update 7(1):161–174

61. De Cherney HA, Russell BJ, Graebe AR, Polan M-L (1986) Resectoscopic management of Mullerian fusion defects. Fertil Steril 45:726–729

62. Valle FR, Sciarra JJ (1986) Hysteroscopic treatment of the septate uterus. Obstet Gynecol 67:253–257

63. March MC, Israel R (1987) Hysteroscopic management of recurrent abortion caused by septate uterus. Am J Obstet Gynecol 156:834–842

64. Perino A, Mencaglia L, Hamou J, Cittadini E (1987) Hysteroscopy for metroplasty of uterine septa: report of 24 cases. Fertil Steril 48:321–323

65. Daly CD, Maier D, Soto-Albors C (1989) Hysteroscopic metroplasty: six years experience. Obstet Gynecol 73:201–205

66. Choe KJ, Baggish SM (1992) Hysteroscopic treatment of septate uterus with neodymium-YAG laser. Fertil Steril 57:81–84

67. Fedele L, Arcaini L, Parazzini F et al (1993) Reproductive prognosis after hysteroscopic metroplasty in 102 women: life-table analysis. Fertil Steril 59:768–772

68. Grimbizis G, Camus M, Clasen K et al (1998) Hysteroscopic septum resection in patients with recurrent abortions and infertility. Hum Reprod 13:1188–1193

69. Horner HA, Li T-C, Cooke ID (2000) The septate uterus: a review of management and reproductive outcome. Fertil Steril 73:1–14

70. Patton PE, Novy MJ, Lee DM, Hickok LR (2004) The diagnosis and reproductive outcome after surgical treatment of the complete septate uterus, duplicated cervix and vaginal septum. Am J Obstet Gynecol 190(6):1669–1675

71. Mollo A, De Franciscis P, Colacurci N, Cobellis L, Perino A, Venezia R, Alviggi C, De Placido G (2009) Hysteroscopic resection of the septum improves the pregnancy rate of women with unexplained infertility: a prospective controlled trial. Fertil Steril 91(6):2628–2631

72. Heinonen PK, Pystynen PP (1983) Primary infertility and uterine anomalies. Fertil Steril 40:311–316

73. Pabuccu R, Gomel V (2004) Reproductive outcome after hysteroscopic metroplasty in women with septate uterus and otherwise unexplained infertility. Fertil Steril 81:1675–1678

74. Nahum GG (1998) Uterine anomalies. How common are they, and what is their distribution among subtypes? J Reprod Med 43:877–887

75. Tomazevic T, Ban-Frangez H, Virant-Klun I, Verdenik I, Pozlep B, Vrtacnik-Bokal E (2010) Septate, subseptate and arcuate uterus decrease pregnancy and live birth rates in IVF/ICSI. Reprod Biomed Online 21:700–705

76. Marabini A, Gubbini G, Stagnozzi R, Stefanetti M, Filoni M, Bovicelli A (1994) Hysteroscopic metroplasty. Ann N Y Acad Sci 734:488–492

77. Pabuccu R, Atay V, Urman B, Ergun A, Orhon E (1995) Hysteroscopic treatment of septate uterus. Gynaecol Endosc 4:213–215

8

Anti-adhesion barrier gels following operative hysteroscopy for treating female infertility

Jan Bosteels · Steven Weyers · Ben W. J. Mol ·
Thomas D'Hooghe

Abstract The aim of this study was to assess the effects of any anti-adhesion barrier gel used after operative hysteroscopy for treating infertility associated with uterine cavity abnormalities. Gynecologists might use any barrier gel following operative hysteroscopy in infertile women for decreasing de novo adhesion formation; the use of any barrier gel is associated with less severe de novo adhesions and lower mean adhesion scores. Nevertheless, infertile women should be counseled that there is at the present no evidence for higher live birth or pregnancy rates. There is a lack of data for the outcome miscarriage. Preclinical studies suggest that the use of biodegradable surgical barriers may decrease postsurgical adhesion formation. Observational studies in the human report conflicting results. We searched the Cochrane Menstrual Disorders and Subfertility Specialized Register (10 April 2013), the Cochrane Central Register of Controlled Trials (*The Cochrane Library* 2013, Issue 1), MEDLINE (1950 to 4 April 2013), EMBASE (1974 to 4 April 2013), and other electronic

J. Bosteels
Department of Obstetrics and Gynaecology, Imeldahospitaal,
Imeldalaan 9, 2820 Bonheiden, Belgium

J. Bosteels (✉)
CEBAM, Centre for Evidence-based Medicine, the Belgian Branch
of the Dutch Cochrane Centre, ACHG, Kapucijnenvoer 33, blok J
bus 7001, 3000 Leuven, Belgium
e-mail: jan.bosteels@med.kuleuven.be

S. Weyers
Universitaire Vrouwenkliniek, University Hospital Gent, De
Pintelaan 185, 9000 Gent, Belgium

B. W. J. Mol
School of Paediatrics and Reproductive Health, The Robinson
Institute, University of Adelaide, 5000 SA Adelaide, Australia

T. D'Hooghe
Leuven University Fertility Centre, KU Leuven, University Hospital
Gasthuisberg, Herestraat 49, 3000 Leuven, Belgium

databases of trials including trial registers, sources of unpublished literature, and reference lists. We handsearched the *Journal of Minimally Invasive Gynecology* (from 1 January 1992 to 13 April 2013); we also contacted experts in the field. We included the randomized comparisons between any anti-adhesion barrier gel versus another barrier gel, placebo, or no adjunctive therapy following operative hysteroscopy. Primary outcomes were live birth rates and de novo adhesion formation at second-look hysteroscopy. Secondary outcomes were pregnancy and miscarriage rates, mean adhesion scores, and severity of adhesions at second-look hysteroscopy. Two authors independently assessed eligible studies for inclusion and risk of bias, and extracted data. We contacted primary study authors for additional information or other clarification. Five trials met the inclusion criteria. There is no evidence for an effect favoring the use of any barrier gel following operative hysteroscopy for the key outcomes of live birth or clinical pregnancy (risk ratio (RR) 3.0, 95 % confidence interval (CI) 0.35 to 26, $P=0.32$, one study, 30 women, very low quality evidence); there were no data on the outcome miscarriage. The use of any gel following operative hysteroscopy decreases the incidence of de novo adhesions at second-look hysteroscopy at 1 to 3 months (RR 0.65, 95 % CI 0.45 to 0.93, $P=0.02$, five studies, 372 women, very low quality evidence). The number needed to treat to benefit is 9 (95 % CI 5 to 33). The use of auto-cross-linked hyaluronic acid gel in women undergoing operative hysteroscopy for fibroids, endometrial polyps, or uterine septa is associated with a lower mean adhesion score at second-look hysteroscopy at 3 months (mean difference (MD) -1.44, 95 % CI -1.83 to -1.05, $P<0.00001$, one study, 24 women; this benefit is even larger in women undergoing operative hysteroscopy for intrauterine adhesions(MD -3.30, 95 % CI -3.43 to -3.17, $P<0.00001$, one study, 19 women). After using any gel following operative hysteroscopy, there are more American Fertility Society 1988 stage I (mild) adhesions (RR 2.81, 95 % CI 1.13 to 7.01,

P=0.03, four studies, 79 women). The number needed to treat to benefit is 2 (95 % CI 1 to 4). Similarly there are less' moderate or severe adhesions' at second-look hysteroscopy (RR 0.25, 95 % CI 0.10 to 0.67, *P*=0.006, four studies, 79 women). The number needed to treat to benefit is 2 (95 % CI 1 to 4) (all very low quality evidence). There are some concerns for the non-methodological quality. Only two trials included infertile women; in the remaining three studies, it is not clear whether and how many participants suffered from infertility. Therefore, the applicability of the findings of the included studies to the target population under study should be questioned. Moreover, only one small trial studied the effects of anti-adhesion barrier gels for the key outcome of pregnancy; the length of follow-up was, however, not specified. More well-designed and adequately powered randomized studies are needed to assess whether the use of any anti-adhesion gel affects the key reproductive outcomes in a target population of infertile women.

Keywords Adhesion prevention · Barrier gel · Operative hysteroscopy · Infertility · Systematic review · Meta-analysis

Background

Intrauterine adhesions (IUAs) are fibrous strings at opposing walls of the uterus. The spectrum of IUA formation may vary from minimal IUAs to the complete obliteration of the uterine cavity. The causes of IUAs are multifactorial; nearly 90 % of cases are associated with postpartum or postabortion dilatation and curettage. The role of infection in the development of IUAs is controversial with the exception of genital tuberculosis [1]. The pathophysiology and the mechanisms of tissue repair in the endometrium are moreover poorly understood despite several theories on the source of cells for human endometrial regeneration [2].

IUA formation is the major long-term complication of operative hysteroscopy in women of reproductive age (Fig. 1). According to a randomized controlled trial (RCT) on the effectiveness of preoperative treatment before operative hysteroscopy, the incidence of postsurgical IUAs at second-look hysteroscopy is 3.6 % after polyp removal, 6.7 % after resection of uterine septa, 31.3 % after removal of a single fibroid, and 45.5 % after resection of multiple fibroids [3]. The investigators of a prospective cohort study in 163 women undergoing operative hysteroscopy conclude that the duration of the endometrial wound healing differs according to the type of pathology treated [4]. At follow-up hysteroscopy 1 month after the surgical intervention, significantly more women achieve a full healing of the endometrial cavity after removal of endometrial polyps (32 of 37 women or 86 %) compared to hysteroscopic lysis of intrauterine adhesions (30 of 45 women or 67 %), treatment of uterine septum (three of 16 women or 19 %), or removal of submucous fibroids (12 of 65 women or 18 %) (*P*<0.05). Significantly more de novo IUAs are detected in women undergoing septoplasty (14 of 16 women or 88 %) or adhesiolysis (34 of 45 women or 76 %) compared to removal of submucous fibroids (26 of 65 women or 40 %) or endometrial polyps (zero of 37 women or 0 %). Women with de novo IUAs are less likely to achieve full endometrial wound healing within 1 month compared with those without de novo IUAs (23 of 74 women or 31 % versus 54 of 89 women or 61 %, *P*=0.0003). The authors conclude that the full recovery of the endometrium varies from 1 month after the removal of polyps to between 2 and 3 months following hysteroscopic myomectomy [4].

Intrauterine adhesions may cause poor reproductive outcome. Firstly, according to a large review of observational studies, 922 of 2,151 women with IUAs (43 %) suffer from infertility [5]. The hypothetical underlying mechanisms for infertility due to IUAs are obstruction of sperm transport into the cervix, impaired embryo migration within the uterine cavity, or failure of embryo implantation due to endometrial insufficiency [1]. Secondly, recurrent miscarriage is often associated with IUAs; the prevalence of IUAs in women suffering from this health problem ranges from 5 to 39 % according to a narrative review of observational studies [6]. Thirdly, the hysteroscopic treatment of severe IUAs may cause long-term major obstetrical complications, such as placenta accreta/increta and higher risks for preterm delivery, uterine rupture, and postpartum hysterectomy [1].

Hyaluronic acid or hyaluronan (HA) is a water-soluble polysaccharide: It consists of multiple disaccharide units of glucuronic acid and *N*-acetylglucosamine, bound together by a β1-3-type glucoside bond. Solutions of HA have interesting viscoelastic properties which have led to interests in developing applications of HA in surgical procedures, for example in eye surgery. HA is not an ideal substance for all procedures, due to its limited residence time when applied to a surgical site. It quickly enters the systemic circulation and is cleared rapidly by catabolic pathways. Attempts to use hyaluronan for preventing postsurgical adhesions have therefore been met with variable success. Several chemically modified derivatives of HA have been developed to circumvent the disadvantages of HA. One such derivative is auto-cross-linked polysaccharide (ACP). It is formed by cross-linking hyaluronan, by direct formation of covalent ester bonds between hydroxyl and carboxyl groups of the hyaluronan molecule. ACP can be prepared with various degrees of cross-linking, which allows tailoring of the viscosity properties of ACP gels [7]. Carboxymethylcellulose (CMC) is a high molecular weight polysaccharide that has a viscosity greater than Dextran 70. CMC can be used for adhesion prevention as a membrane barrier or a gel as a mixture of chemically derivative sodium hyaluronate and carboxymethylcellulose gel (HA–CMC) [8].

Fig. 1 Intrauterine adhesions

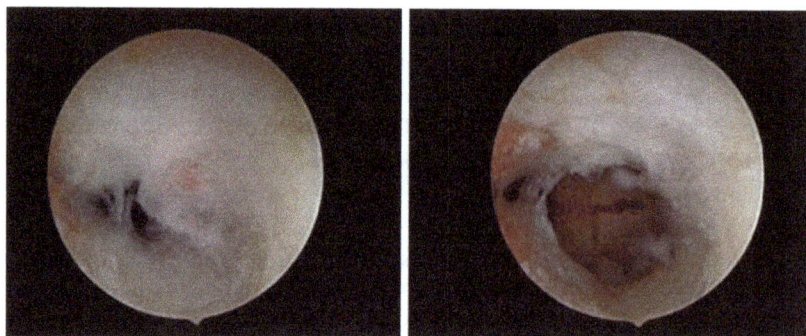

The ideal anti-adhesion barrier following operative hysteroscopy would be the application of a biologically active mechanical separator that achieves the suppression of intrauterine adhesion formation and promotes the healing of the endometrial tissue. The use of the biodegradable gel surgical barriers is based on the principle of keeping the adjacent wound surfaces as mechanically separate [7]. Several preclinical studies in various animal models report the effectiveness of both ACP [9–16] and HA–CMC gels [8, 17] or HA-CMC membranes [18, 19] for preventing postsurgical adhesions. Other preclinical studies in animal models suggest that HA gel remains in situ for more than 5 to 6 days [20, 21]. Similarly, animal studies demonstrate the persistence of HA–CMC for about 7 days after its application [22]. However, most of these studies were done in rodent models, and not in nonhuman primate models with reproductive anatomy similar to humans, like the baboon, a validated model for endometriosis research [23]

The exact mechanisms by which ACP and HA–CMC are able to reduce adhesion reformation are not well known, but may be related to "hydroflotation" or "siliconizing" effects. One French clinical controlled trial ($N=54$ women) studied the effectiveness of the application of ACP gel ($n=30$) versus no gel ($n=24$) at the end of an operative hysteroscopic procedure for treating fibroids, polyps, uterine septa, or IUAs; there are no statistically significant differences for the rate of adhesion formation, the mean adhesion scores, or the severity of the adhesions between both comparison groups [24]. No data are available for the reproductive outcome.

The health burden associated with infertility, abdominal pain, or bowel obstruction due to adhesions is substantial [7, 25, 26]; the total cost of adhesion-related morbidity in the US Health Care system exceeds $1 billion annually [27]. To the best of our knowledge, no economical studies on adhesion prevention after operative hysteroscopy have been conducted in an infertile population.

Postoperative de novo adhesion formation is a determining factor influencing endometrial wound healing [4]. At the present, there is uncertainty whether the use of anti-adhesion barrier gels following operative hysteroscopy affects the pregnancy or live birth rates; this is the main objective of the present systematic review.

Methods

Two reviewers independently searched the Cochrane Menstrual Disorders and Subfertility Specialized Register (10 April 2013), the Cochrane Central Register of Controlled Trials (*The Cochrane Library* 2013, Issue 1), MEDLINE (1950 to 4 April 2013), and EMBASE (1974 to 4 April 2013) using a combination of both index and free-text terms. We used no language restrictions. We searched other electronic databases of trials including trial registers, sources of unpublished literature, and reference lists. We handsearched the *Journal of Minimally Invasive Gynecology* (from 1 January 1992 to 13 April 2013) and contacted experts in the field.

We included only studies that were clearly randomized or claimed to be randomized. Studies were selected if the source population included women of reproductive age suffering from infertility, bound to undergo operative hysteroscopy for suspected or unsuspected intrauterine pathology before spontaneous conception or any infertility treatment. Infertility was defined as "a disease of the reproductive system defined by the failure to achieve a clinical pregnancy after 12 months or more of regular unprotected sexual intercourse" [28]. Studies were excluded if infertility was explicitly reported among the exclusion criteria.

We included the following types of randomized comparisons: any anti-adhesion barrier gel versus placebo, no barrier gel, or another type of barrier gel following operative hysteroscopy. We did not include studies of other anti-adhesion therapies, such as the use of human amnion membrane grafting, insertion of a balloon catheter or IUD, or hormonal treatment; this review focuses exclusively on the effectiveness of anti-adhesion barrier gels.

We selected live birth and de novo adhesion formation at second-look hysteroscopy as primary outcomes. Live birth was defined as a delivery of a live fetus after 20 completed weeks of gestational age that resulted in at least one live baby born. The delivery of a singleton, twin, or multiple pregnancy was counted as one live birth [28]. Ongoing or clinical pregnancy, miscarriage, and mean adhesion scores or severity of adhesions at second-look hysteroscopy were secondary outcomes. Ongoing pregnancy was defined as a pregnancy surpassing the first trimester or 12 weeks of pregnancy; clinical pregnancy was defined as a pregnancy diagnosed by US visualization of one or more gestational sacs or definitive clinical signs of pregnancy [28]. There are at the present seven reported classification systems for scoring the extent or severity of intrauterine adhesions [1]. Some classification systems have incorporated menstrual and obstetric history [29–31]; others rely exclusively on the hysteroscopic evaluation of the uterine cavity [32–35]. None of these systems has been validated or universally accepted [1]. We avoided pooling data from studies using different scoring systems.

One reviewer screened the titles and abstracts from the search to remove the publications which were obviously irrelevant for the research question of the present systematic review. After removing duplicates and after linking multiple reports of the same study together, two reviewers independently assessed the studies by examining the full text reports. This was done without blinding them to the reviewers; studies that appeared to be eligible were included using a pretested data extraction form. We contacted the authors of the primary study report whenever additional information was required. For studies with multiple study reports, we used the main trial report as the primary data extraction source.

Two reviewers independently assessed the risk of bias of the included studies and across studies by using the Cochrane "Risk of bias" tool. The following six items were assessed: random sequence generation, allocation concealment, blinding of participants and personnel, blinding of outcome assessors, selective outcome reporting, and other potential sources of bias. Any disagreements between the reviewers for the selection, data extraction, or risk of bias assessment were resolved through arbitration by a third author; any residual disagreement was reported in the final review.

We used the numbers of events in the comparison groups of each study to calculate the Mantel–Haenszel risk ratios (RR) for the binary data for all the main outcomes; for the secondary outcome "adhesion scores," the mean values and the standard deviations (SD) were used to calculate the inverse variance mean differences (MD) and the 95 % confidence intervals (CI). We used the most recently updated Review Manager 5 software provided by the Cochrane Collaboration for all the calculations, including the 95 % CI.

All main outcomes were expressed as per woman randomized. Multiple live births and multiple pregnancies were counted as one event. We did not attempt to pool any reported data that did not allow a valid analysis, such as "per cycle" data.

We aimed to analyze the data on an intention-to-treat basis (ITT). We tried to obtain as frequently as possible missing data after contacting the primary study authors. If missing data could not be obtained, we undertook imputation of individual values for the primary outcomes only by assuming that live births or de novo adhesions would not have occurred in participants without a reported primary outcome. For all other main outcomes, we used an available data analysis. We subjected any imputation of missing data for the primary outcomes to sensitivity analyses; any substantial difference in the imputed ITT analyses compared to available data analyses was incorporated in the interpretation of the study findings and the discussion.

Meta-analysis was done to provide a meaningful summary whenever enough studies which were sufficiently similar with respect to the clinical and methodological characteristics were available. A formal assessment of statistical heterogeneity was done by using the Q statistic and the I^2 statistic; the combination of both tests is more sensitive to detect the likelihood of substantial statistical heterogeneity. A low P value of the Q statistic ($P<0.10$) means significant heterogeneous results among individual studies. The I^2 statistic describes the percentage of variation across studies that is caused by substantial statistical heterogeneity rather than random chance variation; an I^2 statistic >50 % is the cutoff above which substantial statistical heterogeneity might be present. If there was evidence of substantial heterogeneity, we aimed to explore possible explanations for this observed heterogeneity by performing sensitivity analyses using Review Manager 5 software.

Publication bias, reporting bias, and within-study reporting bias are difficult to detect and correct for. We aimed to do the search for eligible studies as comprehensively as possible and by being alert in identifying duplicated reports of trials in order to minimize the potential impact of reporting and publication bias. Since we retrieved only a limited number of studies, we did not study publication bias or other forms of small study effects by creating a funnel plot.

One reviewer entered the study data and carried out the statistical analysis using Review Manager 5. We considered the outcomes live birth and pregnancy to be positive outcomes of effectiveness and by consequence higher numbers of these events as a benefit. The outcomes miscarriage, de novo adhesion formation, and adhesion scores were on the contrary considered as negative outcomes and higher numbers as harmful. We planned to combine data from primary studies in a meta-analysis with Review Manager 5 using the risk ratio as a summary outcome measure using a random-effects model if enough studies were retrieved and after significant clinical diversity and substantial statistical heterogeneity were confidently ruled out.

We planned to carry out subgroup analyses according to the extent or the severity of the uterine abnormality treated and for studies that reported both "live birth" and "pregnancy" in order to assess any overestimation of the treatment effect. We planned to do sensitivity analyses for the primary outcomes to investigate whether the results and conclusions are robust to arbitrary decisions regarding the eligibility and analysis. These sensitivity analyses included consideration whether conclusions would have differed if the eligibility was restricted to studies without high risk of bias versus all studies or if alternative imputation strategies were adopted, e.g., using odds ratio rather than risk ratio for the summary effect measure or a fixed effect rather than a random effects as the analysis model.

Findings

Description of studies

Results of the search

We identified 203 citations from searching electronic databases. These were combined with 2,826 additional records from other resources. We screened 3,029 records for duplicates by using End Note Web 3.5 and removed 2,823 duplicate citations. The remaining 206 records were assessed for eligibility through checking the titles and/or abstracts. We excluded 76 records as being obviously irrelevant. The remaining 130 full-text articles were assessed for eligibility. We retrieved 14 potentially eligible randomized studies; we included five trials, six trials were excluded, and three are ongoing. See Fig. 2 for the PRISMA flow chart of the search and selection process.

Included studies

Study design and setting Five single-center parallel group RCTs were included in the present systematic review: Four were conducted in Italy [36–39] and one in Israel [40]. All five trials used two comparison groups.

Only one trial [38] reported a statistical power calculation for one of the primary outcomes (incidence of de novo adhesion formation). The protocol of all included trials was approved by the Institutional Review Board. The protocol of the trial from Israel [40] was registered in a clinical trial registry (see NCT01377779 in Clinical Trials.gov). None of the trials reported on funding or other potential conflicts of interest.

Participants Two of the four Italian trials included infertile women: 34 women out of 92 participants [36] and 21 out of 110 participants [38]. The characteristics and data from these infertile women were not available for individual patient data meta-analysis. In the remaining two studies including 60 women [37] and 138 women [39], it is not clear whether and how many participants suffered from infertility. Regrettably we could not obtain any further clarification from the study authors. The study from Israel included 30 women who were

trying to conceive after miscarriage; the proportion of women suffering from infertility was, however, not reported, and this could not be clarified either [40].

Three of the four Italian trials [36, 38, 39] were conducted in the same university hospital; several co-authors participated in the clinical research of all these trials. The in- and exclusion criteria were very similar in these three studies; one trial included only women with intrauterine adhesions [36]; the other trials included women with fibroids, polyps, or uterine septa [39] or women with single or multiple intrauterine lesions except intrauterine adhesions or suffering from dysfunctional uterine bleeding [38]. The description of the source population was not adequate in the fourth Italian study [37]. The fifth included study was conducted in a source population of women with retained products of conception after miscarriage [40].

The mean age of the participants was below 35 years in one study [36]. In two trials, the mean patient age in both comparison groups was above 35 years [38, 39]. The other two studies reported a range between 18 and 65 years [37] or 18 and 50 years [40] without reporting data on the mean ages and SD in both comparison groups.

Interventions Five trials studied the randomized comparison between the intrauterine application of an anti-adhesion gel and no gel following operative hysteroscopy. In three studies, auto-cross-linked hyaluronic acid gel was used [36, 37, 39]; the other two [38, 40] used polyethylene oxide–sodium carboxymethylcellulose gel for the intervention. In three trials, the gel was administered into the uterine cavity through one of the flow channels of the resectoscope; the procedure was judged to be adequate when under hysteroscopic control the gel seemed to have replaced the liquid medium, filling the cavity from the fundus to the internal ostium of the cervix [36, 38, 39]. In one of these three studies [36], ultrasonographic data demonstrated that the anti-adhesive gel was able to keep the uterine walls separated for at least 72 h. In one study [37], the gel was applied using the cannula in a blind way without using hysteroscopic vizualization; for another trial [40], the method of application of the anti-adhesion gel is not clear.

Outcomes The primary outcome of live birth was reported in none of the included studies; the incidence of de novo adhesions was reported in all five studies [36–40]. The following secondary outcomes were reported as follows: clinical pregnancy [40], mean adhesion scores [36, 39], and severity of the adhesions [36–40]. The definition of pregnancy and the time period during which this secondary outcome was assessed in one trial [40] was not described. Four studies [36, 38–40] used the 1988 American Fertility Society (AFS) classification system for scoring intrauterine adhesions at second-look hysteroscopy; one trial [37] used the ASRM modified scoring system. None of these two classifications has been validated since to the best of our knowledge neither of them has been

Fig. 2 Study flow diagram

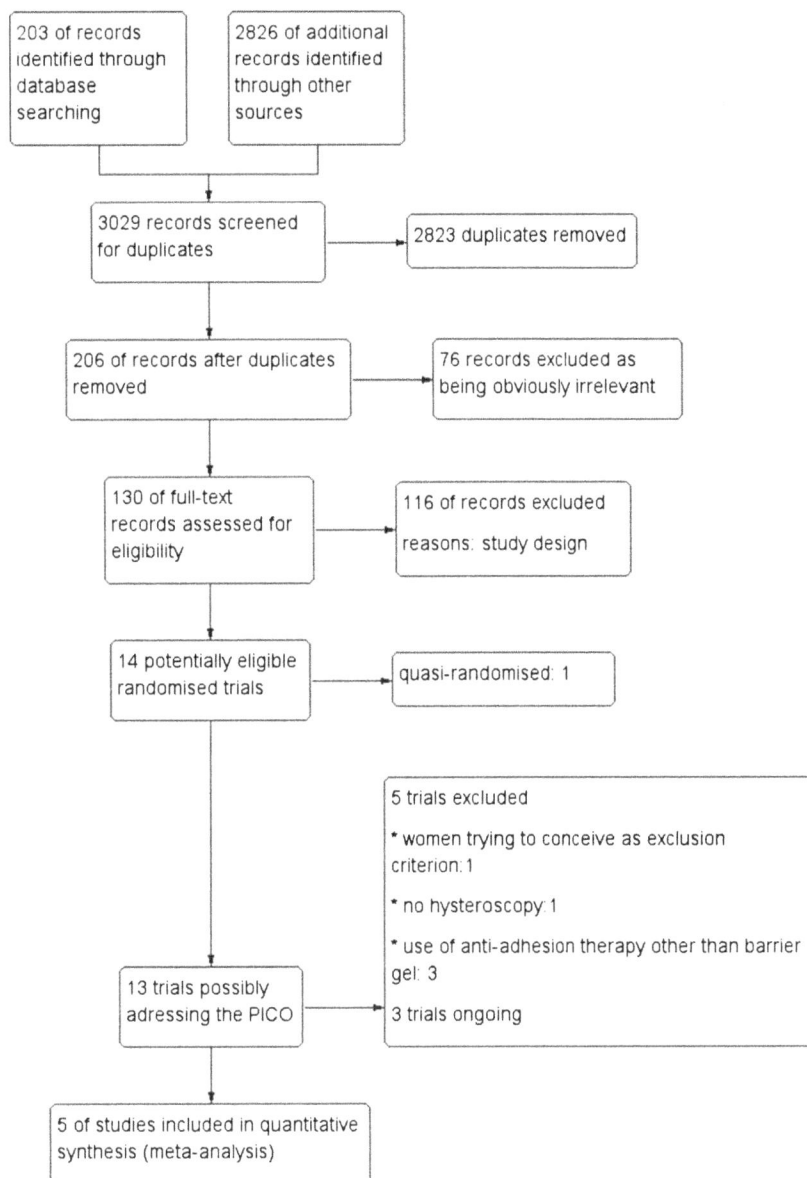

directly linked to reproductive outcome. In all five studies, the incidence and the severity of adhesion formation outcomes were measured at one time point only, ranging from 4 to 12 weeks after the operative hysteroscopy [36–40].

Risk of bias in included studies

Allocation (selection bias)

We judged four of the five trials to be at low risk for selection bias related to random sequence generation [36–39]. One trial [40] did not describe the method of random sequence generation; no further clarification could be obtained. We judged all five studies to be at unclear risk for selection bias related to allocation since they did not adequately describe the method of allocation concealment [36–40].

Blinding (performance bias and detection bias)

In all five trials, the method of blinding of the outcome assessors was not described [36–40]. We judged this risk of bias item to be important for the outcomes incidence of de novo adhesions, mean adhesion scores, and severity of adhesions but less relevant for the outcomes of live birth, ongoing or clinical pregnancy, and miscarriage unless the follow-up period was not long enough.

Incomplete outcome data (attrition bias)

We judged four trials to be at low risk for attrition bias [36, 38–40]. We judged one study to be at high risk for attrition bias related to incomplete outcome data; the loss to follow-up in this study of 33 % (20 out of 60 enrolled women) is sufficiently high and thus very likely to cause substantial attrition bias [37].

Selective outcome reporting (reporting bias)

We judged all trials to be at low risk of reporting bias; no evidence for selective outcome reporting was retrieved in any of the included studies when comparing abstract, methods, and results section [36–40].

Other potential sources of bias

We judged three studies to be at low risk for other potential sources of bias [36, 38, 39]. We judged one study to be at an unclear risk for other potential sources of bias [40]; the other study [37] was judged to be at high risk of bias due to likely imbalance of patient characteristics, imbalanced distribution of co-treatment, and other methodological study flaws (Figs. 3 and 4).

	Random sequence generation (selection bias)	Allocation concealment (selection bias)	Blinding of outcome assessment (detection bias): outcome: live birth or pregnancy	Blinding of outcome assessment (detection bias): outcome: adhesions	Incomplete outcome data (attrition bias)	Selective reporting (reporting bias)	Other bias
Acunzo 2003	+	?	+	?	+	+	+
De Iaco 2003	+	?	+	?	–	+	–
Di Spiezio Sardo 2011	+	?	+	?	+	+	+
Guida 2004	+	?	+	?	+	+	+
Pansky 2011	?	?	+	?	+	+	?

Fig. 3 Risk of bias summary: review authors' judgments about each risk of bias item for each included study

Effects of interventions

Any gel versus no gel

Primary outcomes

1. Live birth

   There were no data for this primary outcome.

2. Incidence of de novo adhesion formation at second-look hysteroscopy

   The use of any gel following operative hysteroscopy decreases the incidence of de novo adhesions (RR 0.65, 95 % CI 0.45 to 0.93, P=0.02, five studies, 372 women). There is no evidence for substantial statistical heterogeneity (chi^2=7.31, df=7 (P=0.40); I^2=4 %) (Fig. 5). The number needed to treat for a benefit is 9 (95 % CI 5 to 33).

Secondary outcomes

3. Pregnancy

   There is no evidence for an effect in favor of the use of polyethylene oxide–sodium carboxymethylcellulose gel following operative hysteroscopy for suspected retained products of conception for the outcome of clinical pregnancy (RR 3.00, 95 % CI 0.35 to 25.68, P=0.32, one study, 30 women) (Fig. 6).

4. Miscarriage

   There were no data for this secondary outcome.

5. Other secondary outcomes

   (a) Mean adhesion score at 3 months in women with fibroids, polyps, or uterine septa

   The use of auto-cross-linked hyaluronic acid gel in women undergoing operative hysteroscopy for myomas, endometrial polyps, or uterine septa is associated with a lower mean adhesion score at second-look hysteroscopy at 3 months (MD −1.44, 95 % CI −1.83 to −1.05, P<0.00001, one study, 24 women). There is no evidence for substantial subgroup differences (chi^2=0.24, df=2 (P=0.88), I^2=0 %) (Fig. 7).

   (b) Mean adhesion score at 3 months in women with intrauterine adhesions

   There are statistically significant differences in the lower mean adhesion scores at second-look hysteroscopy at 3 months in women undergoing operative hysteroscopy for intrauterine adhesions after the use of auto-cross-linked hyaluronic acid gel compared to operative hysteroscopy only (MD −3.30, 95 % CI −3.43 to −3.17, P<0.00001, one study, 19 women) (Fig. 8).

   (c) Severity of adhesions at second-look hysteroscopy when using any gel

Fig. 4 Risk of bias graph: review authors' judgments about each risk of bias item presented as percentages across all included studies

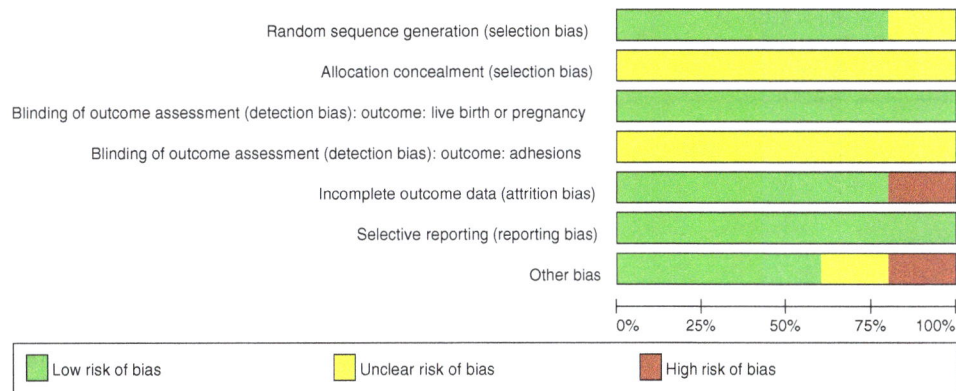

At second-look hysteroscopy, there are more mild adhesions when using any gel following operative hysteroscopy (RR 2.81, 95 % CI 1.13 to 7.01, P=0.03, four studies, 79 women). There is evidence for moderate statistical heterogeneity (chi^2=12.30, df=3 (P=0.006); I^2=76 %) (Fig. 9). The number needed to treat to benefit is 2 (95 % CI 1 to 4).

There is an effect favoring the use of any gel following operative hysteroscopy for the outcome of AFS 1988 stage II (moderate) adhesions at second-look hysteroscopy (RR 0.26, 0.09 to 0.80, P=0.02, three studies, 58 women). There is no evidence for substantial statistical heterogeneity (chi^2=1.43, df=2 (P=0.49); I^2= 0 %) (Fig. 10). The number needed to treat to benefit is 2 (95 % CI 1 to 2).

There is no evidence for a beneficial effect in favor of any gel versus no gel following operative hysteroscopy for the outcome of AFS 1988 stage III (severe) adhesions at second-look hysteroscopy (RR 0.46, 95 % CI 0.03 to 7.21, P=0.58, three studies, 58 women) (Fig. 11). For the composite outcome "moderate or severe adhesions," there are statistically significant differences favoring the use of any gel following operative hysteroscopy (RR 0.25, 95 % CI 0.10 to 0.67, P=0.006, four studies, 79 women). There is no evidence for statistical heterogeneity (chi^2=1.02, df=3 (P=0.80); I^2= 0 %) (Fig. 12). The number needed to treat to benefit is 2 (95 % CI 1 to 4).

Subgroup analyses Since no data were available for the outcome live birth, no subgroup analyses across studies reporting live birth and pregnancy rates or only one of these two key outcomes were done to assess any overestimation of treatment effect. There were enough data available to conduct a subgroup analysis according to the type of pathology treated by operative hysteroscopy. The use of any gel following operative hysteroscopy for fibroids (RR 0.44, 95 % CI 0.17 to 1.14, P=0.09, two studies, 80 women), endometrial polyps (RR 0.32, 95 % CI 0.07 to 1.49, P=0.15, two studies, 109 women), uterine septa (RR 0.26, 95 % CI 0.05 to 1.35, P=0.11, two studies, 29 women), intrauterine adhesions (RR 0.44, 95 % CI 0.18 to 1.05, P=0.06, one study, 84 women), retained products of conception (RR 0.91, 95 % CI 0.57 to 1.45, P=0.69, one study, 30 women), or "not specified" (RR 0.87, 95 % CI 0.33 to 2.29, P=0.78, one study, 40 women) consistently tends to decrease the incidence of de novo adhesions at second-look hysteroscopy; the differences were nevertheless not statistically significant given the limited numbers of women included and the limited numbers of events (Fig. 5). This is a common problem for subgroup analyses, and we should therefore be cautious about the interpretation of the data of this sensible predefined subgroup analysis. There is no evidence for substantial subgroup differences (chi^2=5.69, df=5 (P=0.34), I^2= 12.2 %).

Sensitivity analyses A sensitivity analysis was done to study the impact of the study quality on the direction and magnitude of the treatment effect. If we excluded the single study at high risk of bias [37] in a sensitivity analysis, the use of any gel following operative hysteroscopy was still beneficial for decreasing the incidence of de novo adhesions, but the treatment effect was larger (RR 0.56, 95 % CI 0.35 to 0.90, P=0.02, four studies, 332 women); there is no evidence for substantial statistical heterogeneity (chi^2=7.39, df=6 (P=0.29); I^2= 19 %) nor for substantial subgroup differences in the subgroup analysis according to the type of pathology treated (chi^2= 5.36, df=4 (P=0.25), I^2=25.4 %).

A sensitivity analysis to study the influence of the analysis model for data synthesis (fixed effect rather than random-effects model) did not influence the treatment effect (RR 0.55, 95 % CI 0.38 to 0.79, P=0.001, five studies, 372 women). The choice of the summary effect measure (RR rather than OR) did not influence the treatment effect (OR 0.40, 95 % CI 0.23 to 0.70, P=0.001, five studies, 372 women).

Fig. 5 Any anti-adhesion gel versus no gel, outcome 2: incidence of de novo adhesions at second-look hysteroscopy

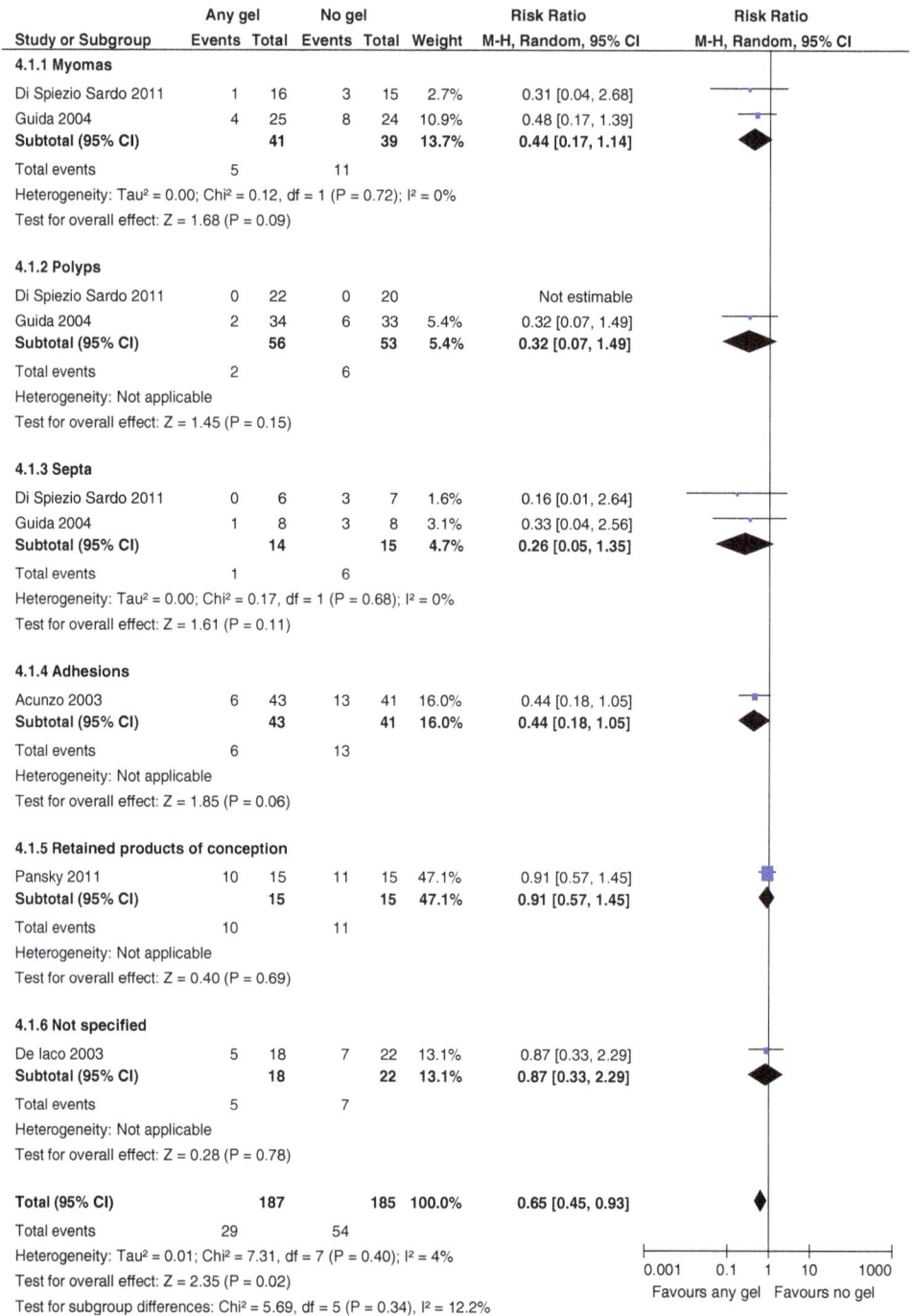

Study or Subgroup	Any gel Events	Total	No gel Events	Total	Weight	Risk Ratio M-H, Random, 95% CI	Risk Ratio M-H, Random, 95% CI
4.1.1 Myomas							
Di Spiezio Sardo 2011	1	16	3	15	2.7%	0.31 [0.04, 2.68]	
Guida 2004	4	25	8	24	10.9%	0.48 [0.17, 1.39]	
Subtotal (95% CI)		41		39	13.7%	**0.44 [0.17, 1.14]**	
Total events	5		11				
Heterogeneity: Tau² = 0.00; Chi² = 0.12, df = 1 (P = 0.72); I² = 0%							
Test for overall effect: Z = 1.68 (P = 0.09)							
4.1.2 Polyps							
Di Spiezio Sardo 2011	0	22	0	20		Not estimable	
Guida 2004	2	34	6	33	5.4%	0.32 [0.07, 1.49]	
Subtotal (95% CI)		56		53	5.4%	**0.32 [0.07, 1.49]**	
Total events	2		6				
Heterogeneity: Not applicable							
Test for overall effect: Z = 1.45 (P = 0.15)							
4.1.3 Septa							
Di Spiezio Sardo 2011	0	6	3	7	1.6%	0.16 [0.01, 2.64]	
Guida 2004	1	8	3	8	3.1%	0.33 [0.04, 2.56]	
Subtotal (95% CI)		14		15	4.7%	**0.26 [0.05, 1.35]**	
Total events	1		6				
Heterogeneity: Tau² = 0.00; Chi² = 0.17, df = 1 (P = 0.68); I² = 0%							
Test for overall effect: Z = 1.61 (P = 0.11)							
4.1.4 Adhesions							
Acunzo 2003	6	43	13	41	16.0%	0.44 [0.18, 1.05]	
Subtotal (95% CI)		43		41	16.0%	**0.44 [0.18, 1.05]**	
Total events	6		13				
Heterogeneity: Not applicable							
Test for overall effect: Z = 1.85 (P = 0.06)							
4.1.5 Retained products of conception							
Pansky 2011	10	15	11	15	47.1%	0.91 [0.57, 1.45]	
Subtotal (95% CI)		15		15	47.1%	**0.91 [0.57, 1.45]**	
Total events	10		11				
Heterogeneity: Not applicable							
Test for overall effect: Z = 0.40 (P = 0.69)							
4.1.6 Not specified							
De Iaco 2003	5	18	7	22	13.1%	0.87 [0.33, 2.29]	
Subtotal (95% CI)		18		22	13.1%	**0.87 [0.33, 2.29]**	
Total events	5		7				
Heterogeneity: Not applicable							
Test for overall effect: Z = 0.28 (P = 0.78)							
Total (95% CI)		187		185	100.0%	**0.65 [0.45, 0.93]**	
Total events	29		54				
Heterogeneity: Tau² = 0.01; Chi² = 7.31, df = 7 (P = 0.40); I² = 4%							
Test for overall effect: Z = 2.35 (P = 0.02)							
Test for subgroup differences: Chi² = 5.69, df = 5 (P = 0.34), I² = 12.2%							

0.001   0.1   1   10   1000
Favours any gel   Favours no gel

Fig. 6 Any anti-adhesion gel versus no gel, outcome 3: pregnancy

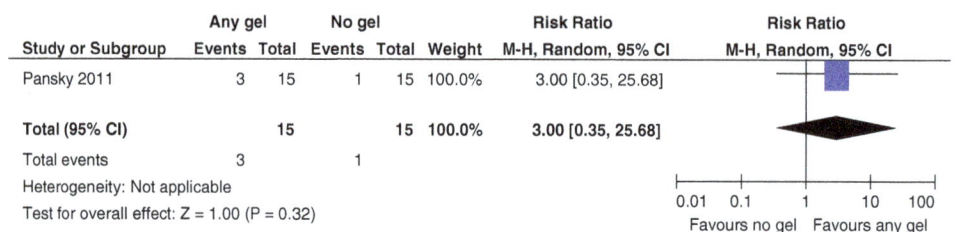

Study or Subgroup	Any gel Events	Total	No gel Events	Total	Weight	Risk Ratio M-H, Random, 95% CI	Risk Ratio M-H, Random, 95% CI
Pansky 2011	3	15	1	15	100.0%	3.00 [0.35, 25.68]	
Total (95% CI)		15		15	100.0%	**3.00 [0.35, 25.68]**	
Total events	3		1				
Heterogeneity: Not applicable							
Test for overall effect: Z = 1.00 (P = 0.32)							

0.01   0.1   1   10   100
Favours no gel   Favours any gel

Fig. 7 Auto-cross linked hyaluronic acid gel versus no gel, outcome 5.1: mean adhesion score AFS 1988 at 3 months in women with myomas, polyps, or uterine septa

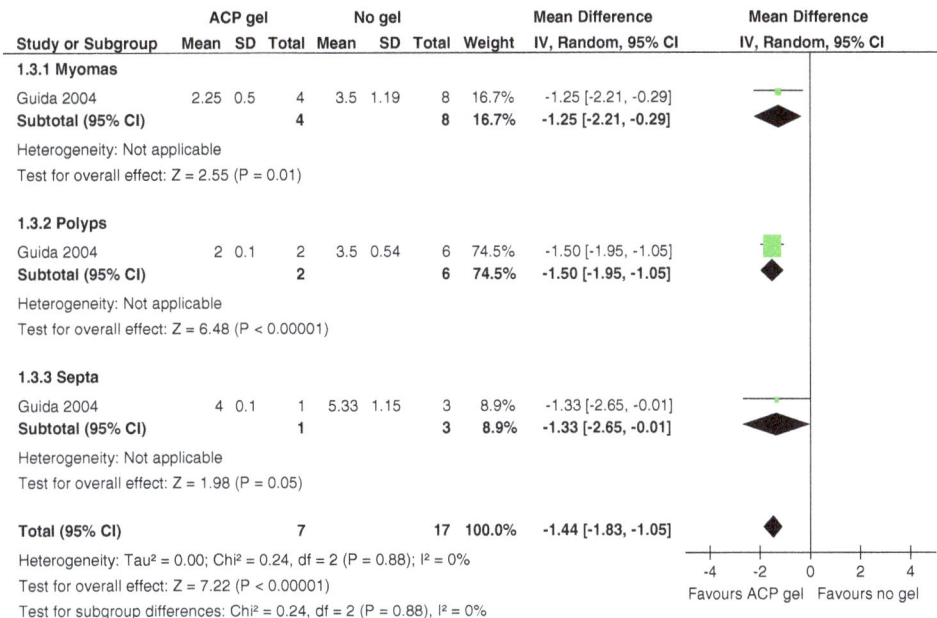

Study or Subgroup	ACP gel Mean	SD	Total	No gel Mean	SD	Total	Weight	Mean Difference IV, Random, 95% CI	Mean Difference IV, Random, 95% CI
1.3.1 Myomas									
Guida 2004	2.25	0.5	4	3.5	1.19	8	16.7%	-1.25 [-2.21, -0.29]	
Subtotal (95% CI)			4			8	16.7%	-1.25 [-2.21, -0.29]	
Heterogeneity: Not applicable									
Test for overall effect: Z = 2.55 (P = 0.01)									
1.3.2 Polyps									
Guida 2004	2	0.1	2	3.5	0.54	6	74.5%	-1.50 [-1.95, -1.05]	
Subtotal (95% CI)			2			6	74.5%	-1.50 [-1.95, -1.05]	
Heterogeneity: Not applicable									
Test for overall effect: Z = 6.48 (P < 0.00001)									
1.3.3 Septa									
Guida 2004	4	0.1	1	5.33	1.15	3	8.9%	-1.33 [-2.65, -0.01]	
Subtotal (95% CI)			1			3	8.9%	-1.33 [-2.65, -0.01]	
Heterogeneity: Not applicable									
Test for overall effect: Z = 1.98 (P = 0.05)									
Total (95% CI)			7			17	100.0%	-1.44 [-1.83, -1.05]	
Heterogeneity: Tau² = 0.00; Chi² = 0.24, df = 2 (P = 0.88); I² = 0%									
Test for overall effect: Z = 7.22 (P < 0.00001)									
Test for subgroup differences: Chi² = 0.24, df = 2 (P = 0.88), I² = 0%									

Favours ACP gel   Favours no gel

Discussion

Summary of main results

This systematic review aimed to appraise critically whether the use of anti-adhesion barrier gels following operative hysteroscopy for suspected or unsuspected intrauterine pathology in women of reproductive age suffering from infertility made a difference to the main outcomes of live birth, incidence of de novo adhesion formation, pregnancy, miscarriage, mean adhesions scores, or severity of adhesions at second-look hysteroscopy. We searched for RCTs on anti- adhesion barrier gels versus other barrier gels, placebo, or no anti-adhesion barrier gels following operative hysteroscopy.

We critically appraised five studies comparing the use of any anti-adhesion gel versus no gel in women of reproductive age treated by operative hysteroscopy for fibroids, polyps, septa, adhesions, or retained products of conception [36–40]. We judged a statistical pooling of the results of these five studies to be sensible given that substantial clinical diversity and statistical heterogeneity could confidently be ruled out.

According to our meta-analysis, there is evidence for an effect in favor of using anti-adhesive gel following operative hysteroscopy for decreasing the incidence of de novo

adhesions at second-look hysteroscopy. By doing a predefined subgroup analysis, the consistency of this beneficial effect for this outcome could be demonstrated across different subgroups according to the type of pathology treated. The beneficial treatment effect for decreasing de novo adhesions at second-look hysteroscopy is robust as demonstrated by multiple sensitivity analyses evaluating the influence of study quality, choice of the analysis model for data synthesis, and the choice of the summary effect measure.

The use of auto-cross-linked hyaluronic acid gel in women undergoing operative hysteroscopy for fibroids, endometrial polyps, uterine septa, or intrauterine adhesions is associated with a lower mean adhesion score at second-look hysteroscopy at 3 months. When de novo adhesion formation is observed at second-look hysteroscopy, there are more mild adhesions and less moderate or severe adhesions by using any anti-adhesion gel after operative hysteroscopy.

There is no evidence for a treatment effect favoring the use of polyethylene oxide–sodium carboxymethylcellulose gel versus no gel in women treated by operative hysteroscopy for suspected retained products of conception for the outcome of pregnancy [40]. Although there was a beneficial trend when using the anti-adhesion gel, the differences between both comparison groups were not statistically significant. This

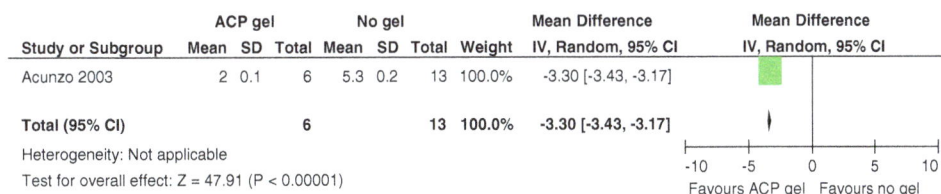

Study or Subgroup	ACP gel Mean	SD	Total	No gel Mean	SD	Total	Weight	Mean Difference IV, Random, 95% CI	Mean Difference IV, Random, 95% CI
Acunzo 2003	2	0.1	6	5.3	0.2	13	100.0%	-3.30 [-3.43, -3.17]	
Total (95% CI)			6			13	100.0%	-3.30 [-3.43, -3.17]	
Heterogeneity: Not applicable									
Test for overall effect: Z = 47.91 (P < 0.00001)									

Favours ACP gel   Favours no gel

Fig. 8 Auto-cross linked hyaluronic acid gel versus no gel, outcome 5.2: mean adhesion score AFS 1988 at 3 months in women with intrauterine adhesions

Fig. 9 Any anti-adhesion gel versus no gel, outcome 5.3: AFS 1988 stage I (mild) adhesions at second-look hysteroscopy

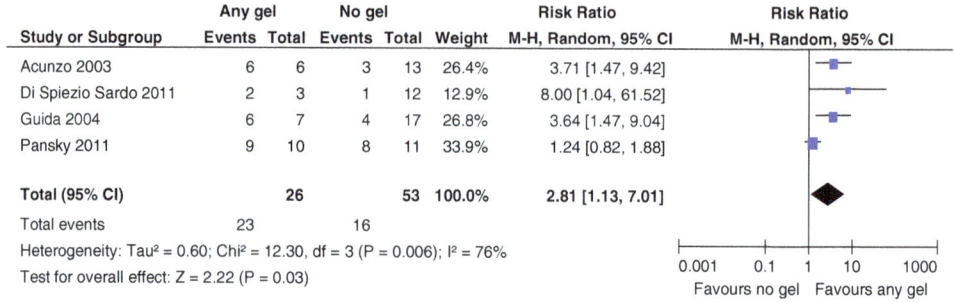

Study or Subgroup	Any gel Events	Total	No gel Events	Total	Weight	Risk Ratio M-H, Random, 95% CI
Acunzo 2003	6	6	3	13	26.4%	3.71 [1.47, 9.42]
Di Spiezio Sardo 2011	2	3	1	12	12.9%	8.00 [1.04, 61.52]
Guida 2004	6	7	4	17	26.8%	3.64 [1.47, 9.04]
Pansky 2011	9	10	8	11	33.9%	1.24 [0.82, 1.88]
Total (95% CI)		**26**		**53**	**100.0%**	**2.81 [1.13, 7.01]**
Total events	23		16			

Heterogeneity: Tau² = 0.60; Chi² = 12.30, df = 3 (P = 0.006); I² = 76%
Test for overall effect: Z = 2.22 (P = 0.03)

0.001　0.1　1　10　1000
Favours no gel　Favours any gel

may be a type II error: To detect a difference between both comparison groups of 13 % in the clinical pregnancy rate with a statistical power of 80 % at a confidence level of 95 % (α= 0.05 and β=0.20), a sample size of 145 women would be needed instead of the much smaller number of 30 participants in this single center study. We refer to Table 1 for a summary of findings for the key outcomes clinical pregnancy and incidence of de novo adhesions at second-look hysteroscopy (Table 1).

Overall completeness and applicability of evidence

The evidence of the effectiveness of using any anti-adhesion gel versus no gel in women of reproductive age treated by operative hysteroscopy for fibroids, polyps, septa, or intrauterine adhesions is limited: No data on live birth, pregnancy, or miscarriage rates were retrieved. In women of reproductive age treated by operative hysteroscopy for retained products of conception, the use of polyethylene oxide–sodium carboxymethylcellulose gel tends to increase the clinical pregnancy rate; the differences between both comparison groups were not statistically significant due to the small statistical power of the trial. Moreover, the proportion of the women suffering from infertility in both comparison groups was not reported, and the trial was at high risk of bias.

There are at the present two ongoing trials on the use of anti-adhesion barrier gels after operative hysteroscopy. The first is a parallel group randomized study on the effectiveness of applying Oxiplex/AP Gel (Intercoat) for preventing intrauterine adhesions in women aged 18 to 50 years following hysteroscopic surgery. This study is at the present not yet recruiting [41]. The second trial will address the effectiveness

of hyaluronic acid gel in women older than 18 years following hysteroscopic surgery; this trial will not answer the research question in the present review since the primary and only outcome measured is the patient satisfaction rate 2 months after the gel application [42].

The applicability of the evidence retrieved is questionable; most trials were conducted in a target population including—but not limited to—women suffering from infertility: Two trials [36, 38] included variable proportions of women suffering from infertility, miscarriage, or risk of preterm delivery; for two studies [37, 39], it is unclear whether and how many participants suffered from infertility while the fifth study [40] included a source population of women with proven fertility trying to conceive after miscarriage. It is unlikely that the mechanisms whereby any of the studied interventions might decrease de novo adhesion formation might differ in infertile versus fertile target populations; nevertheless, we judge the overall applicability of the retrieved best available evidence in a more general source population to a target population of women suffering from infertility to be limited at the best.

Quality of the evidence

We graded the evidence for the randomized comparison between any anti-adhesion barrier versus no gel following operative hysteroscopy for the outcome of pregnancy as very low. For this outcome, only one small study [40] was retrieved with few events. There are some methodological limitations: It is unclear whether and how allocation concealment and blinding of the outcome assessment were done in this study. Although lack of blinding of outcome assessors may

Fig. 10 Any anti-adhesion gel versus no gel, outcome 5.3: AFS 1988 stage II (moderate) adhesions at second-look hysteroscopy

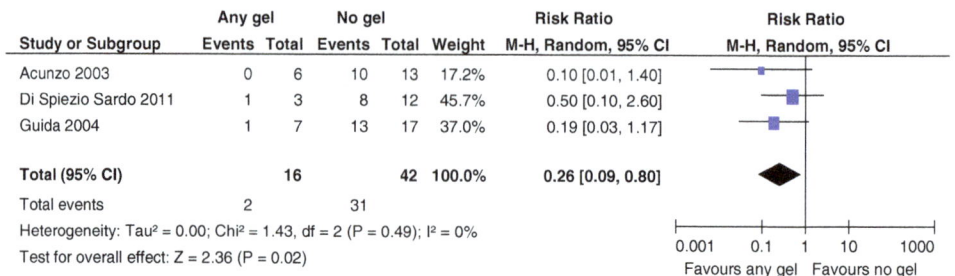

Study or Subgroup	Any gel Events	Total	No gel Events	Total	Weight	Risk Ratio M-H, Random, 95% CI
Acunzo 2003	0	6	10	13	17.2%	0.10 [0.01, 1.40]
Di Spiezio Sardo 2011	1	3	8	12	45.7%	0.50 [0.10, 2.60]
Guida 2004	1	7	13	17	37.0%	0.19 [0.03, 1.17]
Total (95% CI)		**16**		**42**	**100.0%**	**0.26 [0.09, 0.80]**
Total events	2		31			

Heterogeneity: Tau² = 0.00; Chi² = 1.43, df = 2 (P = 0.49); I² = 0%
Test for overall effect: Z = 2.36 (P = 0.02)

0.001　0.1　1　10　1000
Favours any gel　Favours no gel

Fig. 11 Any anti-adhesion gel versus no gel, outcome 5.3: AFS 1988 stage III (severe) adhesions at second-look hysteroscopy

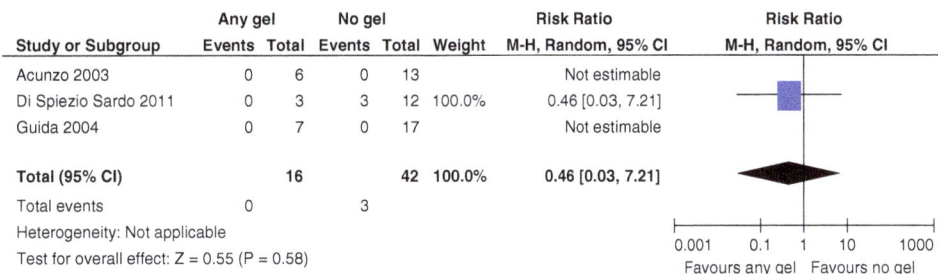

Study or Subgroup	Any gel Events	Total	No gel Events	Total	Weight	Risk Ratio M-H, Random, 95% CI
Acunzo 2003	0	6	0	13		Not estimable
Di Spiezio Sardo 2011	0	3	3	12	100.0%	0.46 [0.03, 7.21]
Guida 2004	0	7	0	17		Not estimable
Total (95% CI)		16		42	100.0%	0.46 [0.03, 7.21]
Total events	0		3			
Heterogeneity: Not applicable						
Test for overall effect: Z = 0.55 (P = 0.58)						

Risk Ratio M-H, Random, 95% CI — scale 0.001 0.1 1 10 1000 — Favours any gel Favours no gel

be less relevant for an unequivocal outcome such as pregnancy, there might be some potential for risk of bias especially since the length of the follow-up period was not adequately described. The women included in this study were treated by operative hysteroscopy for retained products of conception following miscarriage; the proportion and the characteristics of individual women suffering from infertility were not described. The confidence intervals for the point effect estimate were moreover very wide. Formal study of reporting bias was not possible since only one study was retrieved for this outcome; this implies that reporting bias cannot be confidently ruled out.

For the outcome of incidence of de novo adhesions at second-look hysteroscopy, we graded the evidence as very low. We retrieved five studies in 372 women [36–40]. It was unclear whether and how allocation concealment and blinding of the outcome assessment were done in all studies. Lack of blinding of the outcome assessors is very relevant for this outcome since the interpretation of the presence and the hysteroscopic appearance of intrauterine adhesions is to some degree subjective. One study had serious methodological limitations due to high risk of attrition bias [37]. Less than 50 % of the participants of two of the five included studies were infertile women [36, 38] whereas it is unclear whether and how many women from the other three studies [37, 39, 40] suffered from infertility; this questions the applicability of the retrieved evidence in a more general source population including but not limited to women suffering from infertility to a target population of infertile women only. Although we could not

formally investigate reporting bias given the small number of included studies, only studies demonstrating a beneficial effect were retrieved. Therefore, we judged that there might be some potential for reporting bias.

Potential biases in the review process

Our group published a Cochrane review on the effectiveness of hysteroscopy in the treatment of female infertility associated with suspected major uterine cavity abnormalities [43]. Given our prior knowledge of potentially eligible studies, there might have been some potential for detection bias. We therefore aimed to conduct a comprehensive search strategy for the new clinical research question of the present systematic review; this has resulted in finding more studies than would have been detected using the previously developed search strategy.

Agreements and disagreements with other studies or reviews

Two reviews support the use of anti-adhesive gel for reducing de novo adhesion formation following operative hysteroscopy. The first review [1] is a narrative review reporting the results and conclusions of one randomized trial included in the present systematic review [36]. The second review [44] is a systematic review and meta-analysis studying the effectiveness of auto-cross-linked hyaluronan gel for adhesion prevention in laparoscopic and hysteroscopic surgery. The data of three RCTs included in the present systematic review [36, 37, 39] were pooled: The proportion of women with adhesions at second look was significantly lower in women who received auto-cross linked hyaluronan gel than in the control group of women undergoing operative hysteroscopy without ACP gel

Fig. 12 Any anti-adhesion gel versus no gel, outcome 5.3: AFS 1988 stage II (moderate) or stage III (severe) adhesions at second-look hysteroscopy

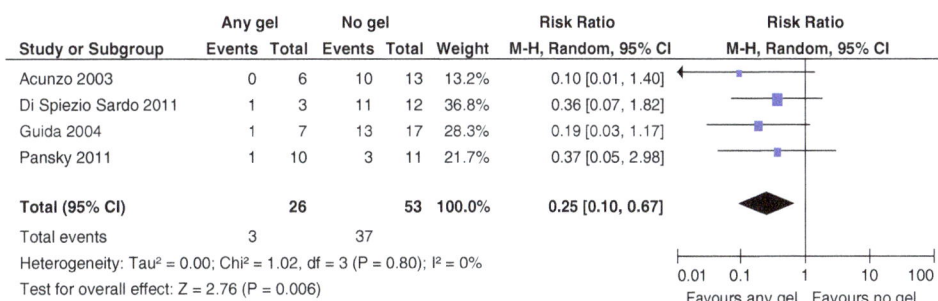

Study or Subgroup	Any gel Events	Total	No gel Events	Total	Weight	Risk Ratio M-H, Random, 95% CI
Acunzo 2003	0	6	10	13	13.2%	0.10 [0.01, 1.40]
Di Spiezio Sardo 2011	1	3	11	12	36.8%	0.36 [0.07, 1.82]
Guida 2004	1	7	13	17	28.3%	0.19 [0.03, 1.17]
Pansky 2011	1	10	3	11	21.7%	0.37 [0.05, 2.98]
Total (95% CI)		26		53	100.0%	0.25 [0.10, 0.67]
Total events	3		37			
Heterogeneity: Tau² = 0.00; Chi² = 1.02, df = 3 (P = 0.80); I² = 0%						
Test for overall effect: Z = 2.76 (P = 0.006)						

Risk Ratio M-H, Random, 95% CI — scale 0.01 0.1 1 10 100 — Favours any gel Favours no gel

Table 1 Summary of findings

Any anti-adhesive gel compared with no gel following operative hysteroscopy

Patient or population: women of reproductive age treated by operative hysteroscopy for myomas, polyps, septa, adhesions, or retained products of conception

Settings: hysteroscopy unit of a tertiary referral center

Intervention: application of auto-cross linked hyaluronic acid or polyethylene oxide–sodium carboxymethylcellulose gel

Comparison: no application of gel

Outcomes	Illustrative comparative risks[a] (95 % CI)		Relative effect (95 % CI)	No. of participants (studies)	Quality of the evidence (GRADE)	Comments: absolute effect
	Assumed risk control	Corresponding risk intervention				
Clinical pregnancy (time period not known)	Average risk population 67 per 1,000	201 per 1,000 (23 to 1,000)	RR 3.00 (0.35 to 25.68)	30 (1 study)	⊕⊝⊝⊝ (very low)	133 more per 1,000 (from 43 fewer to 1,645 more)
De novo adhesions at second look hysteroscopy (1 to 3 months)	Average risk population 292 per 1,000	190 per 1,000 (131 to 272)	RR 0.65 (0.45 to 0.93)	372 (5 studies)	⊕⊝⊝⊝ (very low)	102 fewer per 1,000 (from 20 fewer to 161 fewer)

The corresponding risk (and its 95 % confidence interval) is based on the assumed risk in the comparison group and the relative effect of the intervention (and its 95 % CI). GRADE Working Group grades of evidence: high quality—further research is very unlikely to change our confidence in the estimate of effect, moderate quality—further research is likely to have an important impact on our confidence in the estimate of effect and may change the estimate, low quality—further research is very likely to have an important impact on our confidence in the estimate of effect and is likely to change the estimate, and very low quality—we are very uncertain about the estimate

CI confidence interval, RR risk ratio

[a] The basis for the assumed risk is the pooled risk of the control groups of the five included studies [36–40]

(RR 0.50, 95 % CI 0.31 to 0.85, $P=0.009$, three studies, 256 women). The authors used an older methodological tool (the Jadad scale) for assessing the validity of the included trials. The "scale" methodology is at the present no longer supported by the Cochrane Collaboration which recommends using a more formal assessment by means of the risk of bias tool. This different methodology explains the discrepancy between the statement of Mais et al. [44] that all the included trials in their systematic review were judged to be of a high quality which contrasts with our judgment of "very low quality evidence" for the outcomes of pregnancy and incidence of de novo adhesions.

One French small comparative study ($n=54$ women with uterine pathology) studied the efficacy of auto-cross-linked hyaluronic acid gel in the prevention of adhesions following operative hysteroscopy [24]. Immediately after hysteroscopic surgery, the target population was divided by a non-random process into two groups: In group A, 30 women were treated by the intrauterine application of hyaluronic acid gel whereas the women in group B received no additional treatment (24 women). The key outcomes were the rate of adhesion formation, the mean adhesion score, and the adhesion severity according to the AFS classification, measured by second-look hysteroscopy 2 months after surgery. There are no statistically significant differences for the rate of intrauterine adhesion formation between the two groups (33.3 % for groups A and B) nor for the median adhesion scores (1.30± 2.35 versus 1.42±2.47, $P>0.05$) nor for the severity of the adhesions (70 % stage I adhesions, 20 % stage II adhesions, and 10 % stage III adhesions compared to 62.5 % stage I, 25 % stage II, and 12.5 % stage III in groups A and B, respectively, $P>0.05$). The authors conclude that the use of auto-cross-linked hyaluronic acid gel does not reduce the incidence and the severity of intrauterine adhesions after hysteroscopic surgery. According to a more recent review of the literature [45]—with the first author of the French comparative study [24] as co-author—the majority of the limited published studies until 2008 only evaluated the anatomic efficiency of anti-adhesion agents after hysteroscopic surgery. The authors conclude that the available data for the key reproductive outcomes are not sufficiently convincing to promote the widespread clinical use of anti-adhesive barrier agents as an effective treatment strategy for infertile women treated by operative hysteroscopy, hence their conclusion that additional randomized controlled trials are needed.

Authors' conclusions

Implications for practice

Gynecologists should counsel their patients that intrauterine adhesion formation is the major long-term complication of operative hysteroscopy in women of reproductive age. They might consider using any barrier gel following operative hysteroscopy for suspected uterine cavity abnormalities in infertile women: Its use may decrease de novo adhesion formation (very low quality evidence). If de novo adhesion formation occurs, there are less moderate or severe adhesions and more mild adhesions by using any anti-adhesion gel; the mean adhesion scores at second-look hysteroscopy are lower after using ACP gel. Infertile women nevertheless should be counseled that there is no evidence for higher live birth or pregnancy rates by using any barrier gel following operative hysteroscopy (very low-quality evidence). There are no data at the present of the effects on the miscarriage rates.

Implications for research

The very low-quality evidence retrieved from the limited number of randomized studies in a general source population including, but not restricted to, infertile women is at the present not sufficient to draw robust conclusions in favor of any barrier as an adjunctive therapy following operative hysteroscopy for the key reproductive outcomes; more well-designed pragmatic RCTs are needed to assess whether the use of any anti-adhesion gel affects the live birth, the pregnancy, and miscarriage rates in a target population of infertile women. There are no data on a dose–response relationship between the size, the number, or the severity of the treated pathology and the corresponding magnitude of the increase in effectiveness or decrease in the adverse outcomes that were defined in the present systematic review.

References

1. Deans R, Abbott J (2010) Review of intrauterine adhesions. J Minim Invasive Gynecol 17:555–569
2. Okulicz WC (2002) Regeneration. In: Glasser SR, Aplin JD, Giudice LC, Tabibzadeh S (eds) The endometrium. Taylor and Francis, London, pp 110–120
3. Taskin O, Sadik S, Onoglu A, Gokdeniz R, Erturan E, Burak F, Wheeler JM (2000) Role of endometrial suppression on the frequency of intrauterine adhesions after resectoscopic surgery. J Am Assoc Gynecol Laparoscopists 7(3):351–354
4. Yang JH, Chen MJ, Chen CD, Chen SU, Ho HN, Yang YS (2013) Optimal waiting period for subsequent fertility treatment after various hysteroscopic surgeries. Fertil Steril 99:2092–2096.e3
5. Schenker JG, Margalioth EJ (1982) Intrauterine adhesions: an updated appraisal. Fertil Steril 37:593–610
6. Kodaman PH, Arici A (2007) Intra-uterine adhesions and fertility outcome: how to optimize success? Curr Opin Obstet Gynecol 19(3):207–214
7. Renier D, Bellato PA, Bellini D, Pavesio A, Pressato D, Borrione A (2005) Pharmacokinetic behaviour of ACP gel, an autocrosslinked hyaluronan derivative, after intraperitoneal administration. Biomaterials 26:5368–5374
8. Leach RE, Burns JW, Dawe EJ, SmithBarbour MD, Diamond MP (1998) Reduction of postsurgical adhesion formation in the rabbit uterine horn model with use of hyaluronate/carboxymethylcellulose gel. Fertil Steril 69(3):415–417
9. Belluco C, Meggiolaro F, Pressato D, Pavesio A, Bigon E, Dona M, Forlin M, Nitti D, Lise M (2001) Prevention of postsurgical adhesions with an auto cross linked hyaluronan derivative gel. J Surg Res 100:217–221
10. Binda MM, Molinas CR, Bastidas A, Jansen M, Koninckx PR (2007) Efficacy of barriers and hypoxia-inducible factor inhibitors to prevent CO_2 pneumoperitoneum-enhanced adhesions in a laparoscopic mouse model. J Minim Invasive Gynecol 14(5):591–599
11. Binda MM, Koninckx PR (2009) Prevention of adhesion formation in a laparoscopic mouse model should combine local treatment with peritoneal cavity conditioning. Hum Reprod 24(6):1473–1479
12. Binda MM, Koninckx PR (2010) Hyperoxia and prevention of adhesion formation: a laparoscopic mouse model for open surgery. Br J Obstet Gynaecol 117(3):331–339
13. De Iaco PA, Stefanetti M, Pressato D, Piana S, Donà M, Pavesio A, Bovicelli L (1998) A novel hyaluronan-based gel in laparoscopic adhesion prevention: preclinical evaluation in an animal model. Fertil Steril 69:318–323
14. Koçak I, Unlü C, Akçan Y, Yakin K (1999) Reduction of adhesion formation with cross-linked hyaluronic acid after peritoneal surgery in rats. Fertil Steril 72:873–878
15. Shamiyeh A, Danis J, Benkö L, Vattay P, Röth E, Tulipan L, Shebl O, Wayand W (2007) Effect of hyaluron derivate gel in prevention of postsurgical peritoneal adhesions—an experimental study in pigs. Hepatogastroenterology 54(76):1121–1124
16. Wallwiener M, Brucker S, Hierlemann H, Brochhausen C, Solomayer E, Wallwiener C (2006) Innovative barriers for peritoneal adhesion prevention: liquid or solid? A rat uterine horn model. Fertil Steril 86(4 Suppl):1266–1276
17. Schonman R, Corona R, Bastidas A, De Cicco C, Mailova K, Koninckx PR (2008) Intercoat gel (Oxiplex): efficacy, safety, and tissue response in a laparoscopic mouse model. J Minim Invasive Gynecol 16(2):188–194
18. Kelekci S, Yilmaz B, Oguz S, Zergeroğlu S, Inan I, Tokucoğlu S (2004) The efficacy of a hyaluronate/carboxymethylcellulose membrane in prevention of postoperative adhesion in a rat uterine horn model. Tohoku J Exp Med 204:189–194
19. Rajab TK, Wallwiener M, Planck C, Brochhausen C, Kraemer B, Wallwiener CW (2010) A direct comparison of seprafilm, adept, intercoat, and spraygel for adhesion prophylaxis. J Surg Res 161:246–249
20. Laurent TC, Fraser JRE (1992) Hyaluronan. J Fed Am Soc Exp Biol 6:2397–2404
21. Nimrod A, Ezra E, Ezov N, Nachum G, Parisada B (1992) Absorption, distribution, metabolism and excretion of bacteria-derived hyaluronic acid in rats and rabbits. J Ocul Pharmacol 8:161–172
22. Diamond MP, DeCherney AH, Linsky CB, Cunningham T, Constantine B (1988) Adhesion re-formation in the rabbit uterine horn model: I. Reduction with carboxymethylcellulose. Int J Fertil 33:372–375
23. D'Hooghe TM, Kyama CM, Chai D, Fassbender A, Vodolazkaia A, Bokor A, Mwenda JM (2009) Nonhuman primate models for translational research in endometriosis. Reprod Sci 16(2):152–161
24. Ducarme G, Davitian C, Zarrouk S, Uzan M, Poncelet C (2006) Interest of auto-crosslinked hyaluronic acid gel in the prevention of intrauterine adhesions after hysteroscopic surgery: a case–control study. J Gynecol Obstet Biol Reprod 35(7):691–695
25. DeCherney AH, diZerega GS (1997) Clinical problem of intraperitoneal postsurgical adhesion formation following general surgery and the use of adhesion prevention barriers. Surg Clin North Am 77:671–688
26. diZerega GS (1994) Contemporary adhesion prevention. Fertil Steril 61:219–235
27. Baakdah H, Tulandi T (2005) Adhesion in gynaecology complication, cost, and prevention: a review. Surg Technol Int 14:185–190
28. Zegers-Hochschild F, Adamson GD, de Mouzon J, Mansour R, Nygren K, Sullivan E et al (2009) International Committee for Monitoring Assisted Reproductive Technology (ICMART) and the

World Health Organization (WHO) revised glossary of ART terminology, 2009. Fertil Steril 92(5):1520–1524

29. Wamsteker K, De Block S (1998) Diagnostic hysteroscopy: technique and documentation. In: Sutton C, Diamond M (eds) Endoscopic surgery for gynecologists. Saunders, London, pp 511–524

30. Anonymous (1988) The American Fertility Society classifications of adnexal adhesions, distal tubal occlusion, tubal occlusion secondary to tubal ligation, tubal pregnancies, müllerian anomalies and intrauterine adhesions. Fertil Steril 49:944–955

31. Nasr A, Al-Inany H, Thabet S, Aboulghar M (2000) A clinicohysteroscopic scoring system of intrauterine adhesions. Gynecol Obstet Invest 50:178–181

32. March C, Israel R, March A (1978) Hysteroscopic management of intrauterine adhesions. Am J Obstet Gynecol 130:653–657

33. Hamou J, Salat-Baroux J, Siegler A (1983) Diagnosis and treatment of intrauterine adhesions by microhysteroscopy. Fertil Steril 39:321–326

34. Valle RF, Sciarra JJ (1988) Intrauterine adhesions: hysteroscopic diagnosis, classification, treatment, and reproductive outcome. Am J Obstet Gynecol 158:1459–1470

35. Donnez J, Nisolle M (1994) Hysteroscopic adhesiolysis of intrauterine adhesions (Asherman syndrome). In: Donnez J (ed) Atlas of laser operative laparoscopy and hysteroscopy. Parthenon, London, pp 305–322

36. Acunzo G, Guida M, Pellicano M, Tommaselli GA, Di Spiezio Sardo A, Bifulco G, Cirillo D, Taylor A, Nappi C (2003) Effectiveness of auto-cross-linked hyaluronic acid gel in the prevention of intrauterine adhesions after hysteroscopic adhesiolysis: a prospective, randomized, controlled study. Hum Reprod 18(9):1918–1921

37. De Iaco PA, Muzzupapa G, Bovicelli A, Marconi S, Bitti SR, Sansovini M, Bovicelli L (2003) Hyaluronan derivative gel (Hyalobarrier gel) in intrauterine adhesion (IUA) prevention after operative hysteroscopy. Ellipse 19(1):15–18

38. Di Spiezio Sardo A, Spinelli M, Bramante S, Scognamiglio M, Greco E, Guida M, Cela V, Nappi C (2011) Efficacy of a polyethylene oxide–sodium carboxymethylcellulose gel in prevention of intrauterine adhesions after hysteroscopic surgery. J Minim Invasive Gynecol 18(4):462–469

39. Guida M, Acunzo G, Di Spiezio Sardo A, Bifulco G, Piccoli R, Pellicano M, Cerrota G, Cirillo D, Nappi C (2004) Effectiveness of auto-crosslinked hyaluronic acid gel in the prevention of intrauterine adhesions after hysteroscopic surgery: a prospective, randomized, controlled study. Hum Reprod 19(6):1461–1464

40. Pansky M, Fuchs N, Ben Ami I, Tovbin Y, Halperin R, Vaknin Z, Smorgick N (2011) Intercoat (Oxiplex/AP Gel) for preventing intrauterine adhesions following operative hysteroscopy for suspected retained products of conception—a pilot study. J Minim Invasive Gynecol 18(S21):68

41. Efficiency of INTERCOAT (Oxiplex/AP gel) in preventing intrauterine adhesion formation in hysteroscopic surgery—a prospective double blind randomized study. ClinicalTrials.gov: NCT01637974

42. Use of hyaluronic acid gel to prevent intrauterine adhesions in hysteroscopic surgery. ClinicalTrials.gov: NCT01464528

43. Bosteels J, Kasius J, Weyers S, Broekmans FJ, Mol BWJ, D'Hooghe TM (2013) Hysteroscopy for treating subfertility associated with suspected major uterine cavity abnormalities. Cochrane Database Syst Rev 1, Art. No.: CD009461

44. Mais V, Cirronis MG, Peiretti M, Ferrucci G, Cossu E, Melis GB (2012) Efficacy of auto-crosslinked hyaluronan gel for adhesion prevention in laparoscopy and hysteroscopy; a systematic review and meta-analysis of randomized controlled trials. Eur J Obstet Gynecol Reprod Biol 160:1–5

45. Revaux A, Ducarme G, Luton D (2008) Prevention of intrauterine adhesions after hysteroscopic surgery. Gynecologie, Obstetrique et Fertilité 36(3):311–317

46. Higgins JPT, Green S (eds) (2008) Cochrane handbook for systematic reviews of interventions. Wiley, Chichester

9

Neuropelveological assessment of neuropathic pelvic pain

M. Possover · A. Forman

Abstract The aim of the present report is to emphasize the importance of taking neurological considerations into account in the diagnostic workup of chronic pelvic pain (CPP) of "unknown origin." Based on new knowledge of the functional neuroanatomy of the pelvis and recent developments in the treatment of pelvic neuropathies, we incorporated well-known neurologic diagnostic methods into the classical gynecological workup for CPP. "Neuropelveological" assessment of CPP in women requires a detailed gynecological and neurologic history, a classical gynecological workup, and an adapted "gynecological" examination of the pelvic nerves and plexuses. The present report provides guidelines for "neuropelveological" assessment of chronic pelvic pain in clinical practice. It emphasizes the benefits of taking "neurological" considerations into account when diagnosing chronic pelvic pain.

Keywords Pudendal neuralgia · Vulvodynia · Coccygodynia · Chronic pelvic pain · Genital pain · Neuropelveology

Introduction

Chronic pelvic pain (CPP) afflicts 7 to 24 % of the population and is associated with impaired quality of life and high health care costs. Coccygeal, perianal, perineal, and/or genital pain are frequent complaints that usually occur as a result of common and easily recognizable organic disorders, such as anal fistulae, viral or bacterial infections, thrombosed hemorrhoids, genitoanal cancer, or other dermatologic pathologies. However, they can also occur under circumstances in which no organic cause can be identified. Chronic pelvic pain without any apparently etiology always constitutes a challenge for patients and clinicians. A correct diagnosis is crucial for etiologic treatment of the underlying cause. CPP can occur due to pelvic conditions that affect the nerves or to pathologies of the pelvic nerves and plexuses themselves. Therefore, knowledge beyond the limits of gynecology is required for proper diagnosis. Additional knowledge of pelvic neuroanatomy and clinical neurology is mandatory. This multidisciplinary field, referred to as neuropelveology, focuses on the diagnosis of pathologies and injuries to the pelvic nerves and plexuses responsible for the development of "non-gynecologic" chronic pelvic pain.

Neuro-anatomical considerations

The pelvis contains several parallel nerve systems. The most important nerve groups are the sacral plexus, the inferior hypogastric plexus, and the sensitive branches of the lumbar plexus (genitofemoral and ilioinguinal nerves). The sciatic and gluteal nerves as well as the pelvic splanchnic and pudendal nerves emerge from the sacral plexus.

The *sacral plexus* originates from the lumbosacral trunk (L4, L5, and S1) and the ventral roots of nerves S2 to S4. While most of the fibers originating from L5 and S1 running down into the sciatic nerve, sacral nerve roots S3 and S4 only innervate genito-anal areas without any fibers going to or from the leg. S2 is part of the pudendal nerve and sciatic nerve.

Sensory supply to the vulvar, perineal and perianal skin, and subcutaneous tissue of the lower two-thirds of the vagina is the *pudendal nerve* (PN). The pudendal nerve is a sensory and somatic nerve which originates from the ventral rami of the second to fourth (and occasionally fifth) sacral nerve roots. After branching from the sacral plexus, the nerve leaves the pelvis through the great sciatic notch, re-enters the pelvic cavity through the lesser sciatic notch, and finally travels to three main regions: the gluteal region, the pudendal canal, and the perineum. It accompanies the internal pudendal vessels

M. Possover (✉)
Center of Gynecologic Oncology & Neuropelveology,
Possover International Medical Center,
Hirslanden Clinic, Zurich, Switzerland
e-mail: m.possover@possover.com

M. Possover · A. Forman
Dept of Gynecology & Neuropelveology, University of Aarhus,
Aarhus, Denmark

upward and forward along the lateral wall of the ischiorectal fossa, being contained in a sheath of the obturator fascia termed the pudendal canal (Alcock's canal). The pudendal nerve gives off three distal branches—the inferior rectal nerve, the perineal nerve, and the dorsal nerve of the penis (in males) or the dorsal nerve of the clitoris (in females).

The pudendal nerve innervates not only the external genitalia of both sexes, but also the sphincters of the urinary bladder and rectum. As the bladder fills, the pudendal nerve becomes excited. Stimulation of the pudendal nerve results in contraction of the external urethral sphincter. Contraction of the external sphincter, coupled with that of the internal sphincter, maintains urethral pressure (resistance) higher than normal bladder pressure. The storage phase of the urinary bladder can be switched to the voiding phase either involuntarily (reflexively) or voluntarily. The pudendal nerve causes then relaxation of the levator ani so that the pelvic floor muscle relaxes. The pudendal nerve also signals the external sphincter to open. The sympathetic nerves send a message to the internal sphincter to relax and open, resulting in a lower urethral resistance. The PN is also known to have a potential modulatory effect on bladder function. Somatic afferent fibers of the pudendal nerve are supposed to project on sympathetic thoracolumbar neurons to the bladder neck and modulate their function. This neuromodulatory effect works exclusively at the spinal level and appears to be at least partly responsible for bladder neck competence and urinary continence [1]. Pudendal supply is not significant in the vaginal wall since there is no striated muscle, but efferent supply largely from the pudendal nerve controls the levator muscles that provide support, and influence function of the lower third of the vagina.

The pelvic visceral nerves arise chiefly from the *hypogastric plexus* (T1-L2). Visceral nerve supply is significant for the upper vagina, musculature, and glands. These nerves arise from the inferior hypogastric plexus, which gives rise to three other divisions. One division is the uterovaginal plexus (Frankenhausen's plexus) around the ureter and uterine artery. Fibers from the uterovaginal plexus accompany the vaginal artery and vein to the vagina. Parietal peritoneum in the pouch of Douglas is supplied by the visceral afferent nerves of the uterovaginal plexus. No parasympathetic fibers have been described in association with this hypogastric innervation of the vagina. The chief importance of vaginal parasympathetic efferent fibers (S2-4) is to mediate sexual response in the lower portion of the vagina.

The *ilioinguinal* and *genitofemoral nerves* originate from the upper part of the lumbar plexus of spinal nerves. Both nerves innervate the inguinal skin. In females, the genital branch of the genitofemoral nerve ends in the skin of the mons pubis and the ventral half of the labia majora. These nerves are exclusively sensory except for the genital branch of the genitofemoral nerve, which is responsible for the cremasteric reflex in men.

In view of these anatomical considerations, history-taking must focus on the external genital organs. The vulva and the vagina are the key organs for a proper neuropelveological diagnosis of chronic pelvic pain. Deep vaginal pain corresponds to irritation of the inferior hypogastric plexus and is therefore characterized by visceral pain accompanied by vegetative symptoms. The presence of anterior vulvodynia in combination with groin pain (which may or may not radiate to the thigh) suggests a pathology of the genitofemoral nerve (or lumbar plexus). Pudendal nerve pathology (Alcock's canal syndrome) is always combined with vulvodynia, perineal pain, and perianal pain. The combination of pudendal pain with non-gynecological pain, such as sciatica, gluteal pain, or low-back pain, suggests a pathology of the sacral plexus (sacral radiculopathy). Further pain that radiates to the anterior part of the thigh (lumbar dermatomes) generally corresponds to a spinal cord and/or spinal column disorder.

Neuropelveological assessment of neuropathic pelvic pain

History

Patients are asked a set of questions regarding potential causes (previous surgery, operative vaginal delivery, episiotomy, endometriosis, etc.), time of onset, duration, and severity of pain using a pain intensity scale (visual analog scale, VAS) of 0 (no pain) to 10 (worst imaginable pain) for standardized quantification of pain.

Risk factors for nerve damage Previous pelvic/abdominal surgeries or obstetric events are very important risk factors. All inguinal procedures such as surgical repair for inguinal hernia, low abdominal trocar or drainage incision, and Pfannenstiel incisions are associated with a risk of damage to the genitofemoral and/or ilioinguinal nerves. Laparoscopic and laparotomic approaches to the pelvic side wall or parametric tissues place patients at risk of damage to the somatic pelvic nerves, while central pelvic surgeries (hysterectomy and laparoscopic uterosacral nerve ablation (LUNA)→damage to the inferior hypogastric plexus, and presacral neurectomy→ damage to the superior hypogastric plexus) expose patients to a risk of visceral pelvic pain. Perineal, proctological, and obstetrical interventions expose the pudendal nerve and its branches to a risk of surgical damage.

Pelvic interventions and thrombosis may also promote changes in pelvic vein circulation that may trigger the development of pelvic varicose veins, which are risk factors for vascular entrapment or sacral compartment syndrome. Because the constitution of pelvic and lower limb veins is similar, patients with varicose veins in the legs may also have a higher risk of pelvic varicose veins.

History-taking should also focus on pathologies of the spinal cord, vertebral column, central nervous system (multiple sclerosis, Parkinson's disease, etc.), and peripheral nervous system (polyneuropathy).

Last but not least, the use of pain killers should be thoroughly documented.

Characteristics of pain—quality, location, and radiation Because visceral nerves extend through the pelvic organs like a spider web, visceral pelvic pain is usually described as vague, poorly localized, and dull pain, or as general malaise rather than real pain, which generally radiates to the lower back along midline. Visceral pain is very often associated with vegetative symptoms such as nausea, vomiting, pallor, diaphoresis, and tachycardia.

Somatic pelvic pain occurs due to somatic pelvic nerve damage and is classified as truncular (damage to the sciatic, obturator, femoral, or pudendal nerves) or radicular (damage to the lumbar or sacral plexus). Neuropathic pain causes numerous symptoms, ranging from allodynia, paresthesias, and sensations of electrical discharges to phantom sensations, which are even more confusing when no morphologic correlates are found. Hyperesthesia is usually the result of lesion causing nerve irritation, while hypoesthesia, anesthesia, and phantom pain generally develop after neurogenic nerve damage (axonal nerve damage). Somatic pain is well-described as localized pain with distal radiation in the corresponding dermatome(s) (Fig. 1). Generally, there is a trigger point at the level of irritation. Further symptoms may include increased sensitivity, electric shock-like sensations and/or stabbing, knife-like or aching pain, lump or foreign body sensation, twisting or pinching sensations, abnormal temperature sensations, constipation, pain and straining with bowel movements, straining or burning on urination, painful intercourse, and sexual dysfunction, including hyperarousal or decreased sensitivity.

Aggravating or relieving factors Pudendal neuralgia caused by compression of the pudendal nerve in Alcock's canal (Alcock's canal syndrome) typically induces severe pudendal nerve pain on sitting, which is relieved by standing, and absent when recumbent or when sitting on a toilet seat. Neuropathic pain induced by endometriosis of the pelvic nerves increases during menstruation and may decrease in response to gonadotropin-releasing hormone (GnRH) analogues. In pelvic nerve irritation by vascular entrapment or compression (sacral compartment syndrome), pain is aggravated by all situations that induce an increase in pelvic venous pressure (prolonged standing or sitting, the Valsalva maneuver, etc.) or marked pulsation of the pelvic veins (tricuspid insufficiency, close anatomic relationship with arteries, etc.).

Gynecological examination

The clinical examination focuses on inspection of the genital organs (colposcopy), supported by vaginal culture, urinalysis, vaginal pH testing, Pap smear, and biopsy of abnormal vulvar areas. Recto-vaginal palpation not only focuses on the parametria and rectovaginal space, but also on the pudendal nerves and the low sacral nerve roots (the sacral nerve roots L5 and S1 are not accessible by vaginal or rectal palpation). Direct digital palpation of the pelvic nerves is the key to diagnosis of pelvic nerve dysfunction. The affected patients have exquisite tenderness when digital pressure is applied to the damaged nerve, typically producing Tinel's sign (sensation of tingling or "pins and needles") in the distal distribution of the nerve. The pudendal nerve is accessible to palpation a few millimeters dorsomedial to the sciatic spine, while the low sacral nerve roots are accessible at the sacral bone, a few centimeters left and right of midline (Fig. 1). Selective nerve block is crucial for confirmation of the diagnosis. Pudendal nerve block can be performed via a perineal approach with concomitant vaginal/rectal palpation,

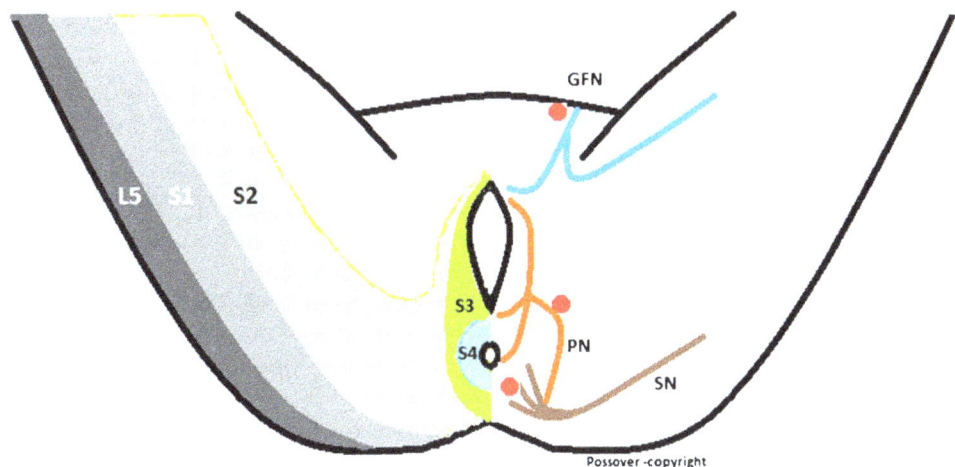

Fig. 1 Neuropelveologic assessment of dermatomes and trigger points of the pelvic nerves. (*L5* fifth lumbar root, *S* sacral nerve root, *PN* pudendal nerve, *SN* sacral nerve roots, *GFN* genitofemoral nerve)

while sacral nerve root block can be achieved by epidural or dorsal transforaminal epidural injection.

Neurologic examination

A full neurological examination includes assessment of both the motor and sensory systems.

Muscle tone and power Ankle clonus is checked by placing the patient's leg turned outwards on the bed, moving the ankle joint a few times to relax it, and then sharply dorsiflexing it. Any further movement of the joint may suggest clonus. The patient is also assessed for possible motor deficits in hip adduction (L3/obturator nerve), knee extension (L1-L4/femoral nerve), ankle dorsiflexion (foot drop—L5), and ankle plantar flexion (S1).

Reflexes The patellar reflex corresponds to the L3 root, whereas ankle jerk corresponds to the S1 root.

Patient walking and Romberg's test When the patient is standing with the feet apart and the eyes closed, any swaying may be suggestive of posterior column pathology.

Sensation The patient is assessed for light touch and pin prick sensation in all lumbosacral dermatomes. Extrinsic lesions (→ nerve irritation) do not cause any loss of sensation or feeling of numbness, while neurogenic nerve damage is accompanied by a loss of sensation or numbness in the corresponding nerve distribution.

Vibration Assessed using a sounding tuning fork placed on the medial malleolus.

Proprioception Assessed by up and down movement of the joint of the great toe (→ joint position sense).

Vaginal ultrasound

Vaginal ultrasound is not only used for assessment of organs and structures within the female pelvis, but also for evaluation of postvoid residual urine volume and bladder wall thickness. Pelvic varicose veins can also be identified directly via transvaginal Doppler ultrasound. Pelvic varicose veins is defined as the presence of dilated (diameter ≥7 mm), tortuous vessels with reflux (presence of bidirectional flow during Valsalva's maneuver).

Renal ultrasound

Routine renal ultrasound may be recommended in all patients with pelvic endometriosis for prevention of silent ureteral stenosis, especially when deeply infiltrating endometriosis is suspected.

Urodynamic testing

Pathologies of sacral nerve roots S2-4 and/or of the pelvic splanchnic nerves induce neuropathic pain as well as lower urinary tract and intestinal dysfunctions. Such disorders may be evaluated by urodynamic testing (cystometry, uroflowmetry, and pressure flow studies), pelvic EMG recording, and video-urodynamic studies. When assessing bladder function, it is very important to differentiate between detrusor hypotonia, which indicates neurogenic damage to the pelvic nerves, and irritation of the pelvic nerves, which is associated with bladder hypersensitivity or overactive bladder (OAB). Urgency, the cardinal symptom of OAB, is defined as a sudden and compelling desire to pass urine that is difficult to defer, while bladder hypersensitivity is a urodynamic diagnosis characterized by an early desire to void without fear of leakage or pain that persists and becomes annoying to the patient. Bladder hypersensitivity may resemble irritation of the pelvic nerves in terms of an incontrollable desire to pass urine without leakage and without a rise in detrusor pressure during filling cystometry, but less so with pathologies of the bladder itself.

Neurophysiological testing

Some of the more commonly used tests include the pudendal nerve terminal motor latency test (PNTML), electromyography (EMG), and magnetic resonance neurography (MRN). EMG studies of the pudendal nerve, often touted as a diagnostic tool, are unreliable since they can be abnormal after vaginal delivery or vaginal hysterectomy. Moreover, they do not define the neurologic level of the pathology.

Most frequent neuropathic pelvic pain

Pudendal neuralgia—Alcock's canal syndrome

The diagnosis of pudendal neuralgia is reserved for patients with allodynia in the entire distribution of the pudendal nerve (vulvar, perineal and perianal area) that does not radiate to other lumbosacral dermatomes The pain is typically more severe when sitting, relieved by standing, and absent when recumbent or when sitting on a toilet seat. Various other symptoms may occur in some cases, for example urinary hesitancy (difficulty starting the flow of urine), frequency (frequent need to pass urine), urgency (sudden sensation to pass urine), constipation/painful bowel movements, reduced awareness of defecation (the process of passing bowel motions), sexual dysfunction including loss of libido. In neurogenic PN damage, loss of sensation or numbness selectively is usually combined with contralateral anal deviation due to homolateral perineal/perianal myoatrophia. Urodynamic testing can show bladder overactivity [2] but may also be normal. Urethral incontinence occurs only in bilateral neurogenic PN damage. By transrectal/vaginal palpation of the pudendal nerve at the sacrospinous ligament, patients have exquisite tenderness with a Tinel's sign in genitoanal area. There are numerous possible causes for pudendal neuropathy. Some of the possible causes are an inflammatory or autoimmune illness, frequently interpreted as infection. After iatrogenic nerve damage, which are frequent in obstetrics and gynecology pudendal neuralgia is common, with etiologies such as compression of the nerve through a postpartum hematoma, fibrosis of the ischiorectal fossa, stretching of the nerve during delivery, or surgical damage during transvaginal sacrospinous colpopexy [3]. Recent interventions using mesh material for sacrospinal fixation [4], sacrocolpopexy, or rectopexy may also expose patients to a risk of pudendal nerve damage [5].

Genitofemoral neuropathy

When the genitofemoral nerve is affected, the pain may be localized in the inguinal area and may radiate to the internal aspect of the thigh and to the genital area. Lesions of the genital branch of the genitofemoral nerve induce vulvodynia or pudendal pain located selectively in the anterior portion of the vulva (clitoris). Surgical access to the inguinal region (appendectomy, herniorrhaphia, introduction of lateral trocar for laparoscopy, etc.) exposes patients to a risk of injury to the genitofemoral nerve. Neurologic symptoms are then restricted to sensory changes located in the groin area, the ventral genital area (as in lesion of the ventral branch of the PN), and/or the internal aspect of the tight (lesion of the femoral branch) but never below the knee. Since the genital branch is only sensitive in females, neither bladder dysfunction nor urinary incontinence occurs. Inguinal nerve block with an anesthetic agent is the diagnostic method of choice.

Sacral radiculopathies

The incidence of sacral radiculopathies is widely underestimated due to the lack of awareness that such lesions exist, but also because of a lack of diagnosis, acceptance, declaration, and reporting, especially when such injuries occur secondary to surgical interventions. Pudendal neuralgia, on the other hand, is often over-diagnosed. In a series of 136 consecutive patients suffering from intractable pudendal pain, only 18 had true PN entrapment, while all of the others had a sacral radiculopathy [6].

Sacral radiculopathy combines "pelvic symptoms" such as pudendal pain, low abdominal pain, vulvodynia, dyspareunia/apareunia, and coccygodynia with non-pelvic symptoms, including low-back-pain, gluteal pain, and sciatica. Massive lesions of the sacral nerve roots (plexopathy) are characterized by a loss of strength in hip extension, knee flexion, and dorsal plantar flexion of the foot. Because the vesical parasympathetic neurons (pelvic splanchnic nerves) are contained in sacral nerve roots S3-5, vesical symptoms are virtually constant. In extrinsic nerve irritation, bladder hypersensitivity is quasi systematic; true bladder overactivity may even be observed. Axonal nerve damage is characterized by loss of sensitivity or even numbness in the corresponding dermatomes, and ultrasound usually reveals postvoid residual urine; urodynamic testing confirms detrusor hypotonia or atonia as well as bladder hyposensitivity and increased bladder capacity.

Uterine myomas, ovarian processes, retroperitoneal vascular abnormalities (vascular entrapment), retroperitoneal fibrosis, and neurogenic tumors are frequent pelvic conditions that may induce pelvic neuropathies. However, the most common causes of sacral radiculopathy are surgical damage, deeply infiltrating endometriosis of the pelvic side wall, and nerve compression/entrapment by pelvic varicose veins [7]. Surgical nerve injuries occur due to coagulation, suturing, ischemia or cutting and induce disorders of sensation, pain, and dysfunction starting immediately after the procedure or within a few days. In contrast, nerve lesions caused by fibrotic tissue or vascular compression/entrapment usually require several months or years to develop. When diagnosing surgically induced sacral radiculopathies, correlation of clinical information with the surgical steps of the procedure permits precise anatomical localization of the neural lesion. This is necessary to adapt the treatment strategy accordingly. Perineal procedures may induce pathologies of the pudendal nerve and abdominal/laparoscopic procedures may affect the sacral nerve roots, while vaginal surgeries can induce both [5]. In a series of 92 consecutive patients with pelvic nerve damage secondary to surgery for pelvic organ prolapse (confirmed by laparoscopic exploration), the most frequent types of nerve damage were injuries to the right S2 nerve root incurred during laparoscopic rectopexy and laparoscopic colpopromontofixation, and injuries to the left S2 nerve root after vaginal uterosacral ligament suspension (McCall procedure). Vaginal mesh implantation for pelvic organ prolapse exposes patients to a risk of secondary nerve entrapment due to scar tissue development, especially when it involves new devices and techniques for blind needle-driving and minimal dissection. The reason is that, when any bleeding occurs, hematomas cannot drain and tend to dissect in retroperitoneal spaces, even in supralevator compartments, resulting in the formation of retroperitoneal fibrotic tissue.

When nerve injuries have occurred, laparoscopic exploration not only provides a tool for anatomic and functional exploration of the nerves, but also for effective neurosurgical treatment using techniques of nerve decompression or reconstruction.

Most pelvic conditions responsible for compression or irritation of the sacral nerve roots can be treated well by laparoscopic surgery. Moreover, neurogenic lesions are accessible to laparoscopic surgery. The "LION procedure" for laparoscopic implantation of neuroprosthesis to the pelvic nerves enables symptomatic pain treatment by selective neuromodulation of damaged nerves [8]. Laparoscopy is therefore an essential and logical step in the management of pelvic nerve pathologies that should be performed as soon as possible, before the nerve damage becomes irreversible and before the pain chronification process has begun.

Conclusions

The main symptom of CPP is chronic pelvic pain, and the main objective of treatment is pain control. Chronic pelvic pain may be caused by gynecologic, dermatologic, or urological disorders as well as by central or peripheral neuropathic conditions. When performing the history and clinical examination, the clinician must consider the combined gynecological, urological, and neurological aspects of pain. For proper diagnosis of CPP, the best way of thinking is to take a neuropelveological approach, which does not initially focus on diagnosing possible pelvic pathologies, but rather on identifying the neurologic pathways responsible for transmission of the pain signals to the central nervous system. Once these have been identified, the next step is to determine the level of the lesion (below, in, or above the pelvis). Determination of the etiology is the last step of neuropelveological diagnosis.

Because neuropelveologic assessment is based on the collection of many small clinical details gathered during careful history-taking and clinical examination, it takes time. Nevertheless, this is simple clinical methodology. An exact neuropelveological diagnosis can be established in most patients suffering from intractable CPP, making it possible to optimally adapt the treatment. Targeted therapeutic options include local injections of local anesthetics, corticoids or botulinum toxin A (Botox), laparoscopic techniques for nerve decompression, neurolysis or neuromodulation (LION procedure), and neurosurgical/orthopedic spinal procedures.

Medical pain treatment is a real option for pain control, and all patients undergoing laparoscopic procedures involving the pelvic nerves must receive such pain management treatment for a certain period. However, if etiological treatment is available, it will have priority over symptomatic treatment. The LION procedure for the implantation of electrodes to pelvic nerves is an innovative treatment option which is indicated only in neurogenic situations with combined pelvic pain and dysfunction. In the past, most patients were subjected to multiple examinations by multiple physicians as well as to strong medications that often caused side effects and reduced quality of life. With the new treatments available today, such problems are now avoidable.

Disclosure   The authors declare that they have no conflict of interest.

References

1. Reitz A, Schmid DM, Curt A, Knapp PA, Schurch B (2003) Afferent fibers of the pudendal nerve modulate sympathetic neurons controlling the bladder neck. Neurourol Urodyn 22(6):597–01
2. Virseda Chamorro M, Salinas-Casdo J, Zarza-Lucianez D, Mendez-Rubio S, Pelaquim H, Esteban-Fuertes M (2012) Participation of the pudendal innervation in the detrusor overactivity of the detrusor and in the overactive bladder syndrome. Actas Urol Esp 36(1):37–41
3. Verdeja AM, Elkins TE, Odoi A, Gasser R, Lamoutte C (1995) Transvagnal sacropsinous colpopexy: anatomic landmarks to be aware of to minimize complications. Am J Obstet Gynecol 173:1468–1469
4. Debodinance P, Amblard J, Fatton B, Cosson M, Jacquetin B (2007) The prosthetic kits in the prolapsed surgery: is it a gadget? J Gynecol Obstet Biol Reprod 36(3):267–275
5. Possover M, Lemos N (2011) Risks, symptoms, and management of pelvic nerve damage secondary to surgery for pelvic organ prolapse: a report of 95 cases. Int Urogynecol J 22(12):1485–1490
6. Possover M (2009) Laparoscopic management of endopelvic etiologies of pudendal pain in 134 consecutive patients. J Urol 181:1732–1736
7. Possover M, Schneider T, Henle KP (2011) Laparoscopic therapy of endometriosis and vascular entrapment of sacral plexus. Fertil Steril 95:756–758
8. Possover M (2010) New surgical evolutions in management of sacral radiculopathies. Surg Technol Int 19:123–128

10

Hysteroscopic myomectomy with the IBS® Integrated Bigatti Shaver versus conventional bipolar resectoscope: a retrospective comparative study

G. Bigatti · S. Franchetti · M. Rosales · A. Baglioni · S. Bianchi

Abstract From June 2011 to June 2013, all hysteroscopic myoma resections at the Ospedale San Giuseppe of Milan were performed using either the IBS® or the Versapoint® bipolar resectoscope. Dilatation time of the cervical canal, resection time, fluid balance, and complete single-stage removal of the myoma have been studied. The outcome was stratified for groups of myomas larger and smaller than 3 cm. Seventy-six myomectomies were performed with the IBS® and 51 with the Versapoint®. Both groups had a similar distribution of difficult cases like G2 and larger than 3 cm myomas. The results show no difference in terms of cervical dilatation, resection time, and fluid deficit between the two groups, but, for myomas less than 3 cm and G2 myomas, the IBS® has been able to treat respectively 93.5 % (p=0.3753) and 62.5 % (p=0.5491) of cases in a single step procedure. The overall number of necessary second procedures has been statistically significantly less in the IBS® Group than in the Versapoint® Group (p=0.0067). Although no significative difference in terms of time of resection, the IBS® has proven to be able to approach all kind of submucosal myomas in a single-step procedure and in a very precise and easy way. The IBS® can be considered a valid alternative to the conventional resectoscope.

Keywords IBS® · Hysteroscopy · Resectoscopy · Shaver · Myomectomy

G. Bigatti (✉) · S. Franchetti · M. Rosales · A. Baglioni
U.O. di Ostetricia e Ginecologia, Ospedale Classificato San
Giuseppe Via San Vittore, 12, 20123 Milan, Italy
e-mail: g.big@tiscalinet.it

S. Bianchi
Direttore dell'Unità Opertiva di Ostetricia e Ginecologia Ospedale
Classificato San Giuseppe Via San Vittore, Università degli Studi di
Milano, 12, 20123 Milan, Italy

Background

The incidence of submucosal myomas in women during their reproductive age ranges from 20 to 25 % [1–3].

Most of submucosal myomas may induce severe clinical symptoms such as abnormal uterine bleeding and menorrhagia with an incidence ranging from 60 to 84 % [3], dysmenorrehea , and infertility [1, 2, 4, 5]. The hysteroscopic treatment of this pathology has shown to be effective in relieving symptoms and in improving on the patients' fertility [6].

Presently, the double-flow bipolar resectoscope is considered the gold standard technique to perform hysteroscopical myomectomy [7, 8]. Unfortunately, the use of a bipolar resectoscope does not prevent overload syndrome and water intoxication [9]. The use of isotonic solutions like 0.9 % sodium chloride prevents dilution hyponatremia and hypocalcaemia [10], but the risk of fluid overload is still present. In addition, the massive absorption of normal saline solution can result in severe hyperchloremic metabolic acidosis and dilution coagulopathy that must be resolved with diuretic therapy [11, 12]. The use of high-frequency current during resection may lead to complications such as uterine perforation with bowel injury and internal and external burns caused by the uncontrolled leakage of current [13–15]. The most important limit of bipolar technique is that, during resection of large myomas, the tissue chips that remain inside the uterine cavity impair the surgeon's visual field, thus increasing the risk of perforation. Tissue pieces must be removed from the uterine cavity in order to complete the procedure under visual control. This makes the operation tiring and increases the overall resection time, thus resulting in a higher risk of intravasation and cervical laceration. Another minor problem is that more than half of the uterine perforations are entry-related because of the conventional resectoscope's large diameter [16].

Due to the above-mentioned features, the Versapoint® resectoscopy has a long learning curve, explaining why, even today, only a few surgeons perform operative hysteroscopy [17, 18]. By removing the tissue chips at the same time as their resection, the Integrated Bigatti Shaver (IBS®) has shown to improve on results of conventional resectoscopy, reducing the complications rate and improving the learning curve time [19]. Our previous study about polypectomy had shown that both resection time and fluid deficit were statistically better when using the IBS®, also because of a much faster learning curve [20]. Unfortunately, randomization has been related only to major pathologies groups and not to each single minor pathological group. Therefore, since myomectomies were unequally randomized, a comparative analysis was not possible. Our study shows that the IBS® is much superior to the Versapoint® in the polypectomy cases, but it is not indicative as to myomectomy.

The present study has been designed to compare 76 myomectomies performed with the IBS® with 51 with the Versapoint®, in order to evaluate whether this new technique offers real advantages.

Materials and methods

Equipment

We have performed all operations using either the IBS® or the conventional bipolar resectoscope (Versapoint® by Gynecare). The choice between one of the two devices was depending on the availability of the IBS®. We could use the IBS® for a 3-month period continuously with a 3-month pause during which the instrument had to be tested by the producing company. During this period of time, we have used only the IBS®. The reseptoscope was alternatively used during the pause period, when the IBS® was not available. The IBS® is made of 90° angulated 6° optics (Karl Storz GmbH of Tuttlingen) provided with a continuous flow sheath and an extra operative channel, into which a rigid shaving system has been inserted (Fig. 1). The continuous flow sheath is connected to a peristaltic pump (Endomat® Karl Storz GmbH of Tuttlingen) to maintain optimal distension and visualization inside the uterine cavity. Two separate stopcocks regulate inflow and outflow. The diameter of the outer sheath is 24 Fr (8 mm). The rigid shaving system consists of two hollow reusable metal tubes fitting into each other. The inner tube rotates within the outer tube, and it is connected to a handheld (Drill cut-x® Karl Storz GmbH of Tuttlingen) motor drive unit (Unidrive® S III Karl Storz GmbH of Tuttlingen) and to a roller pump (Endomat® LC Karl Storz GmbH of Tuttlingen) controlled by a foot pedal (Fig. 2). These two latter units are connected to each other and synchronized. The foot pedal activates simultaneously the shaver tip and the roller pump

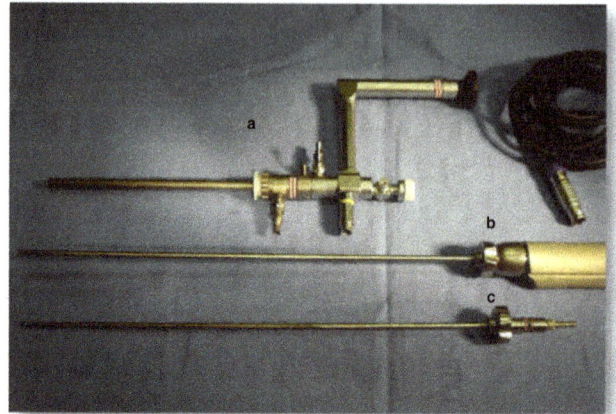

Fig. 1 Integrated Bigatti Shaver (IBS®). a 90° angulated 6° optics (Karl Storz GmbH of Tuttlingen) with a double flow sheath and an extra channel for the insertion of a b Rigid shaving system, c reusable blade

to maintain a continuous suction power on the window tip during the procedure. The first pedal switch activates the roller pump in order to aspirate the pathological site into the window, while the second switch activates the engine of the blades, in order to dissect the pathological tissue. The IBS®

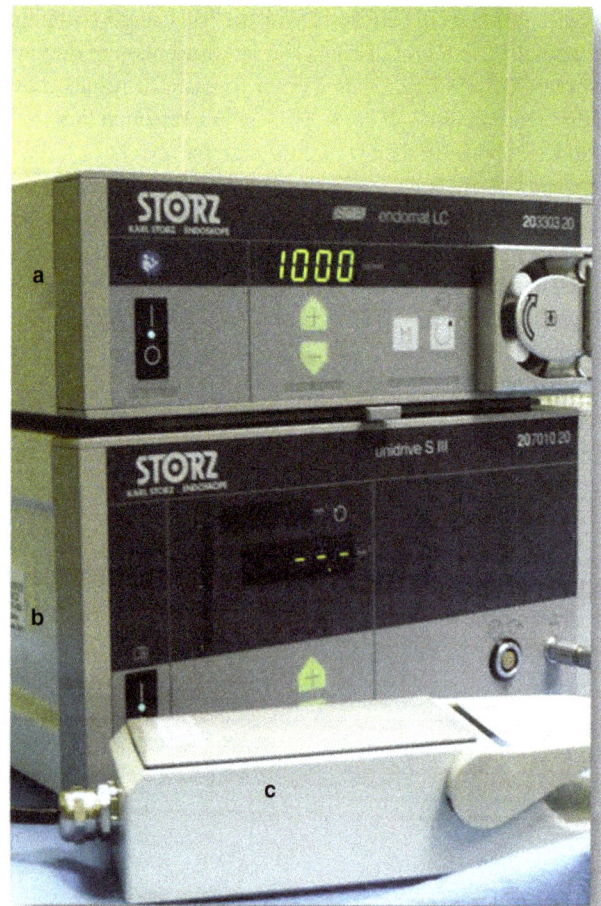

Fig. 2 Integrated Bigatti Shaver (IBS®): a Endomat® LC, b Unidrive® S III, c foot pedal (Karl Storz GmbH of Tuttlingen)

shaver tip is specifically designed in order to be aggressive for any kind of tissue. The inner rotating tube has a double window blade provided with a row of very sharp teeth. At the edge of the outer tube, there is a 25 mm^2 large window provided with teeth, too.

We have used two different shapes of blade: n°6=25 mm^2 flute beak shape and n.7=25 mm^2 elliptically open, similar to shark jaws (Fig. 3).

A power up to 5,000 oscillating rotation power per minute and a 200 to 1,000 ml/min aspiration flow are offered by these units. After dilatation of the uterine cervix internal ostium up to Hegar number 8.5, the panoramic optics (with the in- and outflow channels connected to the Endomat® pump) is inserted into the uterine cavity. A normal isotonic solution, like 0.9 % sodium chloride, is used for the irrigation. The maximum flow setting is 450 ml/min with a <95 mmHg intrauterine pressure. After visualizing the pathological site, the rigid shaving system (connected to the motor drive unit and to the roller pump) is inserted into the operative channel, and the procedure can start. The aspiration is activated only by pressing the roller pump pedal, in order to prevent the massive outflow-related collapse of uterine cavity. The rotating and oscillating movements of the shaving system inner blade cut the tissue. The resected tissue is then aspirated directly into a glass bottle connected to the roller pump (Endomat LC® Karl Storz GMBH of Tuttlingen), in order to be used as histologycal specimens.

Correct fluid balance is calculated by checking the total amount of the fluid aspirated by the Endomat® in addition to the fluid aspirated by the shaving system connected roller pump and to the fluid collected in an underlying graduated plastic bag.

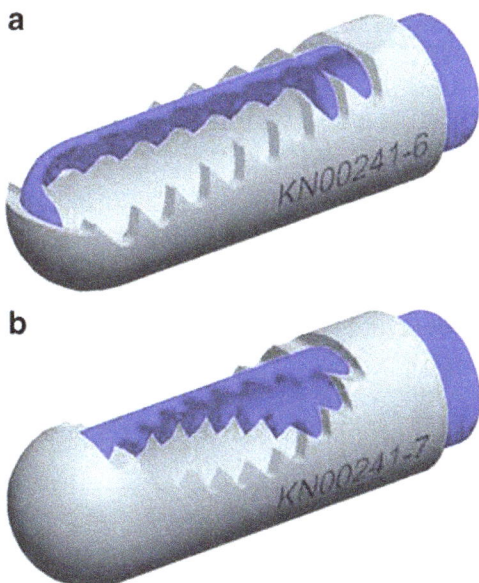

a

b

Fig. 3 Integrated Bigatti Shaver (IBS®) blades: **a** flute beak shape **b** shark jaws shape

The conventional bipolar resectoscope (Versapoint® by Gynecare) consists of a 4-mm wire loop electrode mounted on a working element with hand piece and of a 12° operative optics endoscope. The loop electrode is connected to a Versapoint® unit, automatically supplying a 170 and 80 W bipolar current respectively for cutting and coagulation. The Versapoint® unit is set to VC1 [21]. The operative endoscope has a continuous flow sheath with separate in- and outflow stopcocks connected to a peristaltic pump (Endomat® Karl Storz GmbH of Tuttlingen), to maintain optimal distension and visibility. The continuous flow sheath is rotation-free and has a 27 Fr (9 mm) external diameter.

After dilatation of the internal ostium of the uterine cervix up to Hegar number 9.5, the resectoscope connected to the peristaltic pump is inserted into the uterine cavity. Conventional resection technique is used. A normal isotonic solution, like 0.9 % sodium chloride, is used for the irrigation. The maximal flow setting is 450 ml/min with a lower than 95 mmHg intrauterine pressure. Correct fluid balance is calculated by checking the fluid aspirated by the Endomat® pump, in addition to the fluid collected in a graduated plastic bag placed under the patient.

Source population

The source population includes 238 women undergoing operative hysteroscopy with the IBS® versus 230 women with the Versapoint® over a 2-year period, from June 2011 to June 2013, in our center: Ospedale San Giuseppe of Milan—Italy, a University teaching Hospital. With the IBS®, we have performed 76 myomectomies, 138 polypectomies, 10 mixed pathologies (myomectomies+polypectomies+sinechiolysis), 11 endometrial ablations, and 3 septum resections.

With the Versapoint®, we have performed 51 myomectomies; 157 polypectomies, 6 mixed pathologies (myomectomies+polypectomies+sinechiolysis), 15 endometrial ablations, and 1 septum resection (Table 1).

Oncological cases were excluded from our trial.

Study population

The study population has been selected from the source population (Table 2). Seventy-six patients, of whom 66 (86.8 %) patients with 1 myoma and 10 patients (13.2 %) with more than 1 myoma, undergoing a myomectomy with the IBS® have been included in Group A whereas 51 women, of whom 46 (90.2 %) patients with 1 myoma and 5 patients (9.8 %) with more than 1 myoma, undergoing a myomectomy with the Versapoint® have been included in Group B.

In Group A, a total amount of 88 myomas have been treated, of which 28 (31.8 %) were G0 type myomas, 28 (31.8 %) G1 type, and 32 (36.4 %) G2 type.

Table 1 Source population: IBS® and Versapoint® personal series of a 2-year period, June 2011–June 2013, Ospedale San Giuseppe, Milano, Italy

IBS® and Versapoint® personal series June 2011–June 2013

Indication	IBS® N° of cases	Versapoint® N° of cases
Myomectomies	76	51
• G0	28	18
• G1	28	18
• G2	32	20
Polypectomies	138	157
Myomectomies+polypectomies+ sinechiolysis	10	6
Endometrial ablation	11	15
Septum resection	3	1
Total	238	230

In Group B, a total amount of 56 myomas have been treated, of which 18 (32.1 %) were G0 type myomas, 18 (32.1 %) G1 type, and 20 (35.8 %) G2 type.

Sixty-one (69.3 %) IBS®-treated myomas with a diameter less than 3 cm have been included in Subgroup A1 and 27 (30.7 %) IBS®-treated myomas with a diameter larger than 3 cm have been included in Subgroup A2.

Thirty-five (62.5 %) Versapoint®-treated myomas with a diameter less than 3 cm have been included in Subgroup B1, and 21 (37.5 %) Versapoint®-treated myomas with a diameter larger than 3 cmhave been included in Subgroup B2.

Myomas with a diameter larger than 5 cm, classified according to the Wamsteker classification [22, 23], have been

excluded from this study. Both groups, A and B, were similar as to patients' age, parity, and symptoms (Tables 3, 4, and 5).

Measurement methods

All patients have undergone a general or a regional anaesthesia, and a standard gynaecological set up has been adopted in the operating room. Three skilled surgeons performed all the operations.

The myoma size, type, and position were assessed by vaginal ultrasound and confirmed by diagnostic hysteroscopy.

The time of the cervical canal dilatation, resection time, and the fluid balance have been recorded. The resection time has been measured from the moment the active shaver tip or the resectoscope loop was visible inside the uterine cavity, till resection completion.

The number of second step procedures and device conversions in the two groups has also been evaluated.

Second-step procedures have been referred to those cases, in which, given the fluid deficit or the time limit of the operation, we have had to plan a second procedure, 2 months later, in order to completely remove the myoma. Limits have been referred to a 2,000 ml fluid deficit and to an hour time duration for the whole hysteroscopic procedure.

For conversions, we have considered those operations that started with the IBS® had to be completed with the Versapoint®, for two reasons. The first occurred when the myoma consistency combined with the size was preventing its fast resection with the IBS® [24], the second when, upon reaching of the fluid limit, has made it necessary to remove a

Table 2 Study population: N° of myomas per patient, total N° of myomas per group, type, and size of myomas at myomectomy in Group A (IBS®) and in Group B (Versapoint®) during a 2-year period June 2011–June 2013

N° Myomectomies: June 2011–June 2013

	Group A IBS® (n=76)	Group B Versapoint® (n=51)
N° of myomas per patient		
1	66 (86.8 %)	46 (90.2 %)
>1	10 (13.2 %)	5 (9.8 %)
N° total of myomas	88	56
Type		
G0	28/88 (31.8 %)	18/56 (32.1 %)
G1	28/88 (31.8 %)	18/56 (32.1 %)
G2	32/88 (36.4 %)	20/56 (35.8 %)
Size (mm)		
<30	61/88 (69.3 %) Group A1	35/56 (62.5 %) Group B1
>=30	27/88 (30.7 %) Group A2	21/56 (37.5 %) Group B2

Table 3 Demographic characteristics of the two groups of patients: Group A (IBS®) and Group B (Versapoint®)

	Group A IBS® (n=76)	Group B Versapoint® (n=51)	P value
Age	47.55	48.04	0.8011[a]
Premenopausal age (%)	42 (55.3)	29 (56.9)	0.9966[b]
Postmenopausal age (%)	34 (44.7)	22 (43.1)	
Symptoms			
None	38	27	0.985806[b]
Menorrhagia	18	12	
Pelvic pain	10	6	
Infertility	10	6	
Parity	0.84	0.94	0.5551[a]
Myoma size (mm)	23.12	25.18	0.3567[a]

Normally distributed variables are summarized as mean (95 % confidence interval, SD); non-normally distributed variables are given as median and interquartile range or number (%)

[a] T Student test

[b] Yates corrected chi-square test

Table 4 Group A (IBS®) demographic characteristics, type, and size of myomas, and associated hysteroscopic findings and symptoms

No. of patients	76
No. of myomas	88
Age, mean±SD (95 % CI), years	47.3±10.1 (43.7; 50.9)
Parity, no. (%)	
Nulliparous	36 (47.4)
Pluriparous	40(52.6)
Submucous myomas, no. (%)	
1	66 (86.8)
>1	10 (13.2)
Myomas' size, mm	
Principal myoma, mean±SD (95 % CI)	21.9±10.1 (18.6–25.3)
Second myoma, mean±SD (95 % CI)	23.5±11.4 (12.6–34.4)
Type of principal myomas, no. (%)	
Wamsteker classification	
G0 28 (31.8)	
G1 28 (31.8)	
G2 32 (36.4)	
Associated hysteroscopic findings, no. (%)	
None	66/76 (86.9)
Polyp	9/76 (11.8)
Synechiae	1/76 (1.3)
Symptoms, no. (%)[a]	
None	44/76 (57.9)
Menorrhagia	18/76 (23.6)
Infertility	10/76 (13.1)
Pelvic pain	10/76 (13.1)

Normally distributed variables are summarized as mean and lower and upper quartiles computed at 0.05; non-normally distributed variables are given as median and interquartile range

SD standard deviation, *CI* confidence interval 95 %

[a] Patient may have more than one symptom

Table 5 Group B (Versapoint®) demographic characteristics, type and size of myomas, and associated hysteroscopic findings and symptoms

No. of patients	51
No. of myomas	56
Age, mean±SD (95 % CI), years	48.04±11.4 (44.8–51.3)
Parity, no. (%)	
Nulliparous	23. (45.1)
Pluriparous	28 (54.9)
Sub mucous myomas, no. (%)	
1	46 (90.2 %)
>1	5 (9.8 %)
Myoma size, mm	
Principal myoma, mean±SD (95 % CI)	25.2±14.6 (21.1–29.3)
Second myoma, mean±SD (95 % CI)	20.8±12.1 (18.7–24.9)
Type of principal myoma, no. (%)	
Wamsteker classification	
G0 18 (32.1)	
G1 18 (32.1)	
G2 20 (35.8)	
Associated hysteroscopic findings, no. (%)	
None	45 (88.2)
Polyp	6 (11.8)
Synechiae	0 (0)
Symptoms, no. (%)[a]	
None	27 (52.9)
Menorrhagia	12 (23.5)
Infertility	6 (11.7)
Pelvic pain	6 (11.7)

Normally distributed variables are summarized as mean and lower and upper quartiles computed at 0.05; non-normally distributed variables are given as median and interquartile range

SD standard deviation, *CI* confidence interval 95 %

[a] Patient may have more than one symptom

small portion of a very hard myoma being left in the uterine cavity during the same procedure.

Statistical analyses

No preoperative therapy statistical analysis has been planned.
　Statistical analysis has been based on the Student's *t*test and the Yates corrected chi-square test. Differences between groups have been considered as statistically significant at $p<0.05$. IBM SPSS Statistics 19 (©IBM Corporation 2010, IBM Corporation, Route 100 Somers, NY 1058, USA) statistical software package has been used.

Ethical approval

The institutional ethical committee has approved this research, and all the patients have been provided with informed consent.

Findings

Second-step procedures

Concerning the overall number of second-step procedures (Table 6), there has been a statistically significant difference

Table 6 Comparison of second-step procedures between Group A (IBS®) and Group B (Versapoint®) during a 2-year period June 2011– June 2013

Operative II step procedures

	Group A IBS® (*n*=76)	Group B Versapoint® (*n*=51)	*P* value[a]
N° of II step procedures	7/76 (9.2 %)	15/51 (29.4 %)	0.0067

[a] Yates corrected chi-square test

Table 7 Comparison of second-step procedures and conversions in Group A (IBS®) and second-step procedures in Group B (Versapoint®) during a 2-year period June 2011–June 2013

Operative II step procedures+conversions

	Group A IBS® (*n*=76)	Group B Versapoint® (*n*=51)	*P* value [a]
Operative II step procedures+ conversions	16/76 (21.1 %)	15/51 (29.4 %)	0.6766

[a] Yates corrected chi-square test

between those recorded in the IBS® Group (Group A; 7; 9.2 %) and those recorded in the Versapoint® Group (Group B; 15; 29.4 %; *p*=0.0067).

Second-step procedures and conversions

No statistically significant difference has been shown comparing the overall number of second-step procedures and conversions altogether recorded in the IBS® Group (Group A; 16; 21.1 %) with the number of second-step procedures recorded in the Versapoint® Group (Group B; 15; 29.4 % *p*= 0.6766, Table 7).

N°, type, and size of myomas in the case of second-step procedures and conversions

Four (6.7 %) and six (10 %) patients with one IBS®-treated myoma have, respectively, undergone a second-step procedure and a conversion procedure (Group A; total 10; 16.7 %) against 13 (28.3 %) patients with one Versapoint®-treated myoma (Group B) who have undergone a second-step procedure (*p*=0.2311).

Three (18.8 %) and three (18.8 %) patients with more than one IBS®-treated myoma have respectively undergone a second step and a conversion procedure (Group A; total 6; 37.6 %) against two (40 %) patients with Versapoint®-treated myomas (Group B) who have undergone a second-step procedure (*p*=0.6694).

Two (7.1 %) and four (14.4 %) G0 type myomas have been found in the IBS®-treated Group of patients who have respectively undergone a second step and a conversion procedure (Group A; total 6; 21.5 %), against two (11.1 %) G0 type myomas found in the Versapoint®-treated Group of patients (Group B) who have undergone a second-step procedure (*p*= 0.6153).

Two (7.1 %) and one (14.3 %) G1-type myomas have been found in the IBS®-treated Group of patients who have respectively undergone a second-step and a conversion procedure (Group A; total 3; 21.4 %), against n.3 (16.7 %) G1 type myomas found in the Versapoint®-treated Group of patients (Group B), who have undergone a second-step procedure (*p*= 0.8914).

Five (15.6 %) and seven (21.9 %) G2 type myomas have been found in the IBS®-treated Group of patients who have respectively undergone a second step and a conversion procedure (Group A; total 12; 37.5 %) against 10 (50 %) G2 type myomas found in the Versapoint®-treated Group of patients (Group B) undergoing a second-step procedure (*p*=0.5491).

Three (4.9 %) and one (1.6 %) IBS®-treated myomas with a diameter less than 3 cm(Group A1; tot.4; 6.5 %) have respectively undergone a second-step and a conversion procedure against five (10.52 %) Versapoint®-treated myomas with a diameter less than 3 cm(Group B1) who have undergone a second-step procedure (*p*=0.3753; Odds ratio, 2.38).

Table 8 Comparison of N°, type, and size of myomas in second-step procedures and conversions in Group A (IBS®) and second-step procedures in Group B (Versapoint®) at myomectomy during a 2-year period June 2011–June 2013

Operative II step procedures+conversions

	Group A IBS® II Step P. (no. total=7/76)	Group A IBS® Conversions (no. total=9/76)	Tot.	Group B Versapoint II step P (no. total=15/51)	*P* value [a]
N° of myomas per patient					
1	4/60 (6.7 %)	6/60 (10 %)	10(16.7 %)	13/46 (28.3 %)	0.2311
>1	3/16 (18.8 %)	3/16(18.8 %)	6 (37.6 %)	2/5 (40 %)	0.6694
Type					
G0	2/28 (7.1 %)	4/28 (14.4 %)	6(21.5 %)	2/18 (11.1 %)	0.6153
G1	2/28 (7.1 %)	1/28 (14.3 %)	3(21.4 %)	3/18 (16.7 %)	0.8914
G2	5/32 (15.6 %)	7/32 (21.9 %)	12(37.5 %)	10/20 (50 %)	0.5491
Size (mm)					
<30	3/61 (4.9 %)	1/61 (1.6 %)	4(6,5 %)A1	5/35 (10.52 %) B1	0.3753
>/=30	4/27 (14.8 %)	8/27 (29.6 %)	12(44.4 %)A2	10/21 (43.75 %)B2	0.9418
N° total of myomas	88			56	

[a] Yates corrected chi-square test

Four (14.8 %) and eight (29.6 %) IBS®-treated myomas with a diameter larger than 3 cm, (Group A2; tot.12; 44.4 %) have respectively undergone a second-step and a conversion procedure against ten (43.75 %) Versapoint®—treated myomas with a diameter larger than 3 cm(Group B2) who have undergone a second step procedure (p=0.9418; Odds ratio, 1.14; Table 8).

Resection time, fluid balance, and dilatation time of the cervical canal regarding myomas with a diameter less than 3 cm

As to resection time, fluid used, fluid deficit, and dilatation time of the cervical canal reported during the treatment of myomas with a diameter less than 3 cm, no statistically significant difference has been reported between the IBS® Group (Group A1) and the Versapoint® Group (Group B1) (Table 9).

Resection time, fluid balance, and dilatation time of the cervical canal regarding myomas with a diameter larger than 3 cm

As to the resection time, fluid deficit, and time of dilatation of the cervical canal reported during the treatment of myomas larger than 3 cm no statistically significant difference between the IBS® (Group A2) and the Versapoint® (Group B2) groups have been reported.

For the Versapoint®-treated myomas (Group B2; mean, 5,885 ml; median; 5,100 ml; range, 1,000–17.000 ml; SD, 3,957.84 ml), we have used a statistically significantly smaller fluid volume in comparison with what used for the IBS®-treated myomas (Group A2; mean, 11.583 ml; median, 12.500 min; range, 400–20.000 ml; SD, 4,663.92 ml; p=0.0001, Table 10).

Table 9 Resection time, fluid used, fluid deficit, and cervical dilatation time comparison between Group A (IBS®) and Group B (Versapoint®) in≤3 cm myomas

Outcomes myomas <3 cm	Group A1 IBS® (n=61)	Group B1 Versapoint® (n=35)	P value[a]
Resection time (min)			
Mean (min)	21.12	21.13	0.8715
Median	15	16	
Standard deviation	14.38755	12.3146	
Range	3–60	10–45	
IC 95 %	16.35–25,28	17.12–26.04	
Fluid used (ml)			
Mean (min)	3,765	2,655	0.0998
Median	3,000	1,500	
Standard deviation	3,114.041	2,425.811	
Range	800–15,000	500–10,000	
IC 95	2,843–4,688	1,766–3,544	
Fluid deficit (ml)			
Mean (min)	342	240	0.1486
Median	300	100	
Standard deviation	327.2728	256.3914	
Range	0–1500	0–600	
IC 95	245–439	146–334	
Cervical dilatation (min)			
Mean (min)	1.59	1.60	0.9320
Median	1.5	1.5	
Standard deviation	1.09	0.93	
Range	0–5	0.5–5	
IC 95	1.26–1.91	1.26–1.94	

Normally distributed variables are summarized as mean (95 % confidence interval, SD); non-normally distributed variables are given as median and interquartile range or number (%)

[a] T Student test

Table 10 Resection time, fluid used, fluid deficit, and cervical dilatation time comparison between Group A (IBS®) and Group B (Versapoint®) in ≥3 cm myomas

Outcomes myomas >3 cm	Group A2 IBS® (n=27)	Group B2 Versapoint® (n=21)	P value[a]
Resection time (min)			
Mean (min)	47.19	42.25	0.4333
Median	45	35	
Standard deviation	23.85	17.35	
Range	15–109	25–85	
IC 95 %	38.1–56.26	34.14–50.36	
Fluid used (ml)			
Mean (min)	11,583	5,885	0.0001
Median	12,500	5,100	
Standard deviation	4,663.925	3,957.84	
Range	400–20,000	1,000–17,000	
IC 95	9,807–13,358	4,035–7,735	
Fluid deficit (ml)			
Mean (min)	907	685	0.2352
Median	800	600	
Standard deviation	740.1404	435.6181	
Range	0–1,500	100–1500	
IC 95	625–1189	481–889	
Cervical dilatation (min)			
Mean (min)	1.56	1.57	0.9674
Median	1.5	1.25	
Standard Deviation	0.90	1.08	
Range	0.5–5	0.5–5	
IC 95	1.21–1.90	1.06–1.07	

Normally distributed variables are summarized as mean (95 % confidence interval, SD); non-normally distributed variables are given as median and interquartile range or number (%)

[a] T Student test

Fig. 4 **a** G2 1,5 cm myoma. **b** Integrated Bigatti Shaver (IBS®) in action. **c** With the Integrated Bigatti Shaver (IBS®) myomas are effectively enucleated from their fovea and the myoma intramural site of insertion is removed. **d** The surrounding healthy endometrium is avoided without any thermal injury occurring

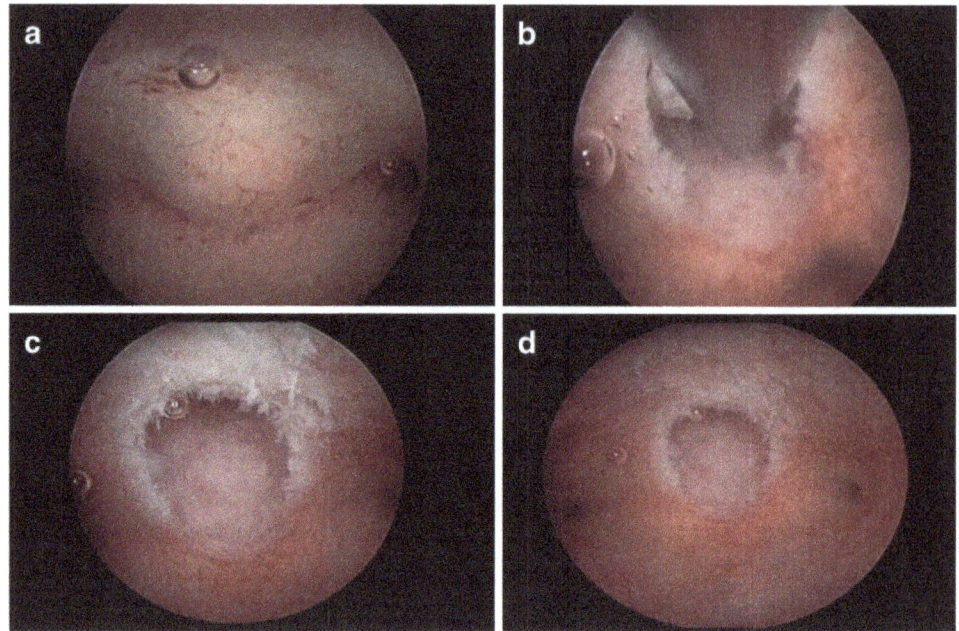

Discussion and conclusion

This study shows that myomectomy performed with the IBS® can be a very easy and precise procedure. It has several well-documented advantages especially for the treatment of myomas up to 3 cm.

First of all, any type of submucosal myoma, including G2 myomas, which had been excluded from similar studies about morcellators, has been included in this study [18]. In addition, one of the main advantages of the IBS® is that it enables the effective enucleation of myomas from their fovea and the removal of its intramural site of insertion (Fig. 4). The surrounding healthy endometrium is protected against any thermal injury; no coagulation is needed, and there are no excessive bleeding problems.

It is worth highlighting that complications like major bleeding, fluid overload, but even more significant postoperative adhesions formation have been reported during myomectomies with the conventional bipolar resectoscope.

Deans and Abbott have reported 31.3 % and 45.5 % adhesions formation after the removal of respectively single and multiple myomas [25].

The continuous cutting capacity always performed under direct visual control together with the immediate removal of the tissue chips at the same time as resection result in a more efficient and safer reduction of the tumor's volume. No bleeding or major complication has been observed in the IBS® group procedures.

Our results show that there is no statistically significative difference in terms of cervical dilatation, resection time, and fluid deficit between the IBS®- and the Versapoint®-treated myomas.

Even if myomas with a less than 3 cm diameter are slightly more represented in the IBS® group compared to the Versapoint® group (69.3 % vs. 62.5 %), this difference is not shown to be significatively in favor of the former group of patients.

However, the data shown in the present study are very promising because they confirm the IBS® ability to treat 93.5 % of myomas with a diameter less than 3 cm and 62.5 % of myomas G2 type ®, in a single procedure without the resectoscope.

With the IBS®, we have reported an overall number of significantly less second step procedures compared to those reported in the Versapoint® Group.

These data are not confirmed when comparing the overall number of second-step procedures and conversions of the IBS ® altogether, with the second-step procedures of the Versapoint®.

On the other hand, a statistically significantly bigger volume of fluid has been used in the IBS® Group, even though the fluid deficit has been the same in both groups.

This is probably due to the double aspiration enabled by the IBS®. One aspiration stopcock is placed in the optical channel while the second aspiration is placed at the back of the drill cut handler and is activated during the resection. With the IBS®, we have used more fluid, but we have also recovered a larger amount of it.

As discussed by Emanuel et al., the diameter of an intra-uterine pathology is strongly related to the operation time and to the complication rate [26]. Considering the tissue volume to be removed according to the $4/34/3\pi r^3$ formula, the conventional monopolar loop-based resection of Ø 2, 3, and 4 cm-sized myomas has respectively taken 8.4, 28.2, and 67.0 min, at a resection speed of 0.5 cm^3/min.

Also in our study, we have reported a 50 % need of second-step procedures in the Versapoint ® group due to the G2 type and to the large diameter of myomas interested by the resection.

Certainly also, the IBS® effectiveness is presently affected by the size rather than the type of myomas, but we think that the IBS® efficacy should be assessed according to the myomas consistency [24].

Regarding the approach of very large myomas some improvements are likely needed to improve our blade system in order to prevent the occurrence of possible drawbacks. Compared with other blind intrauterine applications, the IBS® allows us to perform procedures under visual control and to remove the tissue chips in an automated and straightforward way. As it has been proven in randomized controlled trials [27], the reduction of the instrument diameter improves the accessibility of ambulatory diagnostic hysteroscopy. The absence of complications during the cervical dilatation time enabled by the IBS® indicates that its small size enhances its usability. Although further modifications of the IBS® are necessary, this technique has shown so far very interesting and promising features for the future operative hysteroscopy that can be carried out in a faster and easier way, avoiding major complications.

In conclusion, the IBS® proves to be a promising innovative new instrument for the removal of myomas. This instrument is smaller, thus easier to use than the conventional resectoscope. The fact that surgery is not interrupted by tissue chips removal will likely shorten the total operating time in the future. It is further postulated that electrical current-free resection of myomas could significantly reduce the postoperative adhesions formation and that the IBS® system should preferentially be used in the case of young women, during their reproductive age.

Prospective randomized comparative study should be planned to prove this advantage in the treatment of infertile patients.

Acknowledgments This paper is dedicated to my wife Daniela. Special thanks go to Karl Storz GmbH & Co employees, Storz Italia, for their technical support, and in particular, to Dr. h.c. mult. Sybill Storz and Helmut Wehrstein, who have believed in this project from its beginning. Special thanks are addressed to Prof. Ivo Brosens, Dr. Rudi Campo, Dr. Yves Van Belle, and Prof. Berndt Rudelstorfer maestro di vita.

Translation by Ettore Claudio Iannelli.

Declaration of interest The contracts with Dr. Bigatti and the mutually provided benefits concerning the development and the consultancy on the IBS® are in no way affiliated with any other service or procurement decisions on the part of the contractual parties, including studies like the present one. Therefore, Dr. Bigatti has received no financial compensation for this study.

References

1. Fernandez H, Sefrioui O, Virelizier C, Gervaise A, Gomel V, Frydman R (2001) Hysteroscopic resection of submucosal fibroids in patients with infertility. Hum Reprod 16:1489–1492

2. Valle RF, Baggish M (2007) Hysteroscopic myomectomy. In: Baggish MS, Valle RF, Guedj H (eds) Hysteroscopy. Visual perspective of uterine anatomy. Physiology and pathology diagnostic and operative hysteroscopy, 3rd edn. Lippincott Williams & Wilkins, a Wolters Kluwer Business, Philadelphia, pp 385–404

3. Di Spiezio Sardo A, Mazzon I, Bramante S, Bettocchi S, Bifulco G, Guida M, Nappi C (2008) Hysteroscopic myomectomy: a comprehensive review of surgical techniques. Hum Reprod Update 14(2):101–119

4. Hallez JP (1995) Single stage total hysteroscopic myomectomies: indications, techniques, and results. Fertil Steril 63:703–708

5. Indman PD (2006) Hysteroscopic treatment of submucous fibroids. Clin Obstet Gynecol 49:811–820

6. Somigliana E, Vercellini P, Daguati R, Pasini R, De Giorgi O, Crosignani PG (2007) Fibroids and female reproduction: a critical analysis of the evidence. Hum Reprod Update 13:465–476

7. Mencaglia L, Lugo E, Consigli S, Barbosa C (2009) Bipolar resectoscope: the future perspective of hysteroscopic surgery. Gynecol Surg 6(1):15–20

8. Oona Hamerlynck TW, Dietz V, Schoot BC (2011) Clinical implementation of the hysteroscopic morcellator for removal of intrauterine myomas and polyps. A retrospective descriptive study. Gynecol Surg 8:193–196

9. Witz CA, Silverberg KM, Burns WN, Schenken RS, Olive DL (1993) Complications associated with absorption of hysteroscopic fluid media. Fertil Steril 60(5):745–756

10. Yong Lee G, In Han J, Joo Heo H (2009) Severe hypocalcemia caused by absorption of sorbitol–mannitol during hysteroscopy. J Korean Med 24:532–534

11. Shaafer M, Von Ungern-Sternberg BS, Wight E, Schneider MC (2005) Isotonic fluid absorption during hysteroscopy resulting in severe hyperchloremic acidosis. Anesthesiology 103:203–204

12. Van Kruchten PM, Vermelis JM, Herold I, Van Zundert AA (2010) Hypotonic and isotonic fluid overload as a complication of hysteroscopic procedures: two case reports. Minerva Anestesiol 76(5):373–377

13. Odell R (1993) Electro surgery. In: Sutton CJG, Diamond MP (eds) Endoscopic surgery for gynaecology. WB Saunders, London, pp 51–59

14. Sutton CJG, Mc Donald R (1993) Endometrial resection. In: Lewis BV, Magos AL (eds) Endometrial ablation. Churchill Livingstone, Edinburgh, pp 131–140

15. Pasini A, Belloni C (2001) Intraoperative complications of 697 consecutive operative hysteroscopies. Minerva Ginecol 53(1):13–20

16. Jansen FW, Vredevoogd CB, Van Ulzen K, Hermans J, Trimbos JB, Trimbos-Kemper TC (2000) Complication of hysteroscopy: a prospective, multicenter study. Obstet Gynecol 96(2):266–270

17. Emanuel MH, Wamsteker K (2005) The intrauterine morcellator: a new hysteroscopic operating technique to remove intrauterine polyps and myomas. J Minim Invasive Gynecol 12(1):65–66

18. Van Dongen H et al (2008) Hysteroscopic morcellator for removal of intrauterine polyps and myomas: a randomized controlled pilot study among residents in training. J Minim Invasive Gynecol 15:466–471

19. Bigatti G (2011) IBS® Integrated Bigatti Shaver, an alternative approach to operative hysteroscopy. Gynecol Surg 8(2):187–191

20. Bigatti G, Ferrario C, Rosales M, Baglioni A, Bianchi S (2012) IBS® Integrated Bigatti Shaver versus conventional bipolar resectoscope: a randomised comparative study. Gynecol Surg 9(1):63–72

21. Instruction for Use Versapoint. Official Notification (2001) Gynecare a division of Ethicon. www.ethicon.com.

22. Wamsteker K, Emanuel MH, de Kruif JH (1993) Transcervical hysteroscopic resection of submucous fibroids for abnormal uterine bleeding: result regarding the degree of intramural extension. Obstet Gynecol 82:736–740

23. Salim R, Lee C, Davies A, Jolaoso B, Ofuasia E, Jurkovic D (2005) A comparative study of three-dimensional saline infusion

sonohysterography and diagnostic hysteroscopy for the classification of submucous fibroids. Hum Reprod 20:253–257

24. Bigatti G, Ferrario C, Rosales M, Baglioni A, Bianchi S (2012) A 4-cm G2 cervical submucosal myoma removed with the IBS® Integrated Bigatti Shaver. Gynecol Surg 9: 453–456

25. Deans R, Abbott J (2010) Review of intrauterine adhesions. J Minim Invasive Gynecol 17(5):555–569

26. Emanuel MH, Hart A, Wamsteker K, Lammes F (1997) An analysis of fluid loss during trans cervical resection of submucous myomas. Fertil Steril 68(5):881–886

27. Campo R, Molinas CR, Rombauts L, Mestdagh G, Lauwers M, Braekmans P, Brosens I, Van Belle Y, Gordts S (2005) Prospective multicentre randomized controlled trial to evaluate factors influencing the success rate of office diagnostic hysteroscopy. Hum Reprod 20(1): 258–263

11

Transvaginal endoscopy and small ovarian endometriomas: unravelling the missing link?

S. Gordts · P. Puttemans · Sy. Gordts · M. Valkenburg · I. Brosens · R. Campo

Abstract The incidence of endometriosis in the infertile female is estimated to be between 20 and 50 %. Although the causal relationship between endometriosis and infertility has not been proven, it is generally accepted that the disease impairs reproductive outcome. Indirect imaging techniques and transvaginal laparoscopy now offer the possibility of an early stage diagnosis. Although it remains debated whether the disease is progressive, treatment in an early stage is recommendable as it carries less risk for ovarian damage, hence premature ovarian failure. Under water, inspection with the technique of transvaginal hydrolaparoscopy (THL) accurately shows the invagination of the ovarian cortex as minimal superficial lesions but with the presence of well-differentiated endometrial like tissue at the base, the lateral walls and especially the inner edges of the small endometrioma. An inflammatory environment is responsible for the formation of connecting adhesions with the broad ligament and lateral wall with invasion of endometrial-like tissue and formation of adenomyotic lesions. In around 50 % of the small endometriomas, adhesiolysis is necessary at the site of invagination with opening of the cyst, to free the chocolate content and hereby recognize the underlying endometrioma. The detailed inspection of these early-stage endometriotic lesions at THL reunites the hypothesis of Sampson with the observation of Hughesdon.

Keywords Endoscopy · Transvaginal hydrolaparoscopy · Ovarian endometriosis · Endometrioma · Hydroflotation · Pathogenesis · Surgery

S. Gordts (✉) · P. Puttemans · S. Gordts · M. Valkenburg · I. Brosens · R. Campo
Leuven Institute for Fertility and Embryology (L.I.F.E.),
Tiensevest 168, 3000 Leuven, Belgium
e-mail: Stephan.gordts@lifeleuven.be

Introduction

With an estimated incidence of 2–22 % in the general population, the incidence of endometriosis, diagnosed at laparoscopy in the infertile female, is reported to range between 20 and 50 % [1]. Based on epidemiological data, it is generally accepted that endometriotic implants are related to an impaired reproductive outcome, although the causal relationship between endometriosis (i.e. the implants without adhesions) and infertility has not clearly been proven so far. Treatment of these lesions remains debatable as long as there is no proven causal relationship.

Several hypotheses have been formulated regarding the pathogenesis of endometriosis, the hypothesis of menstrual regurgitation and subsequent angiogenesis and implantation being the most widely accepted [2]. Regurgitated endometrial cells may implant on the ovarian surface, causing local bleeding and adhesions. Hughesdon [3] investigated a series of ovaries with the endometrioma in situ and demonstrated the invaginated cortex with fibrosis and adhesion formation. In contrast with other benign ovarian cysts, the ovarian endometrioma is formed as a pseudocyst. In situ ovarian cystoscopy and selected biopsies by Brosens et al. [4] confirmed these findings. As such the basis and wall of this cyst is formed by inverted ovarian cortex, harbouring primordial and primary follicles. Strictly speaking, this also means the ovarian endometrioma is in fact an extra-ovarian pathology. However, with the aging of the endometrioma, the invaginated cortex gradually thickens by smooth muscle metaplasia and fibrosis and its appearance at cystoscopy changes from pearl-white to yellow-white and finally black and fibrotic [5].

Other theories are the formation of endometriomas by metaplasia of invaginated coelomic epithelium [6] questioning the necessity of the presence of adhesions with the broad ligament as suggested by Hughesdon [3]. In a recent paper, Vercellini et al. [7] conclude that bleeding from a corpus luteum appears to be a critical event in the development of endometriomas and suggest that a possible alternative source of entrapped blood is a cystic corpus luteum developing along an ovarian cortex adherent to the pelvic sidewall. The patients studied in this paper all have been operated previously for endometriosis and were then followed by ultrasound for a period of 2 years. However, Ferrari et al. [8] recently described an ovarian endometriotic cyst in a 26-year-old girl with pre-pubertal hypopituitarism who never ovulated in her life and was treated with hormone replacement therapy.

Follicular growth can start from the basis of the invaginated ovarian cortex and co-exist with the endometriotic cyst. Communicating luteal cysts have been observed by Sampson [9] in 9 % of his cases.

Diagnosis

Transvaginal sonography (TvS) is widely considered as a useful method for early detection of the ovarian endometrioma and seems a reliable technique to exclude significant ovarian endometriosis in infertile patients. However, a recent critical review on the accuracy of ultrasound in the diagnosis of endometriosis found that the available prospective studies all included endometriomas with a diameter of at least 14 mm [10]. So its accuracy in the diagnosis of endometriomas of less than14 mm is not known. In our consecutive series of 169 patients where endometriosis was diagnosed at transvaginal hydrolaparoscopy (THL), preoperative TVU only detected 45 % out of 11 endometriomas smaller than 15 mm (unpublished data).

At laparoscopy, subtle lesions and superficial adhesions are frequently missed as they are masked due to the high abdominal pressure of the CO_2 pneumoperitoneum. The use of hydroflotation [11] prevents the collapse of filmy adhesions and allows the visualization of both subtle lesions and their neovascularization.

Transvaginal hydrolaparoscopy

THL has been described as a more sensitive technique than standard laparoscopy to detect subtle ovarian lesions [12]. The advantages of transvaginal endoscopy are numerous.

First, as distension medium, a pre-warmed Ringer lactate or Hartmann solution is used keeping the organs afloat and enabling visualization of early endometriotic lesions of the peritoneum and ovary such as free-floating adhesions and neoangiogenesis [12]. Secondly, as the visual axis is along the longitudinal tubo-ovarian axis, no extra manipulation is needed for a close inspection of the ovarian fossa avoiding disruption of the adhesions and rupture of the endometrioma by manipulating the ovary [13]. Thirdly, the watery distension

medium enables a clear and highly contrasting visualization of the different planes of cleavage with their vascularisation, allowing a careful dissection and coagulation. Lastly, using 5 Fr instruments and the procedure being performed under water, there is a diminished risk of postoperative adhesion formation. All the procedures are performed in an outpatient hospital setting with patients returning home the same day. In the absence of a panoramic view, there is no place for major operative procedures.

The operative procedure for endometriomata at the time of THL can be performed as described by Gordts et al. [14]. If not detected at ultrasound, the diameter of the endometriotic cyst is estimated during the surgical procedure by comparison to the diameter of the biopsy forceps. Targeted biopsies of endometriomas during hydroflotation are obtained as previously described [14].

The characteristic features, which are identified by the hydroflotation technique, include the retraction and invagination of the cortex, microvascularisation, pigmentation, and free-floating adhesions and in some cases, adhesions with the fossa ovarica. After adhesiolysis and opening of the cyst at the site of invagination by micro scissors and/or a bipolar needle, the wall stays open, typically showing the same pearl-white appearance as the outer cortex, lined by a highly vascularised, polypoidal tissue [15].Targeted biopsies can confirm superficial endometriotic tissue, which usually are found at the edges and cortical tissue at the base of the cyst.

The early stages of invagination of the ovarian cortex can accurately been observed in cases of small endometriotic spots or endometriomata of 5–10 mm. What looks like an endometriotic vesicle implanted at the ovarian surface is in fact hiding an underlying invagination of the ovarian cortex covered by tiny adhesions retaining the typical brownish fluid (Fig. 1a). After the removal of the superficial adhesions and drainage of the fluid, active endometrial-like tissue and neoangiogenesis can be seen at the inside of the extraovarian pseudocyst. This also indicates that the presence of adhesions with the peritoneum of the lateral pelvic wall is not required to result in the development of a small invagination of the cortex, the ceiling of which consists of tiny adhesions. The subsequent shedding of the endometriotic implants at the inside results in the formation of the typical brownish content that is trapped inside the small endometrioma. In the more severe stages of the disease, adhesions with the pelvic sidewall can be formed (Fig. 1b). These adhesions are always connecting the site of invagination with the peritoneum of the pelvic wall (Fig. 2a). Although dealing with small lesions, by careful dissection, there is not only an invagination of the ovarian cortex with the typical lesions insight but also the peritoneal wall opposing the invagination is invaginated itself, and invaded by endometrium like tissue (Fig. 2). There seems to be a continuum between the ovarian endometrioma and the

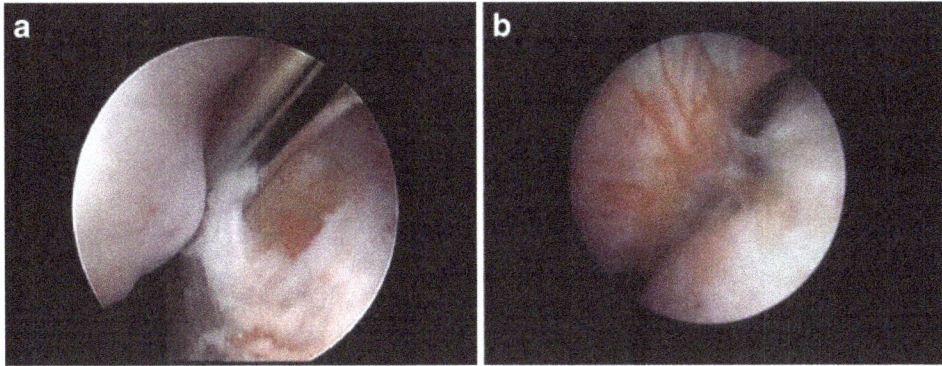

Fig. 1 A A brownish vesicle upon the ovarian surface: after removal of the superficial adhesions and leakage of the brownish fluid small endometrial-like tissue can clearly be seen at the base of this beginning invaginating cortex. **B** Beginning of adhesive process between small ovarian endometriotic lesion and pelvic wall. Remark the neoangiogenesis upon the peritoneal surface

peritoneal lesions covered by adhesions. Once the adhesions are removed, the peritoneal wall lesion can be opened, showing the same pathology as the inside of the ovarian endometrioma. This initially small invading lesion into the pelvic sidewall is probably at the origin of the adenomyotic lesion or so called "silent part" of the disease in a later stage.

Fig. 2 A Fixed adhesion between ovary and pelvic wall at the site of invagination; **B** freed ovary, clearly showing the invagination of the cortex; **C** opening of endometrioma of 1.5 cm with bipolar needle at site invagination; **D** insight view clearly showing the presence of endometrial-like tissue; **E** ablative surgery using bipolar probe; **F** after ablation with bipolar: mark the white color of the base of the cyst like the normal ovarian cortex. No presence of carbonization using the bipolar under water. The image shows clearly the invagination of the cortex

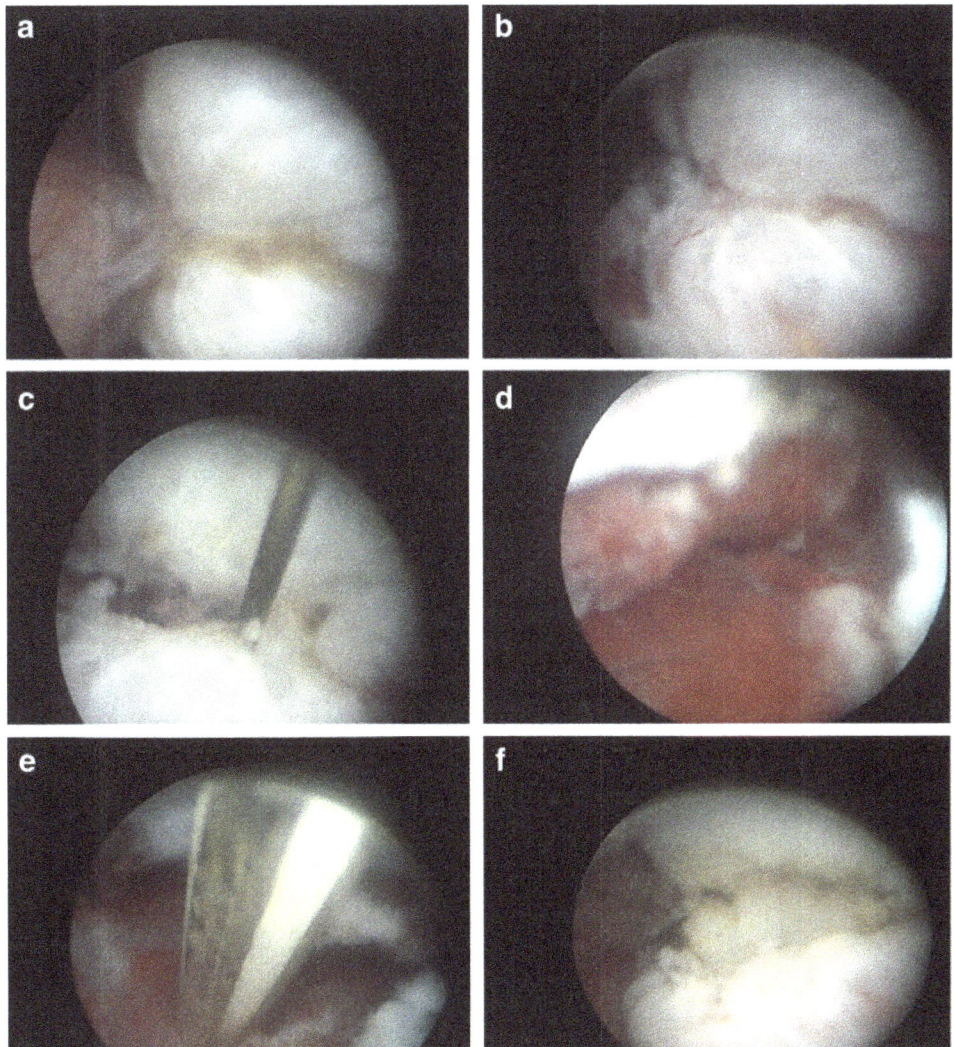

Discussion

THL is an appropriate technique for the detection and surgery of small ovarian endometriomas. Transvaginal endoscopy allows the accurate exploration of the initial stages of ovarian and peritoneal endometriosis. Small endometrioma of 5–10 mm can be formed on the ovarian surface in the absence of connecting adhesions with the pelvic wall. What initially presents as a small superficial lesion without significance, appearing like a small cicatricial line surrounding a brownish spot, can surprisingly hide a much deeper infiltration in the ovarian cortex with the typical inflammatory neovascularization and red endometrial like implants. In approximately half of the cases, active adhesiolysis with micro scissors is needed to discover these deeper invaginations. In the case of connecting adhesions with the pelvic wall, the invagination is more pronounced, with a stronger appearance of the inflammatory reaction and the neoangiogenesis.

Our observational study clearly showed that in cases of small endometriomas the wall is formed by invaginated ovarian cortex, sealed off by fusion and/or adhesions of superficial endometriotic implants at the surface, resulting in an extraovarian pseudocyst. As invagination can clearly be visualized in small ovarian endometrioma without connecting adhesions towards the peritoneum of the lateral pelvic wall, these invaginations and their chocolate content are not due to the fixed adhesion formation preventing endometriotic deposits from escaping, as suggested by Jones et al. [16]. Bleeding originates from the active endometriumal-like tissue covering the inside and mostly the inner edges of the pseudocyst, in the presence of active neoangiogenesis, offering a double target for visually directed endoscopic therapy. The inflammatory reaction originating from the endometrial implants on the ovarian surface initiates the process of small yet strong surface adhesions causing a closure of the invading endometrial tissue with invagination of the cortex. Further inflammatory reaction causes adhesions with the broad ligament originating at the site of invagination and enabling invasion of endometriotic tissue both into the ovary and into the broad ligament.

In none of the operated cases of small ovarian endometriomas, we noticed the presence of a follicular cyst or a connecting corpus luteum, the inside of which has a completely different endoscopic appearance with thick layers of vivid orange-red lutein cells. The hypothesis of Vercellini et al. [7] stating that ovarian endometrioma originates from entrapped tissue in the developing and ovulating follicle cannot be confirmed by our findings.

There is no doubt that from the small brown vesicle on the ovarian surface up to the small endometrioma with or without adhesions towards the pelvic wall, invagination of the ovarian cortex can clearly be demonstrated in each and every case. In contrast with standard laparoscopy, THL allows very detailed inspections of the ovarian endometriotic lesions and as such

provides the missing link in the pathogenesis of the ovarian endometrioma, reuniting the hypothesis of Sampson with the observations of Hughesdon.

Small endometriomas can be treated surgically during a THL procedure [15]. The present experience confirms our previous report that THL provides an atraumatic single access approach for the surgical reconstruction of small ovarian endometriomas. During THL, the whole surface of the floating ovary can be inspected in detail, with special emphasis to its posterior side and the "roof" of the ovarian fossa, without any risk that adhesions are ruptured, start bleeding and collapse before they are inspected. Endometriotic adhesions may contain endometriotic cells and require to be visualized and ablated. The classical steps of ovarian reconstruction are achieved without complex instrumental manipulation by complete adhesiolysis and mobilization of the ovary, followed by opening of the pseudocavity at the site of invagination and rinsing of the chocolate content and finally bipolar ablation of the superficial endometriotic tissue. As the entire procedure is performed under hydro flotation of the ovary, bipolar coagulation is used, minimizing the risk of postoperative adhesion formation.

Indirect imaging techniques and THL now offer the possibility of an early diagnosis of small ovarian endometriotic cysts. The clinical significance of the detection and surgical treatment of small endometriomas in patients with infertility requires further investigation. However, it can be speculated that ablation of an ovarian endometrioma, even small or medium in size, in patients with infertility is as beneficial, if not more, as ablation of minimal or mild endometriosis. The size of the endometrioma is not the only factor determining the severity of the disease. As disease and diameter progresses, the negative impact of fibrosis and smooth muscle metaplasia upon the ovarian reserve are becoming more important [17]. Although today there is growing concern of impaired ovarian function after ovarian endometrioma surgery, surgery in an early stage has the advantage of being less traumatic, and the operative procedure can be performed before the onset of intra ovarian fibrosis and smooth muscle metaplasia [18]. Operating in an early stage carries the potential advantage of a lower risk of recurrence. There is increasing evidence that the diagnosis of endometriosis, whatever its stage, is important in patients with infertility. In a retrospective study of patients with unexplained infertility Akande et al. [19] found that when these patients had minimal or mild endometriosis, which was left untreated, the time to natural conception was significantly prolonged in comparison with patients without lesions. This together with the results of the Canadian Collaborative Group study on ablation of minimal and mild endometriosis [20] supports the view that detecting and treating these lesions as early as possible is beneficial in subfertile women. An Italian study could neither reject nor confirm this observation [21]. A recent review combining the results of both trials into a meta-analysis showed that surgical treatment is more favourable than expectant management (odds ratio for pregnancy 1.7; 95 % confidence interval 1.1–2.5) [22]. As there are at present no specific markers available indicating the aggressiveness of the lesions and the risk of progressivity, treating in this early stage is recommended. More research is needed to evaluate the real risk of progressivity of these lesions.

In conclusion, the visual diagnosis of small ovarian endometrioma at THL is reliable and accurate. It enables to analyse the process of the ovarian endometriosis from his early onset up till the formation of a small endometrioma. The obtained data confirm the extraovarian localization of the endometrioma with the secondary formation of adhesions.

References

1. Moen MH (1987) Endometriosis in women at interval sterilization. Acta Obstet Gynecol Scand 66(5):451–454
2. Sampson JA (1927) Peritoneal endometriosis due to the menstrual dissemination of endometrial tissue into the peritoneal cavity. Am J Obstet Gynecol 14:422–469
3. Hughesdon PE (1957) The structure of endometrial cysts of the ovary. J Obstet Gynaecol Br Emp 44:481–487
4. Brosens IA, Puttemans PJ, Deprest J (1994) The endoscopic localization of endometrial implants in the ovarian chocolate cyst. Fertil Steril 61:1034–1038
5. Darwish AM, Amin AF, El-Feky MA (2000) Ovarioscopy, a technique to determine the nature of cystic ovarian tumors. J Am Assoc Gynecol Laparosc 7:539–544
6. Nisolle M, Donnez J (1997) Peritoneal endometriosis, ovarian endometriosis, and adenomyotic nodules of the rectovaginal septum are three different entities. Fertil Steril 68:585–596
7. Vercellini P, Somigliana E, Vigano P, Abbiati A, Barbara G, Fedele L (2009) 'Blood On The Tracks' from corpora lutea to endometriomas. BJOG 116:366–371
8. Ferrari S, Persico P, Di Puppo F, Garavaglia E, Viganò P, Candiani M (2012) An ovarian endometriotic cyst in a patient with prepubertal hypopituitarism due to a craniopharyngioma: a clue for endometrioma pathogenesis. Eur J Obstet Gynecol Reprod Biol 164(1):115–116
9. Sampson JA (1921) Perforating hemorrhagic (chocolate) cysts of the ovary. Arch Surg 3:245–323
10. Moore J, Copley S, Morris J, Lindsell D, Golding S, Kennedy S (2002) A systematic review of the accuracy of ultrasound in the diagnosis of endometriosis. Ultrasound Obstet Gynecol 20:630–634
11. Laufer MR, Goitein L, Bush M, Cramer DW, Emans SJ (1997) Prevalence of endometriosis in adolescent girls with chronic pelvic pain not responding to conventional therapy. J Pediatr Adolesc Gynecol 10:199–202
12. Brosens I, Gordts S, Campo R (2001) Transvaginal hydrolaparoscopy but not standard laparoscopy reveals subtle endometriotic adhesions of the ovary. Fertil Steril 75:1009–1012
13. Gordts S, Campo R, Rombauts L, Brosens I (1998) Transvaginal hydrolaparoscopy as an outpatient procedure for infertility investigation. Hum Reprod 13:99–103
14. Gordts S, Campo R, Brosens I, Puttemans P (2003) Endometriosis: modern surgical management to improve fertility. Baillieres Best Pract Res Clin Obstet Gynaecol 17:275–287
15. Gordts S, Campo R, Brosens I (2002) Experience with transvaginal hydrolaparoscopy for reconstructive tubo-ovarian surgery. Reprod BioMed Online 4(Suppl 3):72–75, Review
16. Jones KD, Fan A, Sutton CJ (2002) The ovarian endometrioma: why it is so poorly managed? Indicators from an anonymous survey. Hum Reprod 17:845–849
17. Fukunaga M (2000) Smooth muscle metaplasia in ovarian endometriosis. Histopathology 36:348–352
18. Brosens I, Gordts S., Puttemans P, Benagiano P (2013) Pathophysiology of the ovarian endometrioma as a basis for management. RBM online submitted
19. Akande VA, Hunt LP, Cahill DJ, Jenkins JM (2004) Differences in time to natural conception between women with unexplained infertility and infertile women with minor endometriosis. Hum Reprod 19: 96–103
20. Marcoux S, Maheux R, Bérubé S, and the Canadian Colloborative Group on Endometriosis (1997) Laparoscopic surgery in infertile women with minimal or mild endometriosis. N Engl J Med 337: 217–222
21. Parazzini F (1999) Ablation of lesions or no treatment in minimal-mild endometriosis in infertile women: a randomized trial. Hum Reprod 14:1332–1334
22. Olive DL, Pritts EA (2002) The treatment of endometriosis: a review of the evidence. Ann N Y Acad Sci 955:360–372

12

Quality assessment in surgery: where do we stand now and where should we be heading?

S. Weyers · S. Van Calenbergh · Y. Van Nieuwenhove ·
G. Mestdagh · M. Coppens · J. Bosteels

Abstract While surgery is gaining in efficiency it is equally getting more and more complex. Meanwhile patients are getting more and more demanding. In the past decades, safety and quality have become prominent criteria by which surgical care is evaluated. Several important factors can be identified which are influencing the quality of surgical care, in our view these factors can be classified into four major groups: the team of caretakers, the patient, the material, and the procedure. For all of these factors, a high level of knowledge and optimal communication is crucial to guarantee a high standard of care and minimize the chance of complications. Different quality assessment tools are currently used in surgery. Databases of surgical procedures have the potential to offer an enormous amount of information on the quality of care. However, the implementation of comprehensive databases is difficult and expensive, while its value is overshadowed by possible underreporting. Introducing surgical checklists is a cheap yet efficient way to increase both the safety and the quality of surgical care. Nevertheless, its implementation is sometimes opposed since they slow down the patient flow. The risk of complications tends to increase when a new technique is introduced. Therefore, quality assurance (QA) programs have to be implemented. Surgical simulation training is rapidly becoming a necessary adjunct to traditional patient-based training models. Finally, key performance indicators (KPI) can be used for measuring the success of medical interventions such as surgery. For the near future, the introduction of one comprehensive medical file per patient could be a major step in increasing the safety and efficiency of our medical deeds. In parallel, a nationwide prospective registry for surgical interventions should be introduced. Postgraduate surgical training should be organized by the national professional groups and should be adapted to the local needs. A system of accreditation for specific interventions should be introduced guaranteeing their state-of-the-art application.

S. Weyers (✉)
Department of Obstetrics and Gynecology,
Ghent University Hospital, Ghent, Belgium
e-mail: steven.weyers@ugent.be

S. Van Calenbergh
Department of Obstetrics and Gynecology, AZ Turnhout,
Turnhout, Belgium

Y. Van Nieuwenhove
Department of Surgery, Ghent University Hospital, Gent, Belgium

G. Mestdagh
Department of Obstetrics and Gynecology, Ziekenhuis
Oost-Limburg (ZOL), Genk, Belgium

M. Coppens
Department of Anaesthesiology, Ghent University Hospital, Gent,
Belgium

J. Bosteels
Department of Obstetrics and Gynecology, Imelda Hospital,
Bonheiden, Belgium

Keywords Quality indicators · Surgical procedures ·
Education

Background

Safety and quality have become prominent criteria by which surgical care is evaluated. Up till now, due to a tremendous variance in morbidity figures, the interpretation and comparison of surgical results is very difficult. This is mainly caused by the absence of international guidelines on complications: when talking about complications we need to talk the same language, but at the present, no universally accepted classification of surgical complications exists. On the other hand, we have to admit that differences in case mix and observation time might play an important role.

What seems so hard for us to accomplish in surgery has become common practice in private industry for more than six decades: the Japanese car builder Toyota made the pioneering effort to improve quality as early as in the 1950s [1].

In surgery, there are in fact four major determinants of the quality of care: the team of caretakers (physicians, both in hospital and in community, nurses, logistical staff, etc.), patient (including its comorbidity and pathology), material (surgical material, medication, etc.), and procedure.

We aim to address the impact of each of these four factors in the present paper. Moreover, we aim to present an overview of the quality assessment tools that are currently used in surgical practice. Where appropriate, we will try to suggest future applications.

Major determinants of the quality of care in surgery

Team of caretakers

A first prerogative for optimal care consists of a good basic training of all the caretakers involved. Such training should ideally be lifelong; surgeons as well as nurses and logistic personnel should be offered appropriate courses to optimize the patient care in a continuously changing environment. Patient care is becoming more and more demanding and stressful, and as a consequence, the risk of complications gradually increases [2].

Moreover, the principle of medical team training (MTT) has proven to be an important tool to improve surgical efficiency. This consists of a thorough (month-long) planning with all the facilities surgical teams, followed by an on-site learning session with each individual team. MTT is able to improve teamwork, to enhance safety attitudes, and to reduce errors [3]. Moreover, Neily et al. [4] managed to demonstrate that the introduction of such a training was associated with a reduction in surgical mortality rate.

Indeed, optimal communication between different caretakers is a second important factor in patient care: all relevant information on the patient's unique situation should be clearly and fully communicated not only among the treating physicians [organ specialists, surgeons, general practitioners (GPs), anesthesiologists, etc.] but also equally important between surgeons and the other caretakers (nurses, pharmacy, logistics, etc.) in the hospital and between hospital caretakers and those taking care of the patient before and after hospital discharge. The optimization of the patient's condition for surgery should start in primary care: general practitioners can play a major role by identifying potential risks of morbidity (anemia, obesity, suboptimal diabetic control, reduced renal function, etc.). Preoperative correction of even minor anemia can significantly reduce the postoperative need for transfusion (http://www. transfusionguidelines.org.uk). A unique nationwide medical file per patient, accessible by all treating caretakers, would undoubtedly improve communication and transmission of important information between caretakers.

During any intervention, the whole team involved should ensure the best possible treatment not only on the technical point of the intervention itself but also on the level of fluid management (preventing dehydration or overfilling), patient temperature (preventing hypothermia), patient positioning, etc. Surgeons have to ensure that the procedure is as minimally invasive as possible, however, not at the cost of increasing the risks for the patient. All perioperative actions (usage of surgical drains, nasogastric tubes, bladder catheters, analgesic treatment, etc.) should be questioned on their proven benefit and only be used if there is clinical evidence to support their effectiveness [5]. After surgery patients should receive the best possible rehabilitation (early and late recovery) including timely resumption of drinking and eating, addition of nutritional supplements if necessary, early mobilization if possible, adequate analgesia, early removal of drains and catheters, etc.

After discharge, a seamless and continuing care has to be pursued; therefore, all necessary information should be communicated to the patient's family, GP, and other caretakers outside the hospital. Written information on the necessary aftercare (wound care, allowed analgesia, mobilization, etc.), possible complications, and warning signs should be given; moreover, a (temporary) letter of dismissal should be accompanying the patient upon his departure.

Patients

The benefit of preoperative assessment of the surgical patient has been recognized since long and aims at reducing over-all perioperative risks [6]. It is essential to consider patient related factors, social related factors, and the duration and extent of the surgery. Routine gynecological surgery is classified as "low"-risk surgery (cardiac risk< 1 %). Major oncologic surgery is classified as "intermediate" risk (cardiac risk 1–5 %). "High"-risk procedures (cardiac risk>5 %) are aortic surgery and major vascular or peripheral vascular surgery.

Specific preoperative assessment services, performed by trained and competent assessors who can order and/or perform investigations and make referrals if necessary, are fundamental to identifying preoperative risk [7]. Patients are screened with paper or electronically based questionnaires depending on the American Society of Anesthesiologists (ASA) score. Such preoperative assessment services should include direct access to the treating anesthesiologist, surgeon, and other healthcare professionals who are competent to review the findings and agree on management strategies which are to optimize the patient's condition before surgery.

Preoperative exams ideally can be performed 2 to 3 weeks before surgery, thus giving enough time to order additional tests if necessary, while being close enough to the admission date to have up-to-date information. Thus, day-before-surgery admissions can be avoided and nearly all patients can be admitted on the day-of-surgery. Nurses specifically trained to assist in the planning of the surgical procedure can greatly facilitate this process: planning of the necessary preoperative exams, run through the different steps of the procedure indicating possible complications, referring the patient to the hospital social service if assistance upon discharge is necessary, planning of the postoperative checkup, etc.

For ambulatory surgery, the patients should be accompanied by a responsible adult for 24 h. The ambulatory patient should not drive his/her car 24 h postoperatively. There is no evidence regarding the timing of preoperative evaluation on patient outcome. Sufficient time before the planned intervention should allow additional tests (according to local resources and policy) or implementation of preoperative interventions aimed at improving patient outcome. Smoking cessation has shown to be beneficial at 4 to 8 weeks before the surgical procedure. Alcohol abstinence longer than 1 month has positive effects.

All patients should be well informed about the type of surgery and its most common complications and patients should give consent. A true informed consent is based on the knowledge of all the reasonably alternative options, the risks and benefits of each option, and the likelihood that these may occur [8]. In current practice, however, many clinicians, after a very brief oral explanation, request a patient's signature for a specific intervention, and consequently, given the patient–clinician trust relationship, the patient signs. However, since most interventions are elective, assessing the risk–benefit trade-offs is best done in a shared decision-making model. When the patient has a right of say in the decision making, the intervention is planned in true copartnership and the patient will be more understanding in the event of a complication. Of course, this process is only really valuable when there is no distinctive "best" treatment option. Nevertheless, even if there's only one surgical solution, the option of not performing the surgery can be discussed and the patient will at least have the feeling that his opinion is valued.

It is obvious that the complication rate varies according to the pathology, especially if the pathology gives rise to more invasive surgery. A surgical intervention, such as a hysterectomy for an advanced cancer, for example, is more prone to complications than a hysterectomy performed to treat benign gynecological pathology. Postoperative care should therefore be adapted not only to the type of intervention but also to the pathology: in oncological patients, the risk of thromboembolic disease, for example, is much higher and optimal thromboprophylaxis is mandatory.

Material

Surgery nowadays is getting more and more high-tech, implying the use of different energy sources, disposable devices, implantation materials, etc. For surgeons, nurses, and logistic personnel, good knowledge of the material used is essential. Especially in endoscopic surgery, whether it's robotically assisted or not, the technicality is becoming enormous, and endoscopic surgeons nowadays are expected to be genuine technical wizards.

When introducing a new technique and/or material, optimal training should be offered by the manufacturer; moreover, this training should be repeated with regular intervals, especially when new staff is involved. All material used has to be in optimal condition and should only be used for the designed purpose. A hospital or department should consider standardizing equipment as much as possible.

The hospital should have a quality control system to check the operative equipment with regular intervals and replace or repair it when necessary. Complications, such as burns, infections, or left parts of devices in the patient's body, can be due to deficient material. For all routine interventions, checklists have to be available summing up all the necessary material. Before the intervention, all material should be checked on its integrity and function by the operating nurse and should be double checked by the surgeon before use. At the end of the intervention, the surgical material and gauzes should be counted and this is noted in the operative report. The surgical specimen should be correctly labelled and sent to the pathology lab. All unrelated distractions (magazines, mobile phones, etc.) should be removed from the operating theater.

All medication used before, during, and after surgery has to be administered on instruction of the medical doctor and should be noted in the patient's file. Also patient's home medication should be carefully noted and continued if appropriate. When a potentially hazardous product is administered, the correctness of this application should be checked by two people. When the patient is discharged, clear written information has to be provided on the dose and frequency of newly started medication.

Procedure

Sometimes the same pathology can be treated through different interventions: for a woman with bleeding disorders, a hysterectomy can be performed abdominally, vaginally, or laparoscopically. Moreover, a total or subtotal hysterectomy can be chosen; a less invasive procedure, such as an endometrial ablation, can also be considered. The complication rates can vary according to the route or invasiveness of the intervention. If different procedures exist for one and the same pathology, these different options should be discussed with the patient, including differences in complication rates, recovery, recurrence, absence from work, etc.

Quality assurance and assessment tools currently used

Large (national) databases

In the USA as well as in several Nordic countries, large national databases were established to record surgical outcome. The National Surgical Quality Improvement Program (NSQIP) in the USA was established in the early nineties of the previous century to record risk-adjusted surgical morbidity, rate hospital quality, and benchmark surgical performance [9]. These databases have the potential of revealing specific high-risk groups per intervention and could have an influence on decision making. Furthermore, they could give a load of information on the origin of complications. However, such initiatives were slowed down by the changing medicolegal climate (lawsuits) and the enormous costs of data collection. Instead, administrative databases are being increasingly used; however, these are associated with significant lower reliability [10]. Clinical databases, on the other hand (made and controlled by clinicians), might underreport complications [11]; nevertheless, such databases are frequently used for benchmarking between hospitals. However, data recorded in such databases is mostly gathered by residents and trainees, and recent research has showed that outcome assessment by residents is quite unreliable [12]. Therefore self-reported quality reports are likewise largely inaccurate. Moreover, most databases do not record the comorbidity, thus making the outcome hard to compare. Finally, local and national complication registries try to gather information on the encountered complications. However, the weakness of a complication registry is the fact that it only serves when there is a complication, and at that moment, it is easily "forgotten." Postoperative complications are equally underreported, especially if these occur after the patient has been discharged.

Surgical checklists

Checklists are since long widely used in all kinds of professional sectors; in hospitals, however, they have only been introduced recently. In 2009, a study conducted by the "Safe Surgery Safes Lives" study group, using a 19-item surgical safety checklist, was published in the New England Journal of Medicine. This study showed that the use of the checklist improved safety and quality of surgery around the world (both in industrialized as in low-resource countries) [13]. The rate of death declined from 1.5 % before the checklist was introduced to 0.8 % afterwards (P=0.003). Inpatient complications occurred in 11 % of patients at baseline and fell to 7 % after introduction of the checklist (P<0.001).

An important factor is the introduction of a "surgical time out:" a moment of reflection before incision where all members of the team (nurses, surgeons, anesthesiologists, etc.) confirm that they all are aware of each other's functions and responsibilities, the patient's identity, the pathology and intervention, the surgical site, the anticipated blood loss, the necessity of antibiotics, etc. Only when all of these factors have been checked, the intervention is allowed to commence.

Process analysis

The risk of complications increases when a novel technique or approach is introduced without first evaluating the care team's comfort with the change, the team's recognition of potential problems and the team member's understanding of each of their roles. Only rarely proactive steps are taken to identify hazards and design systems to minimize the risk of complications and improves patient outcome. One such program is an initiative for proactive risk analysis by the Department of Veteran Affairs, which uses failure mode and effects analysis (FMEA). The FMEA is a proactive error prevention system designed to identify problems in systems before any adverse events occur. This methodology has been used successfully for reducing errors in medication administration, blood transfusion, and clinical laboratories [14]. However, the application of FMEA in health care delivery is limited.

Important information can be revealed by conducting in situ simulation, i.e., in the same location where actual care takes place, using the same resources and involving actual health-care team members and existing processes (a kind of "mock-procedure").

Even for processes which are already in use a thorough analysis can reveal possible limitations or hazards. Therefore, quality assurance (QA) programs are implemented to monitor and evaluate efficiency and standards of care. In an Australian study, medical students were asked to follow a patient from admission to discharge. Afterwards, these students were very well able to identify QA issues and even to propose solutions [15]. Categories of problems highlighted by these students included inappropriate patient and procedure selection, inadequate pain management, discharge, communication and resource issues. Students made a number of recommendations and they also developed new guidelines and protocols.

Surgical simulation training

Surgical simulation training (both procedural training and surgical team training) are rapidly becoming necessary adjuncts to traditional patient-based training models. Such training provides a safe and ethical acceptable way to acquire the necessary surgical skills before entering an operative theater. Skills acquired through such simulation training seem to be very well transferable to the operative setting. [16]. A systematic review by Cook et al. [17] in the JAMA of 2011 showed that, for health professions education, technology-enhanced simulation training (both computer-assisted and not), in comparison with no intervention, is consistently associated with large effects for the outcomes of knowledge, time skills, process skills, and behaviors.

Key performance indicators

Key performance indicators (KPI) are quantifiable measurements, agreed to beforehand, that reflect the critical success factors of an organization. They can also be used for measuring the success of medical interventions such as surgery. The readmission rate, for example, can be used as a KPI to measure the complication rate of a certain department or even a specific type of intervention. KPIs can also be used to benchmark between different institutions.

In France, every surgeon is expected to register every serious adverse event in a national registry. Analysis of this data showed that very different dynamics occurred, which justifies systematic analysis of different serious events by their nature or context of occurrence. (http://www.drees.sante.gouv.fr).

Future perspectives

Create one comprehensive medical file per patient
and promote the use of it

During the course of his life, each patient will be treated by more than a dozen of physicians on average. In general, each of these physicians will keep his own medical file, and most of these medical files will lack important information on the patient's history. It seems obvious that, as each patient nowadays has an electronic identity (e-ID), the creation of an electronic medical file (e-MF) would have a beneficial effect on the communication between physicians and eventually on the safety of our medical actions. Clinicians would have to access the patient's medical file upon each contact (ambulatory or hospitalization) and fill-in the reasons for encounter, the probable diagnosis and prescribed therapy. This way late onset postoperative complications will not be missed.

Organize nationwide prospective registration of all surgical
interventions

The weakness of a complication registry lies in the fact that it only has to be accessed when a complication occurs, and at that moment, it is easily "forgotten." Therefore, all surgical interventions should be entered into a prospective national registry. A surgical episode should start at the moment that the surgery is planned and should only be closed after a fixed postoperative period (e.g., 6 weeks for a cholecystectomy, 12 weeks after an extra-uterine pregnancy, etc.).

Offer postgraduate training for surgeons

In 2004, the Flemish Society of Obstetrics and Gynecology (VVOG) performed an inquiry into the needs for postoperative training among Flemish gynecologists. From this inquiry,

it became clear that more than 80 % of respondents desired specific endoscopic workshops adapted to their needs. Since then, the Special Interest Group on Gynecological Endoscopy started organizing laparoscopic workshops according to a three level system:

- A first level includes stereotactic exercises and suturing/knotting exercises (dry-lab) plus a simple exercise on tissue handling on a rabbit model.
- A second level includes more suturing and knotting exercises (different types, equally dry-lab), several presentations on the theory plus the practical implementation (video demonstrations) of some more advanced laparoscopic interventions (hysterectomy, myomectomy, and deep infiltrating endometriosis) plus a full-day hands-on training in a pig's lab.
- A third level aims at training the technique of laparoscopic hysterectomy and the dissection of the pelvic sidewall on female Thiel-embalmed corpses [18, 19].

Participants are only allowed to enter a higher level after accomplishing the level below.

Introduce an accreditation system for surgeons for specific
interventions

This is a natural consequence of all of the above: better-trained surgeons will yield less complications and will lead to a cost reduction of our health system. Nowadays, every surgeon is allowed to start using a new technique whenever he/she feels up to it. Up to now, a new surgical technique is largely mastered through apprenticeship and self-study (results from a survey by the Flemish Society of Obstetrics and Gynecology in 2010). However, the introduction of the European Working Time Directive and the pressure to increase surgical productivity have reduced the possibility to learn surgical skills in the operating theater [20]. Moreover, surgery is becoming more and more complex, and a basic specialist training is by far not sufficient to master all interventions. Moreover, basis surgical skills (stereotaxis, knotting skills, etc.) should ideally be acquired before entering the operating theater and performing surgery on patients. Since many years in the UK, there has been an ongoing debate about surgical competence. The majority view is that surgical competence should be based on clinical judgement, operative skills, and cognitive ability. The assessment of technical ability should be based on standardized checklists. Also, the call for competence checks during the professional career of surgeons (e.g., every 5 years) becomes louder [20, 21].

An accreditation system for at least some interventions seems necessary. To get accreditation, surgeons should follow a specific training to make sure that they have the necessary material and perform a minimal number of interventions.

Accredited surgeons will eventually have less complications; moreover, the unnecessary application of some procedures will decrease. The European Society of Gynecological Endoscopy (ESGE), together with the European Academy of Gynecological Surgery, has recently initiated such an accreditation system. This so-called Gynecological Endoscopic Surgical Education and Assessment (GESEA) program is made up of three levels and aims at giving gynecologists a comprehensive endoscopic training based on five pillars of competence: e-learning and self-assessment, training of specific endoscopic skills on pelvic trainers, surgical knowledge assessment (by means of multiple choice tests), surgical practice curriculum (document endoscopic interventions), and continuing medical education (attendance at congresses and workshops; http://www.esge.org/education/guidelines).

Conclusions

Several important factors can be identified which are influencing the quality of surgical care. These factors can be classified into four major groups: the team of caretakers, the patient, the material, and the procedure. For all of these factors, a high level of knowledge and optimal communication is crucial to guarantee a high standard of care and minimize the chance of complications.

Databases of surgical procedures have the potential to offer an enormous amount of information on the quality of care. However, the implementation of comprehensive databases is difficult and expensive, while its value is overshadowed by possible underreporting.

Introducing surgical checklists is a cheap yet efficient way to increase both the safety and the quality of surgical care not only on a local level but also worldwide. Nevertheless, its implementation is sometimes opposed since they slow down the patient flow. However, this so called surgical time-out is in fact its most important mode of action.

The risk of complications tends to increase when a new technique is introduced. But even for processes which are already in use, a thorough analysis can reveal possible limitations or hazards. Therefore, quality assurance programs have to be implemented. Also surgical simulation training is rapidly becoming a necessary adjunct to traditional patient-based training models. Finally, key performance indicators can be used for measuring the success of medical interventions such as surgery.

For the near future, the introduction of one comprehensive medical file per patient could be a major step in optimizing the communication between caretakers and increasing the safety and efficiency of our medical deeds. In parallel, a nationwide prospective registry for surgical interventions should be introduced. The physician's fee could be made partially dependent on the use of the above tools.

As compared to a few decades ago, new surgical techniques are far more rapidly introduced and adopted by surgeons. Therefore, a newly trained specialist can never master all interventions of its discipline, and postgraduate training is becoming more and more important. Such postgraduate training can very well be organized by the national professional groups and should be adapted to the local needs. A system of accreditation for specific interventions should be introduced guaranteeing their state-of-the-art application. In the hands of well-trained surgeons, these specific interventions will generate less complications and will be restrained to its correct applications.

Author's roles All the authors were involved in drafting and revision of article and final approval of submitted manuscript.

Funding No external funding was sought for this study.

References

1. Dindo D, Clavien PA (2010) Quality assessment in surgery: mission impossible? Patient Saf Surg 4:18
2. Arora S, Sevdalis N, Nestel D, Woloshynowych M, Darzi A, Kneebone R (2010) The impact of stress on surgical performance: a systematic review of the literature. Surgery 147:318–330
3. Wolf FA, Way LW, Stewart L (2010) The efficacy of medical team training: improved team performance and decreased operating room delays: a detailed analysis of 4863 cases. Ann Surg 252:477–485
4. Neily J, Mills PD, Young-Xu Y et al (2010) Association between implementation of a medical team training program and surgical mortality. JAMA 304:1693–1700
5. De Hert S, Imberger G, Carlisle J et al (2011) Preoperative evaluation of the adult patient undergoing non-cardiac surgery: guidelines from the European Society of Anaesthesiology. Eur J Anaesthesiol 28:684–722
6. Smith TB, Stonell C, Pukayastha S et al (2009) Cardiopulmonary exercise testing as a risk assessment method in non cardiopulmonary surgery: a systematic review. Anaesthesia 64:883–893
7. Murthy BV (2006) Improving the patient's journey. The role of the preoperative assessment team. R Coll Anaesthesist Bull 37:1885–1887
8. Weinstein JN, Clay K, Morgan TS (2007) Informed patient choice: patient-centred valuing of surgical risks and benefits. Health Aff 26:726–730
9. Rowell KS, Turrentine FE, Hutter MM, Khuri SF, Henderson WG (2007) Use of national surgical quality improvement program data as a catalyst for quality improvement. J Am Coll Surg 204:1293–1300
10. Best WR, Khuri SF, Phelan M et al (2002) Identifying patient preoperative risk factors and postoperative adverse events in administrative databases: results from the Department of Veterans Affairs national surgical quality improvement program. J Am Coll Surg 194:257–266
11. Gunarsson U, Seligsohn E, Jestin P et al (2003) Registration and validity of surgical complications in colorectal cancer surgery. Br J Surg 90:454–459
12. Dindo D, Hahnloser D, Clavien PA (2010) Quality assessment in surgery—riding a lame horse. Ann Surg 251:766–771

13. Haynes AB, Weiser TG, Berry WR et al (2009) A surgical safety checklist to reduce morbidity and mortality in a global population. NEJM 360:491–499

14. Rodriguez-Paz JM, Mark LJ, Herzer KR et al (2009) A novel process for introducing a new intra-operative program: a multidisciplinary paradigm for mitigating hazards and improving patient safety. Anesth Analg 108:202–210

15. Rudkin GE, O'Driscoll MC, Limb R (1999) Can medical students contribute to quality assurance programmes in day surgery? Med Educ 33:509–514

16. Sturm LP, Windsor JH, Cosman PH et al (2008) A systematic review of skills transfer after surgical simulation training. Ann Surg 248: 166–179

17. Cook DA, Hatala R, Brydges R et al (2011) Technology-enhanced simulation for health professions education. A systematic review and meta-analysis. JAMA 306:978–988

18. Thiel W (1992) The preservation of the whole corpse with natural color. Ann Anat 174:185–195

19. Tjalma WA, Degueldre M, Van Herendael B, D'Herde K, Weyers S (2013) Postgraduate cadaver surgery: an educational course which aims at improving surgical skills. Fact Views Vis Obgyn 5:61–65

20. Moorthy K, Munz Y, Sarker SK, Darzi A (2003) Objective assessment of technical skills in surgery. BMJ 327:1032–1037

21. Cuschieri A, Francis N, Crosby J, Hanna GB (2001) What do master surgeons think of surgical competence and revalidation? Am J Surg 182:110–116

13

Oliguria after prophylactic ureteric stenting in gynaecological surgery—a report of three cases and review of the literature

Anita J. Merritt · Ilze Zommere · Richard J. Slade ·
Brett Winter-Roach

Abstract Ureteric injury is one of the most serious complications of gynaecological surgery. Use of prophylactic preoperative bilateral ureteric stents to reduce ureteric injury is established in colorectal surgery and becoming commonplace in complex gynaecological surgery. The safety of the procedure has been questioned due to reports of stent-induced complications including a rare but serious phenomenon of stent-induced transient obstructive oligo-anuria termed reflex anuria, a response to manipulation and irritation of the ureters. A retrospective case-note review of patients who had bilateral ureteric stents placed prior to gynaecological surgery at Salford Royal Hospital, UK, from 2007 to 2011 was performed to identify cases of oligo-anuria post-stenting, which were not related to hypovolaemia, nephrotoxic drugs or a radiologically evident obstruction. All patients had their stents removed immediately at the end of surgery before leaving the operating theatre. Three out of 439 patients (0.7 %), who had preoperative bilateral ureteric stents, developed post-operative oligo-anuria despite relatively normal radiological assessment. In these three cases outlined below, one self-resolved, and two required urgent re-stenting to relieve obstruction. Use of ureteric stents for major gynaecological surgery can expedite intraoperative identification of the ureters to help reduce accidental ureteric injury but can directly cause complications. These three cases have contributed to knowledge of the complications of ureteric stents during major gynaecological surgery. Awareness of reflux anuria as a possible root cause of post-operative acute renal failure is important for guiding appropriate and timely management to preserve renal function.

Keywords Ureteric stents · Catheterization · Reflex anuria · Renal failure

Background

Ureteric injury during gynaecological surgery can be associated with significant morbidity [1]. This injury rate is approximately 1 % but is particularly associated with abdominal hysterectomies and more complex surgery involving exenterative procedures [2]. Preoperative insertion of ureteral catheters/stents to aid identification of the ureters and avoid injury and/or enhance intraoperative recognition of injury and repair is becoming more common in gynaecology and other surgical disciplines.

Whether or not the use of stents actually helps prevent ureteric injury is controversial. Some studies have found that using stents reduced the injury rate [3], whereas others do not find any clear benefit [4, 5]. A large randomised controlled trial of 3,141 women who were randomised to prophylactic bilateral ureteral catheterization versus no catheters showed a similar low incidence of ureteral injury in both groups; however, severe injury was less common in women with ureteral catheterization [5].

The procedure of catheterization and stent insertion *per se* is associated with complications [6]. Urinary tract infection is common but can be reduced by perioperative antibiotics and early stent removal. Macrohaematuria, dysuria, urgency, pain and fever are particularly associated by stents left in for increased time. There are also rare reports of anuria and acute renal failure as a complication of ureteric catheterization.

During a 5-year period from 2007 to 2011, 439 patients had prophylactic ureteric stents prior to major gynaecological surgery at Salford Royal Hospital, UK. All stented patients had the stents removed immediately at the end of the surgery. Of these, three (0.7 %) developed anuria and acute renal

A. J. Merritt (✉) · I. Zommere · R. J. Slade · B. Winter-Roach
Department of Gynaecology, Salford Royal Hospitals NHS Trust,
Stott Lane, Salford M6 8HD, UK
e-mail: anita.merritt@doctors.org.uk

failure not linked to hypovolaemia or acute tubular necrosis, but of a transient obstructive nature, but with relatively normal radiological assessment. These three cases are described.

Case 1

An 82-year-old lady with obesity, hypertension ischemic heart disease and diabetes presented with post-menopausal bleeding. Investigations confirmed an endometrial carcinoma, and she underwent total abdominal hysterectomy and bilateral salpingo-oophorectomy with preoperative bilateral ureteric stenting.

There were no intraoperative complications and no difficulties during stent insertion, but directly after the stents were removed at the end of surgery, gross haematuria was noted. On day 1, post-op haematuria persisted but urine output, vital observations and biochemistry investigations were within normal limits.

On day 2, the patient complained of bilateral groin pain and had persistent haematuria, and despite intravenous fluid challenges, urine output declined to 20 ml/h, (24 h fluid balance: 3,224 ml in/490 ml out). She then developed pulmonary oedema, and investigations revealed metabolic acidosis, urea 7.9 mmol/l, and creatinine 184 µmol/l. A renal tract ultrasound scan showed only mild bilateral hydronephrosis with no site of obstruction or ureteric dilation, and the cause of the oliguria was unclear (Fig. 1b).

Day 3 was a worsening clinical picture (24 h fluid balance: 1,450 ml in/49 ml out, creatinine 339 µmol/l, urea 15.55 mmol/l), and since post-renal obstruction was considered the most likely cause of the acute renal failure, cystoscopy with bilateral ureteric stenting was performed. The stents were inserted with ease and resulted in dramatic diuresis (7 l over 24 h) and much improved renal function tests. The ureteric stents were left in situ for 10 weeks, after which they were removed without further complications.

Case 2

A premenopausal woman with a high grade ovarian malignancy was admitted for total abdominal hysterectomy with right salpingo-oophorectomy with preoperative bilateral ureteric stenting. The stents were removed at the end of surgery. On day 1, post-op urine output was within normal limits (24 h fluid balance: 3,300 ml in/2,310 ml out), and there was no evidence of haematuria. On day 2, post-op urine output decreased (24 h fluid balance: 2,550 ml in/480 ml out), and the patient complained of severe abdominal and back pain, associated with nausea and vomiting, pyrexia, and rise in creatinine to 202 µmol/l and urea to 5 mmol/l. A CT scan of the abdomen and pelvis showed mild prominence of the pelvicalyceal collecting system and proximal ureters bilaterally tapering to normal calibre in the upper third with no evidence of obstruction or extrinsic compression (Fig. 1a).

In light of the clinical and biochemical findings, and experience from case 1 (above), an obstruction of the renal tract was still suspected, and she underwent cystoscopy and bilateral ureteric stents on day 3 post-op, after which the creatinine and urea rapidly decreased to 66 µmol/l and 3.6 mmol/l, respectively, and the normal urine output returned (24 h fluid balance: 3,200 ml in/1,726 ml out). The stents remained in situ for 3 weeks, after which her renal function remained normal.

Case 3

A lady in her 70s' with endometrial cancer was admitted for laparotomy, hysterectomy and bilateral oophorectomy with

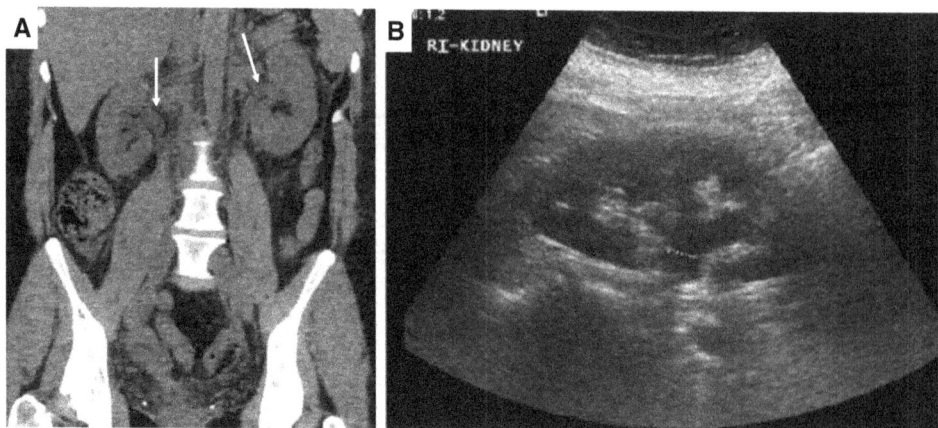

Fig. 1 **a** Computed tomography (CT) of the abdomen and pelvis—unenhanced image, from case 2 showing mild prominence of the pelvicalyceal collecting system and proximal ureters bilaterally (*arrows*), with no evidence of perinephric, peri-ureteric, intra-abdominal or pelvic collections. **b** Ultrasound scan of right kidney from case 1. The right kidney measures 11.3 cm with normal renal parenchyma and no large focal abnormality but with mild dilatation of the pelvicalyceal collecting system. The renal pelvis measures approximately 10.9 mm at the pelvo-ureteric junction (*dotted line*), consistent with mild hydronephrosis. Similar findings were observed for the left kidney (not shown)

preoperative cystoscopy and bilateral ureteric stenting. There were no intraoperative complications, and stents were inserted with ease and removed at the end of surgery. Post-operatively, she passed 1,800 ml of gross haematuria (24 h fluid balance: 2,000 ml in/1,800 ml out) but then became oliguric for 3 days (day 1 post-op 24 h fluid balance: 3,050 ml in/180 ml out, day 2: 2,200 ml in/10 ml out, day 3: 450 ml in/375 ml out), and biochemistry investigations revealed a creatinine of 537 μmol/l and a urea of 16.6 mmol/l. A renal ultrasound performed on day 3 post-op showed no evidence of obstruction and only mild hydronephrosis. Both ureters were not noted to be dilated. She passed 3,700 ml of urine on day 4 (day 4 post-op 24 h fluid balance: 1,300 ml in/3,700 ml out) and 400 ml on day 5 (day 5 post-op 24 h fluid balance: 1,450 ml in/400 ml out) but then again became oliguric for the next 2 days (day 6 post-op 24 h fluid balance: 1,400 ml in/100 ml out, day 7 post-op 24 h fluid balance: 2,500 ml in/0 ml out) (creatinine 602 μmol/l and urea 23.8 mmol/l). Fortunately, she passed 7 l of urine on day 8, and her renal failure was self-resolved without the need for dialysis or further intervention.

Discussion

We describe three case reports of patients who had bilateral ureteric stents placed prior to gynaecological cancer surgery and developed post-operative oligo-anuria with clinically obstructive renal failure despite relatively normal radiological assessment. One case was self-resolved, and two cases required urgent re-stenting to relieve obstruction and regain normal renal function.

Development of oligo-anuria has been occasionally documented as a complication of ureteral catheterization, thought to be caused by transient ureteric obstruction following stent removal [7], and has been estimated as a rate of 0–7.6 % for routine prophylactic ureteric catheterizations [8]. This transient obstructive phenomenon has been described as 'reflex anuria' defined as 'cessation of urine output from both kidneys in response to irritation or trauma to one kidney or ureter or severely painful stimuli to other organs' [9].

The mechanism for the oligo-anuria is not fully understood, but there is evidence that ureteric manipulation can result in reduced renal blood flow and glomerular filtration rate or a reflex spasm of renal arterioles [10]. Other studies suggest ureteric oedema as the cause of uretovesical junction obstruction and resulting anuria [6]. This theory would explain how re-stenting bypasses the oedema, relieves the obstruction and restores renal function. The majority of studies, however, involved colorectal surgery where ureteric stenting has a longer history and such complications are known to those surgeons. There are only two reports of reflex anuria involving

ureteric stents in gynaecological surgery. Abu-Rustum et al. reported that 2 out of 38 hysterectomy cases had a transient rise in post-operative creatinine attributed to distal ureteric oedema and one needed re-stenting to resolve the anuria [3], whereas Wood et al. reported that 7 out of 92 patients had post-operative oligo-anuria [11]. In contrast, Kuno et al. reported 0 out of 469 patients with reflux anuria post-gynaecological surgery [12].

Our case series provides further evidence for transient obstructive renal failure as a complication of ureteric catheterization in gynaecological surgery at a rate of 0.7 %. Whilst we cannot be absolutely certain of the exact aetiology of the oligo-anuria, we consider these to be cases of reflex oligo-anuria as (1) radiologically there was either no abnormality or only mild hydronepthrosis without organic obstruction of the urinary tract, (2) it was rapidly resolved by re-stenting or self-resolving causing a large diuresis, and (3) it was not associated with hypovolaemia or nephrotoxic drugs and did not respond to fluid challenges. As routine prophylactic ureteric stenting prior to gynaecological surgery becomes more widespread, it is crucial that gynaecologists are aware of the more serious complications so as to take appropriate, timely action.

To aid in identification of cases of reflux anuria, post-operative measurement of serum urea and electrolytes may be useful to help evaluate ureteric patency; however, these parameters are commonly affected by factors other than obstruction, such as intraoperative blood loss, fluid replacement and nephrotoxic drugs. It is important to first try to exclude those causes of acute renal failure by fluid challenge and cessation of nephrotoxic drugs.

One way to reduce the possibility of reflux anuria is to use staged removal of stents over a 24-h period or longer [6]. Bothwell used staged removal of stents over 24 h (i.e. removal of the right stent immediately post-operatively and the left stent 24 h later) for 92 colorectal surgery patients and reported no cases of anuria [4], whereas Chou et al. removed bilateral ureteric catheters at the end of surgery for 1,583 patients and reported no complications directly related to the catheters [5]. The timing of stent removal is likely to be an important factor in the development of reflux anuria. Leaving the stents in for longer may indeed reduce complications but may require a longer post-operative stay or readmission for stent removal may incur increased cost and inconvenience for the patient. It may be that time of stent removal should be made on an individual case or individual institution basis taking into account all the above factors.

Whether or not ureteric stents should be used routinely prior to gynaecological surgery is still under debate. Nevertheless, for surgeons using stents either routinely or on a case-by-case basis, awareness of serious complications of stenting such as the oligo-anuria described here is essential to guide appropriate, timely action and preserve renal function.

Declaration of consent All procedures followed were in accordance with the ethical standards of the responsible committee on human experimentation (institutional and national) and with the Helsinki Declaration of 1975, as revised in 2000 (5). Informed consent was obtained from all patients for being included in the study. No identifying information about the patients is included in the article.

Co-author's contributions AJM, IZ and BWR are responsible for the concept and design and execution of the study, AJM wrote the manuscript, and IZ, RJS and BWR were responsible for manuscript editing.

References

1. Carley ME, McIntire D, Carley JM, Schaffer J (2002) Incidence, risk factors and morbidity of unintended bladder or ureter injury during hysterectomy. Int Urogynecol J Pelvic Floor Dysfunct 13(1):18–21
2. Jha S, Coomarasamy A, Chan K (2004) Ureteric injury in obstetric and gynaecological surgery. Obstet Gynaecol 6:203–208
3. Abu-Rustum N, Sonoda Y, Balck D, Chi D, Barakat R (2006) Cystoscopic temporary ureteral catheterization during radical vaginal and abdominal hysterectomy. Gynecol Oncol 103:729–731
4. Bothwell W, Bleicher R, Dent T (1994) Prophylactic ureteral catheterization in colon surgery. Dis Colon Rectum 37:330–334
5. Chou M, Wang C, Lien R (2009) Prophylactic ureteral catheterization in gynaecologic surgery: a 12-year randomized trial in a community hospital. Int Urogynecol J Pelvic Floor Dysfunct 20:689–693
6. Sheik F, Khubchandani I (1990) Prophylactic ureteral catheters in colon surgery – how safe are they? Dis Colon Rectum 33:508–510
7. Levine R, Pollack H, Banner M (1982) Transient ureteral obstruction after ureteral stenting. Am J Roentgenol 138:323–327
8. Bienek J, Meade P (2012) Reflux anuria after prophylactic ureteral catheter removal: a case description and review of the literature. J Endourol 26:294–296
9. Sirota J, Narins L (1957) Acute urinary suppression after ureteral catheterization: the pathogenesis of 'reflex anuria'. N Engl J Med 257:1111–1113
10. Maletz R, Berman D, Peele K, Bernard D (1993) Reflex anuria and uremia from unilateral ureteral obstruction. Am J Kidney Dis 22:870–873
11. Wood EC, Maher P, Pelosi MA (1996) Routine use of ureteric catheters at laproscopic hysterectomy may cause unnecessary complications. J Am Assoc Gynecol Laparosc 3:393–397
12. Kuno K, Menzin A, Kauder H (1998) Prophylactic ureteral catheterization in gynecologic surgery. Urology 52:1004–1008

14

Is pre-operative risk-assessment in laparoscopic treatment of presumed low-risk endometrial cancer effective?

P. A. H. H. van der Heijden · Y. P. Geels ·
S. H. M. van den Berg-van Erp ·
L. F. A. G. Massuger · M. P. M. L. Snijders

Abstract In endometrial (pre)malignancy the pre-operative work-up is primarily based on the histopathological specimen obtained. Total laparoscopic hysterectomy with bilateral salpingo-oophorectomy (TLH + BSO) in presumed low-risk clinical stage I endometrioid endometrial carcinoma (EEC) or atypical hyperplasia (AH), is nowadays considered preferred and sufficient treatment in the Netherlands. To test the effectiveness of this pre-operative work-up, a retrospective cohort analysis was performed. Revised pre- and post-operative histopathology was compared and intra- and post-operative complications registered. In 116 consecutive patients with a pre-operative diagnosis of AH or presumed stage I, grade I or II EEC planned for TLH + BSO. In 24.1 % (28/116) revised endometrial histopathology was upgraded on the definitive hysterectomy specimen. In 3.5 % (4/116) upgrading to high-risk grade III endometrial cancer (EC) was observed. In 9.9 % (8/81) of EC cases a post-operative FIGO stage IG3, II, or III was diagnosed. The major and minor short-term complication rates of TLH + BSO were 12.1 and 7.8 %. In 13.8 % (16/116) of cases conversion to laparotomy was necessary, with a significant higher percentage of obese (68.8 %) patients in the conversion versus the successful TLH + BSO group

(42 %). Clinical relevant inconsistency between pre- and post-operative histopathology or FIGO stage was observed in 9.9 % of EC cases. More extensive pre-operative risk analysis of presumed low-risk EEC may be indicated, especially for the morbid obese, harboring a substantial risk for conversion to laparotomy and complications.

Keywords Endometrial cancer · Total laparoscopic hysterectomy · Complications · Histopathology · Pre-operative · Biopsy

P. A. H. H. van der Heijden · M. P. M. L. Snijders
Department of Obstetrics and Gynaecology, Canisius-Wilhelmina Hospital, Nijmegen, The Netherlands

Y. P. Geels · L. F. A. G. Massuger
Department of Obstetrics and Gynaecology, Radboud University Nijmegen Medical Centre, Nijmegen, The Netherlands

S. H. M. van den Berg-van Erp
Department of Pathology, Canisius-Wilhelmina Hospital, Nijmegen, The Netherlands

P. A. H. H. van der Heijden (✉)
Department of Obstetrics and Gynaecology, Maxima Medical Centre, PO Box 777, Veldhoven 5500 MB, The Netherlands
e-mail: pattyvanderheijden@gmail.com

Background

Annually, 1,900 new cases of endometrial cancer (EC) are diagnosed in the Netherlands. The incidence is increasing due to a rise in obesity and life-expectancy [1, 2]. As women with uterine cancer most often present with abnormal vaginal bleeding as an early symptom, in 75–90 % of the patients, the disease is still confined to the uterine body and classified as Fédération Internationale de Gynécologie Obstétrique (FIGO) stage I [3].

Two different risk types of EC are recognized. Type I carcinomas display well or moderately differentiated endometrioid histology and arise in relatively younger women with obesity, hyperlipidemia, and signs of hyperestrogenism. Hormonally induced atypical endometrial hyperplasia (AH) is observed as a common precursor of and already coexisting with endometrioid endometrial cancer (EEC) type I in the uterine cavity in 30–40 % of patients. Type II carcinomas include poorly differentiated endometrioid, clear cell or serous histology, and carcinosarcoma arising in an atrophic endometrial background, more often arising in non-obese, older women who demonstrate no hormonal risk factors and carry a less favorable course and prognosis [4]. According to the Dutch Guidelines, the pre-operative histopathological diagnosis is obtained using Pipelle or hysteroscopic biopsies to retrieve a representative endometrial specimen. The pre-operative work-up of presumed low-risk EEC includes routine blood testing and chest x-ray, without the use of extra radiological techniques like Magnetic Resonance Imaging (MRI). Thus, in presumed low-risk clinical stage I endometrial (pre)malignancy, i.e., AH or grade I or II EEC, hysterectomy with bilateral salpingo-oophorectomy (BSO) without lymphadenectomy is considered as sufficient surgical treatment (http://www.oncoline.nl/endometriumcarcinoom). Adjuvant radiotherapy, minimizing the risk of loco-regional recurrence, is tailored to post-operative histopathological and well-defined clinical risk factors, the so-called post-operative radiation therapy for endometrial carcinoma (PORTEC) criteria. [5].

Recently, a well-designed prospective randomized Dutch trial comparing total abdominal hysterectomy (TAH) with total laparoscopic hysterectomy (TLH + BSO) revealed superior results for the laparoscopically treated patients. However, as pointed out by Mourits et al., laparoscopic treatment may not be without harm to certain patient groups [6]. In high-risk type II endometrial cancer, a maximal surgical intervention is indicated including pelvic/para-aortic lymphadenectomy and/or omentectomy and/or peritoneal biopsies. This procedure leads to more complete surgical FIGO staging, indicating possible necessary adjuvant chemotherapy and/or radiotherapy. In the Netherlands, this procedure is centralized and performed by well-trained gynecologic oncologists (http://www.oncoline.nl/endometriumcarcinoom).

Thus, correct pre-operative assessment of low- versus high-risk EC including histopathological and clinical aspects appears crucial to individualize the surgical treatment. Pre-operative incorrect diagnosis of tumor histology, grade III, or advanced FIGO stage carries the risk of surgical undertreatment [7]. With respect to the preferred laparoscopic route in low-risk EEC, pre-operative risk analysis of co-morbidity resulting in a potential higher chance for complications may also be of importance.

The purpose of this retrospective analysis on a consecutive series of pre-operatively presumed low-risk AH or EEC patients planned for TLH + BSO is, first, to analyze the level of consistency between pre- and post-operative data on histopathology and presumed FIGO stage I and second, to analyze the operative results of TLH + BSO procedure in terms of short-term major and minor complications.

Methods

A retrospective analysis was conducted on all consecutive patients ($n = 116$), pre-operatively diagnosed with AH or grade I or II clinical FIGO stage I EEC, scheduled for TLH + BSO

between January 2006 and November 2012 at the Canisius-Wilhelmina Hospital, Nijmegen. Patients with pre-operative high-risk EC, i.e., grade III EEC or non-endometrioid type were not included. Clinical data on age, parity, menopausal status, co-morbidity, body mass index (BMI in kilogram per cubic meter), with a BMI of >30 categorized as obese according to World Health Organization criteria, presenting symptoms at time of diagnosis and post-operative FIGO stage of disease were registered from the medical charts (http://www.who.int/gho/ncd/risk_factors/bmi_text/en/).

Pre-operative histopathological diagnosis of AH or grade I or II EEC was based on endometrial biopsy, performed with Pipelle and/or diagnostic hysteroscopy in all patients, according to the national guidelines in the diagnostic work-up of postmenopausal or irregular bleeding (http://nvog-documenten.nl/index.php?pagina=/richtlijn/pagina.php&fSelectTG_62=75&fSelectedSub=62&fSelectedParent=75).

Histopathological review

All histopathological slides of the pre- and post-operative specimens were retrieved from the archive and revised by a gynecopathologist (SvB) and an experienced Ph.D. researcher (YG), unaware of original pathology report and clinical outcome of patients. Review of pre- and post-operative specimens included systematic determination of the endometrium: benign, hyperplasia, or carcinoma, and in case of carcinoma, histological type and tumor grade. When in the initial report only "low-grade" EEC was described, grade II EEC was classified. Review of post-operative specimens included determination of the endometrium as well, and in case of malignancy: histological type, tumor grade, depth of myometrial invasion (>50 or <50 %), lympho-vascular space invasion, and cervical, tubal, or ovarian metastatic growth. In case of discrepancy between the reviewers, consensus was reached reviewing the slides together.

Surgery

The TLH + BSO surgical procedure consisted of laparoscopic hysterectomy with bilateral salpingo-oophorectomy without pelvic and/or para-aortic lymphadenectomy as described by Mourits et al. [6] All data on operative time, estimated blood loss (milliliter), conversion to laparotomy and intra- and post-operative complications were retrieved from the Dutch standardized operation and complication registration documents used (http://www.nvog.nl/vakinformatie/Pati%C3%ABntveiligheid/Complicatieregistratie/Complicatieregistratie+en+bespreking.aspx).

Statistical analysis

Comparisons were made between reviewed pre-operative and post-operative histopathological results. Patient characteristics for the successful laparoscopic group were compared with the patient characteristics of the group who underwent conversion to laparotomy using Pearson's chi-Square (χ^2) test and Fisher's exact test. Occurrence of major and minor complications was compared for the laparoscopic and the conversion group using Fisher's exact test. All statistical analyses were performed using SPSS 19. The P values presented are two-sided and $P < 0.05$ was considered statistically significant.

Ethical approval board

All patient characteristics remained unidentifiable receiving the standard treatment according to the Dutch Guidelines (http://www.oncoline.nl/endometriumcarcinoom), (http://nvog-documenten.nl/index.php?pagina=/richtlijn/pagina.php&fSelectTG_62=75&fSelectedSub=62&fSelectedParent=75). Therefore, approval from the Ethical Approval Board was not necessary.

Findings

Patient characteristics

Patient characteristics are shown in Table 1. Age ranged from 41 to 89 years (median, 62 years). In 53/116 (45.7 %) patients, a BMI of more than 30 was noted.

Histopathology

Table 2 summarizes the differences between the original histopathology and revised histopathology for both pre- and post-operative specimens. Post-operatively, in total, 83 patients were diagnosed with a malignancy, including two patients diagnosed with ovarian malignancy: one with extra/ovarian serous carcinoma showing normal endometrium with serous tumor cells coexisting inside the uterus, and one with an adult granulosa cell tumor of the ovary showing normal endometrium without AH. Of the 81 patients with EC, 79 patients after review were diagnosed with EEC, 1 with grade III mixed clear cell/endometrioid carcinoma, and 1 with grade III mixed serous/endometrioid carcinoma. Twenty-six patients were diagnosed with AH and seven revealed no malignancy nor AH in the hysterectomy specimen.

Post-operative diagnosis was upgraded from AH to EEC and from grades I or II to III in 28/116 (24.1 %) patients. In 4/116 (3.5 %) patients, there was an upgrading to grade III, with

Table 1 Patient characteristics in 116 consecutive patients planned for TLH + BSO

	$N = 116$
Age (years)	
Mean (SD)	61.8 (8.5)
Parity	
Nulliparous (%)	10 (8.6)
Multiparous (%)	106 (91.4)
Median	2
Range	0–6
Missing data	1
Menopausal status	
Premenopausal (%)	8 (6.9)
Climacteric (%)	4 (3.5)
Postmenopausal (%)	105 (90.5)
Co-morbidity factors	
Obesity (BMI>30) (%)	53 (45.7)
BMI mean (SD)	30.0 (6.35)
Diabetes (%)	18 (15.5)
Previous abdominal surgery (%)	37 (31.9)

SD standard deviation, *BMI* body mass index

1 patient being upgraded because of mixed clear cell and 1 patient because of mixed serous histology.

In case of EEC, deep myometrial invasion (extending to outer half of the myometrium, i.e. >50 %) was observed post-operatively in 26/81 (32.1 %) of the patients. In 76/81 (93.8 %) patients, FIGO stage I was diagnosed (54 FIGO stage IA and 22 FIGO stage IB); in 5/81 patients (6.2 %) FIGO stage II or III and in two patients, an ovarian malignancy was diagnosed. All patients were adjuvantly treated according to the PORTEC criteria, i.e., when two of three risk factors were present, patients underwent post-operative radiotherapy [5, 8].

Clinical relevant inconsistencies

Table 3 shows the patient data on clinical relevant post-operative upgrading and/or upstaging occurring in 8/81 (9.9 %) of patients with malignant histopathology (4 because of post-operative upgrading to grade III; 5 because of upstaging to > stage I).

Conversion to laparotomy

In total, 100/116 patients (86.2 %) underwent a successful TLH + BSO, in 16/116 patients (13.8 %) intra-operative conversion to laparotomy was necessary. The reasons not to proceed with laparoscopic surgery mentioned in the operation report were too many adhesions in five patients, too large size of the uterus in three patients to remove the uterus vaginally,

Table 2 Pre-operative versus reviewed post-operative endometrial histopathology and FIGO staging

Histology and grade (%)	Pre-operative $N=116$	Revision	Post-operative	Revision $N=116$
Atrophy/dp	0	2	6	3 (2.6)
Hyperplasia	0	0	5	4 (3.5)
AH	45 (38.8)	36	24	26 (22.4)
EEC G1	41 (35.4)	51	48	55 (47.4)
G2	30 (25.7)	27	28	22 (19.0)
G3	0	0	1	2 (1.7)
Clear cell G3	0	0	1	1 (0.9)
Mixed G3	0	0	1	1 (0.9)
*	0	0	1	1 (0.9)
#	0	0	1	1 (0.9)
Myometrial invasion if endometrial carcinoma present				$N=81$
No invasion				19 (23.5)
$<\frac{1}{2}$				36 (44.4)
$>\frac{1}{2}$				26 (32.1)
FIGO stage after revision of endometrial hysterectomy specimens				$N=81$
IA				**54**
G1				43
G2				9
G3				2
IB				**22**
G1				15
G2				6
G3				1
II				**2**
G1				2
III				**3**
A G1				1
A G2				1
C2G3				1

Dp disordered proliferative, # adult granulosa cell tumor of the ovary, * extra ovarian serous carcinoma

technical in two patients (i.e., strategically in 10/16 patients) besides intra-operative bleeding in three patients, bladder lesion in one patient and anesthesiological problems in two patients (i.e., intra-operative complications in 6/16 patients).

Complications

Fourteen major complications were observed in nine patients (Table 4). The major and minor short-term complication rates of TLH + BSO were 12.1 and 7.8 %, respectively. Nine major complications occurred in five patients who underwent a successful TLH + BSO procedure versus five major complications in four patients who underwent conversion to laparotomy (25 % of 16 patients, $P=0.022$). The minor complication

rate was 50 % in the conversion group, versus 6.0 % in the TLH + BSO group ($P=0.001$). Comparison of co-morbidity factors between the TLH + BSO group and the conversion group reveals a significantly higher percentage (68.8 %) of obese patients compared to the group in whom the TLH + BSO was successful (42.0 %, $P=0.049$).

Conclusions

In this retrospective cohort analysis on daily practice in pre- versus post-operative histopathology and FIGO stage in 116 presumed low-risk endometrial (pre)malignancy-patients planned for TLH + BSO, diagnosis was either changed from AH to EEC, or from EEC grade I or II upgraded to grade III or non-endometrioid histology in 24 % of cases. This figure is somewhat higher than 15–20 % upgrading reported by Daniel et al., however, they only analyzed pre-operative grade I EEC patients [9]. In 32 % of the 81 patients with EC in the current study, deep myometrial invasion (>50 %) was observed. This percentage is also somewhat higher compared to 25 % described by Ben-Shachar et al., but in their study, again, only patients with EEC grade I were included [10]. Of course, grade and absolute depth of myometrial invasion are closely interrelated as described recently by our group [11] Advanced FIGO stage was found in 6.2 % of patients, which is lower than the 10.5 % described by Ben-Shachar et al., however, in our patient cohort information, lymph node status is absent ruling out occult stage III disease.

In the present study, post-operative upgrading and/or upstaging was clinically relevant in 9.9 % of EC patients (three patients because of upgrading to grade III or non-endometrioid histology, five patients because of FIGO > stage I, one patient because of both). These patients were surgically undertreated according to the Dutch guidelines (http://www.oncoline.nl/endometriumcarcinoom). Although surgical restaging including pelvic and para-aortic lymphadenectomy is proposed to these patients, patients and clinicians may be reluctant with repeated abdominal surgery because of an increased risk of complications. Instead, these high-risk patients are most often treated with adjuvant radio- and/or chemotherapy. However, doing so ignorant of pelvic and/or para-aortic lymph node status, adjuvant therapy may in turn be overtreatment, leading to potential unnecessary morbidity. In this respect, a more thorough pre-operative analysis of "clinical behavior markers" may be applied, indicating aggressive tumor biology more exact than histopathology and grade alone. Differences in carcinogenic pathways between the two EC types are already apparent. Type I carcinomas are characterized by diploid tumors, expression of estrogen and progesterone receptors, *PTEN* alterations, microsatellite instability and mutations of *KRas* and *CTNNB1*. Type II carcinomas on the contrary, are often aneuploid, and show over expression of

Table 3 Clinical relevant inconsistencies between pre-operative and reviewed post-operative

Histopathology and FIGO staging in 8 patients

Patients	Pre-operative	Post-operative	Myometrial invasion (%)	FIGO stage
1	EEC G2	EEC G3	<50	IA G3
2	EEC G1	Mixed G3	<50	IA G3
3	EEC G2	EEC G3	>50	IB G3
4	AH	EEC G1	>50	II G1
5	EEC G1	EEC G1	<50	II G1
6	EEC G2	EEC G1	>50	IIIA G1
7	EEC G2	EEC G2	>50	IIIA G2
8	EEC G2	CC G3	>50	IIIC2 G3

p53 and Her2/neu [12–15]. Analysis of aforementioned markers on the pre-operative specimen may lead to more individualized and effective surgical treatment planning for the low- versus high-risk patients. Furthermore, standard pre-operative MRI and/or intra-operative frozen section assessment of myometrial invasion may be useful in assessment of correct FIGO stage. However, as the accuracy of pre-operative MRI assessment may be only 70.7 % [16] and as already 90.1 % of AH and EEC patients in this series was already pre-operatively correct classified as low-risk, standard use of pre-operative radiological imaging techniques may not be cost-effective. On the other hand, as was recently recognized by two large randomized studies comparing surgery for early endometrial cancer with or without lymphadenectomy, there appears no benefit for standard pelvic and/or para-aortic lymphadenectomy in this presumed low-risk patient category [17, 18].

In 116 TLH + BSO procedures, the major complication (12.1 %) and conversion (13.8 %) rates were comparable to the figures of 14.6 and 10.8 % in the prospective study of

Table 4 Number and types of short-term complications and co-morbidity factors in 116 patients with completed TLH + BSO or conversion to laparotomy

	Overall $n=116$	TLH $n=100$	Conversion $n=16$	P value
Co-morbidity factors (%)				
Obese (BMI>30)	53	42 (42.0)	11 (68.8)	0.049
Hypertension	55	45 (45.0)	10 (62.5)	0.207
Diabetes	18	13 (13.0)	5 (31.3)	0.058
Previous abdominal surgery	37	31 (31.0)	6 (37.5)	0.586
Perioperative complication rates (%)				
Patients with major complications	9 (7.8)	5 (5.0)	4 (25.0)	0.022
Type of major complications	14	9	5	
Bowel injury	1 (0.9)	1 (1.0)	0	
Bladder injury	2 (1.7)	1 (1.0)	1 (6.3)	
Infection	3 (2.6)	2 (2.0)	1 (6.3)	
Ileus	2 (1.7)	1 (1.0)	1 (6.3)	
Hemorrhage*	3 (2.6)	1 (1.0)	2 (12.5)	
Hematoma*	3 (2.6)	3 (3.0)	0	
Patients with minor complications (%)				
Type of minor complications	14 (12.1)	6 (6.0)	8 (50.0)	0.001
Urinary tract infection, fever <38	3 (2.6)	1 (1.0)	2 (12.5)	
Urinary retention needing catheter	1 (0.9)	1 (1.0)	0 (0)	
Fever <38	2 (1.7)	0 (0)	2 (12.5)	
Hemorrhage/hematoma without transfusion	7 (6.0)	4 (4.0)	3 (18.8)	
Wound dehiscence without intervention	1 (0.9)	0 (0)	1 (6.3)	

BMI body mass index

*requiring intervention

Mourits et al. [6]. In several prospective controlled studies, it has been shown that TLH is an effective, minimally invasive, safe alternative to total abdominal hysterectomy [19, 20]. Most studies show reduced incidence of treatment-related morbidity, a shorter hospital stay, less blood loss, less pain, and quicker resumption of daily activities with the laparoscopic approach compared to laparotomy. However, most studies are based on healthier populations, bearing benign uterine problems. In contrast, Mourits et al. showed no evidence of a lower major complication rate for TLH + BSO over total abdominal hysterectomy by laparotomy in endometrial (pre)malignancy. In addition, no differences in the quality of life were reported. However, they also did observe a benefit for TLH in the treatment-related outcomes (i.e., less blood loss, shorter operating times, shorter hospital stay) [6].

In our analysis, patients who underwent a conversion to laparotomy showed a significantly higher percentage of major as well as minor complications, post aut propter the conversion. Also, patients with a BM of >30 showed a significantly higher risk for conversion to laparotomy. In recent literature, it is often mentioned that patients with a high BMI and older patients benefit most from TLH [19, 20]. However, the current opinion about TLH for endometrial cancer might be based on overoptimistic reports due to a paucity of randomized trials. In this respect, it is interesting that de Bijen et al. recently reported the opposite, indicating that TLH is not cost-effective in patients with a BMI over 35, based on major complication-free rates as a primary measure of effect. In their opinion, TLH should not be recommended in patients with a BMI of >35 due to a high conversion rate and unfavorable cost effectiveness [21]. Potentially, reference to centers of excellence in operating the morbid obese may be of help. As endometrial cancer incidence is rising in overweight and elderly patients bearing significant co-morbidity, being able to select patients pre-operatively at substantial risks on conversion and complications would help a great deal, counseling the individual patient on risks and benefits of TLH versus TAH.

Although all histopathological specimens were reviewed, this analysis has some limitations; first being retrospective. Second, we did not compare the pre- versus post-operative differences regarding histopathology, FIGO stage, and complication rates in patients treated primarily by laparotomy. Thus, there could be a bias of patient selection on choosing the approach of surgery. However, in this consecutive series, a substantial number of obese patients (45.7 %) and patients with previous abdominal surgery (31.9 %) were included, undergoing a laparoscopic procedure.

In conclusion, 9.9 % of patients with presumed low-risk EEC or AH treated with TLH + BSO were post-operatively diagnosed with high-risk endometrial cancer and thus surgically undertreated. Furthermore, conversion from TLH + BSO to laparotomy (13.8 %) was accompanied by a significantly increased risk of major and minor complications. The chance of conversion appeared significantly higher in obese patients. Centralization of surgery for the morbid obese patients might lead to reduction of these complication rates. Furthermore, a more thorough pre-operative work-up of presumed low-risk EEC is considered by including biomarkers of high-risk tumor behavior and MRI-imaging giving more insight into myometrial invasion and FIGO stage.

References

1. Parazzini F, Negri E, La Vecchia C, Benzi G, Chiaffarino F, Polatti A et al (1998) Role of reproductive factors on the risk of endometrial cancer. Int J Cancer 76(6):784–6
2. Park SL, Goodman MT, Zhang ZF, Kolonel LN, Henderson BE, Setiawan VW (2010) Body size, adult BMI gain and endometrial cancer risk: the multiethnic cohort. Int J Cancer 126(2):490–9
3. Pecorelli S (2009) Revised FIGO staging for carcinoma of the vulva, cervix and endometrium. Int J Gyneacol Obstet 105(2):103–4
4. Geels YP, Pijnenborg JM, van den Berg-van Erp SH, Bulten J, Visscher DW et al (2012) Endometrioid endometrial carcinoma with atrophic endometrium and poor prognosis. Obstet Gynecol 120(5): 1124–31
5. Nout RA, Smit VTHB, Putter H, Jurgenliemk-Schulz IM, Jobsen JJ et al (2010) Vaginal brachytherapy versus pelvic external beam radiotherapy for patients with endometrial carcinoma of high-intermediate risk (PORTEC-2): an open-label, non-inferiority, randomised trial. Lancet 375:816–823
6. Mourits MJE, Bijen CB, Arts HJ, ter Brugge HG, van der Sijde R et al (2010) Safety of laparoscopy versus laparotomy in early stage endometrial cancer: a randomised trial. Lancet Oncol 11(8):763–71
7. Petersen RW, Quinlivan JA, Casper GR, Nicklin JL (2000) Endometrial adenocarcinoma-presenting pathology is a poor guide to surgical management. Aust N Z J Obstet Gynaecol 40:191–4
8. Creutzberg CL, van Putten WL, Koper PC, Lybeert ML, Jobsen JJ et al (2000) Surgery and postoperative radiotherapy versus surgery alone for patients with stage-1 endometrial carcinoma: multicentre randomised trial. PORTEC Study Group. Post Operative Radiation Therapy in Endometrial Carcinoma. Lancet 355:1404–1411
9. Daniel AG, Peters WA (1988) Accuracy of office and operating room curettage in the grading of endometrial carcinoma. Obstet Gynecol 71:612–4
10. Ben-Shachar I, Pavelka J, Cohn DE, Copeland LJ, Ramirez N, Manolitsas T, Fowler JM (2005) Surgical staging for patients presenting with grade 1 endometrial carcinoma. Obstet Gynecol 105(3): 487–93
11. Geels YP, Pijnenborg JM, van den Berg-van Erp SH, Snijders MP, Bulten J et al (2013) Absolute depth of myometrial invasion in endometrial cancer is superior to the currently used cut-off value of 50%. Gynecol Oncol 129(2):285–91
12. Sherman ME (2000) Theories of endometrial carcinogenesis: a multidisciplinary approach. Mod Pathol 13(3):295–308
13. Ellenson HL, Ronnett BM, Kurman RJ (2011) Precursor lesions of endometrial carcinoma. In: Kurman RJ, Ellenson HL, Ronnett BM (eds) Blaustein's Pathology of the Female Genital Tract, 6th edn. Springer, New York, pp 359–91
14. Markova I, Pilka R, Duskova M, Zapletalova J, Kudela M (2010)

Prognostic significance of clinic pathological and selected immuno-histochemical factors in endometrial cancer. Ceska Gynekol 75(3): 193–9

15. Zeimet AG, Reimer D, Huszar M, Winterhoff B, Puistola U et al (2013) L1CAM in early stage type-I endometrial cancer: results of a large multicentre evaluation. J Natl Cancer Inst 105(15):1142–50

16. Sato S, Itamochi H, Shimada M, Fujjii S, Naniwa et al (2009) Preoperative and intraoperative assessments of depth of myometrial invasion in endometrial cancer. Int J Gynecol Cancer 19(5):884–887

17. Kitchener H, Swart AM, Qian Q, Amos C, Parmar MK (2009) Efficacy of systematic pelvic lymphadenectomy in endometrial cancer (MRC ASTEC trial): a randomised study. Lancet 373:125–36

18. Benedetti Panici P, Basile S, Maneschi F et al (2008) Systematic pelvic lymphadenectomy vs no lymphadenectomy in early stage endometrial carcinoma: randomized clinical trial. J Natl Cancer Inst 100:1707–16

19. Lim B, Lavie O, Bolger B, Lopes T, Monaghan JM (2000) The role of laparoscopic surgery in the management of endometrial cancer. BJOG 107(1):24–27

20. Yu CKH, Cutner A, Mould T, Olaitan A (2005) Total laparoscopic hysterectomy as a primary surgical treatment for endometrial cancer in morbidly obese women. BJOG 112(1):115–117

21. Bijen CB, de Bock GH, Vermeulen KM, Arts HJ, ter Brugge HG et al (2011) Laparoscopic hysterectomy is preferred over laparotomy in early endometrial cancer patients, however not cost effective in the very obese. Eur J Cancer 47(14):2158–2165

15

Correlation of laparoscopic and hysteroscopic 30° scope camera navigation skills on box trainers

Juliënne A. Janse · Emilie Hitzerd ·
Sebastiaan Veersema · Frank J. Broekmans ·
Henk W. R. Schreuder

Abstract This study investigated a possible correlation between training of camera navigation skills with a 30° optic in hysteroscopy and laparoscopy by exploring whether 30° camera navigation training in hysteroscopy provides a certain level of expertise in laparoscopic camera navigation. If a correlation exists, training models and programs in gynecology could be simplified. In this prospective, randomized, nonblinded study 34 medical students were divided into two groups. Group A (n=17) performed five exercises on a box trainer for hysteroscopy (HYSTT) and five exercises on a box trainer for laparoscopy (LASTT). Group B (n=17) performed 2×5 exercises on the LASTT model. Both groups performed a LASTT post-test directly afterwards. The outcome parameter recorded was time to correctly perform the exercise. Comparing the results of the LASTT post-test between group A and B, a similar performance of both groups was shown (p=.131). A slightly faster performance in group A is displayed, when comparing the first LASTT exercise between group A (with previous HYSTT training) and group B (without previous HYSTT training); however, this was a nonsignificant finding (p=.114). Both groups display quite similar learning curves, and after five LASTT repetitions, both groups have reached comparable levels for procedure time, despite the earlier HYSTT training of group A. Previous training on the HYSTT model offers some advantage for training on the LASTT model. However, training of 30° camera navigation skills in a hysteroscopic environment does not seem supportive for

obtaining the same level of camera expertise in laparoscopy. Therefore, 30° camera navigation in hysteroscopy and laparoscopy should be trained separately to reach adequate levels of expertise for each procedure.

Keywords Box trainer · Hysteroscopy · Laparoscopy · Training · Camera navigation · Angled optic

Background

Laparoscopy and hysteroscopy have become standard procedures in gynecology. During endoscopic procedures, good visualization of the surgical field is essential and this is achieved by adequate camera navigation [1–3]. Camera navigation is often perceived to be an easy task, but it is far from an innate ability. Psychomotor skills need to be learned to overcome the barriers that are known for endoscopic skills in general, namely the fulcrum effect, loss of binocular vision, a fixed access point, and decreased range of motion [3, 4]. In addition, skills unique to camera navigation include maintaining a correct horizontal axis while centering the operative field, focusing and sizing, maintaining a steady image, and tracking instruments in motion [2, 3]. Especially, angled scopes, by the addition of off-axis viewing, require complex visuospatial skills [5].

In laparoscopy, handling of the camera is often performed by the least experienced person present. Incorrect camera handling results in poor visualization and may cause frustration of the operator, increased operating time and errors [1, 3, 5]. In hysteroscopy, camera navigation is essential due to the decreased range of motion when navigating through the narrow cervical canal and uterine cavity. A 30° angled scope affords an increased view with fewer movements and is increasingly used for vaginoscopic hysteroscopy in the office setting. But when knowledge and skills are lacking, the 30° angled scope can lead to unnecessary damage of the cervical

J. A. Janse (✉) · S. Veersema
Department of Gynecology and Obstetrics, St. Antonius Hospital Nieuwegein, Koekoekslaan 1, 3435 CM Nieuwegein, The Netherlands
e-mail: Julienne.Janse@gmail.com

E. Hitzerd · F. J. Broekmans · H. W. R. Schreuder
Division of Woman and Baby, University Medical Center Utrecht, 3508 GA Utrecht, The Netherlands

canal and endometrium. In a national UK survey among gynecologists, a disappointing percentage of 25.8 of all responders who perform 30° hysteroscopy showed understanding of the principles of 30° angled view [6].

Despite the importance of camera navigation skills, they are not often explicitly addressed in training programs [7, 8]. However, camera navigation skills can be trained easily and effectively outside the operating room [5, 9–11]. During the past years, several models have been developed and validated for camera navigation training in laparoscopy [3, 12, 13] and to a lesser extent in hysteroscopy [14]. The same principles can be observed in urology as well, for laparoscopy and cystoscopy [15]. Even though endoscopy comprises different types of procedures (e.g., laparoscopy and hysteroscopy), they all require mastering of adequate camera navigation skills with a 30° optic. One could question whether a possible correlation exists between the training of camera navigation skills with a 30° optic in hysteroscopy and laparoscopy even though the environments of the abdominal and uterine cavity are fairly different. If this correlation exists, it implies that obtaining 30° camera navigation skills in hysteroscopy also indicates the built up of a certain level of expertise in laparoscopy camera handling. This would mean that training models and programs in gynecology could be simplified. Furthermore, it might also apply for other specialties, for example cystoscopy and laparoscopy in urology. That could lead to a situation in which several endoscopic specialties could train 30° camera navigation on a uniform training model, without a direct relation between the model, a specific organ, cavity or specialty, and the type of endoscopy.

The aim of the present study is to investigate whether 30° camera navigation practice in hysteroscopy also creates a built up of expertise in laparoscopic 30° camera navigation.

Two box trainers have been used in this study: the laparoscopic skills testing and training (LASTT) model and the hysteroscopic skills testing and training (HYSTT) model. Both were designed under auspices of the European Academy for Gynaecological Surgery (Leuven, Belgium). These models train various psychomotor skills including specific exercises for 30° camera navigation training [12, 14].

Methods

Participants and setting

From April to June 2013, 34 novices voluntarily participated in this study. Medical students served as novices and they were invited during or after their gynecology internship via oral and written means, and all agreed to participate. The study was carried out at the University Medical Center Utrecht and at the teaching hospital St. Antonius Ziekenhuis, Nieuwegein, the Netherlands. All participating students filled out a questionnaire which recorded their baseline characteristics. The study was exempt from the institutional review board approval, since no potential harm could be done to humans or nonhumans. All participants gave written consent prior to the start of the study.

Design

This study is a prospective, randomized, nonblinded trial. The participants were divided into two groups by randomization by sealed envelopes. Short series of exercises were designed for the present study, because Molinas et al. observed a plateau phase for the LASTT 30° camera navigation exercise after 5–15 repetitions [12]. Figure 1 displays the scheme of exercises per group. In addition, the scheme shows the two comparative analyses. Analysis 1 addresses the question whether mixed training will lead to the same laparoscopy level as only-laparoscopy training, by comparing the LASTT post-test between both groups. Analysis 2 addresses the question whether prior hysteroscopy training will lead to a higher achievement in laparoscopy in comparison to a short laparoscopy training only. This analysis will compare the first LASTT exercise of group A (with previous HYSTT training) with the first LASTT exercise of group B (without previous HYSTT training).

Both groups received a short standardized introduction on 30° optics and the study protocol. Group A (n=17) was given a specific introduction on hysteroscopy and the HYSTT model, while group B (n=17) received a similar standardized introduction on laparoscopy and the LASTT model. One-minute practice time was given to each participant to obtain familiarization with the model; during this practice time, feedback and instructions were provided. Then, group A performed the HYSTT exercise five times, followed by a 5-min break. During the break, group A received the standardized introduction on laparoscopy and the LASTT model, and 1-minute practice time was provided. After the break, group A performed the LASTT exercise five times, followed by a final LASTT repetition which was recorded as a post-test. Group B performed the LASTT exercise five times, also followed by a 5-min break. After the break, this group repeated the LASTT exercise another five times and performed the post-test on the LASTT model. The post-test, as performed by both groups, consists of a single repetition of the camera navigation exercise on the LASTT model and is performed directly after the training sessions in the same environment. One investigator (E.H.) supervised all exercises and tests to limit intersupervisor bias. During all exercises and tests, no feedback or instructions were provided nor could any questions be asked. After each repetition, the participant could ask questions and feedback was offered.

Materials

The LASTT model consists of a wooden platform (16.5×30 cm) with two modules in the back, two modules in

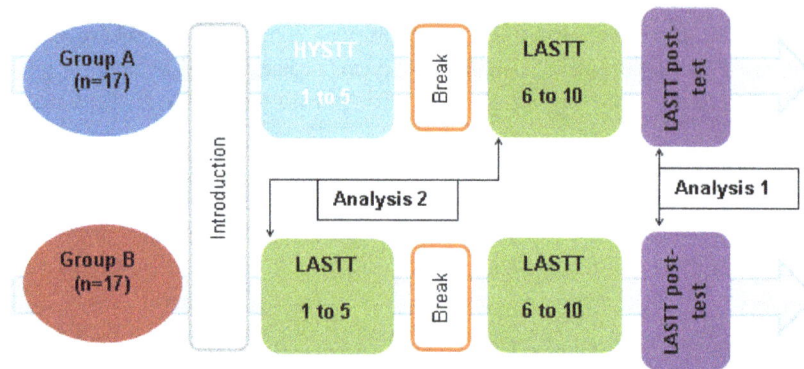

Fig. 1 Study design: scheme of exercises per group. Analysis 1 addresses the question whether mixed training will lead to the same laparoscopy level as only-laparoscopy training under the condition of equal time investment, by comparing the LASTT post-test between both groups. Analysis 2 addresses the question whether prior hysteroscopy training will lead to a higher achievement in laparoscopy in comparison to a short laparoscopy training only, by comparing the first LASTT exercise of group A (with previous HYSTT training) with the first LASTT exercise of group B (without previous HYSTT training)

the middle, and two modules in the front. These modules contain in total of 14 targets. Each target consists of a large symbol, only identifiable from a panoramic view, and a small symbol, only identifiable from a close-up view [12]. The LASTT model was inserted into a Szabo trainer box (Karl Storz, Tutlingen, Germany) (Fig. 2a).

The HYSTT model consists of a white plastic uterus model in which twelve symbols are placed at twelve locations, known as front/mid/back (referring to the depth of the space) combined with anterior/posterior/left/right (referring to the walls of the space). Six models are available in which each location contains a different symbol (models A–F). This plastic uterus is placed in a silicone model of a vulva, which in turn is situated in a plastic pelvis model (Fig. 2b). Originally, the HYSTT model contained 14 target locations with anatomical names as "fundal anterior", "cornual left", "tubal ostium right", and "isthmic posterior". Due to the observation in a pilot study that these anatomical names seem confusing when applied in this simple uterus, the model was adjusted by covering the "cornual" symbols and by renaming the other twelve locations by general terms as front/mid/back.

Both models were designed under auspices of the European Academy for Gynaecological Surgery (Leuven, Belgium). The exercises on the LASTT model were performed with a 10 mm 30° scope and the exercises on the HYSTT model with a 5 mm 30° scope (Karl Storz), both connected to the same straight video camera, light source, and monitor (Telepack, Karl Storz). With regards to the exercises, a black circle (2.5 cm in diameter) was applied in the center of the monitor. The box trainers and the monitor were set up on a large table in line with each other.

Exercises

The participants stood behind the box trainer in the midline, holding the camera with their dominant hand and the fiber optic cable with their nondominant hand for lateral, rotatory, and zoom-in/out navigation. For the LASTT exercise, the scope was inserted through the middle port of the trainer box. At the start of the exercise, the participant had to visualize the first large symbol (i.e., 1) and then identify the small one situated next to it. The small symbol had to be sharply visualized inside the black circle on the screen. This small symbol indicated the next large symbol that had to be visualized. The exercise was finished when the small symbol on the last target (end) was identified correctly. After every run, the targets were ordered differently according to a standardized schedule to prevent memorization.

For the HYSTT exercise, the scope was inserted into the uterus model (model B) through the silicone vulva. The participant had to navigate to a specific location (e.g., mid posterior) as commanded by the investigator and visualize the corresponding symbol inside the black circle on the monitor, after which a new command was given until all 12 symbols were correctly visualized. After every completed session, the sequence of the commands was changed according to a standardized schedule, and after three sessions, another uterus model (model C) was inserted for the last two sessions to prevent memorization.

Outcome measure

The outcome measure for both the HYSTT and LASTT exercises was the total time (recorded in seconds) needed to correctly visualize all the signs.

Statistical analysis

The statistical analysis was performed with SPSS 20.0 for Windows. A power analysis was performed prior to the study to determine the minimal sample size. It showed that a power level of 0.8 with a desired significance level of 0.05 and a difference of 1 SD between groups should be reached at a minimal total sample size of 34 participants. To compare the

Fig. 2 a Set up LASTT model. **b** Set up HYSTT model

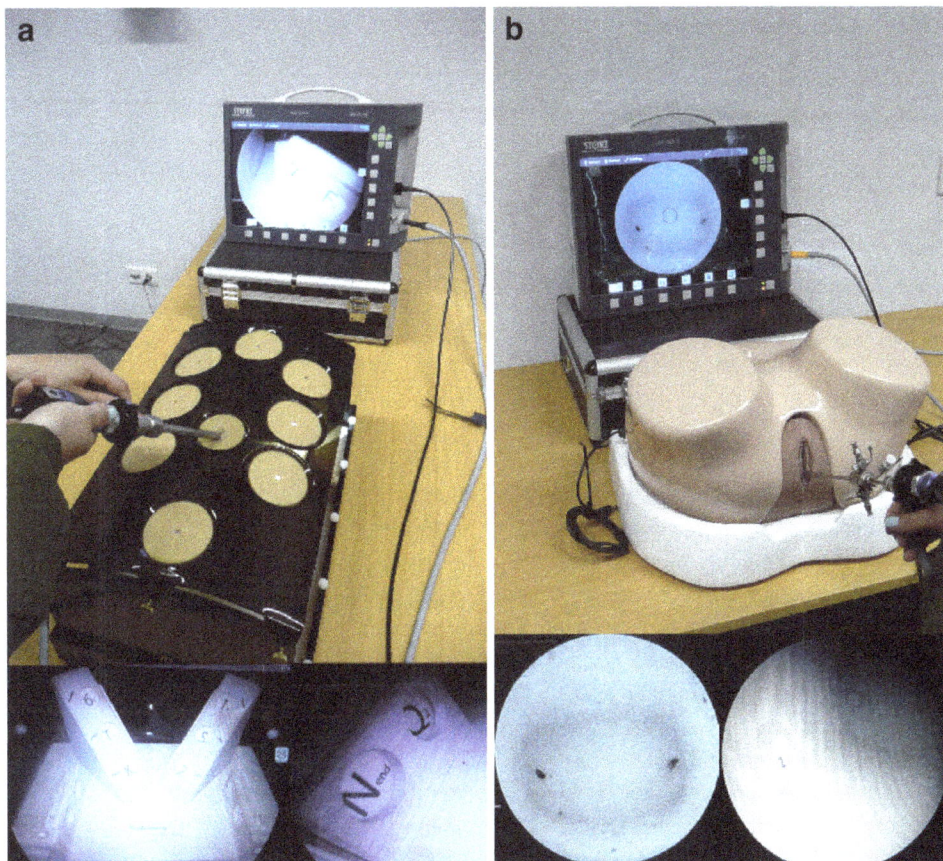

participants' characteristics, the chi-square test was used. Differences in the time measurements between the two groups were analyzed using the nonparametrical Mann–Whitney U test for independent samples. The results are presented as medians with interquartile ranges (IQR) and were considered significant in case of a p value $< .05$.

Findings

The baseline characteristics of the participants are reported in Table 1. The participants were randomized into two groups ($n=17$ per group), and there were no significant differences regarding personal characteristics between these groups. Both groups existed of five men (29.4 %) and 12 women (70.6 %). The median age in group A was 23 years (IQR 22–23) and in group B, 23 years (IQR 23–24). All participants had attended at least one hysteroscopy and/or laparoscopy.

When comparing the results of the LASTT post-test between groups A and B (analysis 1), a similar performance of both groups is shown. The median time needed to complete the post-test was 100.3 (IQR 88.1–121.8)s for group A and 91.1 (IQR 77.2–104.4)s for group B ($p=.131$) (Fig. 3).

Figure 4 displays the median time of both groups per LASTT exercise graphically. It shows that both groups have reached approximately the same level of procedure time during their post-test, and this endorses the results of a similar performance described above. However, despite of their earlier training on the HYSTT model, group A follows more or less the same (steep) learning curve as group B in the first LASTT series instead of following the (flatter) curve in the second LASTT series of group B.

Analysis 2 compares the first LASTT exercise between group A (with previous HYSTT training) and group B (without previous HYSTT training). Group A performed the exercise slightly faster than group B, but this was a nonsignificant finding ($p=.114$). The median performance time of group A was 214.3 (IQR 152.2–261.6)s, while group B recorded a median time of 249.6 (IQR 178.9–307.0)s (Fig. 3).

Both groups display quite similar learning curves, and after five LASTT repetitions, both groups have reached comparable levels for procedure time, despite the earlier HYSTT training of group A.

Discussion

Training programs for endoscopic skills vary throughout institutions worldwide. Furthermore, every specialty has its own training models for specific procedures. As described in the

Table 1 Demographic characteristics of the participants

Characteristics		Group A (*n*=17)	Group B (*n*=17)
Age (years), mean (range)		22.71 (21–26)	23.47 (22–25)
Sex	Male	5	5
	Female	12	12
Dominant hand	Right	13	15
	Left	4	2
Desired future specialty	Surgical	8	10
	Nonsurgical/do not know	9	7
No. of attended hysteroscopy/laparoscopy	1–10	11	8
	>10	6	9

Participants were randomized by sealed envelopes. No statistically significant differences were found between both groups (statistical analysis performed with chi-square test)

introduction, the basic skills required for different endoscopic procedures are fairly similar and endoscopy training outside the operating room could be standardized [7, 12]. This led to the idea that certain general endoscopic skills, such as 30° camera navigation, might be trained on a uniform training model. This study investigated whether a correlation exists between training of camera navigation skills with a 30° optic in hysteroscopy and laparoscopy by exploring whether 30° camera navigation training in hysteroscopy provides a certain expertise in laparoscopic camera navigation.

Firstly, the results show that regardless of training on the HYSTT or the LASTT model, 30° optic skills are easily learned when a standardized explanation and specific exercises for camera navigation are provided. Medical students were able to strongly improve their performance within five repetitions on the LASTT model, reaching a time score of 110 s. This was faster than expected by the results of Molinas et al., where novices (students and inexperienced gynecologists) needed approximately 10 repetitions to reach a procedure time of 110 s [12]. However, in both studies, certain variability between subjects is observed. In the current study, it is not investigated whether this fast performance is lasting.

Secondly, concerning a possible correlation for camera navigation, a similar performance of both groups during the LASTT post-test was found (analysis 1). This might indicate that previous hysteroscopy training does provide built up of expertise in laparoscopic camera navigation. However, after apprehending the fast learning curve in this study, a similar performance after five repetitions can be expected regardless of previous training. And even though group A (with previous HYSTT training) did perform slightly better than group B (without previous HYSTT training) during their first LASTT exercise, this finding was not significant (analysis 2). In addition, the learning curves of both groups were fairly similar when they started performing exercises on the LASTT. Therefore, according to these results, the existence of a pronounced correlation between training of 30° camera navigation skills in hysteroscopy and laparoscopy seems implausible.

A possible explanation for not finding a correlation could be that even though the principles of angled optics are easy to learn when time, attention, and exercises are provided, the abdominal and uterine cavity are too different regarding space and shape. In the uterus and in the corresponding HYSTT model, camera navigation takes place within a small and

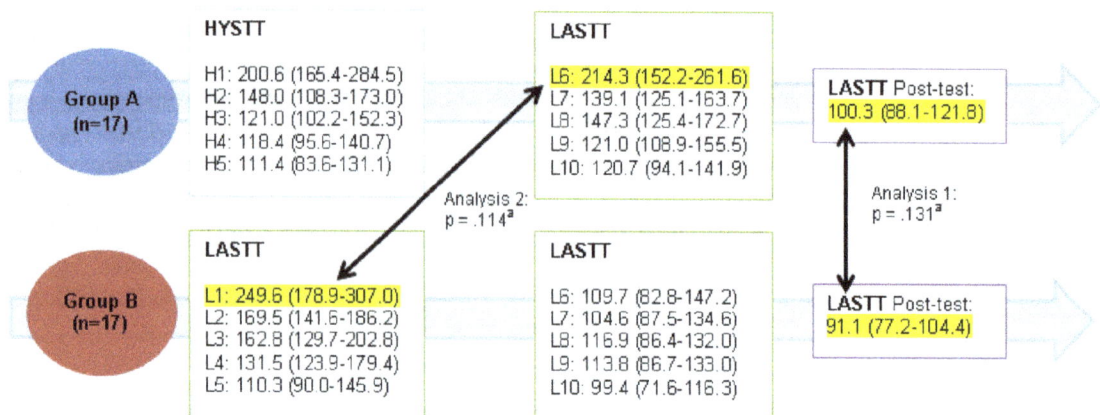

Fig. 3 Median results with interquartile ranges (IQR) in seconds per exercise per group, for both HYSTT and LASTT exercises. Analysis 1 compares the outcome of the LASTT post-test of both groups. Analysis 2 compares the first LASTT exercise of group A (with previous HYSTT training) with the first LASTT exercise of group B (without previous HYSTT training). Statistical analysis performed with Mann–Whitney *U* test

Fig. 4 Median time in seconds of the LASTT repetitions of group A (*blue line*) and group B (*red line*). Interquartile ranges (IQR) are represented by the *vertical gray lines*. Both groups have reached approximately the same level of procedure time at the end of their LASTT exercises. Group A more or less followed the same learning curve as group B in the first LASTT series

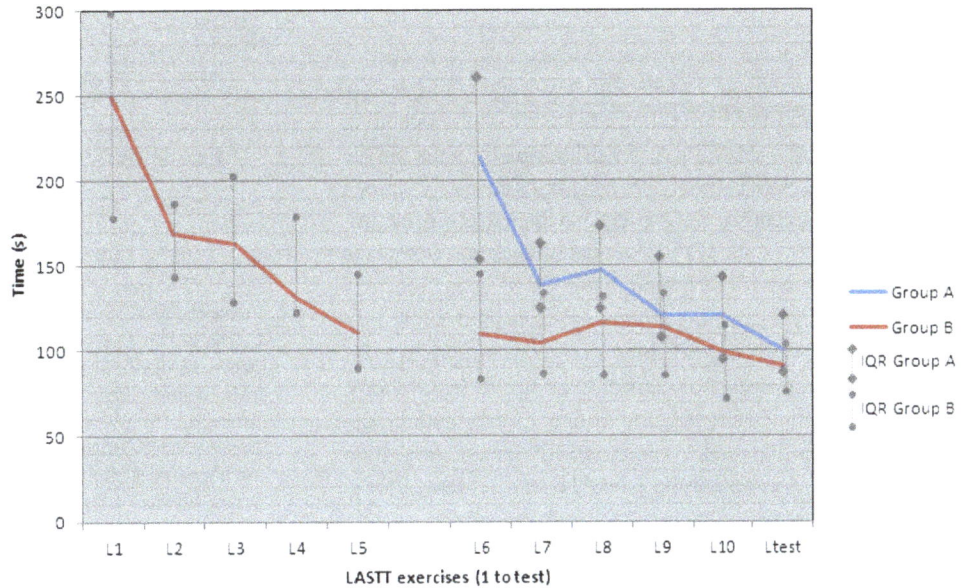

narrow cavity (a specific organ), which requires subtle movements of the scope combined with extensive angled optic use. In the abdomen and in the corresponding LASTT model, a distinctly higher degree of freedom of scope movement is observed. This is due to the wide space after CO_2 inflation during laparoscopy and the environment within the spacious box trainer, respectively. One has to train how to navigate and to apply the principles of angled optics in each different cavity. Camera navigation in hysteroscopy and laparoscopy should be trained separately to reach adequate levels of expertise for each procedure.

Strong points of the present study are the power analysis performed prior to the study and the randomization process, which was executed effectively. The study was nonblinded, because blinding was not possible due to the distinctly different appearances of the two box trainers. Medical students were included in this study as novices, because of their blank training background which gave all participants the same starting point.

The current study design was not established as a proficiency-based training curriculum, since the aim was to investigate a correlation between skills acquisition in two training environments and not to evaluate the efficacy of a curriculum. The number of repetitions was kept small to ensure that participants were not yet fully proficient at the HYSTT model before training at the LASTT box. We wanted to see if the change of environment would alter the ongoing learning curve in comparison to the group that continuously trained at the LASTT model. One could argue that a proficiency-based study design with a 'retention test' performed several weeks to months after the training might provide a better way to investigate our hypothesis, and this presents an area for future research. For clinical use, it should

be emphasized that the design of an efficient training curriculum needs to be proficiency-focused to accommodate the ability and development of each individual [16].

One of the factors that might have influenced the current results is the fact that the exercises per model differ in the way they have to be executed. During the HYSTT exercise, the participants had to follow the investigator's commands, whereas in the LASTT exercise, the visualized sign itself included the next command. Furthermore, time to correctly perform the exercise is the only outcome parameter recorded, and it is recorded by a person. One can imagine that a computerized system as in a virtual reality simulator can offer a more objective scoring and that other factors might affect performance; after all, a faster performance does not automatically mean a better performance. Outcome parameters as the number of errors, path length, camera stability, and number of collisions were not recorded, which is inherent to the design of box trainers. In addition, box trainers in general often lack a realistic display of human anatomy. Even though, box trainers have proven to be simple and relatively cheap models that can effectively train specific psychomotor skills needed for endoscopy [4, 12, 17]. On the other hand, the possibly influencing factors of a box trainer might be overcome by using virtual reality simulators, which objectively record various parameters. The software could provide similar commands for both exercises and record parameters that could display the varying nuances in camera navigation that one has to train when performing both hysteroscopy and laparoscopy. This might provide an area for future research. In addition, it could be an interesting idea for future research to include a test on visuospatial abilities for all participants, in order to retrieve extra information on the training capacity for endoscopic skills.

Conclusion

Correct camera navigation skills with a 30° optic are essential in endoscopy and need to be trained outside of the operating room. This study shows that, regardless of training on the HYSTT or the LASTT model, 30° optic skills are easily learned when specific exercises for camera navigation are provided. Previous training on the HYSTT model offers some advantage for training on the LASTT model, compared to no previous training. However, training of camera navigation skills in a hysteroscopic environment does not seem supportive for obtaining the same level of camera expertise in laparoscopy. The two environments appear too distinct to train both procedures on one unified model. Therefore, 30° camera navigation in hysteroscopy and laparoscopy should be trained separately to reach adequate levels of expertise for each procedure.

Acknowledgments We would like to thank all the participants who voluntarily participated in this study. We would like to thank M.J.C. Eijkemans, Associate Professor in BioStatistics from the Julius Center for Health Sciences and Primary care, University of Utrecht, the Netherlands, for his help with the statistical analysis.

References

1. Conrad J, Shah AH, Divino CM, Schluender S, Gurland B, Shlasko E, Szold A (2006) The role of mental rotation and memory scanning on the performance of laparoscopic skills. Surg Endosc 20:504–510
2. Shetty S, Panait L, Baranoski J, Dudrick SJ, Bell RL, Roberts KE, Duffy AJ (2012) Construct and face validity of a virtual reality-based camera navigation curriculum. J Surg Res 177:191–195
3. Korndorffer JR, Hayes DJ, Dunne JB, Sierra R, Touchard CL, Markert RJ, Scott DJ (2005) Development and transferability of a cost-effective laparoscopic camera navigation simulator. Surg Endosc 19:161–167
4. Schreuder HWR, van den Berg CB, Hazebroek EJ, Verheijen RHM, Schijven MP (2011) Laparoscopic skills training using inexpensive box trainers: which exercises to choose when constructing a validated training course. BJOG 118(13):1576–1584
5. Ganai S, Donroe JA, St. Louis MR, Lewis GM, Seymour NE (2007) Virtual-reality training improves angled telescope skills in novice laparoscopists. Am J Surg 193:260–265
6. Tawfeek S, Scott P (2010) National inpatient diagnostic hysteroscopy survey. Gynecol Surg 7:53–59
7. VanBlaricom AL, Goff BA, Chinn M, Icasiano MM, Nielsen P, Mandel L (2005) A new curriculum for hysteroscopy training as demonstrated by an objective structured assessment of technical skills (OSATS). AJOG 193:1856–1865
8. Kingston A, Abbott J, Lenart M, Vancaillie T (2004) Hysteroscopic training: the butternut pumpkin model. J Am Assoc Gynecol Laparosc 11(2):256–261
9. Paschold M, Niebisch S, Kronfeld K, Herzer M, Lang H, Kneist W (2013) Cold-start capability in virtual-reality laparoscopic camera navigation: a base for tailored training in undergraduates. Surg Endosc 27:2169–2177
10. Franzeck FM, Rosenthal R, Muller MK, Nocito A, Wittich F, Maurus C, Dindo D, Clavien PA, Hahnloser D (2012) Prospective randomized controlled trial of simulator-based versus traditional in-surgery laparoscopic camera navigation training. Surg Endosc 26:235–241
11. Andreatta PB, Woodrum DT, Birkmeyer JD, Yellamanchilli RK, Doherty GM, Gauger PG, Minter RM (2006) Laparoscopic skills are improved with LapMentor™ training. Results of a randomized double-blinded study. Ann Surg 243:854–863
12. Molinas CR, De Win G, Ritter O, Keckstein J, Miserez M, Campo R (2008) Feasibility and construct validity of a novel laparoscopic skills testing and training model. Gynecol Surg 4(5):281–290
13. Yee KA, Karmali S, Sherman V (2009) Validation of a simple camera navigation trainer. J Am Coll Surg 209:753–757
14. Janse JA, Tolman CJ, Veersema S, Broekmans FJM, Schreuder HWR (2013) Hysteroscopy training and learning curve of 30° camera navigation on a new box trainer: the HYSTT. Gynecol Surg. doi:10.1007/s10397-014-0833-9
15. Schout BMA, Ananias HJK, Bemelmans BLH, d'Ancona FCH, Muijtjens AMM, Dolmans VEMG, Scherpbier AJJA, Hendrikx AJM (2009) Transfer of cysto-urethroscopy skills from a virtual-reality simulator to the operating room: a randomized controlled trial. BJUI 106:226–231
16. De Win G, Van Bruwaene S, Allen C, De Ridder D (2013) Design and implementation of a proficiency-based, structured endoscopy course for medical students applying for a surgical specialty. Adv Med Educ Pract 4:103–115
17. Chou B, Handa VL (2006) Simulators and virtual reality in surgical education. Obstet Gynecol Clin N Am 33:283–296

16

A European survey on awareness of post-surgical adhesions among gynaecological surgeons

Markus Wallwiener · Philippe Robert Koninckx · Andreas Hackethal · Hans Brölmann ·
Per Lundorff · Michal Mara · Arnaud Wattiez · Rudy Leon De Wilde ·
for The Anti-Adhesions in Gynecology Expert Panel (ANGEL)

Abstract The present survey was conducted among gynaecological surgeons from several European countries to assess the actual knowledge and practice related to post-surgical adhesions and measures for reduction. From September 1, 2012 to February 6, 2013, gynaecological surgeons were invited to answer an 18-item online questionnaire accessible through the ESGE website. This questionnaire contained eight questions on care settings and surgical practice and ten questions on adhesion formation and adhesion reduction. Four hundred fourteen surgeons participated; 70.8 % agreed that adhesions are a source of major morbidity.

About half of them declared that adhesions represented an important part of their daily medical and surgical work. About two thirds informed their patients about the risk of adhesion. Most cited causes of adhesions were abdominal infections and extensive tissue trauma, and endometriosis and myomectomy surgery. Fewer surgeons expected adhesion formation after laparoscopy (18.9 %) than after laparotomy (40.8 %); 60 % knew the surgical techniques recommended to reduce adhesions; only 44.3 % used adhesion-reduction agents on a regular basis. This survey gives a broad picture of adhesion awareness amongst European gynaecological surgeons, mainly from Germany and the UK. The participants had a good knowledge of factors causing adhesions. Knowledge of surgical techniques recommended and use of anti-adhesion agents developed to reduce adhesions need to be improved.

Keywords Post-surgical adhesions · Gynaecological surgery · Awareness · Prevention

M. Wallwiener (✉)
Department of Obstetrics and Gynaecology, University of Heidelberg, Heidelberg, Germany
e-mail: markus.wallwiener@googlemail.com

P. R. Koninckx
University Hospital Gasthuisberg, Katholieke Universiteit, Leuven, Belgium

A. Hackethal
Queensland Centre for Gynaecological Cancer, Queensland Brisbane, Australia

H. Brölmann
VU University, Amsterdam, The Netherlands

P. Lundorff
Gynecologic Clinic, Private Hospital Molholm, Vejle, Denmark

M. Mara
Charles University, Prague, Czech Republic

A. Wattiez
Hôpital de Hautepierre, Strasbourg, France

R. L. De Wilde
Klinik für Frauenheilkunde, Geburtshilfe und Gynäkologische Onkologie, Universitätsklinik für Gynäkologie, Pius-Hospital, University Oldenburg, Oldenburg, Germany

Background

Post-surgical adhesions—abnormal fibrous connections developing between the peritoneum and organs as a sequel to surgical trauma—are the most frequent complication of abdominal surgery and may represent one of the greatest unmet medical needs of the moment [1].

Yet, many surgeons are still not aware of the extent of the problem and its serious consequences, such as chronic pelvic pain and small bowel obstruction. In addition, post-surgical adhesions are a frequent cause of dyspareunia and secondary infertility.

In a previous survey conducted among gynaecological surgeons in German hospitals, adhesions were believed to develop in 15 % of cases after laparoscopy and 40 % after laparoscopy [2].

In symptomatic patients, removal of post-surgical adhesions requires a new surgical intervention (adhesiolysis). However, adhesiolysis is often followed by adhesion reformation. In this situation, earlier precautions aiming to prevent post-surgical adhesions are of paramount importance.

Developments in adhesion-reduction strategies and new agents now offer a realistic possibility of reducing the risk of adhesions forming and, thus, may improve the outcomes for patients and the associated onward burden.

Based on the fact that for an adhesion to form, there must be a prolonged contact between two areas of injury, two measures are currently recommended to minimise post-surgical adhesions: good surgical practice with minimal tissue trauma, and in addition, anti-adhesion agents used intra-operatively to minimise contact between injured parts of the peritoneum and an adjacent organ [3]. Both measures aim to reduce the abnormal healing process that results in the formation of adhesions.

Epidemiological data have demonstrated that despite these advances in prevention, the burden of adhesion-related complications has not changed [4–8].

In this context, the actual knowledge and practice of gynaecological surgeons with regard to this complication of their interventions was assessed in several European countries. A survey was conducted in order to document the awareness of the risk of post-surgical adhesions amongst gynaecological surgeons, the knowledge of measures to be taken to minimise this complication of surgery, the surgical procedures likely to cause extensive adhesions, the information given to the patients about the risk of post-surgical adhesions during the consenting process, and subsequently the actual practice regarding the prevention of adhesions.

Methods

Gynaecological surgeons were recruited through the micro-website dedicated to post-surgical adhesions developed by

Table 1 Mean and median numbers of interventions performed in 2010 in the gynaecology departments of the survey respondents (all participating countries)

Intervention type	Mean ± SD	Median
Laparotomic	1,213±1,719	700
Laparoscopic	606±710	380
Vaginal	389±1,033	200

the European Society for Gynaecological Endoscopy (ESGE) (http://www.esge.org/index.php?option=com_ surveyforce&view=survey&Itemid=101). Both members and non-members of the ESGE could participate.

Website visitors were invited to fill in an 18-item online questionnaire (Appendix). On top of the questionnaire, the micro-website featured a printable information leaflet for patients about the risk of adhesions and a pictorial version of the ESGE expert consensus position on the prevention of post-surgical adhesions [9].

No financial incentives were proposed to the survey participants.

Due to the nature of the survey, the statistics were purely descriptive and expressed in percentages. Means and standard deviations, medians, minimum, and maximum were calculated where applicable. These calculations were not corrected for missing data.

Results

Between September 1, 2012 and February 6, 2013, 233 gynaecological surgeons completed the whole questionnaire; another 181 participated in the survey but left at least one question unanswered.

Out of the 414 participants, 356 (86 %) downloaded the ESGE expert consensus position paper on adhesions.

Fig. 1 Distribution of survey respondents per type of hospitals

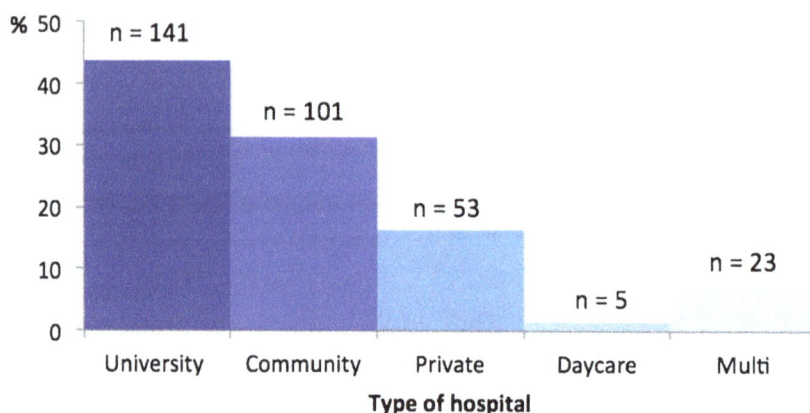

Fig. 2 Number of laparoscopic interventions performed by each gynaecological surgeon

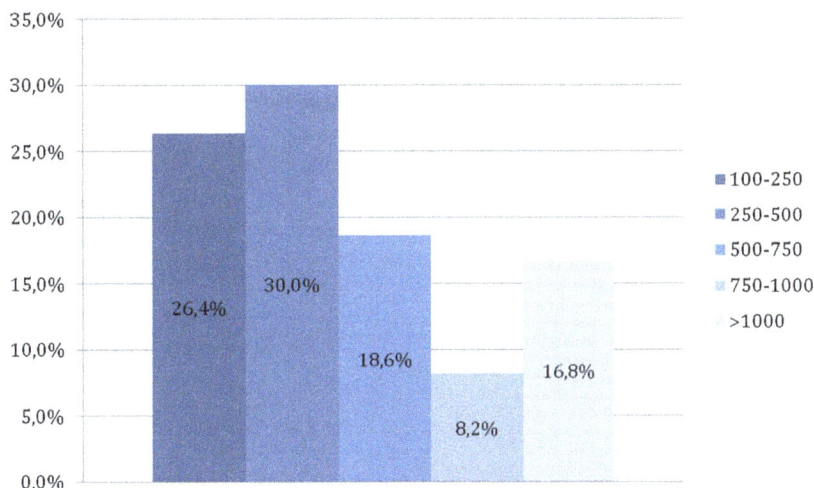

Fig. 2 Number of laparoscopic interventions performed by each gynaecological surgeon

Care settings and levels of activity

Although the survey participants worked in a variety of care settings, a majority (75 %) worked exclusively or partially in a university or a community hospital (Fig. 1). The two main countries represented were the UK (20.6 % of participants) and Germany (20.0 %), followed by Italy (16.2 %) and the Netherlands (7.5 %).

Owing to the 265 participants who answered this question, the mean number of laparotomic, laparoscopic, and vaginal interventions performed per gynaecology department in 2010 was 1,213, 606, and 389, respectively. However, the actual numbers reported for each department varied widely (Table 1).

The number of laparoscopic interventions performed by each gynaecological surgeon during the previous 5 years was also variable (Fig. 2).

Table 2 summarizes the number of surgical interventions performed in 2010, per hospital type, in the two main participating countries (UK and Germany).

Among 253 responders, 70.8 % agreed that post-surgical adhesions are a source of major morbidity. They were 50.4

and 57.0 %, respectively, to declare that patients with adhesions represented an important to very important part of their daily medical work outside of the operating room and of their daily surgical work (Fig. 3).

Patient consenting

Out of 244 responders to the inquiry regarding the daily practice of consenting their patients about adhesions, 64.3 % declared they provide information about the risk of adhesion formation. Further, 65.6 % declared to provide information regarding possible complications of adhesions and 52.5 % declared to provide information regarding treatment options for adhesions (Table 3).

Surgical procedures leading to intra-abdominal adhesion formation

For 40.8 ± 22.1 % of the survey participants, laparotomic interventions were associated with a risk of post-surgical adhesions; they were fewer to associate this risk with laparoscopic interventions (18.9 ± 16.3 %), vaginal surgery

Table 2 Summary of the number of surgical interventions performed in 2010 per hospital type: Germany and UK data

Type of hospital	Country	Percentage of participants providing data on number of interventions % (n/N)	Laparotomies mean number ± SD	Laparoscopies mean number ± SD	Vaginal route mean number ± SD
University hospital	Germany	66.6 (24/36)	1,236.7±1,344.8	1,624.7±1,730.0	998.7±1,390.2
	UK	87.5 (42/48)	1,649.4±1,086.6	827.6±512.9	437.4±333.2
Community hospital	Germany	83.3 (25/30)	409.5±302.2	750.0±589.7	298.0 ±264.9
	UK	78.9 (15/19)	1,518.2±1,647.2	622.7±562.7	265.9±208.6
Private hospital	Germany	78.5 (11/14)	155.9 ±132.5	780.3±819.8	383.1±796.4
	UK	87.5 (7/8)	1,155.8±1,214.1	1,192.7±1,425.4	748.3±1,163.7
Daycare hospital	Germany	100 (2/2)	0.0 ±0.0	1,650.0 ±1,202.	1,200.0±1,131.4
	UK	0	–	–	–

Fig. 3 Importance of patients with post-surgical adhesions in a gynaecologist's daily work

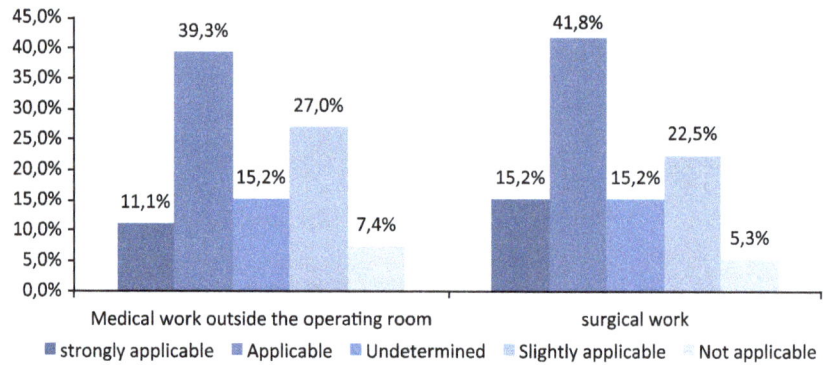

Medical work outside the operating room   surgical work

■ strongly applicable ■ Applicable ■ Undetermined ■ Slightly applicable ■ Not applicable

(22.1±17.1 %) or natural orifice transluminal endoscopic surgery (NOTES) (17.6±16.9 %). The difference between laparotomy and laparoscopy was independent from the type of surgical intervention considered (Table 4).

Among the different gynaecological operations, endometriosis surgery and myomectomy were thought to be the most likely to be associated with adhesions (Table 4). The risk was considered low with caesarean section and only occasionally associated with ectopic pregnancy, single port, and NOTES.

Table 3 Selected results of the present survey, presented after Hackethal et al [2]

Entry	% of participants
Adhesions considered as a major source of morbidity	70.8
Adhesions considered as an important part of daily medical work	50.4
Adhesions considered as an important part of daily surgical work	50.7
Estimated incidence of adhesions post-laparotomy	40.8
Estimated incidence of adhesions post-laparoscopy	18.9
Patients informed of risk of adhesions during consenting	64.3
Regular use of anti-adhesion agents	44.3
Anti-adhesion agents considered as cost-effective	77.5
Anti-adhesion agents considered as too expensive	71.6
Anti-adhesion agents considered as insufficiently refunded	75.8
Consider themselves as well informed about adhesions	60.0
Source of adhesion knowledge	
Scientific publications	85.6
Personal experience	82.6
Discussions with colleagues	75.8
Continuous medical education	84.7
Consensus paper	66.5
ESGE conferences	61.5

Considerations regarding surgical adhesion induction

Table 5 indicates the characteristics thought to have a high impact on the formation of adhesions. Intra-abdominal infections and extensive tissue trauma were quoted as having the highest impact.

Virtually all the gynaecological surgeons (94.8 % of 238 responders) considered that good surgical practice was important to prevent post-surgical adhesions. They were 60.5 and 55.3 %, respectively, to consider antiadhesive barriers and peritoneal conditioning as important.

The relevant elements of peritoneal conditioning identified by 247 respondents were temperature, gas environment, and the type of irrigation fluid (Fig. 4). Additional preparation of the rinsing fluid had an undetermined effect for heparin and for vitamin C (Fig. 4).

Indications for surgical adhesiolysis

The main reasons for adhesioysis were symptoms (95.0 % of the responders), infertility (93.7 %), young age (73.5 %), and previous surgery (68.9 %); 53.4 % of the responders declared that adhesiolysis was performed in all patients.

Table 4 The type of surgery in benign conditions leading to intra-abdominal adhesions with the estimated likelihood on a scale from 0 (unlikely) to 4 (highly likely)

Type of surgery	Median score ± SD of 5-point Likert rating scale	
	Laparotomy	Laparoscopy
Endometriosis surgery	3.6±0.6	2.8±0.8
Myomectomy	3.4±0.7	2.6±0.9
Adhesiolysis	3.3±0.7	2.5±0.9
Adnexal surgery	2.9±0.8	2.6±0.8
Hysterectomy	3.1±0.6	2.0±0.7
Ectopic pregnancy	2.2±0.8	
Caesarean section	2.5±0.8	

Table 5 Parameters influencing adhesion formation and the estimated likelihood on a scale from 0 (unlikely) to 4 (highly likely)

Characteristic	Median score ± SD of five-point Likert rating scale
Infections within abdomen	3.7±0.7
Extensive tissue trauma	3.7±0.6
Postoperative infections	3.6±0.8
Previous surgeries	3.6±0.6
Foreign body incompatibility	3.2±1.0
Quantity of sutures/staples/meshes	3.2±0.9
Blood in abdomen	3.2±0.9
Extensive coagulation	3.2±0.9
Chronic inflammatory bowel diseases	3.1±1.0
Affinity to reduce wound healing	2.8±0.9

Awareness of anti-adhesion agents

The survey participants were asked whether they knew and utilized the currently available anti-adhesion agents. Although the formation of adhesions was a topic of major interest for 90.3 % of 236 responders, no single agent was known by more than 60 % of them; Ringer lactate was the anti-adhesive barrier most frequently used and additionally considered as most important anti-adhesive barrier (Table 6).

Anti-adhesion agents were used on a regular basis (at least twice in the previous month) by 44.3 % of 253 responders (Table 6). Figure 5 suggest that except for Ringer lactate, use of antiadhesive barriers was positively influenced by the importance given to adhesions in daily medical and surgical work.

For 77.5 % of 236 responders, adhesion prevention was deemed cost-effective because it eliminates further adhesion-related interventions. However, a majority declared that antiadhesive barriers are too expensive and insufficiently refunded by health insurance systems (71.6 and 75.8 %, respectively).

More than 60 % of the survey participants estimated they were adequately informed about the pathogenesis of adhesions and the techniques recommended and agents proposed to prevent adhesions.

Table 3 indicates the relative importance of sources of this knowledge.

Intraoperative adhesion assessment

The criteria useful for a classification of the risk of adhesions in routine practice were the area coverage for 95.3 % of the 236 responders, the location for 93.2 %, the macroscopic evaluation for 92.4 %, the organs involved for 91.5 %, and the lysis characteristics for 79.7 %.

Discussion

This survey reflects a strong interest of participating European gynaecological surgeons in post-surgical adhesions and their prevention measures. More than 90 % of participants declared their awareness on adhesions and over 95 % agreed that good surgical practice may reduce the formation of adhesions. In line with conventional knowledge, they were a majority to consider that laparoscopic interventions are associated with a much lower incidence of adhesions than laparatomic interventions, although strong evidence supporting this assertion is lacking.

The survey participants had a good knowledge on factors associated with a high risk of post-surgical adhesion formation, similar to those quoted in the literature [10]. Surgery for endometriosis was thought to be majorly associated with the formation of adhesions, followed by myomectomy, adhesiolysis, and adnexial surgery. These results were independent of the type of surgical approach, laparotomy or laparoscopy. However, the assumption that laparoscopic adnexal surgery was associated only occasionally with a limited risk of adhesion formation, would need to be confirmed by a wider scale study.

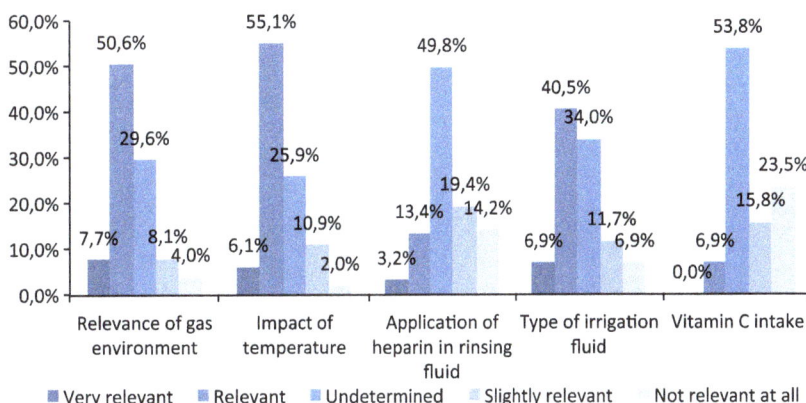

Fig. 4 Significance of some aspects of the peritoneal conditioning in the adhesions prevention (N=247)

Table 6 Summary of different adhesion prophylaxis products, knowledge of their existence, use, and importance rated on a scale from 0 (do not know this agent) to 2 (used it within the last 6 months)

Adhesion prophylaxis products	Known (% of participants)	Used (% of participants)	Importance
Ringer lactate	53.8	38.2	1.3 ± 0.6
Adept/Icodextrin 4 %	55.5	26.5	1.1 ± 0.7
Interceed®	56.3	23.9	1.0 ± 0.7
Hyalobarrier Gel®	56.3	19.3	0.9 ± 0.7
Humidified/warm CO_2	55.5	18.1	0.9 ± 0.7
Intercoat®	48.3	9.7	0.7 ± 0.6
SprayShield®	56.3	9.7	0.8 ± 0.6
Seprafilm®	63.8	4.6	0.6 ± 0.6

Most of our data are in agreement with those of a previous survey performed in 2010 among heads of gynaecological departments in Germany (Table 3) [2]. In particular, the estimated risks of post-surgical adhesions are similar in both surveys and confirm that laparoscopic procedures are commonly believed to be less adhesiogenic and cause fewer de novo adhesions compared to open surgery [11]. However, for complex laparoscopic procedures, the comparative risk of adhesion-related complications following open and laparoscopic gynaecological surgery is similar [5, 10].

The rate of information about post-surgical adhesions given to the patients (Table 3) was markedly lower in our survey than in the Hackethal survey [2]. Conversely, we report here a more frequent use of anti-adhesion agents (44.3 vs 22.0 %). Elucidating whether these differences are linked to the mode of recruitment of the two surveys (open to all gynaecological surgeons visiting the ESGE website or through a direct contact with the heads of gynaecological departments in Germany) is beyond the scope of the present work.

The data presented here suggest that efforts should be made to increase awareness of the risk of post-surgical adhesions

and knowledge of the preventive measures. About one third of surgeons considered themselves as not adequately informed about the pathogenesis of adhesions and the preventive measures. Consistent with this finding, about 40 % ignored the existence of one or more of the antiadhesive barriers currently marketed and utilization of these agents was clearly suboptimal.

Furthermore, we noted a distinct discrepancy between the knowledge of the existence of adhesion prophylaxis products of nearly more than half of the respondents (ranging from 48.3 to 63.8 %)compared to low percentage of participants routinely using barriers (ranging from 4.6 to 38.2 % regarding the usage in the last 6 months). Some products such as Seprafilm ® had an inverse ratio with the highest awareness (63.8 %) compared to low routine usage (only 4.6 %). In addition, barriers such as Icodextrin were rated as important by a large number of participants, despite the scientific evidence.

This could be explained by contortioned perception due to lack of awareness of scientific sources such as the ESGE consensus paper [9].

The fact that lactated Ringer's solution was considered as the most frequently used prevention method and ranked as most important could be explained by cost-driven considerations due to a lack of reimbursement as well clearly shows the need for evidence based education.

There is also a need for improvement of patient information and consenting about the risk of post-surgical adhesions. It has been shown in a population of patients from Germany and the UK that less than 50 % were aware of adhesions and even fewer were informed about the possible complications of adhesions; 46 % of patients cited the surgeon lack of knowledge as the reason for not informing them [12]. Comparatively, the higher rate of patient information reported by our survey participants seems encouraging—but might be due to a selection bias: the majority of surgeons that volunteered to answer our questionnaire had probably a strong interest in adhesion-related issues.

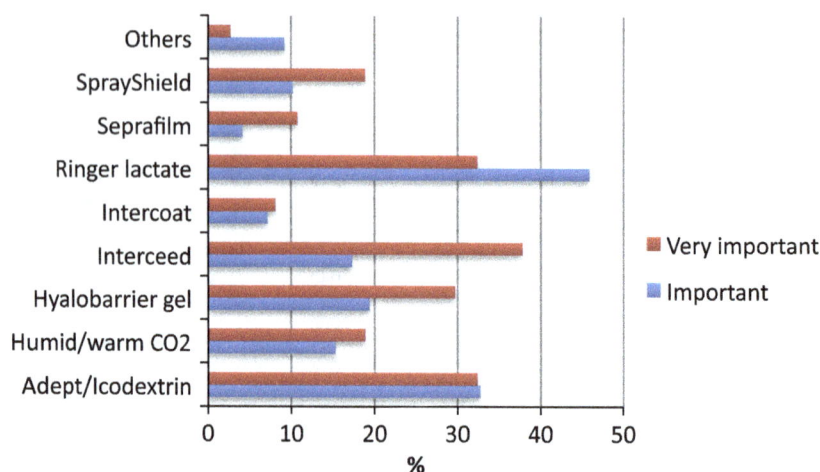

Fig. 5 Use of adhesion-reduction agents within the six previous months, as a function of importance given to adhesions in daily surgical work

Cost considerations may contribute to the limited regular use of antiadhesive barriers. These survey participants considered such barriers as too expensive and insufficiently refunded by health systems. These opinions were already expressed by the German survey participants [2]. Thus, regarding the economical impact of intraoperative utilization of antiadhesive barriers, there seems to be a gap between the opinion of gynaecological surgeons and that of decision-makers who shape national public health policies. While the former are sensitive to the potential long-term benefits of antiadhesive barriers, the latter are most probably motivated by immediate reduction of healthcare-related expenses. Furthermore, the evidence for the use of antiadhesion barriers is limited. Though, in experimental and clinical studies, adhesion reduction works in reducing adhesions, there is a lack of efficacy in terms of clinical benefits (i.e. reduction of pain and improved fertility).

Limitations of this survey should be taken into account when interpreting its results.

As all surveys, this one was based on self-reporting of information by the participants and the data were not censored. Many participants did not answer all questions and no methodology was planned to recover the missing data. Also, whether our survey describes accurately the opinions of the whole community of European gynaecological surgeons is questionable. However, the wide variation in the number of interventions performed would suggest that the participants were at least representative of the different levels of experience of European gynaecologists in current practice.

In summary, the present survey gives a broad picture of awareness of post-surgical adhesions and their reduction among European gynaecological surgeons. Results are generally encouraging but emphasize the necessity to continue educational activities in order to optimize the rate of practitioners applying the measures recommended to reduce this common complication of gynaecological surgery. In particular, a widespread dissemination of the field guidelines on the prevention of adhesions in gynaecological surgery published in 2012 [13] is warranted. An information leaflet has also been published to help surgeons inform their patients about the risk of adhesions, their potential complications, and their reduction measures [14].

Reducing the personal and economical burden of post-surgical adhesions should become a common goal for all gynaecological surgeons. The present survey shows that further efforts should be made to ensure that all women—in particular those wishing to conceive—can benefit from the solutions designed to reduce post-surgical adhesions and their complications.

Conflict of interest This study was supported by an unrestricted grant of Nordic Pharma. Michal Mara, Arnaud Wattiez, Hans Brölmann and Per Lundorff declare no conflict of interest. Philippe Robert Koninckx is stockholder of Endosat NV. Andreas Hackethal consults NordicPharma, Ethicon, Fisher&Paykel, Olympus and Terumo. Markus Wallwiener consults Nordic Pharma. Rudy Leon De Wilde consults Karl Storz, Nordic Pharma, Terumo, Actamax and Bayer. This article does not contain any studies with human or animal subjects performed by the any of the authors

References

1. Trew G, Lower A (2004) Consensus in adhesion reduction management. Obstet Gynaecol 6:1–16
2. Hackethal A, Sick C, Brueggmann D, Tchartchian G, Wallwiener M, Muenstedt K, Tinneberg HR (2010) Awareness and perception of intra-abdominal adhesions and related consequences: survey of gynaecologists in German hospitals. Eur J Obstet Gynecol Reprod Biol 150:180–189
3. DeWilde RL, Trew G, on behalf of the Expert Adhesions Working Party of the European Society of Gynaecological Endoscopy (ESGE) (2007) Postoperative abdominal adhesions and their prevention in gynaecological surgery. Expert consensus position. Gynecol Surg 4:161–168
4. Monk BJ, Berman ML, Monitz FJ (1994) Adhesions after extensive gynecologic surgery: clinical significance, etiology and prevention. Am J Obstet Gynecol 170:1396–1403
5. Diamond MP, Freeman ML (2001) Clinical implications of postsurgical adhesions. Hum Reprod Update 7:567–576
6. Kössi J, Salminen P, Rantala A, Laato M (2003) Population-based study of the surgical workload and economic impact of bowel obstruction caused by postoperative adhesions. Br J Surg 90:1441–1444
7. Brüggmann D, Tchartchian G, Wallwiener M, Münstedt K, Tinneberg HR, Hackethal A (2010) Intra-abdominal adhesions: definition, origin, significance in surgical practice, and treatment options. Dtsch Arztebl Int 107:769–775
8. Trew G, Pistofidis G, Pados G, Lower A, Mettler L, Wallwiener D, Korell M, Pouly JL, Coccia ME, Audebert A, Nappi C, Schmidt E, McVeigh E, Landi S, Degueldre M, Konincxk P, Rimbach S, Chapron C, Dallay D, Röemer T, McConnachie A, Ford I, Crowe A, Knight A, Dizerega G, Dewilde R (2011 Aug) Gynaecological endoscopic evaluation of 4 % icodextrin solution: a European, multicentre, double-blind, randomized study of the efficacy and safety in the reduction of de novo adhesions after laparoscopic gynaecological surgery. Hum Reprod 26(8):2015–2027
9. DeWilde RL, Trew G, on behalf of the Expert Adhesions Working Party of the European Society of Gynaecological Endoscopy (ESGE) (2007) Postoperative abdominal adhesions and their prevention in gynaecological surgery. Expert consensus position. Part 2—steps to reduce adhesions. Gynecol Surg 4:243–253
10. Lower AM, Hawthorn RJ, Clark D, Surgical and Clinical Research (SCAR) Group et al (2004) Adhesion-related readmissions following gynaecological laparoscopy or laparotomy in Scotland: an epidemiological study of 24 046 patients. Hum Reprod 19:1877–1885
11. Lower AM, Hawthorn RJS, Ellis H, O'Brien F, Buchan S et al (2000) The impact of adhesions on hospital readmissions over ten years after 8489 open gynecological operations: an assessment from the Surgical and Clinical Adhesions Research Study. Br J Obstet Gynaecol 107:855–862
12. Kraemer B, Birch JC, Birch JV, Petri N, Ahmad U, Marikar D, Wallwiener M, Wallwiener C, Foran A, Rajab TK (2011) Patients' awareness of postoperative adhesions: results from a multi centre study and online survey. Arch Gynecol Obstet 283:1069–1073

17

Routine vaginoscopic office hysteroscopy in modern infertility work-up: a randomized controlled trial

Atef M. Darwish · Ahmad I. Hassanin ·
Mahmoud A. Abdel Aleem · Ibraheem I. Mohammad ·
Islam H. Aboushama

Abstract This study aims to estimate the safety, efficacy, and patient acceptability of adding vaginoscopic office hysteroscopy (VOH) to the routine infertility diagnostic work-up for evaluation of the endometrial cavity. This study is a prospective comparative diagnostic trial. This study was conducted in a tertiary care referral facility and university hospital. This study comprised a total of 156 infertile patients scheduled for laparoscopy. Seventy-eight patients had VOH on one stop bases in addition to the usual infertility work-up and were assigned as group B while a similar number was examined by the usual diagnostic work-up and assigned as group A. The main outcome measure is the diagnostic accuracy of VOH alone in comparison to hysterosalpingography (HSG) and diagnostic laparoscopy (DL) and assessment of combined VOH and HSG in diagnosing intrauterine abnormalities. There was insignificant difference between both groups regarding socio-demographic and HSG data. Abnormal DL findings were more significant in group A. VOH detected 50 % abnormal endometrial cavity in group B with a significant superiority over HSG. There was a high percentage of agreement in the diagnosis of uterine abnormalities between HSG and VOH (96 %). Generally, VOH was an acceptable procedure with mild pain and feasible in most cases. Adding VOH to the routine diagnostic work-up of infertile couples prior to laparoscopy seems to be a feasible, safe, simple, tolerable, and quick outpatient procedure. It can diagnose intrauterine abnormalities in about a quarter of infertile women with normal HSG. VOH has an additional value to HSG and DL in diagnosing uterine. Nevertheless, whether its use would increase pregnancy rate among infertile women requires a further longitudinal comparative study.

Keywords Vaginoscopic · Office hysteroscopy · Infertility · Hysterosalpingography · Laparoscopy

Introduction

Diagnosis of infertility causes requires comprehensive testing on both partners. On the female side, infertility testing usually involves hormonal testing to determine the patient's ovarian reserve, diagnostic imaging to see if there are any anatomical problems (such as blocked fallopian tubes or uterine fibroids), and immunological testing to rule out any maternal autoimmunity. Knowing the root cause of a couple's infertility is the first step toward successful fertility treatment.

Unexplained infertility is infertility that is idiopathic in the sense that its cause remains unknown even after an infertility work-up, usually including semen analysis in the man and assessment of ovulation and fallopian tubes in the woman. The available diagnostic tools for intrauterine causes of infertility include transvaginal ultrasonogragoy, hysterosalpingography (HSG), or sonohysterography [1]. Manifest uterine causes may include intrauterine adhesions, polypi, or uterine cavity malformations. Hidden uterine factors may include infections, thin endometrium, poor endometrial receptivity, and immunological incompatibility which have received the most attention in recent years. Most of the uterine causes of infertility can be easily diagnosed using hysteroscopy. Moreover, we frequently predict tubal patency at hysteroscopy by noticing suction of air bubbles by the patent ostium.

Office hysteroscopy is an exciting modern diagnostic tool with expanding popularity all over the world [2]. Adding vaginoscopic approach to office hysteroscopy is an extra simplification of the procedure with elimination of pain during

A. M. Darwish (✉) · A. I. Hassanin · M. A. A. Aleem ·
I. I. Mohammad · I. H. Aboushama
Department of Obstetrics and Gynecology, Woman's Health
University Center, Assiut University, P.O. Box (1) Assiut,
Assiut 71111, Egypt
e-mail: atef_darwish@yahoo.com

examination [3]. Delicate instrumentation of operative office hysteroscopy enabled successful operations even through an intact hymen [4].

Regarding the role of vaginoscopic office hysteroscopy (VOH) in infertility, a lot of the published work on VOH demonstrates the feasibility of the procedure and highlights the possible advantages and the skills of the surgeons. The question is not whether the procedure is feasible or not, but whether VOH is superior to and beneficial to a particular patient as well as cost effective for the community at large. This study aims to estimate the safety, efficacy, and patient acceptability of adding VOH to the routine infertility diagnostic work-up for evaluation of the endometrial cavity.

Patients and methods

After obtaining the acceptance of the ethics committee of Assiut Faculty of Medicine, this study was conducted in the outpatient hysteroscopy unit of the Woman's Health University Hospital from February 2011 to December 2012. It included infertile women referred for diagnostic/operative laparoscopy. Patients were randomly classified into two groups using a computer-generated numbers in sealed envelops with 1/1 ratio. Dr. Islam was the one responsible for the process of randomization and patient allocation. Group A included usual infertility work-up in the form of normal hormonal profile, basic transvaginal ultrasonography (TVS), normal husband' semen analysis, and a recent HSG. Group B included the same diagnostic tools in addition to VOH. Sample size was estimated utilizing (PS) computer program. For detecting assumed 15 % difference in the rate of abnormal intrauterine findings between group A (10 %) and group B (25 %) with 80 % power at 5 % significance level, it was found that 78 patients are required in each group. Exclusion criteria included suspected pregnancy, active pelvic infection, severe co-morbidity, e.g., severe cardiac, neurologic, or chest disease, other medical contraindications to pregnancy, male factor, or abnormal hormonal profile of both couples. All patients had clear description of the study and were asked to participate. An informed consent was taken from those who agreed.

The included patients were subjected to complete history taking and meticulous physical examination. VOH was done using a 2.9-mm 30° rigid scope with 4-mm single flow sheath (Promis, Tutlingen, Germany), and the uterus was distended with normal saline at 100 mmHg generated from a pneumatic cuff of sphygmomanometer. We used a 250-W Xenon light source for the video OH. The scope was introduced gently through the vulva, vagina, and then the cervical canal without previous dilatation using the saline to expand the way in front of the scope. The cervical canal was examined for polypi, Nabothian cysts, or micropolypi suggestive of chronic cervicitis. The best view of the entire uterus cavity is obtained when the hysteroscope is placed at the junction of the lower

uterine segment and upper cervical canal. The uterine cavity was examined systematically starting by its anterior and posterior walls, the fundus, and the borders, and examination was considered complete if the both tubal ostia were reached describing any gross pathology, e.g., septum, adhesions, polyp, myoma, growth, etc. The primary outcome measure was the feasibility and ability for the diagnosing intrauterine abnormalities by VOH versus HSG. Secondary measures included the accuracy of combination of methods in diagnosing the cause of infertility and patient acceptance of VOH.

Categorical date were described as percentages and compared with chi square and exact Fischer tests. Continuous data were described as mean±SD or median (according to data distribution) and compared using t test, Mann-Whitney test, and ANOVA test with LSD post hoc test when appropriate. Correlation was used when appropriate. Simple agreement was calculated as a percentage of the number of cases agreed by both methods as positive plus those agreed by both methods as negative and divided by the total number of cases. A probability value (P value) less than 0.05 was considered statistically significant. All statistical calculations were done using computer programs Microsoft Excel version 7 (Microsoft Corporation, NY, USA) and SPSS 16 (Statistical Package for the Social Science; SPSS Inc., Chicago).

Results

We examined 659 patients referred for diagnostic/operative laparoscopy. Of those, 215 had abnormal semen parameter(s), 201 had an ovulation, 63 had no HSG, and 48 refused to participate (some women had more than one cause for exclusion).

This study comprised 156 infertile women who were divided into two groups (78 each), and all completed all examinations. Group A included patients without VOH, while group B included women with VOH. There was no statistically significant difference between both groups regarding age distribution ($P=0.26$), type and duration of infertility ($P=0.73$), or sociodemographic data ($P=0.32$). The same insignificant difference was applied for HSG findings in both groups (Table 1). However, laparoscopic findings were evidently abnormal in group A than group B with a statistically significant difference as shown in Table 2. VOH detected 50 % abnormal endometrial cavity in group B with a significant superiority over HSG (Table 3). Diagnostic indices of VOH and HSG are shown in Table 4. There was agreement in the diagnosis of uterine abnormalities between HSG and VOH in 80 %. Generally, VOH was an acceptable procedure with mild pain and feasible in all except two cases as shown in Table 5.

Table 1 HSG findings of both groups

	Group A (n=78)		Group B (n=78)		P value
	No.	%	No.	%	
Normal cases	52	66.7	50	64.1	0.736
Abnormal cases:	26	33.3	28	35.9	0.736
Uterine abnormalities					
Unicornuite uterus	1	1.3	0	0.0	
Uterine septum	0	0.0	8	10.3	
Arcuate uterus	0	0.0	1	1.3	
Intrauterine adhesions	0	0.0	1	1.3	
Tubal abnormalities:					
Bilateral tubal block	13	16.7	5	6.4	
Unilateral tubal block	9	11.5	3	3.8	
Filling defect	0	0.0	5	6.4	
Pelvic adhesions	3	3.8	5	6.4	

Discussion

There is a general consensus but not evidence-based agreement that basic tests of infertility work-up should include normal semen analysis, ovulation detection test, tubal patency testing, and hormonal profile. Some authors add postcoital test [5]. Non-universal agreement on the steps and stratification of diagnostic tools can be attributed to wide variations of the infertile population regarding age, duration of marriage, primary or secondary infertility, psychologic status of the couple, and the interest of the infertility team. It has been noticed that some centers interested in ART push patients to try IUI or IVF/ICSI without prior laparoscopy or even HSG. Many subsequent failures can be attributed to abnormal uterine cavity or distended hydrosalpingeal tubes which are unfortunately diagnosed too late in many cases. These alarming data call for more strict infertility work-up that should be supported by big infertility societies.

Table 2 Laparoscopic findings of the studied groups

	Group A (n=78)		Group B (n=78)		P value
	No.	%	No.	%	
Normal cases	34	43.6	57	73.1	<0.0001*
Abnormal cases	44	56.4	21	26.9	<0.0001*
Tubal block	11	14.1	9	11.5	
Ovarian abnormalities	14	17.9	6	7.7	
Uterine abnormalities	6	7.7	2	2.6	
Endometriosis	8	10.3	4	5.1	
Extensive adhesions	5	6.4	0	0.0	

*Means highly significant

Table 3 The appearance of endometrial cavity by HSG and VOH among group B population (78 cases)

	HSG		Office hysteroscopy		P value
	No.	%	No.	%	
Normal cases	60	76.9	38	50.0	0.001*
Abnormal cases	18	23.1	38	50.0	0.001*
Endometrial hyperplasia	0	0.0	5	6.6	
Polyp	5	6.4	11	14.5	
Fibroid	0	0.0	4	5.3	
Adhesions	5	6.4	7	9.2	
Septum	8	10.3	11	14.5	
Total	78	100.0	76[a]	100.0	

[a] Two cases were invisible by office hysteroscopy

*Means highly significant

Infertility related to uterine cavity abnormalities has been estimated to be the causal factor in as many as 10 to 15 %. Moreover, abnormal uterine findings have been found in 34 to 62 % of infertile women. This had been traditionally carried out using HSG. Hysteroscopy despite being a well-known standard diagnostic tool for intrauterine lesions was not widely used for this purpose due to technical difficulties [6,7]. The concept of office outpatient hysteroscopy is expanding worldwide with a lot of publications. In this study, we carried out an infertility work-up algorithm based on four cornerstone steps: semen analysis, HSG, and laparoscopy±office hysteroscopy in 78 women (group B) to judge the value of the latter method. The prevalence of abnormalities was remarkable (50 %). Of these, 14.5 % were uterine or cervical polypi. Similarly, polpi were diagnosed in 21.96 % [8]. We diagnosed uterine septa, submucous tiny myomata, and adhesions in 14.5, 5.3, and 9.2 % of cases, respectively. These figures are more or less similar to other studies [8]. Finally, we found thickened endometrium in 6.6 % women in this study. Detection of delicate endometrial lesions is a marvelous advantage of OH over other diagnostic tools. In a previous study, this team could diagnose endometrial lesions that could not be seen by other tools [2].

Table 4 Diagnostic accuracy of single versus combined tests for assessment of uterine factor among group B

	HSG Vs VOH[a]	VOH+HSG
Sensitivity	39.47	97.4 %
Specificity	100.00	56.2 %
Positive predictive value	100.0	80.9 %
Negative predictive value	62.3	90 %
Accuracy	69.7	59.2 %
AUC	0.697	0.521

[a] Agreement between both tests was 80 %

Table 5 Pain grading, acceptability, and feasibility of VOH

	No. (n=78)	Percent
Pain grading		
Mild painful	5	6.4
Moderate painful	3	3.8
Severe painful	1	1.3
Painless	69	88.5
Acceptability		
Tolerable	78	100.0
Not tolerable	0	0.0
Feasibility		
Feasible	76	97.4
Not feasible	2	2.6

In about two third of infertility cases, hysteroscopy findings were not correlated with those found on HSG [9]. Moreover, they reported that 54.3 % of intrauterine adhesions diagnosed on HSG were not found on direct hysteroscopic examination. Diagnosing some missed intrauterine abnormalities with the aid of VOH despite normal HSG would highlight the central role of this outpatient procedure in eliminating unneeded lengthy induction of ovulation and even IVF/ICSI repeated trials. Furthermore, VOH allows the exact localization of intrauterine lesions and provides a better way than the blunt curettage to ensure complete excision of such lesion. Most importantly, VOH would save money and omit stress for the patient and will improve health care services for the community. Practically, vaginoscopic approach with elimination of speculum insertion and traction on the cervix with a tenaculum had made hysteroscopy as simple as vaginal examination with high patient acceptability of this procedure in this study. Nevertheless, whether adding VOH to the infertility workup prior to DL is better than performing concomitant conventional 4-mm hysteroscopy at the time of DL routinely has not yet been studied. Based on our experience, pre-DL VOH has the advantage of diagnosing any intrauterine abnormalities that would require operative hysteroscopy with proper preparation of the cervix, informing an experienced hysteroscopist, and preparing a suitable operative hysteroscopy set at the time of DL.

In this study, there was 81.6 % of normal laparoscopy that were also normal in HSG and this seems to be logical based on

Fig. 1 CONSORT 2010 flow diagram

CONSORT 2010 Flow Diagram

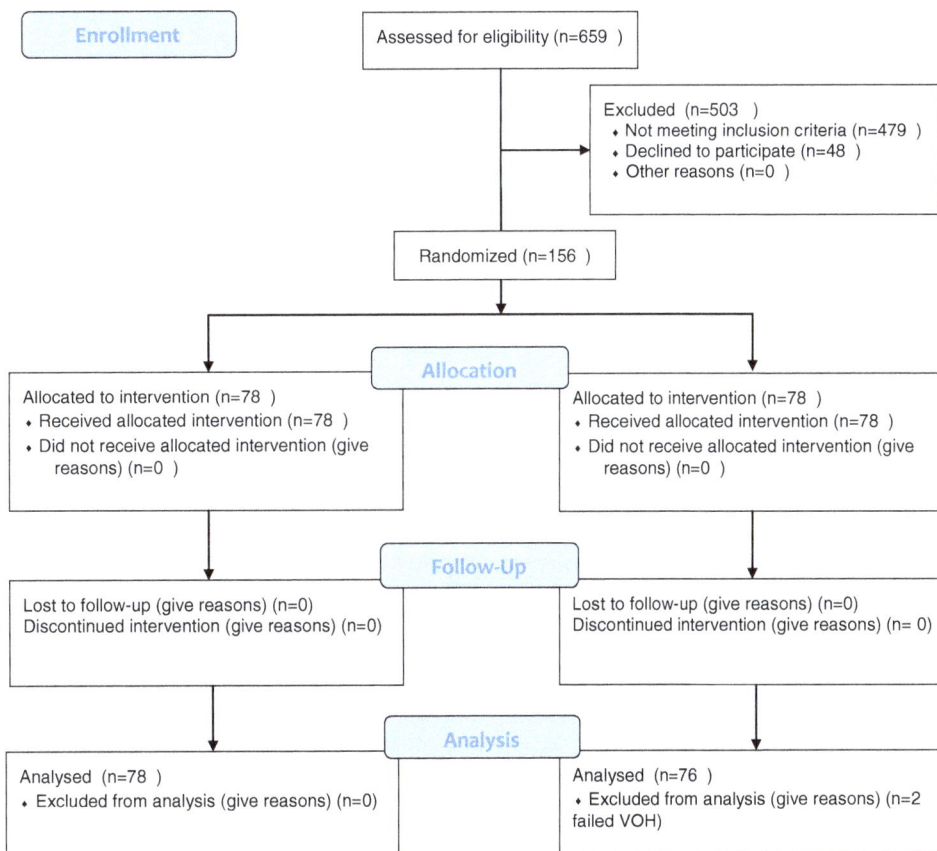

the different view they demonstrate (external versus internal). When VOH is combined with HSG, the accuracy is 59.2 %. The degree of agreement was as high as 80 % between VOH and HSG in this conclusion regarding the uterus. Small sample size as well as heterogeneity of infertile women without classification into primary and secondary infertility is a clear drawback of this study. Lack of another group of patients with concomitant conventional hysteroscopy and laparoscopy to be compared with preoperative VOH is an evident disadvantage of this study. From this study, VOH seems to be a feasible, safe, simple, tolerable, and quick outpatient procedure. It can diagnose intrauterine abnormalities in 23.7 % of infertile women with normal HSG. VOH achieves marvelous agreement with HSG in diagnosing uterine abnormalities (96 %). We recommend adding VOH to the routine diagnostic work-up of infertile couples prior to laparoscopy. Nevertheless, whether its use would eventually increase pregnancy rate among infertile women requires a further longitudinal comparative study (Fig. 1).

Informed consent All procedures followed were in accordance with the ethical standards of the responsible committee on human experimentation (institutional and national) and with the Helsinki Declaration of 1975, as revised in 2000 [5]. Informed consent was obtained from all patients for being included in the study.

References

1. Darwish AM, Youssef AA (1999) Screening sonohysterography in infertility. Gynecol Obstet Invest 48(1):43–47
2. Darwish AM, Sayed EH, Mohammad SA, Mohammad II, Hassan HI (2012) Reliability of out-patient hysteroscopy in one-stop clinic for abnormal uterine bleeding. Gynecologic Surgery 9(3):289–295
3. Emanuel MH. New developments in hysteroscopy. Best Pract Res Clin Obstet Gynaecol. 2013 Feb 2. pii: S1521-6934(13)00005-9.
4. Joseph N, Al Chami AG, Musa AA, Nassar AH, Kurdi A, Ghulmiyyah LH. Vaginoscopic Resection of vaginal septum. Surg Technol Int. 2012 Dec 30;XXII. pii: sti22/41.
5. Eimers JM, te Velde ER, Gerritse R, van Kooy RJ, Kremer J, Habbema JD (1994) The validity of the postcoital test for estimating the probability of conceiving. Am J Obstet Gynecol 171(1):65–70
6. Dechaud H, Daures JP, Hedon B (1998) Prospective evaluation of falloposcopy. Hum Reprod 13:1815–1818
7. Glatstein IZ, Sleeper LA, Lavy Y, Simon A, Adoni A, Palti Z, Hurwitz A, Laufer N (1997) Observer variability in the diagnosis and management of hysterosalpingogram. Fertil Steril 67:223–237
8. Bettocchi S, Nappi L, Ceci O, Selvaggi L (2004) Office hystroscoy. Obstet Gynecol Clin North Am 31(3):641–654
9. Kessler I, Lancet M (1986) Hysterography and hysteroscopy: a comparison. Fertil Steril 46:709–710

18

Hysteroscopic diagnosis and excision of myometrial cystic adenomyosis

S. Gordts · R. Campo · I. Brosens

Abstract In 1908, Cullen described the first cases of cystic adenomyosis in his textbook on adenomyomata. Although not very common, with the introduction of noninvasive imaging techniques such as magnetic resonance imaging (MRI) and 3-D transvaginal ultrasound, an increasing number of cases have been reported. Patients primarily complain of severe dysmenorrhea, chronic pelvic pain, and dysfunctional uterine bleeding. Currently, it is unclear whether adenomyosis and, more specifically, cystic adenomyosis can be an underlying reason for impaired fertility and reproductive outcome. With the postponement of childbearing, the number of patients with adenomyosis and cystic adenomyosis seeking fertility treatment is increasing. Therefore, in these patients, uterine exploration should include not only the evaluation of the endometrial cavity but also the exploration of the sub-endometrial zone. Indirect imaging techniques, combined with office mini-hysteroscopy, offer the possibility of complete uterine exploration. Two patients with cystic adenomyosis are described in this paper: one had the chief complaint of menorrhagia and the other was referred for evaluation of infertility and severe dysmenorrhea. The aim of these case reports is to present hysteroscopic dissection and ablation of adenomyotic cysts as an alternative procedure for the surgical management of this condition.

Keywords Adenomyosis · Cystic · Hysteroscopy · Diagnosis · Treatment

Background

The uterine adenomyotic cyst is a cystic structure lined with endometrial tissue and surrounded by myometrial tissue that, in most cases, contains hemorrhagic material. Cullen [1] described the first cases in 1908 in his textbook on adenomyomata, in which he distinguished submucosal and subperitoneal cystic adenomyomata. In contrast to diffuse adenomyosis, the disease primarily occurs in adolescents and women younger than 30 years and is not associated with diffuse uterine adenomyosis [2].

The clinical symptoms are nonspecific and include dysmenorrhea starting at an early age around the time of menarche, chronic pelvic pain, and dysfunctional uterine bleeding. The dysmenorrhea tends to progressively increase and is resistant to therapy with analgesics or cyclic oral contraceptives. When viewed with ultrasound, the cyst increases in size at the time of menstruation and hormonal suppression with continuous oral contraceptive pills results in a partial regression [3].

Since the introduction of imaging techniques, an increasing number of cases have been described in adolescents and young adult women with untreatable dysmenorrhea. Currently, the diagnosis is primarily based on magnetic resonance imaging (MRI) criteria or 3-D ultrasound; it appears as a cystic structure with an internal diameter of ≥ 10 mm, with hemorrhagic content surrounded by myometrial tissue. The disease has received significant attention in Japan where more than 11 cases of cystic adenomyomata have been described [4, 5].

In a review of cystic adenomyosis of the uterus, Brosens et al. [2] defined three subtypes (A, B, and C) according to the location of the cyst and complexity of the lesion: subtype A1 includes the submucous or intramural cystic adenoma, subtype A2 includes cases with a cystic polypoid lesion, subtype B1 includes subserous cystic adenomyosis, subtype B2

S. Gordts (✉) · R. Campo · I. Brosens
Leuven Institute for Fertility & Embryology, Tiensevest 168, 3000 Leuven, Belgium
e-mail: stephan.gordts@lifeleuven.be

includes cases with exophytic growth, and subtype C comprises uterine-like masses.

Medical treatment in adolescents includes the continuous use of an oral contraceptive [2, 4]. The use of a progestogen-loaded intrauterine device has been suggested for subtype A cystic adenomyosis [6]. In young women under menstruation-suppression therapy, the cyst has been shown to regress [3].

In most cases, surgical excision is performed via laparotomy; however, in recent years, laparoscopy has been employed [4, 5]. Hysteroscopy is commonly used for exploring the uterine cavity [7–9]. The cyst may bulge into the uterine cavity, and changes, such as abnormal vascularization or fibrosis, may be observed in the endometrium at the site of the cyst. Lowering the intrauterine pressure is helpful for a better identification of the submucosal cystic structures.

Ryo et al. [10] used a radio-frequency needle inserted via the cervix under ultrasound guidance for ablation of the cyst. Giana et al. [11] described hysteroscopic removal of a polypoid adenomyotic cyst. The 2-cm cystic mass arising from the posterior right lateral wall of the uterus was surrounded by hemorrhagic endometrium and a thin layer of myometrium. The cyst did not appear to communicate with the endometrial cavity, and it was deflated by aspiration of a brownish yellow dense fluid. The cyst wall was removed. Microscopic examination revealed that the cyst was lined by endometrial epithelium and several adenomyotic foci. The aim of these two case reports is to highlight the possible use of operative hysteroscopy, using mechanical dissection and ablative bipolar current, as an alternative surgical option for the treatment of cystic adenomyosis.

Material and methods

Mini-hysteroscopes are commonly used for the exploration of the uterine cavity. Through a gliding system, the Trophy° hysteroscope (Karl Storz, Germany) offers the possibility to change from a diagnostic 2.9-mm hysteroscope to an operative 4.4-mm scope without the need to remove the hysteroscope. Through the operative channel, 5-Fr instruments (scissors, bipolar needle, and bipolar coagulation probes) are used for dissection or coagulation.

In addition to the direct visualization of the uterine cavity, the hysteroscopic approach offers the possibility of obtaining endometrial/myometrial biopsies under visual control and/or ultrasound guidance. The biopsy of focal endometriotic lesions and/or a hyperplastic junctional zone is technically difficult, if not impossible, to perform. A new device, the Utero-Spirotome (Fig. 1), offers the possibility of a direct and frontal (D&F) tissue harvest. This procedure allows the biopsy of endomyometrial layers. Significant experience with this biopsy system exists in breast applications where efficacy and safety have been fully documented (12, 13). The Utero-

Spirotome operates with two devices in tandem: the receiving needle with a cutting helix at the distal end, and a cutting cannula as an outer sheet. The correct direction and position of the helix point is under continuous ultrasonographic imaging and hysteroscopic control. Under ultrasound guidance, the spirotome can be directed towards any intramural localized lesion such as cystic adenomyosis, thus creating a visible hysteroscopic channel that allows access to the cystic cavity.

Both patients gave their written informed consent.

Case 1

A 44-year-old woman was referred to our unit with a history of secondary infertility of 12-month duration. Hysteroscopy revealed the presence of an intracavitary 2-cm myoma, which was removed at that time by an operative hysteroscopic procedure. After the second IVF cycle, the patient became pregnant; however, the pregnancy was terminated as a missed abortion at 8-week gestation. Because of her age, she had no further desire for pregnancy. In 2007, the patient, now 51 years old, was again referred to us for evaluation of menorrhagia.

Using a mini-hysteroscope and fluid as a distension medium, hysteroscopy was performed; it revealed the presence of a small opening in the fundus and a bulging area of abnormal vascularization on the anterior wall (Fig. 2). The abnormal vascularization became clearly visible after lowering the intrauterine pressure. Opening of the cystic bulging at the place of abnormal vascularization with 5-Fr scissors resulted in the outflow of a brownish fluid. An internal view of the cyst showed the presence of a somewhat fibrotic wall and areas of endometrial-like tissue. The lesion was completely resected with 5-Fr scissors.

Histologic examination revealed a cystic structure lined by endometrial epithelium and surrounded by myometrium, compatible with benign cystic adenomyosis (Fig. 3).

Case 2

A 38-year-old woman was referred to our center with a history of primary subfertility of 3-year duration. Previously, at another facility, a laparoscopic left salpingo-oophorectomy had been performed for severe endometriosis. An intramural cyst was diagnosed via MRI preoperatively, and the cyst was punctured and aspirated under ultrasound guidance during the operative laparoscopy. Because of recurrence of this intramural cyst, patient was referred to our center for hysteroscopic treatment.

Vaginal ultrasound imaged the persistence of a cystic adenomyotic cyst at the isthmic level of the uterus (Fig. 4). At hysteroscopy, the endometrial cavity had a normal appearance and there were no direct visible signs of the presence of this cystic structure. Using the hysteroscope with ultrasound guidance, the cystic lesion was localized. After removal of the

Fig. 1 Utero-Spirotome mounted in outer sheet of Trophy° hysteroscope

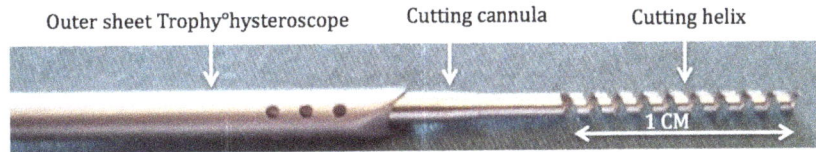

endoscope, the spirotome was inserted in the outer hysteroscopic sheet, and under ultrasound guidance, it was directed towards the cystic structure. A turning movement inserts the helix of the spirotome into the cystic structure. After withdrawal of the spirotome, the hysteroscope was reinstalled in the outer sheet. The spirotome created a clearly visible channel at hysteroscopic examination, allowing access to the cystic structure. Endometrial-like tissue was visible within the cyst. The inner cystic wall was coagulated using the small bipolar resectoscope and the bipolar coagulating probe. Another hysteroscopy 10 weeks after the first showed a normal uterine cavity with no adhesions and a slightly inflamed endometrial cavity. The patient underwent 2 months of GnRha therapy and was referred to our IVF program. Because a pregnancy did not develop following three IVF cycles and the patient suffered a recurrence of menorrhagia, another MRI was performed that revealed a focal enlargement of the junctional zone present at the mid-third of the uterine corpus. Another 3-month cycle of GnRha was planned before another IVF attempt.

Discussion

The present cases illustrate the possibility of hysteroscopy for diagnosis and resection or ablation of intramural cystic adenomyosis. Although diagnostic hysteroscopy does not reveal the pathognomonic signs of adenomyosis, some studies suggests that an irregular endometrium with endometrial defects, altered vascularization, and cystic hemorrhagic lesion are possibly associated with adenomyosis [9].

With the use of MRI imaging and 3-D ultrasound adenomyosis, junctional zone hyperplasia and adenomyotic cysts can now be detected in younger patients during their reproductive years. The use of 3-D vaginal ultrasound for the diagnosis of a junctional zone abnormality or adenomyotic pathology has been extensively described by Exacoustos et al. [14] and can now be implemented in patients seeking fertility treatment. As patients are postponing their desire to conceive, we can expect an increasing incidence of adenomyotic pathology in patients with fertility problems.

Fig. 2 Case no. 1. **a** Cystic adenomyotic lesion at transvaginal ultrasound. **b** Abnormal vascularization and detail of the opened cyst after outflow of the brownish fluid. **c** Inside view of the cystic structure. **d** Dissection of cyst using 5-Fr scissors

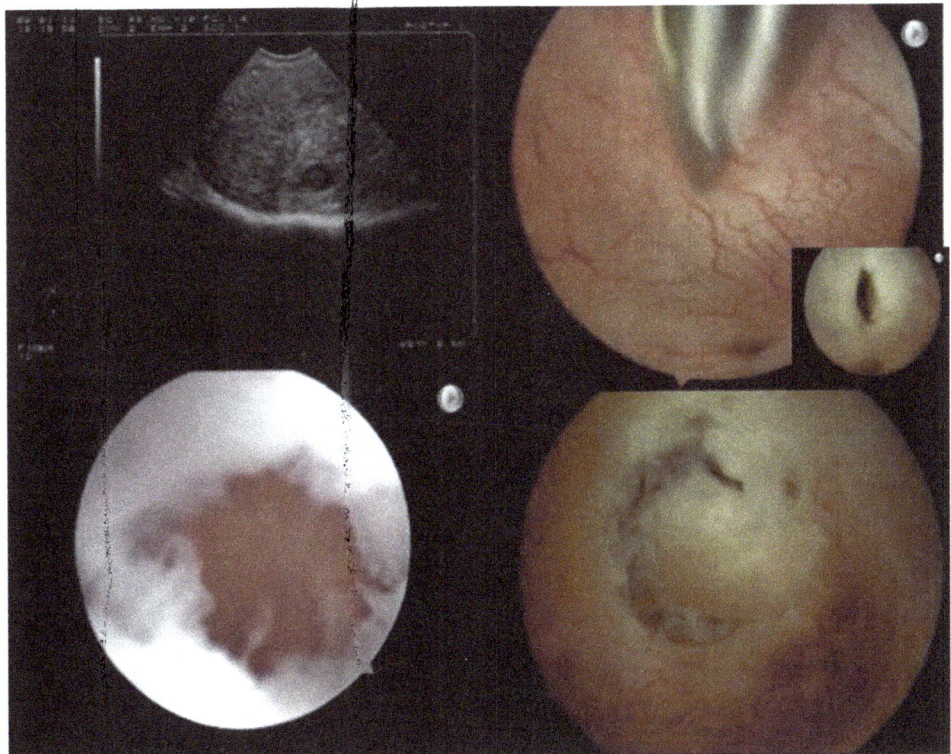

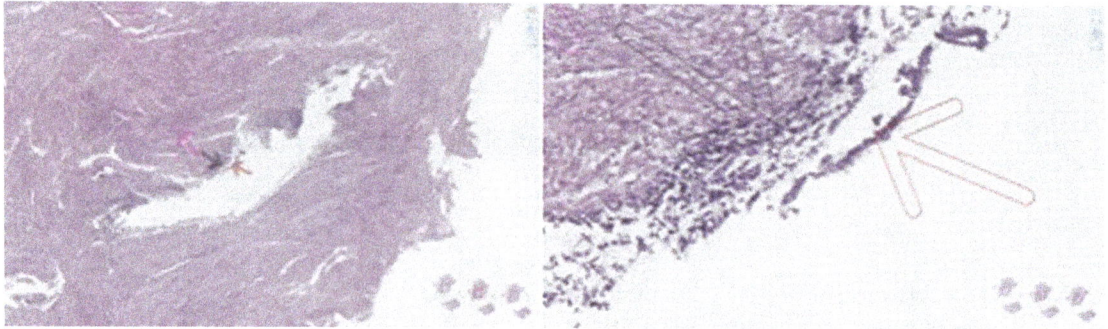

Fig. 3 Histologic image. *Red arrow* endometrial epithelium. *Black arrow* stroma. *Purple arrow* myometrium

Brosens et al. [2] suggested the acronym MUSCLE for the classification of the cystic adenomyosis: M= myometrial location (intramural, submucous, subserous), U= uterine site (midline, paramedian, lateral); S= structure (cystic, mixed, polypoid), C= contents (clear, hemorrhagic), L= level (fundus, body, cervix), and E= endometrial or inner lining (endometrium,

Fig. 4 Case no. 2. **I** Ultrasound and MRI image of cystic lesion right isthmic part. **II** *a* Access to cystic structure after ultrasound-guided creation of channel to intramural cyst, *b* widening of access to cyst using a bipolar resectoscope, *c* insight view of cyst, *d* coagulation of insight cyst using a bipolar loop resectoscope

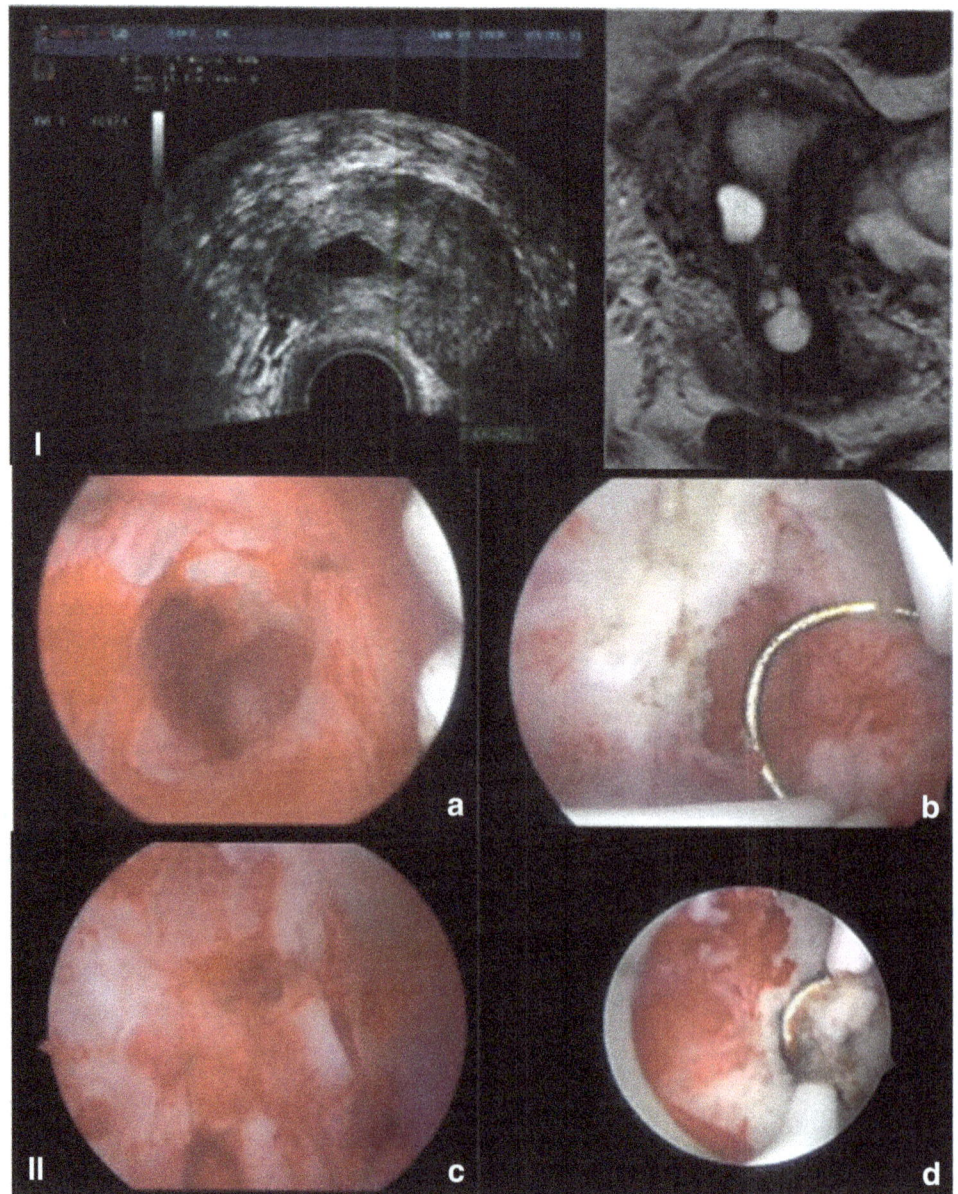

metaplastic). The first patient can be classified as M(2)U(2)S(1) C(2)L(2)E(1) and the second as M(1)U(2)S(1)C(2)L(2)E(1). To distinguish the condition from other intramural cysts, histologic diagnosis is necessary to identify the endometrial inner layering and the presence of outer myometrium.

In cases of submucous cystic adenomyotic lesions or an adenomyoma bulging into the uterine cavity, direct hysteroscopic access is possible. Using 5-Fr scissors during hysteroscopy allows a clear dissection of the myometrial wall of the cyst from the surrounding myometrium. Instead of dissection with scissors, an ablative technique that destroys the inner cystic wall is a possible treatment option. We believe that this ablative approach is preferable for those cysts localized deeper in the intramural portion. In contrast to the healing process after hysteroscopic myomectomy, where a normal uterine cavity is expected, resection or ablation of adenomyotic cysts bulging into the uterine cavity results in a visible defect of the myometrium.

In cases in which intramural cystic structures are present, ultrasound guidance is mandatory for localization of the cystic structure. The spirotome offers the possibility of penetrating the cyst and leaving behind a visible channel allowing hysteroscopic entrance into the cystic structure for an ablative procedure using bipolar current.

It is currently unclear whether cases of intramural cystic adenomyosis, which do not communicate with the endometrial cavity, can be adequately treated with an ablative procedure or should be managed by enlarging the cyst opening to allow communication with the endometrial cavity.

The hysteroscopic technique has the advantage of leaving the outer myometrium intact and avoiding an abdominal scar. Because the incidence of adenomyosis is increasing with age and women are postponing their childbearing, increases of incidence of adenomyotic pathology in those patients referred for fertility treatment can be expected. Therefore, uterine exploration should not only focus on a careful inspection of the endometrial cavity but also entail an evaluation of the uterine wall with special attention to the junctional zone. This can routinely be performed in an office setting using 3-D vaginal ultrasound and office mini-hysteroscopy.

Cystic adenomyosis represents a specific entity of adenomyosis and has to be distinguished from other intramural cystic structures. The diagnosis necessitates a histologic examination showing endometrial epithelial lining of the inner cystic wall with surrounding outer myometrium. The differential diagnosis in adolescents includes the congenital anomaly of a hematometra in a non-communicating horn; therefore, hysteroscopy is indicated to observe both tubal openings and the presence of a normal endometrial cavity [15]. In younger women, Acien et al. [16] have described comparable cystic structures as accessory cavitated uterine masses (ACUMs). The lesions were primarily isolated cysts located at the insertion of the round ligament without infringement on the uterine cavity. He suggested that these lesions might arise from persistence of ductal Müllerian tissue near the round ligament. At present, there is no consensus regarding the most appropriate way to treat these lesions and the need of treatment for infertility patients. Thalluri and Tremelen [17] reported an impaired clinical pregnancy rate in patients with adenomyosis (23.6 versus 44.6 % in controls) undergoing IVF treatment using an antagonist ovarian stimulation protocol. A lower clinical pregnancy rate and higher spontaneous abortion rate are also reported in the meta-analysis of Vercellini et al. [18]. A conservative fertility-sparing technique is preferable. A laparoscopic cystectomy for a limited number of patients has been described in the Japanese literature [4, 5, 19, 20]. Takeuchi [4] described the use of laparoscopic cystectomy in nine cases with a reduction of pain postoperatively; two of three patients who desired to conceive became pregnant afterwards; however, the time between intervention and conception was 2 and 7 years. Also, Kriplani [21] reported on the laparoscopic treatment of four patients who experienced a reduction of pain postoperatively. Akar [22] described the use of robotics for performing a resection of cystic adenomyosis. Reduction of pain has been described after simple transvaginal aspiration of the fluid content [23].

If larger cystic adenomyotic structures localized in the outer intramural third are present, a laparoscopic approach is preferable. Although the cyst is unencapsulated (unlike the myoma), complete removal is possible, in contrast to focal or diffuse adenomyosis. Of the reported adenomyotic cysts [2], only 13 % had a diameter greater than 50 mm and 40 % were smaller than 25 mm. In these smaller structures, laparoscopic identification can be difficult. In these cases, laparoscopic access can cause significant trauma to the myometrial wall. Most laparoscopic resections have been performed for severe dysmenorrhea and/or dysfunctional uterine bleeding. Fertility was not a major factor in these patients. For patients desirous of pregnancy, a procedure with the highest fertility preservation and minimal trauma must be chosen. As in cases of a small adenomyoma, our experience showed that when smaller cystic structures were present in the inner third of the intramural part or submucosally, a minimally invasive hysteroscopic approach is possible. Some of the lesions are directly recognizable at hysteroscopy because they bulge into the endometrial cavity, thus favoring a minimally invasive dissection. For lesions localized deeper in the intramural portion, the spirotome can be introduced under ultrasound guidance; it creates a channel and provides hysteroscopic access to the cystic structure. Treatment by resection or ablation can then be performed.

Giana et al. [11] described the use of a bipolar resectoscope for the treatment of a cystic adenomyosis in a 46-year-old woman. In a report by Kumar [24], an intramural cyst was inadvertently opened during an ablative procedure for dysfunctional uterine bleeding. After exclusion of the possibility of uterine perforation, the procedure was continued. Histology confirmed the diagnosis of an adenomyotic cyst.

Conclusions

The incidence of adenomyosis in patients with infertility is unclear. An estimated prevalence in patients with endometriosis has been reported to be approximately 70 % [25], and Brosens et al. [26] reported an incidence of 50 % in patients with subfertility, dysmenorrhea, and dysfunctional uterine bleeding. Cystic adenomyosis is a somewhat rare form of adenomyosis; however, with more women delaying pregnancy and with the availability of accurate and easy accessible indirect imaging techniques such as 3-D ultrasound, we can expect that more women seeking assisted reproduction will be diagnosed with adenomyosis and cystic adenomyosis. Together with office mini-hysteroscopy, a complete exploration of the uterus can now be performed including the endometrial cavity and the myometrial layers. Hysteroscopy offers the possibility of clear visualization of intracavitary lesions with a direct access to cystic adenomyosis. Treatment can be performed by mechanical dissection or bipolar ablative surgery. The spirotome allows performing a direct forward biopsy, and under ultrasound guidance, access is gained to intramural cystic lesions without visible intracavitary components. Hysteroscopy offers an alternative access for the treatment of cystic adenomyosis while producing minimal tissue damage. Further research is needed to better understand the impact of cystic adenomyosis on fertility and the possible beneficial effect of surgical removal.

Ethical standard   All procedures followed were in accordance with the ethical standards of the responsible committee on human experimentation (institutional and national) and with the Helsinki Declaration of 1975, as revised in 2000 (5). Informed consent was obtained from all patients for being included in the study.

References

1. Cullen TS (1908) Adenomyoma of the uterus. W.B. Saunders, Philadelphia
2. Brosens I, Gordts S, Habiba M, Benagiano G (2014) Uterine cystic adenomyosis: a disease of younger women. J Pediatr Adolesc Gynecol (accepted and in press)
3. Fisseha S, Smith YR, Kumetz LM, Mueller GC, Hussain H, Quint EH (2006) Cystic myometrial lesion in the uterus of an adolescent girl. Fertil Steril 86:716–718
4. Takeuchi H, Kitade M, Kikuchi I, Kumakiri J, Kuroda K, Jinushi M (2010) Diagnosis, laparoscopic management, and histopathologic findings of juvenile cystic adenomyoma: a review of nine cases. Fertil Steril 94:862–868
5. Takeda A, Sakai K, Mitsui T, Nakamura H (2007) Laparoscopic management of juvenile cystic adenomyoma of the uterus: report of two cases and review of the literature. J Minim Invasive Gynecol 14:370–374
6. Branquinho MM, Marques AL, Leite HB, Silva IS (2012) Juvenile cystic adenomyoma. BMJ Case Rep 19
7. Dobashi Y, Fiedler PN, Carcangiu ML (1992) Polypoid cystic adenomyosis of the uterus: report of a case. Int J Gynecol Pathol 11:240–243
8. Steinkampf MP, Manning MT, Dharia S, Burke KD (2004) An accessory uterine cavity as a cause of pelvic pain. Obstet Gynecol 103:1058–1061
9. Molinas CR, Campo R (2006) Office hysteroscopy and adenomyosis. Best Pract Res Clin Obstet Gynaecol 20(4):557–567
10. Ryo E, Takeshita S, Shiba M et al (2006) Radiofrequency ablation for cystic adenomyosis: a case report. J Reprod Med 51:427
11. Giana M, Montella F, Surico D, Vigone A, Bozzola C, Ruspa G (2005) Large intramyometrial cystic adenomyosis: a hysteroscopic approach with bipolar resectoscope: case report. Eur J Gynaecol Oncol 26:462–463
12. Cusumano P, Lucani G, Verjans M, Belleza G, Janssens J (2008) Direct frontal core biopsy in breast cancer detection. Ann Oncol 19:132
13. Cornelis A, Verjans M, Van den Bosch T, Wouters K, Van Robaeys J, Janssens J, Working Group on Hormone Dependent Cancers, The European Cancer Prevention Organization (2009) Efficacy and safety of direct and frontal macrobiopsies in breast cancer. Eur J Cancer Prev 18:280–284
14. Exacoustos C, Luciano D, Corbett B, De Felice G, Di Feliciantonio M, Luciano A, Zupi E (2013) The uterine junctional zone: a 3-dimensional ultrasound study of patients with endometriosis. Am J Obstet Gynecol 209(3):248
15. Jain N, Goel S (2012) Cystic adenomyoma simulates uterine malformation: a diagnostic dilemma: case report of two unusual cases. J Hum Reprod Sci 5:285–288
16. Acien P, Acien M, Fernandez F et al (2010) The cavitated accessory uterine mass: a Mullerian anomaly in women with an otherwise normal uterus. Obstet Gynecol 116:1101
17. Thalluri V, Tremellen K (2012) Ultrasound diagnosed adenomyosis has a negative impact on successful implantation following GnRH antagonist IVF treatment. Hum Reprod 27:3487–3492
18. Vercellini P, Consonni D, Dridi D, Bracco B, Frattaruolo MP, Somigliana E (2014) Uterine adenomyosis and in vitro fertilization outcome: a systematic review and meta-analysis Hum. Reprod 29:964–977
19. Nabeshima H, Murakami T, Terada Y et al (2003) Total laparoscopic surgery of cystic adenomyoma under hydroultrasonographic monitoring. J Am Assoc Gynecol Laparosc 10:195–199
20. Kumakiri J, Kikuchi I, Sogawa Y, Jinushi M, Aoki Y, Kitade M, Takeda S (2013) Single-incision laparoscopic surgery using an articulating monopolar for juvenile cystic adenomyoma. Minim Invasive Ther Allied Technol 22:312–315
21. Kriplani A, Mahey R, Agarwal N, Bhatla N, Yadav R, Singh MK (2011) Laparoscopic management of juvenile cystic adenomyoma: four cases. J Minim Invasive Gynecol 18:343–348
22. Akar ME, Leezer KH, Yalcinkaya TM (2010) Robot-assisted laparoscopic management of a case with juvenile cystic adenomyoma. Fertil Steril 94:55
23. English DP, Verma U, Pearson JM (2012) Uterine cyst as a cause of chronic pelvic pain: a case report. J Reprod Med 57(9–10):446–448
24. Kumar A, Kumar A (2007) Myometrial cyst. J Minim Invasive Gynecol 14:395
25. Kunz G, Beil D, Huppert P, Noe M, Kissler S, Leyendecker G (2005) Adenomyosis in endometriosis—prevalence and impact on fertility. Evidence from magnetic resonance imaging. Hum Reprod 20:2309–2316
26. Brosens JJ, de Souza NM, Barker FG (1993) Uterine junctional zone: function and disease. Lancet. 16; 341(8838): 181–2

19

Dilemmas in management of bilateral ectopic pregnancies—report of two cases

Arpita Ghosh · Daniel Borlase · Tosin Ajala ·
Anthony James Kelly · Zaky Ibrahim

Abstract Simultaneous bilateral ectopic pregnancies occurring spontaneously or following assisted conception techniques, although rare, present the clinician with diagnostic uncertainty and management dilemmas which may have an implication on the patient's future fertility. A review of available literature suggests that there is no universally accepted management strategy towards this condition, and care needs to be tailored to the needs of the patient, patient's preferences and the clinical picture. We report two such rare cases of simultaneous bilateral ectopic pregnancies with different management and outcomes highlighting the fact that these cases not only pose diagnostic and management challenges but also has complex ethical issues associated with it.

Keywords Bilateral ectopic · Salpingostomy · Salpingectomy

Introduction

Simultaneous bilateral ectopic pregnancies occurring spontaneously or following assisted conception techniques are rare, with an incidence reported to be between 1 in 725 to 1 in 1,580 of all extrauterine pregnancies Rondeau et al. [1].

A. Ghosh (✉) · D. Borlase · T. Ajala · A. J. Kelly
Brighton and Sussex University Hospitals NHS Trust, Brighton, UK
e-mail: arpitagmc@yahoo.com

D. Borlase
e-mail: danielborlase@hotmail.com

T. Ajala
e-mail: Tosin.Ajala@bsuh.nhs.uk

A. J. Kelly
e-mail: Tony.kelly@bsuh.nhs.uk

Z. Ibrahim
Western Sussex Hospitals NHS Trust, West Sussex, UK
e-mail: Zaky.Ibrahim@wsht.nhs.uk

Management of these rare cases presents the clinician with diagnostic and management dilemmas. This is primarily due to rarity of the condition posing diagnostic difficulties with ultrasonography and implication of its treatment on fertility of the women.

We report two such rare cases of simultaneous bilateral ectopic pregnancies with different management and outcome, highlighting the fact that these cases not only pose diagnostic and management challenges but also has complex ethical issues associated with it.

Case reports

Case 1

History

A 37-year-old lady self-referred to the Early Pregnancy Assessment Unit (EPAU) at our local hospital at approximately 6 weeks into a planned pregnancy (Fig. 1). She presented with vaginal spotting which self resolved 7 days before attending. She denied any abdominal pain. Her previous obstetric history was that of a forceps-assisted delivery in 2008 and an early miscarriage in 2012. There was no history of previous tubal problems, gynaecological surgery or pelvic inflammatory disease. Her Abdominal and pelvic examination was unremarkable.

A transvaginal ultrasound scan on the day she presented revealed an empty uterus with an endometrial thickness of 7 mm. The right ovary showed two small haemorrhagic cysts of about the same size (18 mm × 12 mm × 16 mm). Adjacent to the left ovary was a solid cystic lesion approximately 34 mm × 33 mm × 19 mm in size (Fig. 2). This lesion demonstrated no colour Doppler flow.

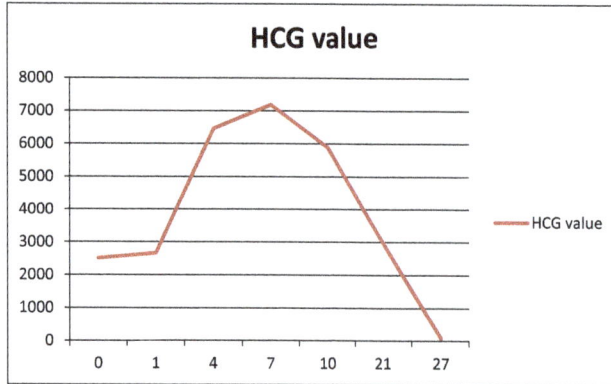

Fig. 1 Trend of HCG level in IU plotted against number of days

In view of her scan findings, particularly the empty uterus, blood was taken for serum levels of β-human Chorionic Gonadotrophin (β-hCG), progesterone and a full blood count. Her β-hCG was reported to be 2,512 IU with progesterone of 56.3 IU. Her Haemoglobin level was normal.

In view of her β-hCG level and scan findings, the decision was made to perform a diagnostic laparoscopy with a possibility of proceeding to salpingectomy as an emergency procedure. This was in line with the local guideline according to which laparoscopy is indicated in women with B-hCG more than 1,500 with no evidence of intrauterine gestation.

Laparoscopy revealed a 20-mm swelling in the mid-ampullary region covered with inflammatory material, suggestive of a chronic ectopic pregnancy. On further assessment, a smaller bean-shaped swelling of approximately 10 mm size in the mid-ampulla of the right tube was noticed (Fig. 3). This had the appearance of an acute tubal ectopic pregnancy. The options at this point were to do bilateral salpingectomy, salpingectomy and salpingostomy salpingectomy and methotrexate management or only methotrexate management. Due to the facts that the patient was asymptomatic, bilateral ectopic

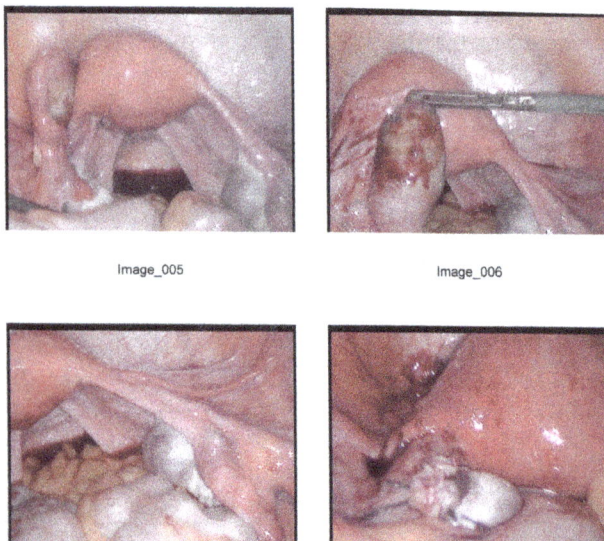

Fig. 2 Pictures showing left chronic tubal ectopic pregnancy case 1

pregnancy was an incidental finding, patient was not consented for further surgery, right tubal pregnancy was less than 3 cm in size and serum HCG was less than 3,000; the decision was made to perform salpingectomy only on the left side. Further management of right acute unruptured tubal pregnancy was deferred pending discussion with the patient pertaining to implications on her future fertility.

Postoperatively, the findings were explained to the patient, and the options were discussed which included conservative management, medical management with methotrexate and further laparoscopic surgery with a view to do salpingostomy. After a detail discussion, it was decided to manage this patient with methotrexate, which was given the day after her initial surgery. In line with the local protocol, plan was made to monitor her β-hCG levels on days 1, 4, 7 and 10 following methotrexate treatment.

Patient was clinical assessed after it was noted that β-hCG levels were rising on day 4 (see Fig. 1) after treatment with methotrexate. She was pain free and well. She was then treated with oral mifepristone 200 mg stat and was allowed home pending her further β-hCG level on day 7.

On day 7, her β-hCG levels were still rising, but she remained asymptomatic. At this point, the option of surgical management was re-discussed, and it was decided to continue to manage her conservatively. By day 10, 18 % decline in her HCG levels was noted. The mifepristone was repeated, and she was reviewed again 7 days later. Her β-hCG was still declining but not at a satisfactory rate. As the patient was still not complaining of any symptoms, it was decided to repeat the methotrexate regime. A steady decline in HCG levels was noted after the second cycle of Methotrexate treatment. The levels dropped down to 72 on day 10 following second cycle of methotrexate.

She was followed up in gynaecology outpatient clinic, and arrangements were made for her to under a go a laparoscopy and dye to test for tubal patency. At laparoscopy, the right tube had an appearance of chronic ectopic but her serum HCG at this point was less than 1. Hydrotubation revealed a free spillage of dye from the right tube confirming its patency.

Case 2

A 34-year-old woman with a BMI of 26 was referred to the infertility clinic with a 2-year history of primary infertility. No identifiable risk factors for sub-fertility were present in her and her partner. Her hormone profile did not reveal any abnormality. Hysterosalpingogram revealed bilaterally patent tubes with normal uterus.

Following the cycle of IUI, she presented at 5 weeks of gestation to the early pregnancy clinic with light per-vaginum bleeding and mild left iliac fossa pain. Pelvic ultrasound did not show any intrauterine gestation sac and reported the endometrial thickness of 10 mm with two small cystic areas

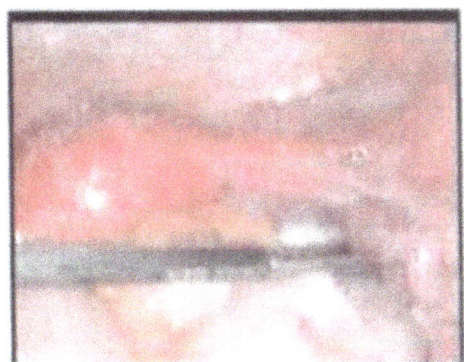

image_002

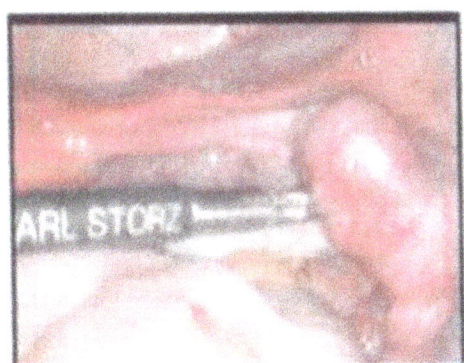

image_003

Fig. 3 Pictures showing right acute tubal ectopic pregnancy case 1

near both ovaries suggestive of either a corpus luteal cyst or ectopic pregnancies. Her serum HCG level was 9,691 IU and she was haemodynamically stable. She was admitted to the hospital with a provisional diagnosis of 'pregnancy of unknown location', and the possibility of ectopic pregnancy was explained to her. A diagnostic laparoscopy was planned the following day, and the patient was counselled and consented for a possible salpingectomy.

Laparoscopy revealed bilateral haemorrhagic masses with a small amount of blood in the pouch of Douglas. As the patient was already seeking fertility treatment for unexplained infertility and the option of IVF was available to the couple if IUI treatment failed, the decision was made to perform bilateral salpingectomies and thereafter plan further IVF treatment. Histology confirmed the diagnosis of bilateral ectopic pregnancies. She and her partner were then offered IVF to help attain pregnancy. A year later, she had a successful intrauterine pregnancy following IVF treatment.

Discussion

Ectopic pregnancy is an important cause of maternal mortality and morbidity. Every 11 in 1,000 pregnancies are reported to be an ectopic (CEMACH report 2003–2005). The latest CEMACH report from 2003-2005 emphasise the importance of early recognition and diagnosis of such pregnancies to save mothers' lives. There has been a persistent failure to recognise ectopic pregnancy and hence one of the 'top ten' key recommendations from the latest CEMACH report is that there should be national guidelines for the management of pain and bleeding in early pregnancy. Comprehensive clinical guidelines for the treatment of ectopic pregnancy have been published by the Royal College of Obstetricians and Gynaecologists. Because of its rarity, bilateral ectopic pregnancy is not referred to in the guidelines, but the same principles of management can still be applied.

The main purpose of reporting these two cases of bilateral ectopic pregnancy is to highlight the two different management approaches for the same condition and to discuss the challenges and dilemmas faced by the clinicians while diagnosing and managing such rare cases. In both the above cases, the noninvasive diagnostic methods with transvaginal ultrasonography and serial serum HCG monitoring failed to establish conclusively the presence of bilateral ectopic pregnancy. Given the rarity of the condition, difficulties in interpretation of serum HCG and the limitations of ultrasonography, timely diagnosis can be difficult. However, its early diagnosis is imperative in preservation of future fertility of the woman.

A review of available literature reveals that in most cases, preoperative investigations with serum HCG and ultrasonography fail to diagnose the presence of bilateral ectopic pregnancy [2]. It is commonly diagnosed intraoperatively at the time of laparoscopy. In the majority of the cases, ultrasonography will diagnose the presence of ectopic pregnancy in one tube, with the subsequent unexpected finding of bilateral ectopics during laparoscopy. This emphasises the importance of maintaining a high index of suspicion and the importance of examining the contralateral tube carefully during the laparoscopy. It can be specially challenging for the clinicians making these complex decisions during an emergency procedure with limited time to discuss and think about the implications of different management options with regards to the women's future chances of conception and the desire for preservation of fertility.

A diagnosis of bilateral tubal ectopic pregnancy at laparoscopy presents the clinician with the dilemma that the curative approach, which is to perform a bilateral salpingectomy, will render the women infertile. Thereafter, the only option of conceiving is through assisted conception technique. This is an important consideration especially as in majority of the cases the condition is found incidentally at laparoscopy giving no time for a detailed discussion with the women regarding its implications. Most of the clinicians choose to attempt conserving at least one tube if not both. In the cases where both tubal ectopic pregnancies are found to be ruptured and patient is haemodynamically compromised, it may be reasonable to perform a bilateral salpingectomy as a lifesaving measure. Also, in cases where a woman is already considering an IVF treatment and performing a conservative tubal surgery would increase her risk of further ectopic pregnancy, bilateral salpingectomy can be considered as a treatment of choice provided that this has been discussed with the women. Loo et al. [3] reported the rare occurrence of spontaneous synchronous bilateral ectopic pregnancy in a haemodynamically unstable patient needing bilateral salpingectomy. Martinez J et al. reported one such case where bilateral salpingectomy was performed, and Marasinghe JP et al. reported a case where the patient needed emergency laparotomy in view of ruptured ectopic pregnancy.

However, in majority of the cases, it is either both ectopic pregnancies are unruptured or there is a unilateral ruptured ectopic pregnancy. Stamatellos I.et al. described a case of unrecognised bilateral ampullary ectopic pregnancy, and bilateral salpingostomy was performed for this. Eze JN et al. reported a case of spontaneous bilateral ectopic pregnancy with one ruptured and one unruptured ectopic pregnancy needing both salpingectomy and salpingostomy.

Conservative management poses further dilemma between performing a salpingostomy and opting for a medical management with methotrexate postoperatively. In haemodynamically stable patients with unruptured tubal pregnancy, systemic methotrexate and laparoscopic salpingostomy are both successful in treating the majority of cases, and there is no significant difference between the treatments in the homolateral patency rate. (Dr PJ Hajenius et al.).

Salpingostomy is a conservative tubal surgery, but it carries the risks of incomplete evacuation and persistence of gestational tissue post procedure. Moreover, salpingostomy is performed less frequently and consequently in the present system of training most of the clinicians are not trained enough to perform this competently, especially so in an emergency situation. This also re-emphasises the importance of pre-empting this rare condition so that the surgery could be as planned as possible with appropriate expertise available. Rammah A.M. reported a case of bilateral unruptured ectopic pregnancy following assisted conception technique, and the women had bilateral salpingostomy performed.

There was one report (Marcovici I.et al.) where methotrexate management was opted for bilateral ectopic pregnancy, but it failed and authors questioned the optimal dose of methotrexate to treat bilateral ectopic pregnancy. Methotrexate management postoperatively needs further monitoring of the patient with serial HCG and the risk of needing further surgery persists. However, it gives the clinician an opportunity to discuss treatment options with the women and have an informed consent to proceed with management decisions. While managing such rare but fatal cases, the clinician should carefully consider and weigh the risks and benefits of each of the treatment option in the light of individual patient's condition.

The incidence of simultaneous bilateral ectopic pregnancies is between 1 in 725 and 1 in 1,580 of all extrauterine pregnancies (Rondeau JA et al.) Although spontaneous bilateral ectopic pregnancies have also been reported, these are rare. The majority of such cases happen as a consequence of assisted conception techniques primarily with IVF. Reddy et al. [2] and Shetty JP et al. report cases of spontaneous bilateral ectopic pregnancy highlighting the diagnostic pitfalls and treatment options. Wali AS et al. also describe a similar case with diagnostic challenges and state that occurrence of bilateral ectopic pregnancies is on increase.

With the advent of artificial reproductive techniques, the risk of ectopic pregnancies has increased in the last few years. The risk of developing unilateral ectopic pregnancy following intrauterine insemination with ovarian stimulation is well recognised and is quoted to be between 4 and 8 % in literature (Azantee et al. [4] and Chang et al. [5]). However, simultaneous bilateral ectopic pregnancies following IUI is rare, and to our knowledge, there are only very few cases reported. Plotti et al. in [6] reported bilateral ovarian pregnancy after IUI. Shiau et al. in [7] reported a case of severe ovarian hyperstimulation syndrome with simultaneous bilateral tubal pregnancy following intrauterine insemination. Burgos San Cristobal D.J et al. and Woo I et al. each reports similar cases after IUI treatment. Khong et al. [8] and Mathew et al. [9] reported such cases after clomiphene ovulation induction.

Majority of bilateral ectopic pregnancies are reported after ART treatments like IVF and ICSI (intra cytoplasmic sperm injection). Bustos Lopez HH et al. reported two such cases and stated that attempts should be made to diagnose these rare conditions preoperatively using available noninvasive methods. Campo s et al. report a case of bilateral ectopic pregnancies after IVF treatment. These were the only two cases where a preoperative diagnosis of bilateral ectopic pregnancy was made based on transvaginal scan report. Sergent F et al., through their case report, have attempted to explain the reasons for an increase in rate of bilateral ectopic pregnancies in recent years and highlights the importance of thorough pelvic examination at the time of laparoscopy to avoid missing such rare condition. Klipstein S et al. and Reyad R.M. et al. report similar cases after IVF and ICSI treatment, respectively.

In summary, once bilateral ectopic pregnancies have been diagnosed, the management options include the following:

(a) Bilateral salpingectomy
(b) Salpingostomy and salpingectomy
(c) Salpingectomy and methotrexate management
(d) Bilateral salpingostomy
(e) Methotrexate management only

Therefore, the management option has chosen needs to be tailored to the needs of the patient, patient's preferences and the clinical picture, preferably after a detailed discussion with the patient.

Conclusion

Bilateral ectopic pregnancies occurring spontaneously or following assisted conception techniques, although rare, present the clinician with diagnostic uncertainty and management dilemmas. Available literature review suggests that most clinicians opt for a more conservative approach with salpingostomy if the ectopic pregnancy is unruptured, whereas the decision to perform bilateral salpingectomy is noted more in cases where patient is haemodynamically compromised with unilateral or bilateral ruptured ectopic pregnancies. Maintaining a high index of suspicion and examination of the contralateral tube carefully during the laparoscopy is imperative, as it can significantly influence management decisions that can have a long-term influence on the patient's fertility.

Informed consent taken from both patients discussed above This article does not contain any studies with human or animal subjects performed by the any of the authors.

References

1. Rondeau JA, Hibbert ML, Nelson KM (1997). Combined tubal and cornual pregnancy in a patient without risk factors. A case report. J Reprod Med 42(10):675–677
2. Reddy AP, Chowdhary S, Saxena RK, Venkatesh S, Pandey P (2012) Spontaneous bilateral ectopic pregnancy. BJOG: Int J Obstet Gynaecol 119(151):1470–0328
3. Loo CY, Ng S, Rouse AM (2012) Spontaneous synchronous bilateral tubal ectopic pregnancy: a tale of caution. BJOG: Int J Obstet Gynaecol 119:217–218, 1470-0328
4. Azantee YW, Murad ZA, Roszaman R, Hayati MY, Norsina MA (2011) Associated factors affecting the successful pregnancy rate of intrauterine insemination at International Islamic University Malaysia (IIUM) Fertility Centre. Med J Malaysia 66(3):195–198
5. Chang MY, Huang HY, Lee CL, Lai YM, Chang SY, Soong YK (1993) Treatment of infertility using controlled ovarian hyperstimulation with intrauterine insemination: the experience of 343 cases. J Formos Med Assoc 92(4):341–348
6. Plotti F, Di Giovanni A, Oliva C, Battaglia F, Plotti G (2008) Bilateral ovarian pregnancy after intrauterine insemination and controlled ovarian stimulation. Fertil Steril 90(5):2015.e3–5
7. Shiau CS, Chang MY, Chiang CH, Hsieh CC, Hsieh TT (2004) Severe ovarian hyperstimulation syndrome coexisting with a bilateral ectopic pregnancy. Chang Gung Med J 27(2):143–147
8. Khong SY, Dimitry ED (2005) Bilateral tubal ectopic pregnancy after clomiphene induction. J Obstet Gynaecol 25(6):611–612
9. Mathew M, Saquib S, Krolikowski A (2004) Simultaneous bilateral tubal pregnancy after ovulation induction with clomiphene citrate. Saudi Med J 25(12):2058–2059

Further Reading

10. Aziz S, Al Wafi B, Al Swadi H (2011) Frequency of ectopic pregnancy in a medical centre, Kingdom of Saudi Arabia. J Pak Med Assoc 61(3):221–224
11. Martínez-Varea A, Hidalgo-Mora JJ, Payá V, Morcillo I, Martín E, Pellicer A (2011) Retroperitoneal ectopic pregnancy after intrauterine insemination. Fertil Steril 95(7):2433.e1–3
12. Bugatto F, Quintero-Prado R, Kirk-Grohar J, Melero-Jiménez V, Hervías-Vivancos B, Bartha JL (2010) Heterotopic triplets: tubal ectopic and twin intrauterine pregnancy. A review of obstetric outcomes with a case report. Arch Gynecol Obstet 282(6):601–606
13. Svirsky R, Maymon R, Vaknin Z, Mendlovic S, Weissman A, Halperin R, Herman A, Pansky M (2010) Twin tubal pregnancy: a rising complication? Fertil Steril 94(5):1910.e13–6
14. Ibrahim AG, Badawi F, Tahlak M (2009) Heterotopic pregnancy: a growing diagnostic challenge. BMJ Case Rep
15. Zadehmodarres S, Oladi B, Saeedi S, Jahed F, Ashraf H (2009) Intrauterine insemination with husband semen: an evaluation of pregnancy rate and factors affecting outcome. J Assist Reprod Genet 26(1):7–11
16. Childs AJ, Royek AB, Leigh TB, Gallup PG (2005) Triplet heterotopic pregnancy after gonadotropin stimulation and intrauterine insemination diagnosed at laparoscopy: a case report. South Med J 98(8):833–835
17. Chueh HY, Cheng PJ, Wang CW, Soong YK (2002) Inadvertent superovulation and intrauterine insemination during pregnancy: a lesson from an ectopic gestation. J Assist Reprod Genet 19(2):87–89
18. Berliner I, Mesbah M, Zalud I, Maulik D (1998) Report of a case with successful twin intrauterine gestation. J Reprod Med 43(3):237–239
19. Bontis J, Grimbizis G, Tarlatzis BC, Miliaras D, Bili H (1997) Intrafollicular ovarian pregnancy after ovulation induction/intrauterine insemination: pathophysiological aspects and diagnostic problems. Hum Reprod 12(2):376–378
20. Kably Ambe A, Garza Rios P, Serviere Zaragoza C, Delgado Urdapilleta J (1992) [Heterotopic pregnancy in intrauterine insemination. Presentation of a case]. [Article in Spanish]. Ginecol Obstet Mex 60:110–111
21. Marcovici I, Scoccia B (1997) Spontaneous bilateral tubal ectopic pregnancy and failed methotrexate therapy: a case report. Am J Obstet Gynecol 177/6(1545-1546):0002–9378
22. Bustos Lopez HH, Rojas-Poceros G, Barron Vallejo J, Cintora Zamudio S, Kably Ambe A, Valle RF (1998) Conservative laparoscopic treatment of bilateral ectopic pregnancy. 2 case reports and review of the literature. [Spanish] Tratamiento laparoscopico conservador del embarazo ectopico bilateral. Informe de dos casos y revision de la literatura. Ginecol Obstet Mex 66(13-7):0300–9041, 0300-9041
23. Klipstein S, Oskowitz SP (2000) Bilateral ectopic pregnancy after transfer of two embryos. Fertil Steril 74/5(887-8):0015–0282, 0015-0282
24. Reyad RM, Aboulghar MA, Serour GI, Mansour RT, Amin YM, Momtaz M, Youssry I (1998) Bilateral ectopic pregnancy with an intact intrauterine pregnancy following an ICSI procedure. Middle East Fertil Soc J 3/1:1110–5690
25. Sergent F, Verspyck E, Marpeau L (2003) Management of ectopic pregnancies complicating in vitro fertilization: a remarkable case of bilateral ectopic pregnancy with independent courses of the pregnancies. [French] Prise en charge des grossesses extra-uterines apres fecondation in vitro: a propos d'un cas remarquable d'une grossesse extra-uterine bilaterale dont chacune des grossesses a evolue independamment. J Gynecol Obstet Biol Reprod 32/3 Pt 1(256-60):0368–2315, 0150-9918
26. Stamatellos I, Anagnostou E, Stamatopoulos P, Bontis I (2006) Unrecognized spontaneous bilateral ampullary pregnancy treated by laparoscopy. Gynecol Surg 3/3(218-219):1613–2076, 1613-2084

27. Burgos San Cristobal DJ, Agirregoikoa JA, Albisu M, Mieza J, Corcostegui B, Prieto B, Ramon O, Matorras R (2004) Simultaneous bilateral ectopic pregnancy after IUI [Spanish] Embarazo ectopico bilateral simultaneo tras IAC. Rev Iberoam Fertilidad Reproduccion Humana 21/5(349-353):1132–0249

28. Altinkaya SO, Ozat M, Pektas MK, Gungor T, Mollamahmutoglu L (2008) Simultaneous bilateral tubal pregnancy after in vitro fertilization and embryo transfer. Taiwan J Obstet Gynecol 47/3(338-40): 1028–4559, 1875-6263

29. Issat T, Grzybowski W, Jakimiuk AJ (2009) Bilateral ectopic tubal pregnancy, following in vitro fertilisation (IVF). Folia Histochem Cytobiol 47/5(S147-8):0239–8508, 1897-5631

30. Marasinghe JP, Condous G, Amarasinghe WI (2009) Spontaneous bilateral tubal ectopic pregnancy. Ceylon Med J 54/1(21-2):0009–0875, 0009-0875

31. Martinez J, Cabistany AC, Gonzalez M, Gil O, Farrer M, Romero JA (2009) Bilateral simultaneous ectopic pregnancy. South Med J 102/10(1055-7):0038–4348, 1541-8243

32. Shetty JP, Shetty B, Makkanavar JH, Chandrika (2011) A rare case of bilateral tubal pregnancy. J Indian Med Assoc 109/7(506-7):0019–5847, 0019-5847

33. Wali AS, Khan RS, Jcpsp NO (2012) Spontaneous bilateral tubal pregnancy. J Coll Physicians Surg Pak 22/2(118-9):1022–386X, 1681-7168

34. Woo I, Christianson M, Swelstad B, Yates M, Garcia J (2012) Bilateral ovarian ectopic pregnancies following intrauterine insemination after unsuccessful oocyte retrieval. Fertil Steril 97/3 SUPPL. 1(S31), 0015-0282

35. Rammah AM, Al Hijji JY, Amen AM, Chibber R, Ali SA (2012) Bilateral tubal ectopic pregnancy case presentation and review of literature. Int J Gynecol Obstet 119(S707-S708):0020–7292

36. Eze JN, Obuna JA, Ejikeme BN (2012) Bilateral tubal ectopic pregnancies: a report of two cases. Ann Afr Med 11/2(112-5): 0975–5764, 0975-5764

37. Hajenius PJ, Engelsbel S, Mol BWJ, van der Veen F, Ankum WM, Bossuyt PMM, Hemrika DJ, Lammes FB (1997) Randomised trial of systemic methotrexate versus laparoscopic salpingostomy in tubal pregnancy. Lancet 350(9080):774–779. doi:10.1016/S0140-6736(97)05487-1

38. Gazvani MR, Baruah DN, Alfirevic Z, Emery SJ (1998) Mifepristone in combination with methotrexate for the medical treatment of tubal pregnancy: a randomized, controlled trial. Hum Reprod 13(7):1987–1990. doi:10.1093/humrep/13.7.1987

20

Laparoscopic ovarian reconstruction without suturing after cystectomy for endometrioma

P. G. Paul · Harneet Kaur · Dhivya Narasimhan · Gaurav Chopade · Dimple Kandhari

Abstract The primary aim of this study is to evaluate the technique of ovarian reconstruction without suturing after laparoscopic cystectomy of endometrioma. The secondary aim is to find the pregnancy rate following this technique. The study is a prospective observational study (Canadian Task Force classification II-3). The interventions used in the study are laparoscopic ovarian cystectomy and reconstruction without suturing. Laparoscopic ovarian cystectomy was performed in 240 patients between May 2007 and April 2012 of which 182 consecutive patients who met the selection criteria were enrolled in the study. Intraoperatively, the cyst wall is completely enucleated. Ovarian tissue is kept apposed together with a bowel grasper for 5 min to reconstruct the ovary. No sutures are used for approximation of ovarian edges. The median (range) operating time for cystectomy and reconstruction was 22 min (15–75), and estimated blood loss was 50 ml (30–200). The ovarian reconstruction was good in 84.6 % of the cases, average in 10 % and poor in 5.4 % of the patients. Postoperative scan on day 1 showed pelvic collection (blood) in five cases (20–50 ml). 9.89 % had intraovarian haematoma of 2–3 cm which resolved spontaneously. All patients were followed at 1 month and pregnancy rate was calculated after a minimum follow up of 12 months. Pregnancy rate was 50.7 % (33 patients) in our study. Approximation of ovarian surface for ovarian reconstruction was associated with shorter operating times, good morphological ovarian reconstruction and comparable pregnancy outcome. This technique requires further well-designed randomized controlled trials.

Keywords Laparoscopic cystectomy · Endometrioma · Ovarian reconstruction

Introduction

Endometriotic cysts are among the most common ovarian cysts encountered during surgery [1]. Endometriomas can cause pelvic pain, infertility and dyspareunia, and the most preferred treatment is surgical [2]. Various laparoscopic techniques have been described for the treatment of ovarian endometriomas: cyst wall laser vaporization preceded or not by medical therapy, drainage and bipolar coagulation of the cyst wall and stripping of the cyst wall [3–5]. Laparoscopic stripping is the preferred and safer technique [6]. After stripping of the cyst wall, bleeding from the ovarian wound is controlled by bipolar coagulation, suturing, or tissue sealants [7, 8]. Each of these is associated with its own advantages and disadvantages.

We believe that the ovaries should be reconstructed after cystectomy for better functional outcome and reduced postoperative adhesions. We have been reconstructing the ovaries by approximating the ovarian edges with a bowel grasper for few minutes. This technique used minimal diathermy and avoided suturing, thus achieving shorter operating times without requiring endosuturing expertise. Without washing of the residual blood, we keep the adjacent surface of the ovary approximated with pressure for a few minutes and this helps in the reconstruction. The primary aim of this study is to evaluate the technique for ovarian reconstruction after

P. G. Paul (✉) · H. Kaur · D. Narasimhan · G. Chopade · D. Kandhari
Centre for Advanced Endoscopy and Infertility Treatment, Paul's Hospital, Vattekkattu road, Kaloor, Cochin, Kerala 682 017, India
e-mail: drpaulpg@gmail.com

H. Kaur
e-mail: harneet.dmc@gmail.com

D. Narasimhan
e-mail: drzesto6666@yahoo.com

G. Chopade
e-mail: hschopade@rediffmail.com

D. Kandhari
e-mail: dimple.kandhari@yahoo.co.in

Fig. 1 Preoperative ultrasound—
endometrioma

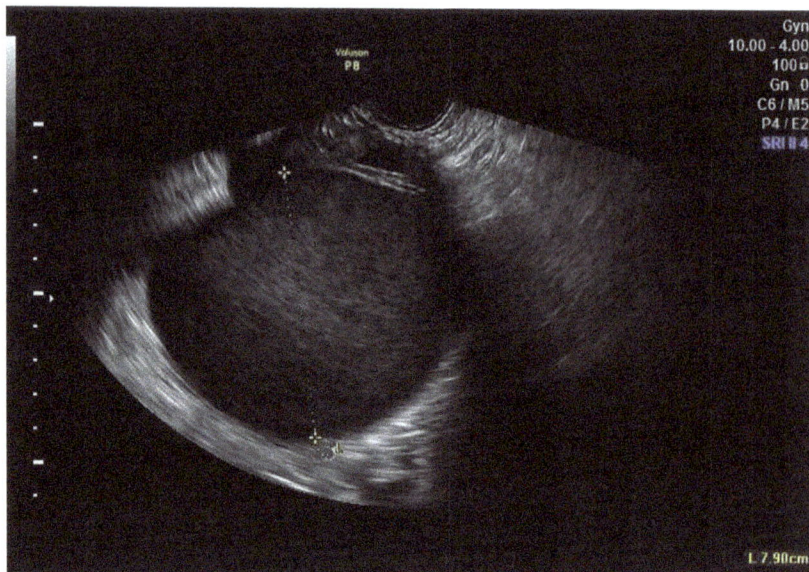

laparoscopic cystectomy of the endometrioma. The secondary aim is to find the pregnancy rate following this technique.

Materials and methods

This is a prospective observational study done at Paul's Hospital. A total of 240 patients underwent laparoscopic cystectomy for endometriosis between May 2007 and April 2012 at Paul's Hospital. Of these, 182 consecutive patients with endometriotic cyst >3 cm in size were included in the study.

The exclusion criteria are the following:

1. Preoperative clinical diagnosis of non-endometriotic cyst
2. Severely distorted pelvic anatomy at surgery (i.e., large size uterine fibroids, severe adhesions, congenital abnormalities) which required additional surgical procedure

with consequent increase of operating times and possible conversion to laparotomy

3. Previous surgery for endometriosis
4. Patients treated with gonadotropin-releasing hormone (GnRH) analogues in the past 6 months

The institutional ethical committee of Paul's Hospital approved the data collection, aggregation, identification and analysis for this study. Informed consent is obtained from all patients. Data regarding patient characteristics like age, body mass index, parity, previous surgeries and intraoperative details like duration of surgery, complications, estimated blood loss, duration of hospital stay and postoperative events are evaluated. The outcome is evaluated as complete reconstruction, complications, symptomatic relief and pregnancy rate. Patients were excluded from data analysis if endometriosis was not confirmed at histopathology.

Fig. 2 Left endometrioma of
8 cm

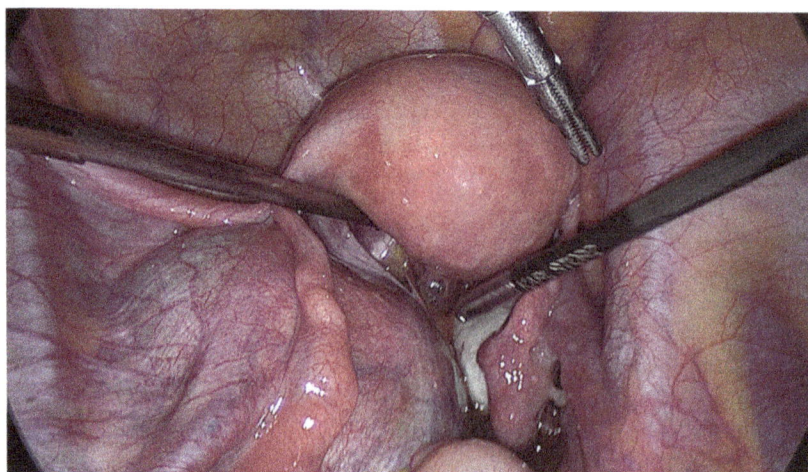

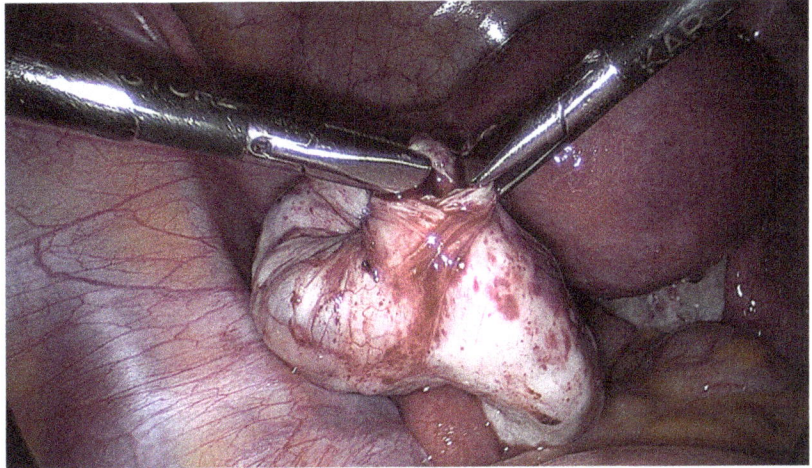

Fig. 3 Controlled tear on the edges of the cyst by traction with two graspers

Patient evaluation

All patients are submitted to a detailed history regarding severity of abdominal pain, dysmenorrhoea, dyspareunia, bowel symptoms, previous abdominopelvic infections and surgeries. Clinical examination and transvaginal ultrasonography are done by the operating surgeon prior to surgery (Fig. 1). In celibate patients, transabdominal ultrasound is done. MRI is not routinely done.

Patients are admitted to the hospital on the day of surgery and kept nil per orally for 6 h prior to surgery. Bowel preparation is performed using sodium phosphate solution enema. Antibiotic prophylaxis is given at the time of induction of anaesthesia. Procedures are performed under general anaesthesia. All surgical procedures are carried out by the first author.

The patients are discharged on postoperative day 1 of surgery, and ultrasound examination is done for any pelvic or intraovarian haematoma before discharge (Fig. 6). All patients are followed up at 1 and 12 months and evaluated for any symptoms, and pregnancy rate was calculated. Postal questionnaires are sent to all patients, and telephonic enquiries are made at the end of the study. Minimum follow-up period is 1 year.

Surgical technique

Pneumoperitoneum is created using Veress needle at the umbilicus or at the Palmer's point. Peritoneal entry is done by direct trocar insertion or visual entry technique using Ternamian EndoTIP (Karl Storz, Tuttlingen) at the umbilicus or supraumbilical in patients with large abdominal masses. Abdominopelvic inspection is done for omental and bowel adhesions and to confirm the preoperative diagnosis (Fig. 2). Three accessory port techniques are used, two ports in the lower quadrants lateral to the inferior epigastric artery and the third port in the suprapubic area. Endometriosis is staged according to the revised American Fertility Society (rAFS) classification [9].

Since 2 years, we have been using dilute vasopressin for generalized vasoconstriction in the pelvis which helps in achieving initial haemostatic dissection of the adnexa and

Fig. 4 Separation of cyst wall from the ovarian tissue

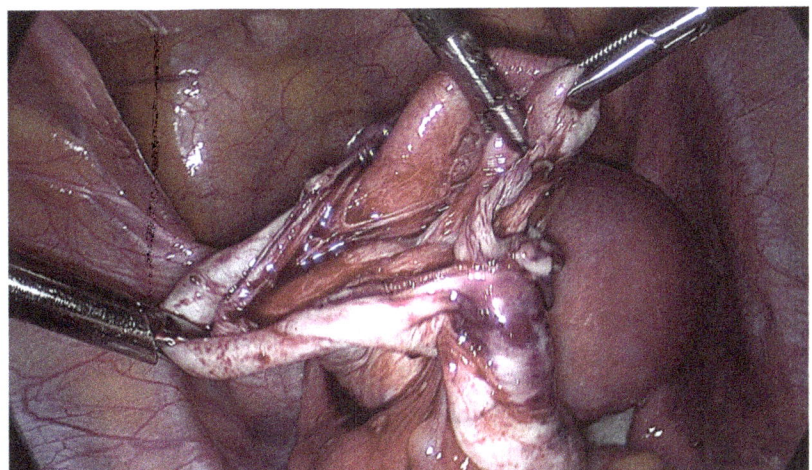

Fig. 5 Approximation of the
edges with bowel grasper

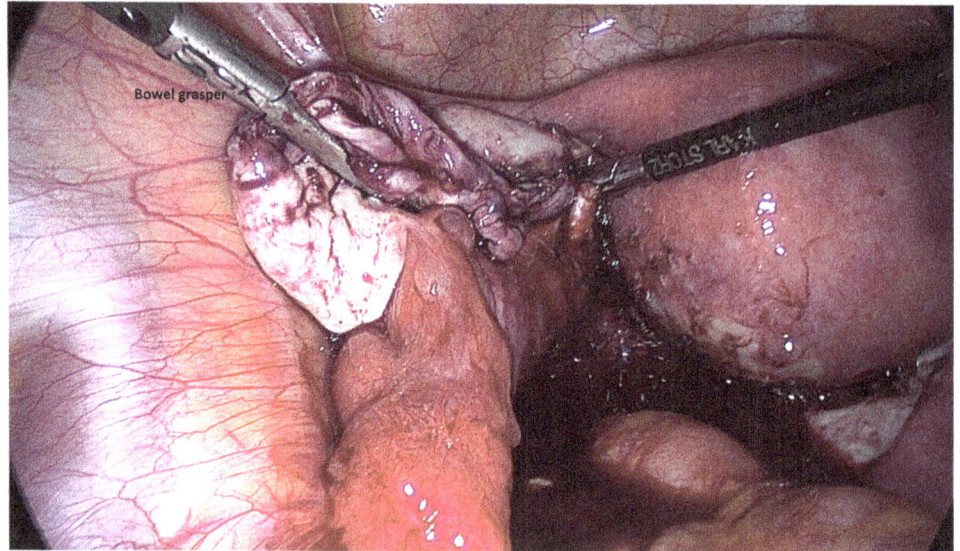

rectosigmoid. Twenty units of vasopressin is diluted in 100 ml
of normal saline, and 40 to 60 ml of this solution is injected
into the myometrium till the uterus is blanched. After
anteverting the uterus with a Spackman cannula, salpingo-
ovariolysis is done with sharp dissection. All fleshy adhesions
from the uterus and pouch of Douglas are excised. All superficial endometriosis implants are coagulated, and deep ones
are excised.

The ovary with small endometrioma is mobilized from the
pelvic ovarian fossa, and when the chocolate material invariably leaks out, the leaked out contents are aspirated, followed
by complete irrigation and aspiration of the cyst. For large
endometrioma, we puncture the cyst with trocar and aspirate
the chocolate material. We make a controlled tear of 1 cm on
the edge of the cyst by traction with two graspers, rather than
using sharp cutting (Fig. 3). This step separates the cyst wall
from the ovarian tissue. After identification of the cleavage
plane, the cyst wall is enucleated through traction exerted in
opposite directions with two grasping forceps. The cyst wall is

held with a toothed grasper, and ovarian tissue is held with an
atraumatic grasper. Traction and countertraction are done to
separate the cyst from the ovarian tissue (Fig. 4). Complete
removal of the cyst wall is done. Enucleation is done gently
near the ovarian ligament and hilum to avoid bleeding and
injury. Any residual endometriosis on the edges of the ovary is
excised. At the end of the procedure, only the active bleeding
vessel is controlled with bipolar coagulation. No sutures are
used for approximation of the ovarian edges. The ovarian
edges are held together with three graspers, and by trial and
error, the best symmetrical approximation of the edges is
achieved. Ipsilateral grasper is replaced with the bowel grasper to achieve the maximal approximation of the ovarian edges.
The suprapubic grasper is released once the bowel grasper is
in proper position. The specimen is removed through the 10-
mm primary trocar after changing the camera to a 5-mm
telescope introduced through the suprapubic port. Large cysts
were removed with an endobag after enlarging the primary
port. The vaginal assistant holding the bowel grasper keeps

Fig. 6 Large ovarian
endometrioma (19×6 cm)

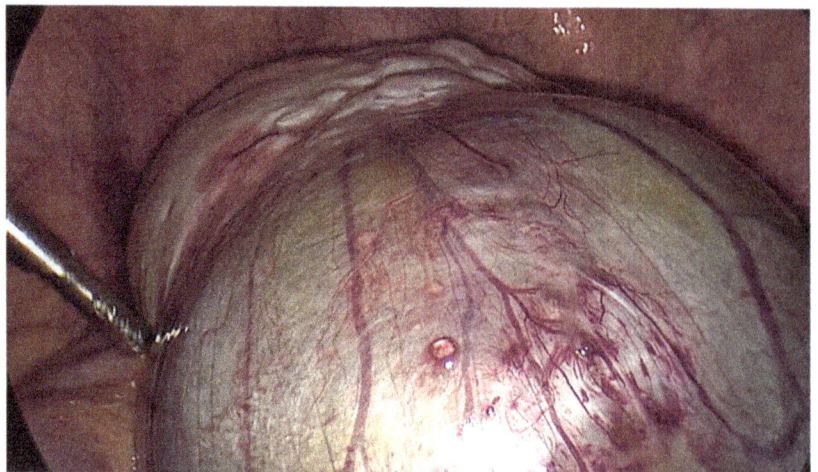

Fig. 7 Large ovarian endometrioma reconstructed after cystectomy with bowel graspers

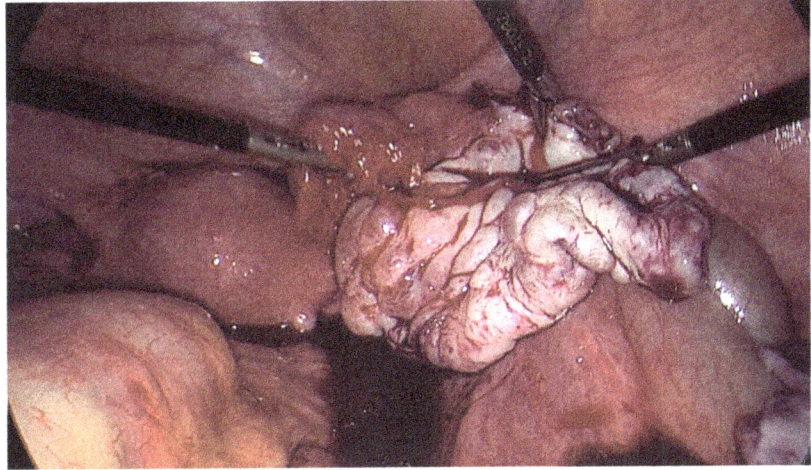

the forearm rested on the corresponding thigh of the patient and is not involved in specimen retrieval. The edges are hence approximated, and the tissue is held together for 5 min (Fig. 5). Trimming of the ovarian edges is rarely needed and done only to excise endometrial implants. For very large cysts, the bowel grasper is applied more towards the edges and rotated laterally to get a better approximation of the inner wall of the ovary (Figs. 6 and 7). The uterus can be deviated laterally with the manipulator to compress the ovary against the pelvic side wall. Rarely, ovarian reconstruction cannot be achieved due to a persistent bleeder from the cystectomy site. In such a situation, the ovary has to be reopened and the offending bleeding is controlled, and the aforementioned steps are repeated to achieve ovarian reconstruction. The ipsilateral bowel grasper and the contralateral graspers are released, and the ovary is inspected whether it is fully reconstructed (Fig. 8). The morphological appearance of the ovary is described as good reconstruction if the surface apposition was >75 %, average if the surface apposition was 50–75 % and poor if the surface apposition was <50 %.

Findings

Laparoscopic ovarian cystectomy was performed in 240 patients with endometriosis between May 2007 and April 2012. Of these patients, 33 patients had previous surgery for endometriosis, 7 patients were previously treated with GnRH analogues, 15 patients had severely distorted pelvic anatomy at surgery requiring additional surgical procedures and 5 patients were detected with non-endometriotic cysts and hence excluded from the study. Hence, 182 patients were enrolled in the study. Patients' data are shown in Table 1. The mean±standard deviation (SD) age of patients was 30.37±5.7 years; body mass index was 23.8±4.2. Fifty-nine patients had previous abdominal surgery (laparotomy, laparoscopy for indications other than endometriosis and did not have severely distorted pelvic anatomy). Out of the total, 16 patients were celibate, 124 were nulliparous and 42 were parous, of which 20 had previous caesarean section. The presenting complaints of patients were dysmenorrhoea in 68 patients and abdominal pain in 47. In 101 patients presented with infertility (duration

Fig. 8 Ovary after reconstruction

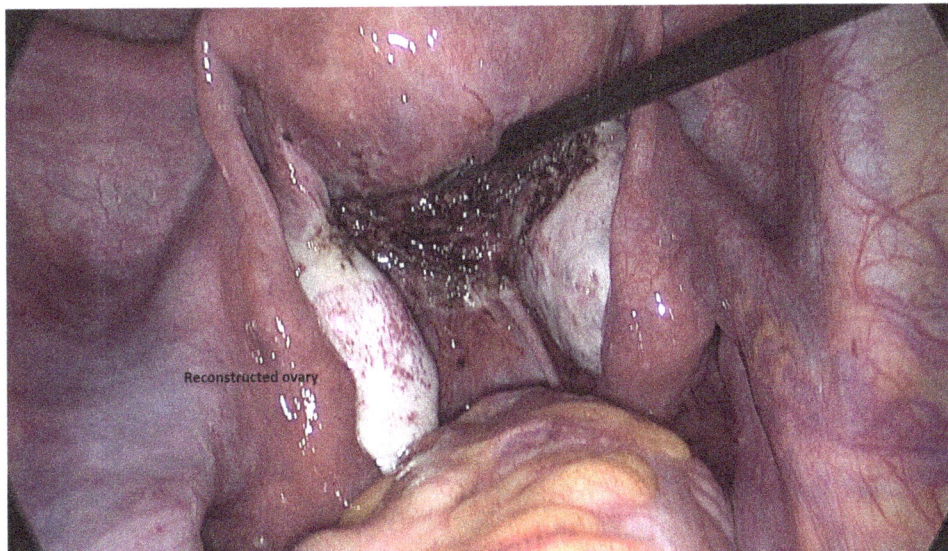

Table 1 Demographic characteristics/patient details

Variable	No. of cases
Age	30.37±5.7
BMI	23.8±4.2
Presenting complaints	
Dysmenorrhoea	68
Pain abdomen	47
Primary in fertility	72
Secondary infertility	29
Dyspareunia	2
Deliveries	
Vaginal	20
Caesarean section	20
Parity	
Celibate	16
0	124
1	35
≥2	7
Previous surgeries	59
1	18
2	41

of infertility ranging from 1 to 5 years), out of these patients, 31 had fibroid uterus and 5 had adenomyosis of the uterus with endometriosis and hence excluded from the pregnancy rate calculation to avoid multiple variables.

Preoperative sonography findings are tabulated in Table 2. The size and localization of endometriomas were documented.

Intraoperative findings and type of surgery are mentioned in Table 3. Seventy-five patients had bilateral cystectomy, and five patients who were not desirous of future fertility and had severe pelvic pain underwent unilateral adnexectomy of the relatively severely affected ovary and cystectomy of the remaining ovary. The median (range) operating time for cystectomy and reconstruction was 22 min (15–75) (from the beginning of cystectomy to removal of bowel grasper), and the estimated blood loss was 50 ml (30–200). Since cystectomy was done as the last step, the suction aspirate was measured separately to evaluate the blood loss. Ovary

Table 2 Preoperative ultrasound findings

Size	Localization		
	Right adnexa	Left adnexa	Bilateral
1–3 cm	18	13	40
3–7 cm	23	28	42
>7 cm	5	7	6
Total	46	48	88

Table 3 Operative details

rAFS score median (range) 24 (16–94)	No. of cases
Stage III	68
Stage IV	114
Type of surgery	
Unilateral cystectomy	66
Right	32
Left	34
Bilateral cystectomy	75
Cystectomy with unilateral adnexectomy	5
Unilateral cystectomy with myomectomy	21
Unilateral cystectomy with hysteroscopic polypectomy	2
Bilateral cystectomy with myomectomy	10
Bilateral cystectomy with hysteroscopic polypectomy	2
Bilateral cystectomy with hysteroscopic myomectomy	1
Duration of cystectomy and reconstruction	22 min (15–75)
Blood loss	50 ml (30–200)
Morphological appearance of reconstructed ovary	
Good (>75 % reconstructed)	154 (84.6 %)
Average (50–75 %)	18 (10 %)
Poor (<50 %)	10 (5.4 %)

rAFS revised American Fertility Society

reconstruction was good in 84.6 % of the cases, average in 10 % and poor in 5.4 % of the patients (Table 3).

Suturing of the ovarian edges was required in two patients as the ovarian tissue had irregular edges, and reconstruction was not possible otherwise. None of the patients required conversion to laparotomy. No intraoperative or postoperative complication occurred. Length of postoperative stay was 1 day (1–4).

Postoperative scan reports are tabulated in Table 4. Postoperative ultrasonography on day 1 showed pelvic collection (blood) in five cases (20–50 ml) (Fig. 9). Ninety percent of the patients had no intraovarian haematoma. Haematoma in the ovary greater than 2 cm was seen in 18 cases (2–3 cm). None

Table 4 Postoperative ultrasound findings

Ultrasound—size of the ovary	No. of cases
3–6 cm	160 (87.9 %)
>6 cm	22 (12.1 %)
Intraovarian haematoma	
<2 cm	164 (90.10 %)
2–3 cm	18 (9.89 %)
Pelvic collection	
<20 ml	177 (97.25 %)
20–50 ml	5 (2.75 %)

Fig. 9 Postoperative day 1 ultrasound showing the reconstructed ovary

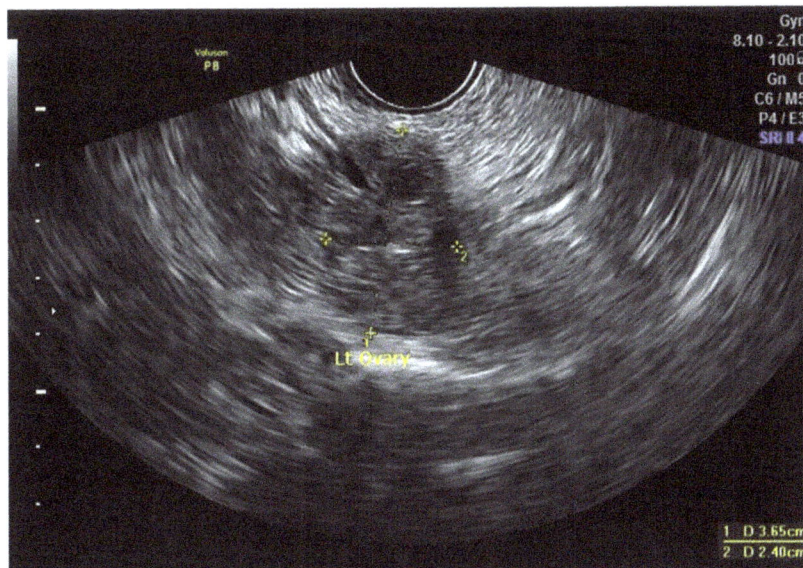

of these patients required any intervention and haematoma resolved on serial ultrasound scans.

Of the 65 patients desiring fertility, 21 % of male partners had moderate oligoasthenozoospermia and 8 % had severe oligoasthenozoospermia. Thirty-three patients (50.7 %) conceived and 22 conceived spontaneously and 11 after assisted reproductive technology (ART).

Discussion

In recent years, laparoscopy has become the gold standard for the treatment of ovarian endometriotic cysts [10, 11]. Laparoscopic stripping is the most preferred procedure [6]. Good haemostasis is important after laparoscopic stripping of the cyst wall, and techniques like bipolar coagulation, sutures, fibrin sealants and direct pressure are used [8]. Bipolar coagulation of the ovarian stroma is effective but damages the healthy ovarian tissue. When the ovarian capsule is left open after bipolar coagulation, it is associated with more adhesions as compared to the reconstruction of the ovary [12]. In contrast, sutures are useful but also cause additional damage to the healthy tissue [13]. Though suturing technique has been shown to cause less adhesions as compared to bipolar coagulation by various studies, sutures cause more postoperative adhesions as seen in the myomectomy studies and suturing is technically more demanding [7, 14]. Thus, avoiding suturing will be a simpler technique for the reconstruction. In this study, we used compression with bowel grasper for ovarian reconstruction after laparoscopic cystectomy of endometrioma.

Our technique of laparoscopic stripping is similar to other studies, except that vasopressin is injected on the uterus rather than on the endometrioma [6, 15]. On injecting vasopressin on the uterus, we get a generalized vasoconstriction of the pelvis which helps in maintaining a clear view without much bleeding during adhesiolysis.

With approximation of the adjacent surfaces of the ovary using the bowel graspers, the ovaries maintained its shape after removal and this is possibly due to the fibrin formed from the oozing ovarian surface. The empirical usage of 5 min correlates with the average clotting time of blood. Though the fibrinogen concentration of sealants is 15–25 times higher than the circulating plasma, the endogenous fibrin was sufficient to stick the tissues in our study. Tissue sealants like FloSeal (gelantine thrombin matrix) sealant have been used to control bleeding following the ovarian stripping, but patients had postoperative pelvic pain with its use [8]. Fibrin sealants have been used in various urological procedures for controlling bleeding [16]. Fibrin glue has been used after laparoscopic excision of large endometriomas by Takeuchi et al. and had reduced postoperative adhesions as compared to the use of bipolar [12].

In our study, the ovarian reconstruction was good in 84.6 %, average in 10 % and poor in 5.4 % of the patients. Suturing of the ovarian edges was required in two patients only. We could not find any study describing the morphological appearance of the ovary after laparoscopic cystectomy.

Table 5 Pregnancy rate

Outcome	No. of cases
Pregnancy	33 (50.7 %)
Spontaneous conception	22 (66.6 %)
Assisted reproductive technology (ART)	11 (33.2 %)
Abortions	5 (15.1)
Term deliveries	28 (84.9 %)

In our study, postoperative scan on day 1 showed pelvic fluid collection in five cases (20–50 ml). In 18 cases, haematoma in the ovary was greater than 2 cm (2–3 cm). Ninety percent of the patients had no intraovarian haematoma. None of these patients had evidence of infection and did not require any intervention. The pelvic collection and intraovarian haematoma resolved on serial ultrasound scans. In a case report by Ebert et al. using FloSeal for intraovarian haemostasis following cystectomy, day 2 ultrasound revealed a residuum of 10 mm within the ovary and residual fluid of less than 5 ml in cul-de-sac [8]. Hence, the failure rate in our technique considering both morphological appearance (5.4 %) and postoperative ovarian haematoma >2 cm (10 %) was 15.4 %.

Pregnancy rate in our study was 50.7 % (33 patients). Twenty-two patients had spontaneous pregnancy and 11 after ART (Table 5). Out of the 33 patients who conceived, 28 delivered and 5 had abortions. Vercellini et al. observed an overall crude pregnancy rate of 41 % after primary surgery for endometriosis similar to our study [10].

The limitation of the present study is that it is an observational study, with no randomization, and we did not do a second look laparoscopy. Thus, further prospective randomized control trial studies are needed to validate our results.

Conclusion

Different techniques for haemostasis and ovarian reconstruction following cystectomy are use of bipolar coagulation, sutures, fibrin sealants and direct pressure. We reconstructed the ovaries by approximating the ovarian surface with a bowel grasper for few minutes, and it was associated with a successful outcome. Though this is a simpler technique, further well-designed randomized controlled trials are needed.

Informed consent All procedures followed were in accordance with the ethical standards of the responsible committee on human experimentation (institutional and national) and with the Helsinki declaration of 1975, as revised in 2000(5). Informed consent was obtained from all patients for being included in the study.

References

1. Loh FH, Tan AT, Kumar J, Ng SC (1999) Ovarian response after laparoscopic ovarian cystectomy for endometriotic cysts in 132 monitored cycles. Fertil Steril 72:316–321
2. Valle RF, Sciarra JJ (2003) Endometriosis: treatment strategies. Ann N Y Acad Sci 997:229–239. doi:10.1196/annals.1290.026
3. Brosens IA, Van Ballaer P, Puttemans P, Deprest J (1996) Reconstruction of the ovary containing large endometriomas by an extraovarian endosurgical technique. Fertil Steril 66(4):517–521
4. Beretta P, Franchi M, Ghezzi F, Busacca M, Zupi E, Bolis P (1998) Randomized clinical trial of two laparoscopic treatments of endometriomas: cystectomy versus drainage and coagulation. Fertil Steril 70:1176–1180
5. Canis M, Mage G, Wattiez A, Chapron C, Pouly JL, Bassil S (1992) Second look laparoscopy after laparoscopic cystectomy of large ovarian endometriomas. Fertil Steril 58:611–619
6. Muzii L, Bellati F, Palaia I, Plotti F, Manci N, Zullo MA et al (2005) Laparoscopic stripping of endometriomas: a randomized trial on different surgical techniques. Part I: clinical results. Hum Reprod 20:1981–1986
7. Pellicano M, Bramante S, Guida M, Bifulco G, Di Spiezio SA, Cirillo D, Nappi C (2008) Ovarian endometrioma: postoperative adhesions following bipolar coagulation and suture. Fertil Steril 89(4):796–799
8. Ebert AD, Hollauer A, Fuhr N, Langolf O, Papadopoulos T (2009) Laparoscopic ovarian cystectomy without bipolar coagulation or sutures using a gelantine-thrombin matrix sealant (FloSeal): first support of a promising technique. Arch Gynecol Obstet 280:161–165
9. (1997) American, Society for Reproductive Medicine Revised classification of endometriosis: 1996. Fertil Steril 67:817–21
10. Vercellini P, Somigliana E, Viganò P, De Matteis S, Barbara G, Fedele L (2009) The effect of second-line surgery on reproductive performance of women with recurrent endometriosis: a systematic review. Acta Obstet Gynecol Scand 88(10):1074–1082
11. Yeung PP, Shwayder J, Pasic RP (2009) Laparoscopic management of endometriosis: comprehensive review of best evidence. J Minim Invasive Gynecol 16(3):269–281
12. Takeuchi H, Awaji M, Hashimoto M, Nakano Y, Mitsuhashi N, Kuwabara Y (1996) Reduction of adhesions with fibrin glue after laparoscopic excision of large ovarian endometriomas. J Am Assoc Gynecol Laparosc 3(4):575–579
13. Fedele L, Bianchi S, Zanconato G, Bergamini V, Berlanda N (2004) Bipolar electrocoagulation versus suture of solitary ovary after laparoscopic excision of ovarian endometriomas. J Am Assoc Gynecol Laparosc 11(3):344–347
14. Dubuisson JB, Fauconnier A, Chapron C, Kreiker G, Nörgaard C (1998) Second look after laparoscopic myomectomy. Hum Reprod 13(8):2102–2106
15. Saeki A, Matsumoto T, Ikuma K, Tanase Y, Inaba F, Oku H, Kuno A (2010) The vasopressin injection technique for laparoscopic excision of ovarian endometrioma: a technique to reduce the use of coagulation. J Minim Invasive Gynecol 17(2):176–179
16. Pursifull NF, Morey AF (2007) Tissue glues and nonsuturing techniques. Curr Opin Urol 17(6):396–401

21

Cryptomenorrhea with cervicovaginal aplasia: endoscopic transfundal development of the lower genital tract

Ali M. El Saman · Magdi M. Amin ·
Mohamad T. Khalaf · Dina M. Habib ·
Omar M. Shaaban · Alaa M. Ismail

Abstract The current case series was done to evaluate the feasibility of transfundal hysteroscopy (TFH) in helping the development of new cervical canal in cases with cervical aplasia. Five cases with obstructive cervicovaginal agenesis with hematometra were included in this report. Laparoscopic-guided TFH was done in conjunction with endoscopic canalization to all cases. Additional retropubic balloon vaginoplasty (BV) was needed in three cases with associated vaginal aplasia. The hysteroscope was passed through the uterine fundus. After complete washing, the endometrial lining was inspected, and a properly located intrauterine catheter coming out from the vagina or vaginal dimple was used to drain the uterine cavity and maintain the cervical tract. The procedure was done successfully in all cases with adequate drainage of hematometria. Additional time needed for TFH was between 4 to 15 min. Second-look hysteroscopy revealed adequate canalization in all cases. The five cases had regular menstrual cycles up to the sixth postoperative month. In conclusion, TFH is a safe and feasible procedure as a harmonizing technique during endoscopic canalization of cervical atresia with or without BV in cases of obstructive Müllerian anomalies. The procedure accelerates the drainage of uterine contents and localizes the correct site of draining catheter.

Condensation Laparoscopic transfundal hysteroscopy was performed for patients with cervical/cervicovaginal aplasia to examine uterine cavity, facilitate washing of uterine contents, and decide the proper location of the draining catheter

A. M. El Saman · M. T. Khalaf · D. M. Habib ·
O. M. Shaaban (✉) · A. M. Ismail
Department of Obstetrics and Gynecology, Faculty of Medicine,
Assiut University, P.O. Box 174, Assiut, Egypt
e-mail: omshaaban2000@yahoo.com

M. M. Amin
Department of Obstetrics and Gynecology, Faculty of Medicine,
Sohag University, Sohag, Egypt

Keywords Balloon vaginoplasty · Neovagina · Laparoscopy · Vaginal aplasia · Cervical aplasia · Hysteroscopy · Hematometra · Transfundal hysteroscopy

Introduction

Müllerian aplasia represents a wide spectrum of disorders, which are occasionally associated with functioning uterus and menstrual retention. Balloon vaginoplasty (BV) was introduced by El-Saman and coworkers as scar-free procedure for construction of a new sexual port that mimics the normal vagina in several ways [1–3]. The patients with isolated vaginal or cervicovaginal aplasia and functioning uteri are often treated by laparotomies or advanced laparoscopic operations. In our previous reports, such patients were successfully treated by BV in conjunction with endoscopically monitored introduction and fixation of a silicon catheter through the vaginal dimple. The catheter drains the retained bloody contents of the uterus for 6-month period required for complete establishment of a communicating tract [4–6]. In these cases, the proper placement of the intrauterine catheter/drain is the key of success.

The present report represents the first trial to use the conventional rigid hysteroscopy in a transfundal visualization of the uterine cavity and localization of the proper site of catheter or the silicon drain insertion in women with vaginal or cervicovaginal aplasia with functioning uteri.

Patients and methods

This is a case series performed in the Women's Health Hospital of the Assiut Medical School during the period from May 2012 to May 2013. The study had obtained the ethical clearance of the Institutional Ethical Review Board. The study comprised five adolescent patients. They all had complete vaginal and/or cervical aplasia; two of them were classed as U0C4V0 and three as U0C4V4 according to ESHRE/ESGE classification system [7]. All patients presented with cyclic pains secondary to menstrual retention. Complete history was taken and a vigilant examination with objective measurements of the depth of the vaginal dimple. We counseled our participants for having the balloon vaginoplasty and endoscopic canalization (BV-EC) with inspection of the uterine cavity via transfundal hysteroscopy (TFH). This is in a trial of creation of new cervical or cervicovaginal tract to correct their congenitally malformed lower genital tract and to establish their reproductive functions.

A written consent was obtained from each participant after reading the patient's information sheet that includes detailed explanation of the procedure including benefits and possible risks. Laparoscopically guided TFH was done in conjunction with canalization to all cases in this series. The procedure was carried out under general anesthesia with endotracheal tube. The patients were sterilized and draped in a dorsal lithotomy position and thoroughly examined. Preoperative antibiotic was given in all cases. The procedure started by laparoscopy in all cases using a 5-mm intra-umbilical port. Detailed examination of the abdominal and pelvic organs was performed to confirm the diagnosis and the exact localization of the site of aplasia and estimate the missing aplastic portion of the genital tract.

A specially designed reusable sterilized inserter, which was designed to perforate the vaginal dimple in cases of BV in women with Müllerian agenesis, was used to make a uterine fundal hole. The inserter is 35 cm long and 4 mm girth and is made of stainless steel. It has a sharp penetrating pyramidal tip with a long double strand silk suture (DSSS) threaded into its fenestrated caudal end. After penetrating the uterine fundus with the inserter under laparoscopic guidance, the inserter passes across the distended uterine cavity to pass through the atretic segment of the cervix to be finally extracted through the vagina in cases with isolated cervical atresia or through vaginal dimple in cases with concomitant vaginal aplasia. A silicon catheter is then inserted from the vaginal side through the hole made by the inserter and manipulated into the uterine cavity as described in our original procedure. The catheter was pulled up into the uterine cavity via the DSSS. The inserter and the technique used in BV-EC was previously described [5].

Then, under laparoscopic guidance, a 4-mm rigid hysteroscopy was passed across an ancillary midline port then through the same puncture of the inserter across the uterine fundus to inspect the uterine cavity as shown in Fig. 1. Continuous irrigation of the uterine cavity was made using saline solution pushed through the TFH until clear fluid came out through the intrauterine catheter coming out from the vaginal side (Fig. 2). Detailed hysteroscopic inspection of the uterine cavity was done including visualization of the tubal ostia when 70° hysteroscopic lens was used. The position of the balloon was ascertained to confirm its accurate intrauterine placement. After confirmation of the intrauterine location of the catheter, the hysteroscopy was withdrawn. Laparoscopic inspection of the access site at the uterine fundus was done for detection of and management of any bleeding from the edges.

The three cases with associated vaginal aplasia (U0C4V4) required additional retropubic balloon vaginoplasty (previously described in our early series) [8] to increase the length of the vaginal dimple and carry it up to meet the newly formed cervix.

The above-described inserter was passed again just behind the symphysis pubis carrying a catheter on its caudal end. The catheter was passed across the retropubic space until the balloon-bearing segment appears at the vaginal dimple (Fig. 3a). The balloon was distended with 20 mm saline and traction was initiated until disappearance of the balloon within the vaginal introitus. Support of the catheter in place after traction was done using a supporting plate placed over a dressing on the abdominal wall retained in its place by sterile umbilical cord clamp (Fig. 3b). This is followed by 1–2 cm daily increase in the traction exerted on the catheter by adding another proximal clamp. Pulling up on the retropubic balloon was coupled with pulling down on the uterine catheter until the two balloons become in contact, a process that was monitored via transrectal ultrasound (Fig. 4). More details about retropubic BV can be found in a previous publication [8]. When vaginal depth increased to 9–10 cm on days 6–7, the retropubic catheter was removed and uterine catheter was exchanged with new silicon one. The uterine catheter was changed every 30 to 40 days during that change; office hysteroscopy was done to ensure the patency of the cervical track. The catheter was finally removed after 4 to 6 months of the procedure and complete epithelization of the cervical tract had been visualized through the hysteroscopy.

Results

The mean age of the five patients was 13.1±1.1 years. Their main complaint was recurrent cyclic lower abdominal pains and amenorrhea. None of them was married at the time of operation. One of them had two previous attempts of uterovestibular anastomosis and had severe abdominal pain and fever with lower abdominal tenderness. Details of patients' clinical and operative data are summarized in Table 1. The canalization procedure was performed successfully in the five cases. Endoscopic transfundal canalization was done alone in cases with isolated cervical aplasia with rather adequate vaginal length. However, the canalization was done in conjunction with retropubic BV in three cases with cervicovaginal aplasia.

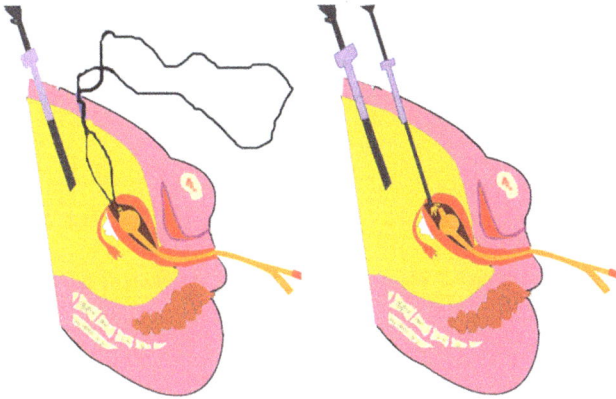

Fig. 1 A long metal inserter with a long double strand of silk suture is being inserted transfundal under laparoscopic monitoring

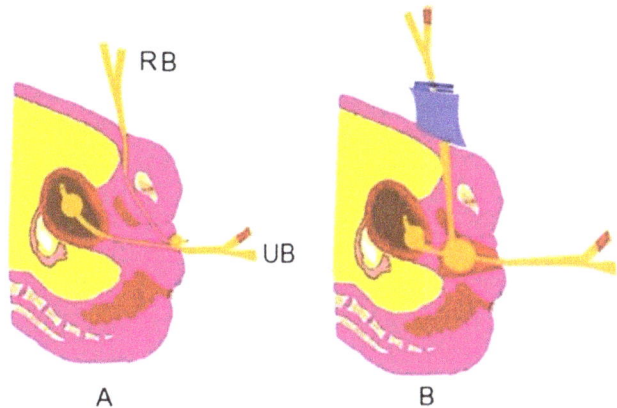

Fig. 3 Combined TFH canalizations with intrauterine catheter draining the uterine cavity coming out from the vaginal dimple, and retropubic vaginoplasty with the catheter coming out from the anterior abdominal wall in cases with cervicovaginal aplasia. **a** Catheters before traction. **b** Catheters after traction. *UB* uterine balloon, *RB* retropubic balloon

Transfundal hysteroscopy was successfully performed for the five cases. The operative time of TFH ranged between 5 and 14 min. Most of the time was spent in drainage and washing out the uterine contents. The uterine contents were thick chocolate blood in two cases, liquid dark blood in two cases, and creamy colored infected contents in one case. The endometrium was healthy in four cases and covered with pyogenic membrane in the infected case. The irrigation was continued until most of the pyogenic membrane was detached and washed out. The intrauterine location of balloon was confirmed in all cases. Tubal ostia were visualized in three cases (when the 70° telescope was available); in the other two cases, 30° telescope was used which not allowing visualization of the ostia. Inspection of the access site at the fundus was done for all cases and confirmed the absence of any significant

bleeding. None of the cases required suturing of the fundal puncture. Bladder or rectal injuries have not occurred during any of the procedures.

In the cases with vaginal aplasia (U0C4V4), combined upward and downward traction was monitored via transrectal ultrasound until the uterine and retropubic balloons became in contact; kissing balloons was achieved (Fig. 4).

Day 7 second-look transvaginal office hysteroscopy was done across the new vagina and via the catheter tract during catheter change in three cases. The puncture site at the fundus was invisible and the whole fundus was lined by healthy endometrium. Uterine silicone catheters were changed three to five times and were retained for 3–6 months. Hysteroscopic examination of the communication tract and uterine cavity revealed epithelization of the tract from the first postoperative menstrual period. One case got married 6 months after the procedure, her follow-up data as regard the sexual penetration and satisfaction scores were give in Table 1.

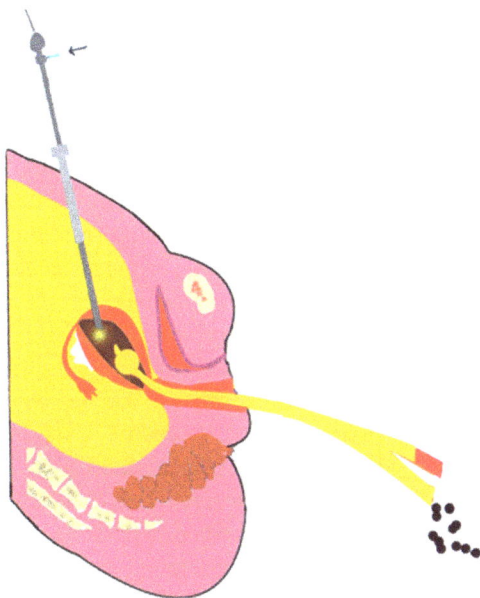

Fig. 2 Transfundal hysteroscopy is being passed through the already present fundal puncture; intrauterine contents going to be washed under vision. A probably placed intrauterine catheter is draining the uterine cavity and establishing the cervical canal

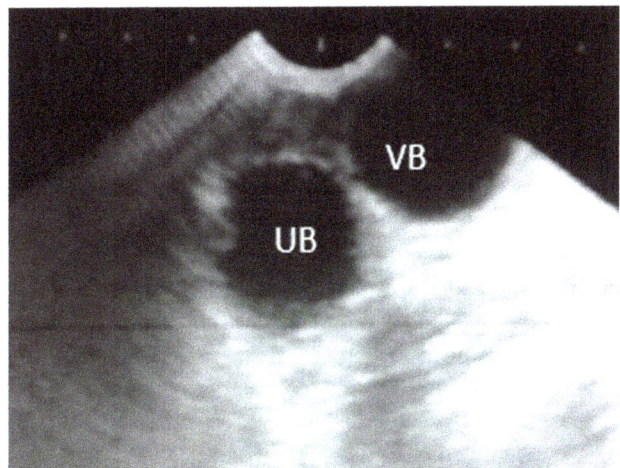

Fig. 4 Transrectal ultrasounds scan showing the uterine balloon (*UB*) in close contact with retropubic balloon (*VB*)

Table 1 Clinical findings, type of the procedure, and outcomes in the five cases undergone transfundal hysteroscopy

Findings	Infected hematometra (1 case)	Thick chocolate blood (2 cases)	Thin chocolate blood (2 cases)
Presentation	Fever, pains, and tenderness	Cyclic pains	Cyclic pains
Previous surgeries	2 conventional trials of utero-vestibular anastomosis	Appendectomy	Appendectomy 1 case Laparoscopy in the other
Type of anomaly	Cervicovaginal aplasia (U0C4V4)	Cervicovaginal aplasia (U0C4V4)	Isolated cervical aplasia (U0C4V0)
Type of procedure	Canalization + RBV	Canalization + RBV	Canalization only
Operative time (min)			
Total	70	55 and 65	40 and 35
TFH	14	13 and 12	5 and 6
Endometrium	Covered with pyogenic membrane	Healthy	Healthy
Menstrual flow during follow-up	6 months Regular menstruation	18 and 25 months Regular menstruations	22 and 28 months Regular menstruations
Cyclic pains	Dramatic relive	Dysmenorrhea	Relived
Neovaginal depth (cm.)	9	9 and 10	–
Penetration scores (…/100 points)			
Husband	–	80	–
Wife		80	
Satisfaction scores (…/100 points)			
Husband	–	90	–
Wife		90	

TFH transfundal hysteroscopy, *RBV* retropubic balloon vaginoplasty

Discussion

In the present work, we describe the use of rigid hysteroscopy through a transfundal approach during the endoscopic managements of cervical and or cervicovaginal atresia. The procedure was performed alone in women with isolated cervical atresia and in conjunction with retropubic BV in cases associated with vaginal aplasia. The procedure was done successfully in the five cases reported in this case series. The operations were followed by resumption of regular menstruation, relive of pain in all operated cases, and by normal sexual relations in one of the cases who got married.

Obstructive Müllerian anomalies (OMAs) represent a challenging category of Müllerian duct anomalies [7, 8]. In this case series, OMAs cases secondary to isolated cervical atresia/aplasia were treated with a simple endoscopic canalization technique without laparotomy or any dissection at the lower pole of the uterus or at the vaginal apex.

Compared to open surgical procedures [9–11] that were either performed via exploratory laparotomy or assisted by laparoscopy, the present procedure does not entail any dissection. Absence of dissection may be an important attributing factor to the long-lasting success that was achieved [5, 6]. Cases with OMAs associated with vaginal aplasia (U0C4V4) on the other hand were treated with endoscopic canalization using TFH in conjunction with retropubic BV [6]. In both circumstances, placement of intra-cervical stent was crucial

for success. Silicone catheters gauge 24–25 have a good caliber and less compressible stem that was used as a self-retaining cervical stent after inflation of its intrauterine placed balloon. Precise balloon placement inside the uterine cavity is an important key point for successful outcome.

In the present report, confirmation of accurate balloon placement was done via transfundal hysteroscopic examination. The visualization of whole circumference of balloon inside the uterine cavity was considered as an adequate evidence of its correct intrauterine location. Furthermore, the introduction of hysteroscopy with its pressurized fluid distention media allowed expedite and complete drainage of all thick retained menstrual blood that might minimize the chances of subsequent infection. In the single patient with concurrent infection, hysteroscopy distention media allowed not only rapid and complete drainage of pus and infected blood but also allowed detachment and washout of the pyogenic membrane. Dramatic relief of fever and improvement of the associated pain followed the procedure.

At the first glance, TFH can be considered as an invasive procedure since it was carried out through an intentional fundal perforation. However, the procedure itself did not add any invasive steps as the puncture of the myometrium was already created during the process of canalization and catheter placement. Therefore, the intended uterine puncture was a fundamental step of the original canalization procedure and the hysteroscopy was just passed through the preformed passage.

There are several other described successful procedures for management of cervicovaginal aplasia [9–13]. However, dissection either abdominal or vaginal is a fundamental part of these procedures. Therefore, subsequent scar formation is an anticipated consequence. If contracture of the scar develops, long-term failure of the procedure might result. In addition, subsequent surgeries will be more difficult. On contrast, our scalpel-free endoscopic procedures are not associated with any dissection and expected to have an expanding role for future management of OMAs.

The weakness point of the present report is the limited number of cases. However, there are some favorable points beside the aforementioned immediate benefits. This endoscopic development of lower genital tract opens new perspective for lesser invasive surrogate access to the uterine cavity whenever the natural access is impossible.

Informed consent All procedures followed were in accordance with the ethical standards of the responsible committee on human experimentation (institutional and national) and with the Helsinki Declaration of 1975, as revised in 2000. Informed consent was obtained from all patients for being included in the study.

References

1. El Saman AM (2010) Retropubic balloon vaginoplasty for management of Mayer-Rokitansky-Kuster-Hauser syndrome. Fertil Steril 93: 2016–2019
2. El Saman AM, Fathalla MM, Nasr AM, Youssef MA (2007) Laparoscopically assisted balloon vaginoplasty for management of vaginal aplasia. Int J Gynaecol Obstet 98:134–137
3. El Saman AM, Fathalla MM, Zakherah MS, Shaaban OM, Nasr A (2009) Modified balloon vaginoplasty: the fastest way to create a natural: minor changes in technique eliminate the need for customized instruments. Am J Obstet Gynecol 201(546):e1–e5
4. El Saman AM, Habib DM, Othman EE, Tawfik RM (2011) Successful canalization of a noncommunicating uterine horn by horn-vaginal anastomosis: preliminary findings of a novel approach for an unclassified anomaly. J Pediatr Surg 46:1464–1468
5. El Saman AM (2010) Endoscopically monitored canalization for treatment of congenital cervical atresia: the least invasive approach. Fertil Steril 94:313–316
6. El Saman AM (2009) Combined retropubic balloon vaginoplasty and laparoscopic canalization: a novel blend of techniques provides a minimally invasive treatment for cervicovaginal aplasia. Am J Obstet Gynecol 201(333):e1–e5
7. Grimbizis GF, Gordts S, Di Spiezio Sardo A, Brucker S, De Angelis C, Gergolet M, Li TC, Tanos V, Brolmann H, Gianaroli L, Campo R (2013) The ESHRE/ESGE consensus on the classification of female genital tract congenital anomalies. Hum Reprod 28:2032–2044
8. El Saman AM, Nasr A, Tawfik RM, Saadeldeen HS (2011) Mullerian duct anomalies: successful endoscopic management of a hybrid bicornuate/septate variety. J Pediatr Adolesc Gynecol 24:e89–e92
9. Roberts CP, Rock JA (2011) Surgical methods in the treatment of congenital anomalies of the uterine cervix. Curr Opin Obstet Gynecol 23:251–257
10. Rock JA, Roberts CP, Jones HW Jr (2010) Congenital anomalies of the uterine cervix: lessons from 30 cases managed clinically by a common protocol. Fertil Steril 94:1858–1863
11. Grimbizis GF, Tsalikis T, Mikos T, Papadopoulos N, Tarlatzis BC, Bontis JN (2004) Successful end-to-end cervico-cervical anastomosis in a patient with congenital cervical fragmentation: case report. Hum Reprod 19:1204–1210
12. Deffarges JV, Haddad B, Musset R, Paniel BJ (2001) Utero-vaginal anastomosis in women with uterine cervix atresia: long-term follow-up and reproductive performance. A study of 18 cases. Hum Reprod 16:1722–1725
13. Fliegner JR, Pepperell RJ (1994) Management of vaginal agenesis with a functioning uterus. Is hysterectomy advisable? Aust N Z J Obstet Gynaecol 34:467–470

22

Proposal of a modified transcervical endometrial resection (TCER) technique for menorrhagia treatment. Feasibility, efficacy, and patients' acceptability

Pietro Litta · Luigi Nappi · Pasquale Florio ·
Luca Mencaglia · Mario Franchini · Stefano Angioni

Abstract The aim of this study is to evaluate the feasibility, efficacy, safeness, and patients' acceptability of a modified transcervical endometrial resection (TCER) technique for the treatment of menorrhagia. Eighty-four premenopausal women with menorrhagia after careful investigation and 2 months therapy with GnRHa underwent a modified TCER. It was performed with a standard dual channel, 26 French irrigating resectoscope (Karl Storz, GmbH, Germany) after cervix dilatation to 10 mm and sorbitol mannitol solution used as distension medium. The modified technique was based on the resection of the endometrium and of the first myometrial layers only on the anterior and posterior walls, without treating fundus and cornual areas as usually performed. Endometrial resection was performed to a depth of 4 to 5 mm. Clinical and hysteroscopic follow-up was performed for 60 months. Early and late complications, changing in bleeding patterns, and patients' satisfaction were recorded. Sixty-four out of 73 patients that completed the 60 months improved. Eumenorrhea was achieved in 68.5 %, hypomenorrhea in 5.5 %, and amenorrhea in 13.7 %. Most of the patients (86.3 %) showed satisfaction at the follow-up interview. Control hysteroscopy showed that post modified TCER uterine cavity maintained the possibility of macroscopic and histopathology investigation during follow-up. Modified TCER is a technique easy to perform and effective in the long-term resolution of menorrhagia. In particular, it avoids the formation of synechiae and the shrinkage of the uterine cavity that may be the cause of various long-term complications, such as the delay in the diagnosis of endometrial carcinoma onset.

Keywords Menorrhagia · AUB · Endometrial resection · Minimally invasive surgery · Hysteroscopy

P. Litta
Department of Gynecological Science and Human Reproduction, University of Padua, Padua, Italy

L. Nappi
Department of Medical and Surgical Sciences, Institute of Obstetrics and Gynaecology, University of Foggia, Foggia, Italy

P. Florio
U.O.C. Obstetrics & Gynecology, "San Giuseppe" Hospital, Empoli, Italy

L. Mencaglia
Section of Gynecology, Centro Oncologico Fiorentino, Sesto Fiorentino, Italy

M. Franchini
Palagi Freestanding Unit, Florence, Italy

S. Angioni (✉)
Department of Surgical Sciences, Section of Obstetrics & Gynecology, University of Cagliari, Azienda Ospedaliero Universitaria, Blocco Q, SS554, Monserrato, Cagliari, Italy
e-mail: sangioni@yahoo.it

Introduction

Hysteroscopic transcervical endometrial resection (TCER) is a minimally invasive surgical technique developed in recent years with the purpose of removing the entire thickness of the endometrium lining of the uterus [1]. Indeed, to suppress menstruation successfully, it is essential to remove the full thickness of this lining together with the superficial myometrium, including the deep endometrial basal glands which are believed to be the primary foci for endometrial regrowth [1, 2]. However, TCER is not always completely successful and, in some cases, additional surgical treatment is required, thus limiting the benefits related to the reduced trauma and post-operative complications to the woman. The risk of failure and the expense of multiple treatments opened a debate whether endometrial ablation should replace or not hysterectomy [3], or if it might be an effective therapy for women with hyperplasia, with abnormal uterine bleeding, with high risk for medical therapy or hysterectomy [4]. The emerging clinical opinion is that TCER is an effective and safe alternative to hysterectomy that should be offered to women with menorrhagia for the relief of their heavy menstrual bleeding, together with the caution that there should be the possibility of further surgery, either repeat endometrial ablation or hysterectomy [5].

Matter of discussion related to TCER is also the putative occurrence of other problems related to the endometrial injury, as in the case of immediate (vascular or metabolic type complications (fluid overload) and perforation), or delayed complications (as in the case of the development of partial intrauterine dense adhesions and/or total obliteration of the cavity) [5–12]. Therefore, the ideal method of TCER associating high efficacy to nice tolerability and low incidence of complications is still far from being achieved. In the present study, we evaluated short- and long-term outcomes associated with a new TCER technique to treat menorrhagia that differ from the standard one in the fact that uterine fundus and cornual areas are not removed in the modified technique.

Materials and methods

Subjects

For this prospective cohort study, we consecutively enrolled from October 2, 2000 to September 24, 2005 all women suffering of menorrhagia who referred to our tertiary centers of women health care. The diagnosis of menorrhagia was performed by means of a pictorial blood loss assessment chart, adjusted to our needs in patients describing a history of heavy menstrual blood loss over several consecutive cycles [13]. A scoring system ranging from 1 to 10 was used, with 1=slightly soiled tampon, 5=moderately soiled, and 10=heavily soiled. Sanitary napkins were assigned ascending scores from 1 to 20. A total score more than 100 for each pictorial chart was meant as a confirmed diagnosis of menorrhagia [14]. We considered for the study only patients who had performed a full clinical evaluation including colposcopy and Papanicolaou test, transvaginal ultrasonography, and hysteroscopy with endometrial biopsy [15]. Exclusion criteria were the following: not confirmed diagnosis of menorrhagia, uterine size >12 cm, presence of large organic intrauterine lesions (endometrial polyp >3 cm, submucous myomas G0>2 cm or submucous myomas G1 and G2); desire of future pregnancy, cervical and endometrial pre- and malignant conditions or adnexal pathologies; and debilitating medical condition. Any medical hormonal treatment was suspended at least 1 month before enrollment. All procedures followed were in accordance with the ethical standards of the responsible committee on human experimentation (institutional and national) and with the Helsinki Declaration of 1975, as revised in 2000. Informed consent was obtained from all patients for being included in the study.

Surgical procedure: modified TCER

All the women underwent therapy with GnRH analogs (Leuprolide Acetate 3.75 mg) for 2 months (every 28 days) before surgery, as in standard practice [6]. All procedures were performed under general anesthesia, with induction by propofol 2 mg kg^{-1} and spontaneous ventilation with a mixture of 60 % nitrous oxide and 40 % oxygen isofluothane, or spinal anesthesia in selected patient [16]. Hysteroscopic MTCER was performed with a standard dual channel, 26 French irrigating resectoscope (Karl Storz, GmbH, Germany) after that cervix was dilated to 10 mm. The uterine cavity was distended with sorbitol mannitol solution used as distension medium, and a suction-irrigating unit (Endomat, Karl Storz, GmbH, Germany) was used to provide positive pressure (120 mmHg) and continuous outflow suction control (0.5 bar). Fluid balance was carefully monitored throughout the procedure that was interrupted if fluid deficit was over 1,000 cm^3. Surgical time was recorded starting at resectoscope introduction inside the uterus and ending at its last removal.

Compared to the technique described by Wortman and Dagget [2], our modified TCER began on either anterior or posterior uterine wall and was based on the resection of the anterior cardinal strip of tissue followed by resection of the posterior and the two lateral cardinal strips without treating fundus and cornual areas (Fig. 1). The conventional TCER approach consists in the treatment of fundal and cornual areas by the equatorial loop and/or the use of the rollerball electrode. Endometrial resection was performed to a depth of 4 to 5 mm, and endomyometrial strips were removed from the cavity and sent for histological assessment. The procedure was scheduled for a 1-day surgery.

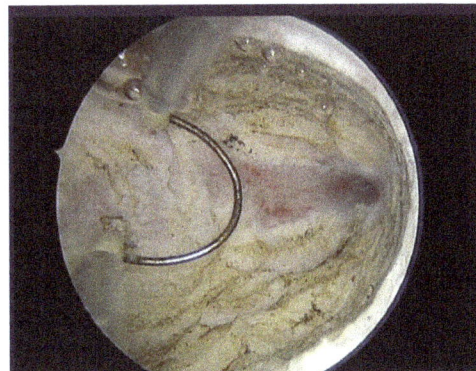

Fig. 1 Resection of the anterior cardinal strip of tissue followed by resection of the posterior and the two lateral cardinal strips without treating fundus and cornual areas

Office hysteroscopy

Control hysteroscopy was scheduled at 3, 12, 24, and 60 months after the surgery. It was performed by using vaginoscopic approach, with a continuous-flow hysteroscope using Telescope 2.9 mm (HOPKINS II Forward-Oblique Telescope 30°; Karl Storz, Tuttlingen, Germany) [17, 18]. The uterine cavity was distended with temperate saline solution and irrigated using an electronic irrigation pump (Hysteromat, Karl Storz®, Karl Storz, Tuttlingen, Germany). Examination was performed in an office setting, without anesthesia or cervical dilatation.

Main outcomes of the study

Outcome measures referred to changes in bleeding patterns, safeness, and patients' acceptability. In details, after modified TCER, women underwent office hysteroscopy for uterine cavity evaluation (with endometrial biopsy) 3, 12, 24, and 60 months after TCER, and simultaneously, patients were asked about the amelioration or persistence of bleeding, duration of amenorrhea, improvement of dysmenorrhea, and if they need any hormonal or surgical treatment for heavy bleeding after modified TCER.

Modified TCER was considered successful when it was associated with amenorrhea, hypomenorrhea, and eumenorrhea. A women was defined as amenorrheic when reporting persistent ceasing of menstruation after surgery. Eumenorrhea referred to regular menstrual cycle with average length of 28 days (range, 21–35 days), lasting on average for 4 days (range, 1–8 days) and of normal quantity (flowing less than 80 mL per cycle). Hypomenorrhea referred to menstruations regular in frequency but poor in quantity and/or lasting less than 2 days [1]. Resection was considered non-effective when the patient reported persistence or relapse of menorrhagia.

Interviews were done at the time of every follow-up hysteroscopy, and data were related to patients' subjective experiences related/consequent to modified TCER and their health status concerning endometrial status.

Statistical analysis

All data were analyzed with Prism software (GraphPad Software Inc., San Diego, CA, USA) and expressed as mean ±SD. The Kolmogorov-Smirnov test was used to evaluate whether values had a Gaussian distribution, in order to choose between parametric and non-parametric statistical tests. Therefore, the unpaired t test was used to compute statistical significance, and χ-square and Fisher exact test to analyze differences between proportions. Statistical significance was assumed for values of $P<0.05$.

Results

Some patients were not included in the study. Exclusion criteria were the following: not confirmed diagnosis of menorrhagia (26 women), uterine size >12 cm (10 patients), presence of large organic intrauterine lesions (endometrial polyp >3 cm, submucous myomas G0 >2 cm, and submucous myomas G1 and G2) (15 patients); desire of future pregnancy (eight patients), cervical, and endometrial pre- and malignant conditions or adnexal pathologies (10 patients).

Eighty-four patients out of 153 (age 45.37±4.02) entered the study. The clinical study protocol consisted of modified TCER, followed by the assessment of endometrial cavity by office diagnostic hysteroscopy 3, 12, 24, and 60 months after the surgery. Table 1 shows clinical and demographic details of the population evaluated in the study. Endometrial resection was successfully performed in all patients enrolled. No one of the patients had early or late complications. In 24 out of 84 patients, endometrial resection was associated with the simultaneous removal of small polyps ($n=15$) or myomas ($n=9$) (data not shown). In any case, the time required for endometrial resection with associated polypectomy (13.31±6.09 min) or myomectomy (14.7±8.2 min) did not differ when compared to the endometrial resection alone (11.91±4.15 min; $P>0.05$), as well as the time spent for cervical dilatation and the infusion volume needed for uterine distension (data not shown). In 11 cases (13 %), adenomyosis was evidenced by histopathologic examination.

Follow-up outcomes: clinical findings

Eleven women dropped out (13.1 %) and did not complete the first year of follow-up, while 73 (86.9 %) patients completed the follow-up for at least 60 months (Table 2) and 61 (83.6 %) of these reached a 84-month follow-up. During the observational time interval, bleeding patterns were observed in eumenorrhea in 50 out of 73 women (68.5 %), hypomenorrhea in four patients (5.5 %), and amenorrhea in 10 subjects (13.7 %) (Table 2). None of them reported spotting, neither dysmenorrhea onset or worsening, nor medium-/

Table 1 Anthropometric and surgical data related to the population prospectively evaluated

Age (years)	45.37±4.02
Gravida	2.3±1.2
Parity	2.4±1.2
BMI (kg/m²)	28.7±3.3
Mean operating time (min)	12.4±1.8
Cervical dilatation (min)	1.4±0.4
Infusion volume (mL)	2,500±550
Fluid deficit (mL)	250±110

Data are reported as mean±SD

Table 2 Data related to the clinical findings retrieved at follow-up after modified TCER in women prospectively evaluated

Patients underwent MTCER (n; %)	84 (100 %)
Follow-up completed after 3 months (n; %)	84 (100)
Follow-up completed after 60 months (n; %)	73 (86.9)
Bleeding patterns after TCER	
Eumenorrhea (n; %)	50/73 (68.5)
Hypomenorrhea (n; %)	4/73 (5.5)
Amenorrhea (n; %)	10/73 (13.7)
Menorrhagia (n; %)	7/73 (9.6)
Recurrence of AUB/DUB (n; %)	2/73 (2.7)

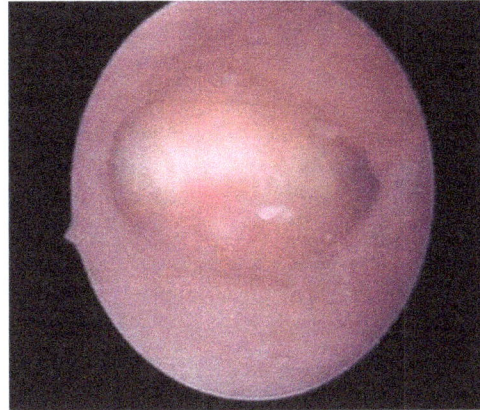

Fig. 2 Hysteroscopic appearance of endometrial cavity at 3-month follow-up after MTCER. None of the patients were found to have intrauterine adhesions

long-term complications such as pregnancy or complications putatively related to the development of intra-cavitary adhesions, such as hematometra and/or cornual hematometra, as observed at diagnostic office hysteroscopy.

Seven (9.6 %) patients continued to have menorrhagia, and among them, two of the 11 cases were with adenomyosis (18.2 %). Three patients underwent laparoscopic hysterectomy (n=3) after an average interval of 6 months (range, 1–11 months), two patients underwent hormonal treatment by means of levonorgestrel-based intrauterine device, and the remaining two women underwent 4-month GnRH analog administration (n=2) (data not shown). In these patients, a second modified TCER was not performed because patients refused such a type of treatment.

In addition, AUB recurred in two women (2.7 %) after 12 and 60 months after endometrial resection (Table 2). They underwent a new modified TCER or laparoscopic hysterectomy (for the women in whom recurrence occurred 60 months after modified TCER) (data not shown).

Follow-up outcome: data from interview

At the end of 3-month follow-up, 63 women (86.3 %) stated they were satisfied by the surgery so much that they would recommend it to women with menorrhagia, whereas the remaining 10 patients (13.7 %) would not, for reasons mainly related to the fear of general anesthesia (n=8; 80.0 %) or office hysteroscopy in the follow-up (n=2; 20 %). None of the patients had symptoms or conditions invalidating and/or limiting their quality of life (data not shown).

Follow-up outcome: hysteroscopic findings

Considering findings recorded at hysteroscopic follow-up, none of the patients was found to have intra-uterine adhesions or cavity contracture after 3 months. It was possible to evaluate the entire cavity, including the cornual area and the tubal ostia in all patients (Fig. 2). The same findings were obtained

at all time points in the follow-up, even if the uterine cavity at the hysteroscopic evaluation performed after 12, 24, and 60 months from endometrial resection was markedly reduced to a narrow tube as a result of fibrosis and contracture (Fig. 3). In any case, the entire uterine cavity, including the cornual areas, was found to be open and the tubal ostia were visualized at all time points of follow-up. In addition, histological evaluation of endometrial biopsy annually performed failed to found cancerous or pre-cancerous endometrial lesions (data not shown).

Discussion

The present study first refers on the clinical efficiency and patients' perception of a new endometrial resection technique, by using which menorrhagia was resolved in the majority of patients, without surgical complications, no intrauterine adhesions formation in the follow-up, no fluid overload syndrome, short operative time, and a high degree of patients' satisfaction.

The reasons that led us to devise such a new technique are related to the fact that the *conventional* hysteroscopic TCER is

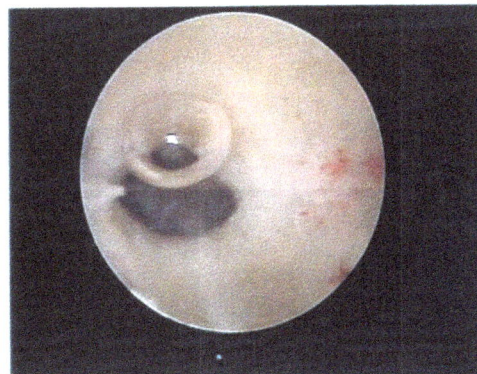

Fig. 3 A narrowing of the cavity is evidenced at 60 months but it does not hinder to evaluate the entire cavity, including the cornual area

sometime associated to clinical problems, like surgical (perforation of the uterus), vascular complications or fluid overload syndrome [5–12]. Moreover, like resectoscopic myomectomy, TCER is a surgical procedure suggested only to experienced surgeons [19]. Consequently, our aim was to simplify and to accelerate the procedure maintaining the success rate and possibly decreasing the complications in order to make it accessible even to less experienced gynecologists. In addition, we intended to decrease the occurrence of intrauterine adhesions, contractures, and/or hematometra [12, 20–22]. These last side effects are due to the fact that after the endometrium is destroyed or resected, the myometrium is exposed and intrauterine walls, collapsing on each other, have a natural tendency to grow together. The final result is the intrauterine contracture and marked reduction of the endometrial cavity to a narrow tubular structure as a result of fibrosis that often obstructs the cornual area. This mechanism is responsible for the occurrence of synechiae in 40 % of women submitted to total TCER [2] that may limit the access to the uterine cavity, hematometra, that usually localizes in the fundus of the uterus, or obstruction of the cornual area in 13 % of cases [11, 22, 23]. The persistence in these obstructed areas of islands of endometrial tissue may cause retrograde menstruation or symptomatic cornual hematometra, with an incidence of even 18 %, causing painful distension of the uterus [24]. The potential of all these complications may limit the clinical efficacy of hysteroscopic TCER and can require hysterectomy. In our technique, the resection of the endometrium and of the first myometrial layers was limited only on the anterior and posterior and lateral walls, without treating fundal and cornual areas by using the rollerball, as usually performed [1, 2] The initial hypothesis was that preserving endometrial mucosa of the fundal and cornual areas could decrease the risk of synechiae or focal hematometra facilitating the long-term uterine inspection [15, 25]. The possibility that this approach could result in menorrhagia or bleeding persistence due to the endometrial mucosa not removed was not shown by our study. Moreover, in our case series, we failed to detect intrauterine adhesions at all evaluated time points after 12, 24, and 60 months and it was possible to carry out an endometrial biopsy sampling for histological evaluation despite the presence of some cavity contracture in the long-term follow-up. As possible explanation, one may propose that the integrity of corneal and fundal areas might sustain intrauterine walls.

On this regard, the work of McCausland and McCausland was pioneering, since recommending ablation of only one wall of the uterine cavity and avoiding the cornual areas reduced the incidence of adhesions formation after TCER [26]. Moreover, other authors have already proposed the resection of the entire upper uterine fundus, but sparing the isthmus and the immediate supraisthmic region to prevent hematometra caused by stenosis at the level of the cervical isthmus [27].

Findings obtained in the long-term follow-up of the present study showed the absence of intrauterine adhesions and/or hematometra: no patient reported, both in the hysteroscopic and clinical verification, the appearance or worsening of dysmenorrhea, and none of them had long-term complications ascribable to the development of intrauterine synechiae such as cornual hematometra. These findings lead us to suggest that the modified TCER we are proposing is able to avoid the formation of synechiae or shrinkage of the uterine cavity.

The second clinical matter that merits discussion refers to the absence in our study of intra- and peri-operative complications (uterine perforation, hemorrhage, excess fluid absorption, and thermic damages to peri-uterine structures). Cornual myometrium is indeed notoriously thin and thus with low resistance, therefore representing the critical area for any procedure performed at uterine fundus. Deciding not to treat such zone, we simplified the procedure making uterine perforations or thermic damages to peri-uterine structures improbable or at least less frequent compared to the conventional technique. Nevertheless, in modified TCER, the exposure of a smaller surface of the myometrium and the short operating time needed may together contribute to reduce absorption of hypotonic, electrolyte-free non-conductive distention solution, consequently not allowing the development of the overload syndrome [28].

It could be criticized that the residual endometrial tissue not removed in uterine fundus and cornual areas may be the site of putative pre- or markedly malignant lesions. We took care of this criticism, and so, we submitted our patients to an endometrial surveillance by endometrial biopsy under hysteroscopic guidance. Our follow-up hysteroscopies consented to visualize and collect samples from fundus and corneal areas in every patient. On the contrary, in the conventional TCER technique, the habitual collapse of the uterine walls and the formation of synechiae may hinder endometrial biopsy. Whether such a problem does not seem to affect low-risk population (i.e., patients with pre-ablation biopsy negative for hyperplasia and negative medical history for common risk factors for uterine neoplasia) [29], modified TCER may represent a valid therapeutic option for those patients considered at increased risk of developing hyperplasia and endometrial carcinoma. The unquestionable advantage of TCER, as opposed to new-generation destructive ablation methods, is to provide additional tissue for histological examination of the endometrium so that it is possible to detect any presence of micro foci of neoplasia or a high risk for it in the resected material previously not diagnosed in pre-surgical biopsy [30]. On the other hand, patients with increased risk of hyperplasia or endometrial neoplasia frequently are also at higher risk for major surgery, such is hysterectomy. Indeed, cardiovascular diseases, severe obesity, chronic nephropathies, coagulopathies, and hepatopathies are often co-existent with a history of meno- or metrorrhagia and also imply a high surgical and anesthesiological risks. The modified TCER we propose can be even more suitable for those "complex" patients, since it would have the advantage to be performed more quickly, with less intra- and peri-operative complications that the endometrial resection used so far.

In conclusion, despite the limitation due to the small sample size, our data on complications and the low (11.3 %) prevalence of bleeding persistence after operative hysteroscopy would suggest that modified TCER is a technique easy to perform, effective in the resolution of long-term menorrhagia and useful in patients with high surgical and anesthesiological risks. In addition, this new approach allows avoiding the formation of synechiae and the shrinkage of the uterine cavity that may be the cause for various long-term complications, such as the delay in the diagnosis of endometrial carcinoma onset.

Informed consent All procedures followed were in accordance with the ethical standards of the responsible committee on human experimentation (institutional and national) and with the Helsinki Declaration of 1975, as revised in 2000. Informed consent was obtained from all patients for being included in the study.

References

1. Magos AL, Baumann R, Lockwood GM, Turnbull AC (1991) Experience with the first 250 endometrial resection for menorrhagia. Lancet 337:1074–1078

2. Wortman M, Daggett A (1994) Hysteroscopic endomyometrial resection: a new technique for the treatment of menorrhagia. Obstet Gynecol 83:295–299

3. Farquhar CM, Steiner CA (2002) Hysterectomy rates in the United States 1990–1997. Obstet Gynecol 99:229–234

4. Vilos GA, Harding PG, Ettler HC (2002) Resectoscopic surgery in women with abnormal uterine bleeding and nonatypical endometrial hyperplasia. J Am Assoc Gynecol Laparosc 9:131–137

5. Lethaby A, Penninx J, Hickey M, Garry R, Marjoribanks J (2013) Endometrial resection and ablation techniques for heavy menstrual bleeding. Cochrane Database Syst Rev 8, CD001501

6. Litta P, Merlin F, Pozzan C, Nardelli GB, Capobianco G, Dessole S, Ambrosini A (2006) Transcervical endometrial resection in women with menorrhagia: long-term follow-up. Eur J Obstet Gynecol Reprod Biol 125:99–102

7. MacLean-Fraser E, Penava D, Vilos GA (2002) Perioperative complication rates of primary and repeat hysteroscopic endometrial ablations. J Am Assoc Gynecol Laparosc 9:175–177

8. Papadopoulos NP, Magos A (2007) First-generation endometrial ablation: roller-ball vs loop vs laser. Best Pract Res Clin Obstet Gynaecol 21(6):915–929

9. Paschopoulos M, Polyzos NP, Lavasidis LG, Vrekoussis T, Dalkalitsis N, Paraskevaidis E (2006) Safety issues of hysteroscopic surgery. Ann N Y Acad Sci 1092:229–234

10. Perino A, Castelli A, Cucinella G, Biondo A, Pane A, Venezia R (2004) A randomized comparison of endometrial laser intrauterine thermotherapy and hysteroscopic endometrial resection. Fertil Steril 82(3):731–734

11. Boujida VH, Philipsen T, Pelle J, Joergensen JC (2002) Five-year follow-up of endometrial ablation: endometrial coagulation versus endometrial resection. Obstet Gynecol 99(6):988–992

12. Propst AM, Liberman RF, Harlow BL, Ginsburg ES (2000) Complications of hysteroscopic surgery: predicting patients at risk. Obstet Gynecol 96(4):517–520

13. Higham JM, O'Brian PMS, Shaw RW (1990) Assessment of menstrual blood loss using a pictorial chart. Br J Obstet Gynaecol 97:734–739

14. De Angelis C, Carnevale A, Santoro G, Nofroni I, Spinelli M, Guida M, Mencaglia L, Di Spiezio Sardo A (2013) Hysteroscopic findings in women with menorrhagia. J Minim Invasive Gynecol 20(2):209–214

15. Angioni S, Loddo A, Milano F, Piras B, Minerba L, Melis GB (2008) Detection of benign intracavitary lesions in postmenopausal women with AUB. A prospective study on outpatients hysteroscopy and blind biopsies. J Minim Invasive Gynecol 15(1):87–91

16. Florio P, Puzzutiello R, Filippeschi M, D'Onofrio P, Mereu L, Morelli R, Marianello D, Litta P, Mencaglia L, Petraglia F (2012) Low-dose spinal anesthesia with hyperbaric bupivacaine with intrathecal fentanyl for operative hysteroscopy: a case series study. J Minim Invasive Gynecol 19(1):107–112

17. Di Spiezio Sardo A, Bettocchi S, Spinelli M, Guida M, Nappi L, Angioni S, Sosa Fernandez LM, Nappi C (2010) Review of new office-based hysteroscopic procedures 2003–2009. J Minim Invasive Gynecol 17:436–448

18. Daniilidis A, Pantelis A, Dinas K, Tantanasis T, Loufopoulos PD, Angioni S, Carcea F (2012) Indications of diagnostic hysteroscopy, a brief review of the literature. Gynecol Surg 9(1):23–28

19. Litta P, Conte L, De Marchi F, Saccardi C, Angioni S (2014) Pregnancy outcome after hysteroscopic myomectomy. Gynecol Endocrinol 30(2):149–152

20. Overton C, Hargreaves J, Maresh M (1997) A national survey of the complications of endometrial destruction for menstrual disorders: the MISTLETOE study. Minimally Invasive Surgical Techniques–Laser, EndoThermal or Endoresection. Br J Obstet Gynaecol 104(12):1351–1359

21. Hart R, Magos A (1997) Endometrial ablation. Curr Opin Obstet Gynecol 9(4):226–232

22. Wortman M, Daggett A (2001) Reoperative hysteroscopic surgery in the management of patients who fail endometrial ablation and resection. J Am Assoc Gynecol Laparosc 8(2):272–277

23. Tapper AM, Heinonen PK (1995) Hysteroscopic endomyometrial resection for the treatment of menorrhagia–follow-up of 86 cases. Eur J Obstet Gynecol Reprod Biol 62(1):75–79

24. McCausland AM, McCausland VM (2002) Frequency of symptomatic cornual hematometra and postablation tubal sterilization syndrome after total rollerball endometrial ablation: a 10-year follow-up. Am J Obstet Gynecol 186:1274–1280

25. Litta P, Merlin F, Saccardi C, Pozzan C, Sacco G, Fracas M, Capobianco G, Dessole S (2005) Role of hysteroscopy with endometrial biopsy to rule out endometrial cancer in postmenopausal women with abnormal uterine bleeding. Maturitas 50(2):117–123

26. McCausland AM, McCausland VM (1999) Partial rollerball endometrial ablation: a modification of total ablation to treat menorrhagia without causing complications from intrauterine adhesions. Am J Obstet Gynecol 180:1512–1521

27. Perino A, Cittadini E, Colacurci N, De Placido G, Hamou J (1990) Endometrial ablation: principles and technique. Acta Eur Fertil 21(6):313–317

28. Witz CA, Silverberg KM, Burns WN, Schenken RS, Olive DL (1993) Complications associated with the absorption of hysteroscopic fluid media. Fertil Steril 60(5):745–756

23

Transvaginal hysterotomy for cesarean scar pregnancy in 40 consecutive cases

Zhang Huanxiao · Chen Shuqin · Jiang Hongye ·
Xie Hongzhe · Niu Gang · Xu Chengkang ·
Guan Xiaoming · Yao Shuzhong

Abstract To propose a novel procedure as a safe and effective treatment for cesarean scar pregnancy (CSP), a cohort study was initiated in patients diagnosed with CSP and treated with transvaginal hysterotomy from December 2009 to March 2013, either as a primary or secondary therapy. All diagnoses were confirmed by both sonography and pathology, either a gestational sac or residual tissue after termination of pregnancy or miscarriage in the cesarean section scar. Basic clinical characteristics and perioperative data were collected and analyzed. A total of 40 patients were included. The mean age was 32.88 ± 4.55 years. The mean size of gestational sacs of the CSP mass at diagnosis was 33.78 ± 13.14 mm. Mean serum β-hCG level at diagnosis was 47379.73 ± 45285.10 IU/L. Mean operative time was 57.25 ± 24.52 min. Mean postoperative hemoglobin drop was 1.635 ± 0.906 g/dL. Complications were one case of bacteremia and two cases of hematoma. Mean hospital stay after surgery was 4.95 ± 2.62 days. Mean serum β-hCG levels decreased by 88.5, 93.5, and 96.5 % at postoperative day 2, 4, and 6, respectively. All patients' β-hCG levels returned to normal range within 1 month after surgery. Transvaginal hysterotomy with removal of ectopic pregnancy tissue and repair of cesarean scar defect is a promising approach to manage CSPs, with a short hospital stay, low postoperative pain, blood loss, and cost.

Keywords Cesarean scar pregnancy · Treatment · Transvaginal hysterotomy

Introduction

As a rare form of ectopic pregnancy, cesarean scar pregnancy (CSP) refers to the implantation of a pregnancy within the myometrium at the site of a prior cesarean scar. If not detected early and managed properly, CSP can result in life-threatening complications, such as massive hemorrhage, uterine rupture, disseminated intravascular coagulation, and even maternal death [1]. Once diagnosed, therapy is strongly recommended to avoid subsequent life-threatening complications. However, no obvious most effective therapeutic strategy has been established to date. Removal of the ectopic pregnancy tissue is usually done. By following the concepts of minimally invasive surgery, we designed and carried out the first case of hysterotomy by transvaginal approach for the treatment of CSP in 2009. A preliminary report of six cases was published in 2011 with encouraging results [2]. Since 2009, we have successfully completed 40 transvaginal CSP cases without significant complications. Herein, we summarize our experience with this novel surgical approach for CSP and propose the procedure as a safe, effective, and minimally invasive treatment modality.

Z. Huanxiao · C. Shuqin · J. Hongye · X. Hongzhe · N. Gang ·
X. Chengkang · Y. Shuzhong (✉)
Department of Gynecology & Obstetrics, The First Affiliated
Hospital of Sun Yat-sen University, No. 58 2nd Zhongshan Road,
Guangzhou, Guangdong Province, China
e-mail: yszlfy@163.com

G. Xiaoming
Baylor College of Medicine, Houston, USA

Patients and methods

All patients diagnosed with CSP and consented to have a transvaginal surgery were enrolled in this study from

December 2009 to March 2013. The study protocol was approved by the institutional ethics committee of the university, and all patients provided written informed consent before enrollment.

Diagnosis and grouping

Cesarean scar pregnancy was diagnosed by ultrasonography and β-human chorionic gonadotropin (β-hCG) level. The diagnostic criteria for transvaginal ultrasound were as follows: (1) an empty uterine cavity and cervical canal with a clearly demonstrated endometrium and (2) a gestation sac, with or without fetal cardiac activity, embedded in and surrounded by the myometrium and the fibrous tissue of the cesarean section scar in the anterior part of the uterine isthmus, that was separated from the endometrial cavity or fallopian tube, with a diminished or absent myometrial layer between the bladder and the sac [3–5]. Patients with residual in the cesarean scar tissue following spontaneaous miscarriage, termination of pregnancy, or previous treatment of CSP were also included as a subgroup. These were patients in whom the diagnosis was made based on prolonged vaginal bleeding, elevated β-hCG level, and a heterogeneous mass at the same site as the gestational sac described above. Previous treatments were considered unsatisfactory if the level of β-hCG failed to decrease 1 week after treatment, or massive vaginal bleeding developed.

To confirm the diagnosis, morphologic and pathological information were collected during and after surgery.

Treatment protocol

Preoperative preparation was the same as for other transvaginal surgical procedures. All patients were placed in a dorsal lithotomy position, and the bladder was emptied. General anesthesia was applied. After a pair of vaginal retractors was placed into the vagina, the cervix was grasped and manipulated with a toothed tenaculum. Adrenaline solution (1.5 μg/mL; 10–20 mL) was injected submucosally for hydrodissection and hemostasis before an incision was made at the anterior cervicovaginal junction (Fig. 1a). The bladder was dissected away until the anterior peritoneal reflection was identified. The anterior retractor was inserted into the vaginal incision to lift up the bladder. The CSP was identified as a bluish bulge located in the anterior wall of the lower uterine segment (Fig. 1b). A transverse incision was made on the lower margin of the most prominent area of the bulge. Ectopic pregnancy tissue was removed with sponge forceps or suction through the incision on the uterus isthmus (Fig. 2). Thorough curettage was done through the incision or cervical canal. The edges of the incision were trimmed with scissors to remove all of the scar tissue (Fig. 3). The myometrial (Fig. 4) and vaginal

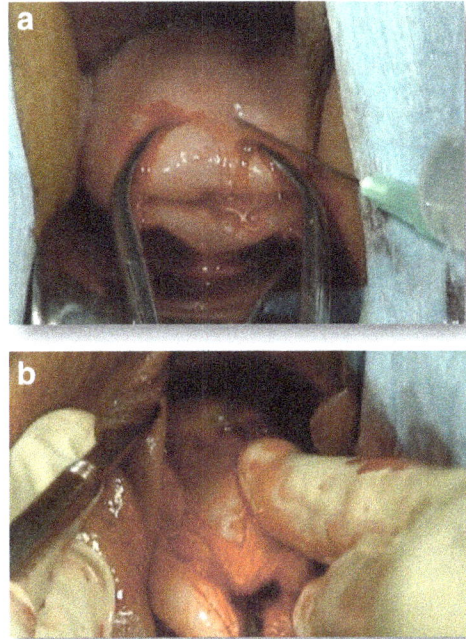

Fig. 1 **a** Adrenaline solution was injected submucosally for hydrodissection and hemostasis. **b** The bladder was dissected away and the CSP (*arrow*) was identified as a bluish bulge located in the anterior wall of the lower uterine segment

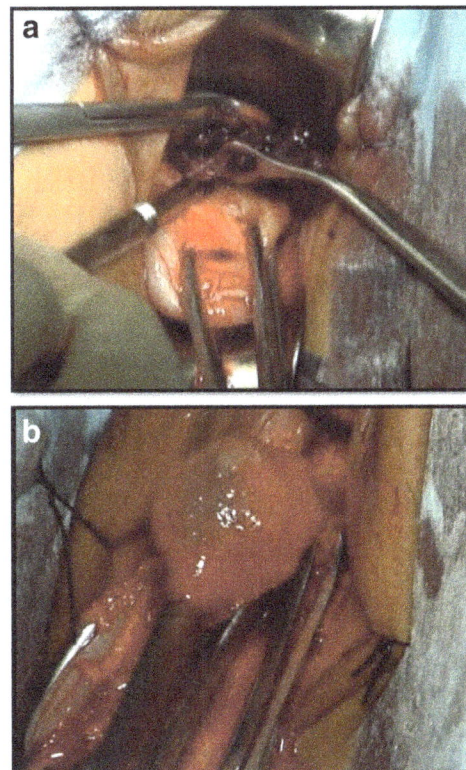

Fig. 2 Ectopic pregnancy tissue was removed with sponge forceps (**a**) or suction (**b**) through the incision on the uterus isthmus

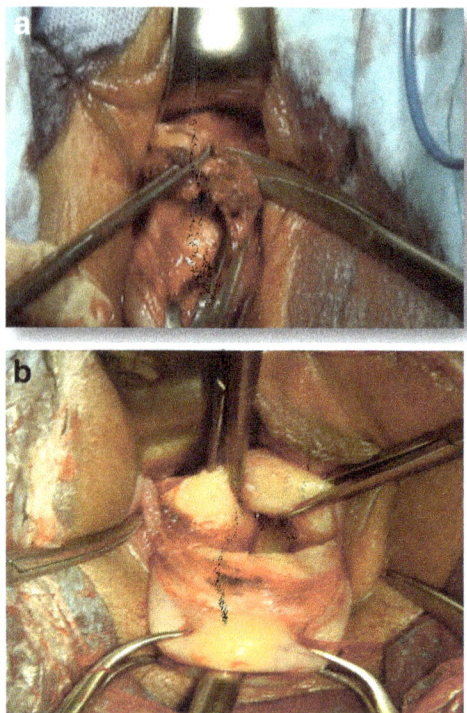

Fig. 3 The edges of the incision were trimmed with scissors to remove all scar tissue

(Fig. 5) incisions were closed with continuous locking sutures using 2–0 absorbable sutures.

Postoperative assessment

Perioperative parameters included operating time, blood loss, blood transfusion, conversion to laparotomy, complications related to surgery, course of serum β-hCG titers, length of hospital stay after surgery, and other adverse effects.

Follow-up assessments included remission of symptoms, monitoring decrease of serum β-hCG titer, and resumption of menstruation thereafter. Serum β-hCG level was monitored

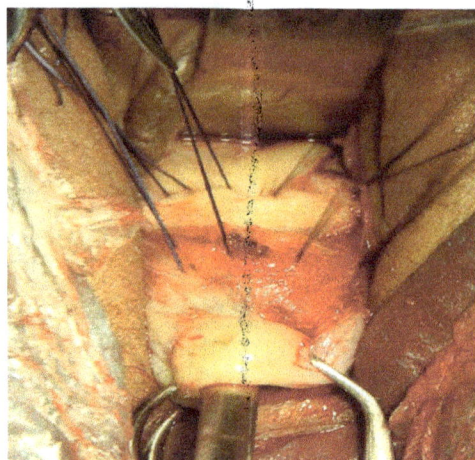

Fig. 4 The myometrial incision was closed with interrupted suture and then continuous locking sutures

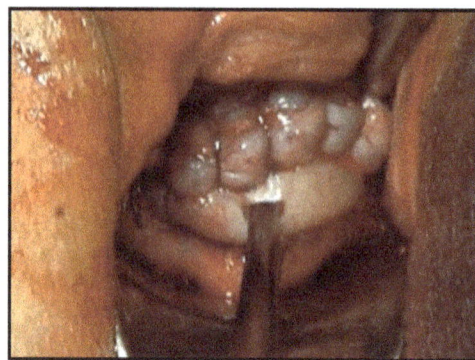

Fig. 5 The vaginal incision was closed with continuous locking sutures

every other day in the first week after the surgery and weekly thereafter until the titers returned to normal levels.

Statistical analysis

Data were collected and evaluated for parametric analysis. Mean±standard deviations (SD) are reported for continuous data, whereas categorical data are presented as the absolute count and percentage. ANOVA test was used to compare the mean differences. $P<0.05$ was considered statistically significant. SPSS 13.0 software was used to perform statistical analysis.

Results

A total of 40 consecutive patients with CSP who underwent vaginal surgery were enrolled in the study. The baseline clinical characteristics are presented in Table 1. Twenty-five patients presented with vital pregnancy (Group A), 23 of which had fetal heart activity at the moment of surgery. Eight patients underwent medical treatment or embolization prior to admission (Group B), including two cases of uterine artery embolization (UAE) combined with local methotrexate (MTX) injection, three cases of systemic MTX injection, and three cases who received mifepristone treatment. All of

Table 1 The baseline clinical characteristics of 40 patients [a]

Characteristic	Mean±SD (range)[a]
Age (yr)	32.88±4.55 (24–43)
Interval from last cesarean section to surgical treatment (month)	68.61±45.34 (9–188)
Gestational age (day)	58.59±16.48 (41–120)
Serum β-hCG level (IU/L)	47,379.73±45,285.10 (9.2–188,942)
Diameter of gestational sac (mass) on ultrasound scan (mm)	33.78±13.14 (12–60)

[a] Data are given as mean±SD (range)

Table 2 Perioperative evaluation of the surgical procedure

Variable	Mean±SD (range)[a]
Duration of surgery, (min)	57.25±24.52 (20–120)
Estimated blood loss during surgery, (mL)	47.88±35.71 (10–200)
Length of hospital stay after surgery, (day)	4.95±2.62 (2–17)
Hemoglobulin decreased after 24 h, (g/L)	16.35±9.06 (2–41)

[a] Data are given as Mean±SD (range)

these were considered unsatisfactory. The other seven patients presented with residual products of conception in the cesarean scar on ultrasound scan after spontaneous or elective abortion (Group C). One patient had undergone three previous lower segment transverse cesarean sections. Fourteen patients had two previous cesarean sections. The remaining 25 patients had one previous cesarean section. Twelve patients were asymptomatic. Twenty-eight patients complained of various patterns of vaginal bleeding, including one case of hemorrhagic shock.

Perioperative data on vaginal surgery is presented in Table 2. None of the patients required conversion to laparotomy. Blood transfusion was needed only for the single patient who presented with hypovolemic shock at admission. No excessive bleeding or injury to adjacent organ was observed. Only one patient developed postoperative gram negative septicemia as demonstrated by hemoculture. The patient completed a 7-day course of antibiotic treatment and was subsequently discharged without further signs of infection. Two patients developed a local hematoma that resolved spontaneously after 3 months with no further complications. The mean serum β-hCG level decreased by 88.5, 93.5, and 96.5 % at postoperative day 2, 4, and 6, respectively, comparing to baseline. In all patients, trophoblast and scar tissue

within the uterine smooth muscle confirmed the pathologic diagnosis of CSP.

Gestational age, β-hCG level, and size of gestational sac were not associated with operating time, hemoglobin decrement, or length of hospital stay after surgery. The subgroup of patients who underwent other treatment for CSP before vaginal surgery had significantly longer operating time than those without previous treatment (73.1±28.2 vs. 52.2±23.2). Hemoglobin drop and length of hospital stay after surgery were not significantly different among the subgroups (Table 3).

Finally, patients were categorized into two cohorts of 20 by chronological order. Their age, gestational age, serum β-hCG level, and size of gestational sac were comparable. Hospital stay after surgery significantly decreased in the second group (6.0±3.20 vs. 3.90±1.25). Though there was a trend for shorter operating time (60.0±20.33 vs. 54.5±28.37) and hemoglobin drop (18.25±8.69 vs. 14.45±9.23), this was not significant.

Follow-up data were obtained from all patients between 2 and 36 months after surgery. Vaginal bleeding stopped around 1 week after transvaginal surgery. The serum β-hCG level in all the cases resolved to normal range within 1 month after surgery. All patients recovered without complications, no subsequent treatment was needed, and there was no further report of abnormal menstrual pattern.

Discussion

As CSP is an iatrogenic complication of cesarean section, the incidence of CSP is likely to rise dramatically in the near future due to the increase of cesarean section rates as well as the increased utilization of diagnostic ultrasound. Since first

Table 3 Comparison of subgroups[b]

	Sub-group[a]		
	Group A (vital CSPs without previous treatment)	Group B (CSPs with previous conservative treatment)	Group C (CSPs with pregnant tissue residues)
No. of cases	25	8	7
Age, (yr)	33.6±4.4	31.0±4.8	32.4±4.7
Serum β-hCG level (IU/L)	58,160.4±46,189.4[d]	40,481.4±36067.2	16,761.0±40,457.9[b]
Size of gestational sac (mass) on ultrasound scan before surgery, (mm)	34.8±10.9	28.0±14.2	38.0±20.5
Duration of surgery, (min)	52.2±23.2[c]	73.1±28.2[b]	57.1±19.5
Hemoglobulin decrement within 24 h, (g/L)	17.0±10.1	13.3±7.4	17.7±6.7
Length of hospital stay after surgery, (day)	5.48±3.0	4.13±1.2	4.0±1.7

[a] Data are given as mean (SD). The mean difference is significant at the 0.05 level

[b] Significantly different from Group A

[c] Significantly different from Group B

[d] Significantly different from Group C

being reported by Larsen and Solomon in 1978 [6], the number of cases of CSP showed an exponential increase. Between 1978 and 2001, only 18 cases of CSP were reported in the English literature [3]. In a later review in 2007 [4], 161 cases of CSP from 58 citations were included. Jurkovic et al. and Seow et al. have estimated the prevalence of CSP in their local population attending the early pregnancy assessment unit to be 1:1800 [7] and 1:2216 [8], respectively.

As a tertiary center in southern China, we have been dealing with CSP for a long time. Our data through 2011 showed that CSPs constituted 2.2 % of ectopic gestations in our hospital [2]. Before 2009, most of CSPs were managed by UAE and MTX administration. Since the first transvaginal hysterotomy in 2009, this treatment was explained to every patient diagnosed with CSP as well as UAE. All patients agreed to have vaginal surgery and provided informed consent. It had been successfully performed in 40 cases of CSP.

In patients with prior cesarean section, transvaginal hysterotomy through the vesicouterine fold has met conceptual hurdles mainly because of concerns for adhesions from prior cesarean section scar and for injury of the bladder during surgery. We have treated patients with β-hCG level as high as 188,942 U/mL, gestational sac as large as 60 mm in diameter, or gestational age as advanced as 10 weeks. The mean operating time was no more than 1 h, and the mean decrease in hemoglobin within 24 h was 1.635 g/dL, which is tolerable for most patients. No major complications such as massive bleeding or bladder injury were reported for any of the cases. Mean hospital stay after surgery was less than 5 days, which could be further reduced to 3 or 4 days without compromising safety. Serum β-hCG titers decreased by more than 90 % before postoperative day 4 and resolved to normal range within 1 month after surgery.

Based on our observations that prior conservative treatment did not reduce operating time or hemoglobin loss, we do not recommend prior medical treatment or UAE to improve safety or efficacy of transvaginal surgery. There was both a difference in operating time or hemoglobin drop between vital pregnancy and those with residual tissue. Although in this series there was no relationship between gestational age, β-hCG level and size of gestational sac, and safety of surgery, it is probable that it is more likely to encounter difficulties in more advanced gestation. Therefore, it would seem logical to recommend early diagnosis by transvaginal ultrasound in pregnant women with previous cesarean section, though our data cannot contribute to the risk/benefit analysis of such strategy.

Although the exact pathogenetic mechanism of CSP is unknown, a potential predisposing factor is a microtubular tract between the cesarean section scar and the endometrial canal. [3]. By removing the cesarean scar together with the pregnancy tissue, we tried to avoid such persistent canal, hence may reduce recurrence—though this cannot be proved by the current study.

Before transvaginal surgery was described, MTX administered either systemically or locally with UAE was the primary management method in our hospital. Lian et al. [15] published a series of 21 patients who received MTX (2005–2009). All patients received systemic MTX (50 mg/m^2) as initial therapy. Only nine showed a rapid decrease of serum b-hCG within a week, while MTX failed in the remaining 12. They had additional UAE combined with local MTX. Although eventually all patients responded to MTX treatment with or without UAE, it took 2 months to achieve serum β-hCG resolution and 6 months for the masses to disappear on ultrasound. Moderate elevation of liver enzymes was documented in three patients receiving systemic MTX, low grade fever (<38 °C) in five, and low abdominal pain in three with UAE combined with local MTX. In summary, MTX administration was associated with slower recovery and more adverse effects.

Based on our experience, we suggest the following for transvaginal hysterotomy approach to CSP management. Cervical injection of diluted adrenaline solution is performed before dissecting the vesicocervical gap to reduce bleeding. This step may also help avoid injuring the bladder and urethra and prevent the occurrence of vesicovaginal fistula formation. We used suction and curettage for complete removal of the products of conception as completely as possible. Continuous yet locking sutures were used to repair the incision of the anterior uterine wall under the guidance of a probe.

Prompt hysterectomy may be warranted only for dramatic cases presenting with massive bleeding or shock. Most other therapeutic options for CSPs have been adapted from protocols used for the treatment of other locations of ectopic pregnancies. The medical therapies include systemic and local administration of methotrexate (MTX), KCl, or the combination of these agents. The surgical treatments include dilatation and curettage, selective UAE, operative hysteroscopy, laparoscopy, and laparotomy. In cases of CSPs with decreasing serial serum β-hCG levels, expectant management may be offered. However, some reports showed that expectant management was associated with a high risk of uterine rupture and, therefore, could not be recommended in most cases [8–10]. Despite the effectiveness of MTX in decreasing the serum β-hCG levels, systemic or local injection of MTX requires close monitoring for a longer period of time. MTX sometimes requires repeat injection that can be associated with chemotherapy-induced side effects, slowly decreasing serum β-hCG levels and longer hospitalization [4, 11]. Moreover, there is often incomplete reabsorption of the gestational sac with ongoing irregular vaginal bleeding. Many of these women need additional and sometimes more aggressive methods to surgically remove the persistent gestational sac and resolve the bleeding [11–13]. Uterine artery embolization has been shown to carry risks of postoperative fever and abdominal pain [14], as well as being associated with longer duration of close monitoring and hospitalization [15].

Surgery has the advantage of offering the possibility of immediate remission. Hysteroscopy can be used to observe the distribution of blood vessels at the implantation site and to separate the gestational sac from the uterine wall directly. However, these procedures require good control of hysteroscopic instruments, excellent orientation within the uterine cavity, and clear visualization, which may not always be achievable [16]. In addition, hysteroscopic resection carries a risk for bladder injury, including delayed bladder perforation by thermal injury [17]. According to Fylstra's review [3], termination of the pregnancy with repair of the accompanying uterine scar dehiscence is probably the best treatment for the cesarean scar pregnancy. Laparoscopy is a minimally invasive option for resection of the scar, with preservation of the woman's reproductive capacity. Although laparoscopic and laparotomy approaches have already been successfully applied in CSPs [18, 19], a case report of CSP showed that the lower edge of the uterine defect was not accessible abdominally during emergency laparotomy. An additional vaginal approach was needed to achieve hemostasis [20]. This observation supports the feasibility of transvaginal repair of the uterine defect after cesarean section. Furthermore, compared to laparoscopy, transvaginal hysterotomy has the advantage of avoiding trocar insertion, therefore reducing the risks associated to this modality [21]. In addition, transvaginal hysterotomy may decrease cost associated with the use of equipment. As transvaginal hysterotomy requires only conventional equipment and the general skills of vaginal surgery, it is more convenient and more feasible to be conducted in most hospitals at lower cost than other surgical approaches. Since our first description, several other institutions employed this protocol successfully [22].

Conclusion

In summary, this transvaginal hysterotomy approach allows for removal of ectopic pregnancy tissue and repair of uterine defect. It is safe and effective, associated with a short hospital stay, low postoperative pain, blood loss, and cost.

Authors' contribution Zhang Huanxiao and Yao Shuzhong designed this study and carried out most of the data collection; Xie Hongzhe, Niu Gang, and Xu Chengkang took part in several surgeries, respectively; and Chen Shuqin, Jiang Hongye, and Guan Xiaoming contributed to the preparation of this manuscript.

Informed consent All procedures followed were in accordance with the ethical standards of the institutional committee on human experimentation and with the Helsinki Declaration of 1975, as revised in 2000. Informed consent was obtained from all patients for being included in the study.

References

1. Einenkel J, Stumpp P, Kosling S et al (2005) A misdiagnosed case of caesarean scar pregnancy. Arch Gynecol Obstet 271:178–181. doi:10.1007/s00404-004-0683-1
2. He M, Chen MH, Xie HZ et al (2011) Transvaginal removal of ectopic pregnancy tissue and repair of uterine defect for caesarean scar pregnancy. BJOG 118:1136–1139. doi:10.1111/j.1471-0528.2011.02891.x
3. Fylstra DL (2002) Ectopic pregnancy within a cesarean scar: a review. Obstet Gynecol Surv 57:537–543. doi:10.1097/01.OGX.0000025517.33346.1E
4. Ash A, Smith A, Maxwell D (2007) Caesarean scar pregnancy. BJOG 114:253–263. doi:10.1111/j.1471-0528.2006.01237.x
5. Zhuang Y, Huang L (2009) Uterine artery embolization compared with methotrexate for the management of pregnancy implanted within a cesarean scar. Am J Obstet Gynecol 201:151–152. doi:10.1016/j.ajog.2009.04.038
6. Larsen JV, Solomon MH (1978) Pregnancy in a uterine scar sacculus—an unusual cause of postabortal haemorrhage. A case report. S Afr Med J 53:142–143
7. Jurkovic D, Hillaby K, Woelfer B et al (2003) First-trimester diagnosis and management of pregnancies implanted into the lower uterine segment Cesarean section scar. Ultrasound Obstet Gynecol 21:220–227. doi:10.1002/uog.56
8. Seow KM, Huang LW, Lin YH (2004) Cesarean scar pregnancy: issues in management. Ultrasound Obstet Gynecol 23:247–253
9. Herman A, Weinraub Z, Avrech O et al (1995) Follow up and outcome of isthmic pregnancy located in a previous caesarean section scar. Br J Obstet Gynaecol 102:839–841
10. Condous G (2009) Ectopic pregnancy: challenging accepted management strategies. Aust N Z J Obstet Gynaecol 49:346–351. doi:10.1111/j.1479-828X.2009.01032.x
11. Sadeghi H, Rutherford T, Rackow BW et al (2010) Cesarean scar ectopic pregnancy: case series and review of the literature. Am J Perinatol 27:111–120. doi:10.1055/s-0029-1224874
12. Deb S, Clewes J, Hewer C et al (2007) The management of Cesarean scar ectopic pregnancy following treatment with methotrexate—a clinical challenge. Ultrasound Obstet Gynecol 30:889–892. doi:10.1002/uog.5149
13. Hwu YM, Hsu CY, Yang HY (2005) Conservative treatment of caesarean scar pregnancy with transvaginal needle aspiration of the embryo. BJOG 112:841–842. doi:10.1111/j.1471-0528.2004.00533.x
14. Takeda A, Koyama K, Imoto S et al (2010) Diagnostic multimodal imaging and therapeutic transcatheter arterial chemoembolization for conservative management of hemorrhagic cesarean scar pregnancy. Eur J Obstet Gynecol Reprod Biol 152:152–156. doi:10.1016/j.ejogrb.2010.05.032
15. Lian F, Wang Y, Chen W et al (2012) Uterine artery embolization combined with local methotrexate and systemic methotrexate for treatment of cesarean scar pregnancy with different ultrasonographic pattern. Cardiovasc Intervent Radiol 35:286–291. doi:10.1007/s00270-011-0097-y
16. Wang CJ, Chao AS, Yuen LT et al (2006) Endoscopic management of cesarean scar pregnancy. Fertil Steril 85:491–494. doi:10.1016/j.fertnstert.2005.07.1322
17. Robinson JK, Dayal MB, Gindoff P et al (2009) A novel surgical treatment for cesarean scar pregnancy: laparoscopically assisted operative hysteroscopy. Fertil Steril 92:1413–1497. doi:10.1016/j.fertnstert.2009.07.996
18. Wang YL, Su TH, Chen HS (2006) Operative laparoscopy for unruptured ectopic pregnancy in a caesarean scar. BJOG 113:1035–1038. doi:10.1111/j.1471-0528.2006.01031.x
19. Halperin R, Schneider D, Mendlovic S et al (2009) Uterine-preserving emergency surgery for cesarean scar pregnancies: another medical solution to an iatrogenic problem. Fertil Steril 91:2623–2627. doi:10.1016/j.fertnstert.2008.03.021

24

Efficacy of ovarian suspension to round ligament with a resorbable suture to prevent postoperative adhesions in women with ovarian endometrioma: follow-up by transvaginal hydrolaparoscopy

**Massimiliano Pellicano · Pierluigi Giampaolino ·
Giovanni Antonio Tommaselli · Ursula Catena ·
Carmine Nappi · Giuseppe Bifulco**

Abstract The aim of this study was to assess the effect of ovarian suspension to the round ipsilateral ligament with a resorbable suture, performed during laparoscopic surgery for endometrioma, on postoperative ovarian adhesion formation. The tool used to assess this effect was not conventional laparoscopy but outpatient transvaginal hydrolaparoscopy. Fifty women with single ovarian endometrioma were divided in two groups (group A, 24 and group B, 26). All patients underwent laparoscopic ovarian cystectomy for endometriosis. In group A, the ovary was suspended to the ipsilateral round ligament. In group B, ovarian suspension was not performed. All patients underwent transvaginal outpatient hydrolaparoscopy as follow-up. A significantly lower rate of postsurgical ovarian adhesion in group A in comparison with group B (33.3 vs 80.8 %—$p=0.001$) was observed. Operative time and postoperative pain were similar in both groups. Ovarian suspension to the ipsilateral round ligament with a resorbable suture during surgery for endometrioma is associated with a lower rate of postoperative ovarian adhesion formation.

Keywords Endometrioma · Laparoscopy · Ovarian suspension · Adhesion prevention · Transvaginal hydrolaparoscopy

M. Pellicano · P. Giampaolino · G. A. Tommaselli · U. Catena (✉) ·
C. Nappi · G. Bifulco
Department of Obstetrics and Gynaecology, University of Naples,
"Federico II", Via Pansini 5, 80131 Naples, Italy
e-mail: ursula.catena@gmail.com

Background

Ovarian endometriomas are a form of ovarian endometriosis, classified as cysts within the ovaries [1] accounts for 35 % of benign ovarian cysts [2], and are present in 17–44 % of patients with endometriosis. Expectant management is not an option for women with endometrioma because of severe symptoms [1].

Operative laparoscopy is the first-line treatment option available to the general consensus in the treatment of endometriomas >3 cm. However, debate still continues on the type of laparoscopic procedure. The main point of debate is excision or ablation of the cyst capsule [3, 4]. Since the ovarian endometrioma is a pseudocyst, excisional surgery involves the removal of ovarian cortex with primordial follicles, reducing the fertility potential of the affected ovary, especially when extensive hemostasis irreversibly diminishes or impairs the blood supply towards the affected ovary. Ovarian cystectomy for endometriomas seems to cause significant damage to ovarian reserve with up to 40 % fall in serum AMH concentration [5, 6]. According to Donnez et al., cystectomy may be destructive for the ovary, whereas ablation may be incomplete with a greater risk of recurrence [7]. With the combined technique (excision of a large part of endometrioma wall with vaporization of the remaining 10–20 % of endometrioma wall close to the hilus), we achieve the benefits of stripping on symptoms and recurrence, and a less harmful effect of ablation on ovarian reserve.

Adhesions formation rate after laparoscopic endometriosis surgery has been reported in more than 80 % cases [8–11]. The most common site of postoperative adhesions formation is between the ovary and the pelvic wall [12]. Notwithstanding the advances in surgical techniques [13] and the use of surgical anti-adhesive agents, the incidence of adhesion-related complications do not seem to have significantly declined [14].

The aim of this study was to assess the effect of ovarian suspension to the round ipsilateral ligament with a resorbable suture, during laparoscopic surgery for endometrioma in terms of postoperative ovarian adhesions after surgical procedure evaluated with office transvaginal hydrolaparoscopy.

Methods

This study was performed in the Infertility Clinic of our Department. During the period from March 2010 to March 2012, 185 women affected by endometriosis were evaluated for inclusion in the study. Inclusion criteria were: age between 18 and 40 years; history of infertility >2 years; single endometrioma cysts ≥4 or ≤7 cm [15] on preoperative ultrasound screen. Patients with smaller endometriomas were excluded because treatment of endometriomas of 1–3 cm was recommended only for the treatment of pain. When endometriosis is identified at laparoscopy, it is recommended to surgically treat endometriosis, as this is effective for reducing endometriosis-associated pain [16]. In these cases, we performed drainage and coagulation of the endometrioma wall because of the possible difficulty in the removal of very small cysts, due to the absence of a clear surgical plane.

Exclusion criteria were: masses occupying the Douglas pouch; previous surgery for endometriosis or additional concomitant surgical procedure planned during the laparoscopic procedure; current pregnancy, including ectopic pregnancy; serum glutamic-oxaloacetic transaminase (sgot), serum glutamate pyruvate transaminase (sgpt), and/or bilirubin >20 % above the upper limit of the normal range; azotemia and creatinine >30 % above the upper limit of the normal range; concurrent use of systemic corticosteroids, antineoplastic agents, and/or radiation; and active pelvic or abdominal infection.

The study was approved by the Institutional Review Boards of our Institution and all patients gave informed consent to participate in the study. Eighty-three patients matched the inclusion criteria and agreed with the study protocol, 21 however refused to participate to the study. Sixty-two patients were divided into two groups (group A, $n=31$; group B, $n=$ 31). Patients in group A underwent ovarian suspension to round ligament, while patients in group B did not undergo additional procedures other than that indicating laparosocopy. Both patients and surgeons performing THL were blinded with regard to which cases had their ovaries suspended and which cases did not.

The laparoscopic procedure was performed in the modified dorso-lithotomic position under endotracheal general anesthesia. After pneumoperitoneum induction with a Veress needle and introduction of a 10-mm laparoscope (Karl Storz—

Tuttlingen, Germany) in the standard umbilical position, three 5-mm trocars were placed in the following positions: suprapubic, left iliac fossa, and right iliac fossa. After careful exploration of the pelvic organs and upper abdomen, patients with single endometrioma adherent to the ipsilateral fossa were included, while patients with clinical evidence of cancer, rectovaginal endometriosis or bilateral endometriosis were excluded.

Light adhesions on the controlateral adnexa and/or small subserosal uterine myomas observed at first surgery were not considered as exclusion criteria. Ovarian endometriomas were removed following the technique described by Donnez [7]. Briefly, the ovarian cyst was opened and its content drained, the cleavage plane was found and the pseudo-capsule was separated from the ovarian parenchyma by means of repeated diverging traction applied with atraumatic forceps. Light coagulation with bipolar forceps was performed only if necessary, exclusively inside the ovarian parenchyma, before closure of the ovary. The suture was performed using a single running suture with an absorbable monofilament suture (Vicryl Rapid 2.0, CT-1 needle, Sommerville, NJ, USA, Ethicon) with intraovarian knots. Ovarian suture was performed so that no coagulated tissue was detectable outside as previously reported [13]. In group A, the ovary was suspended to the ipsilateral round ligament using an absorbable monofilament suture (Vicryl Rapid 2.0, CT-1 needle, Sommerville, NJ, USA, Ethicon). The suture was performed approximately 1 cm from the inguinal canal, to separate the ovary approximately 1.5–2 cm from the ovarian fossa (Fig. 1). In group B, ovarian suspension was not performed.

The operation time was calculated from the induction of pneumoperitoneum to desufflation. Blood loss during surgery was estimated by measuring the aspirated blood volume. Surgery was performed with an indwelling Foley catheter in situ that was removed as soon as the patient could independently reach the toilet. Twenty-four hours after the procedure,

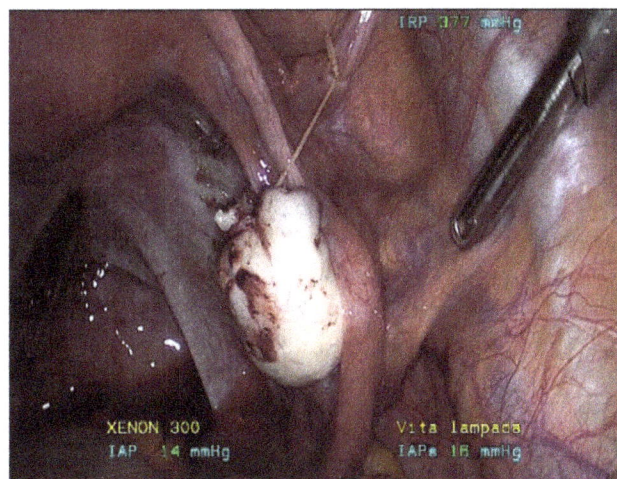

Fig. 1 Ovarian suspension to round ligament

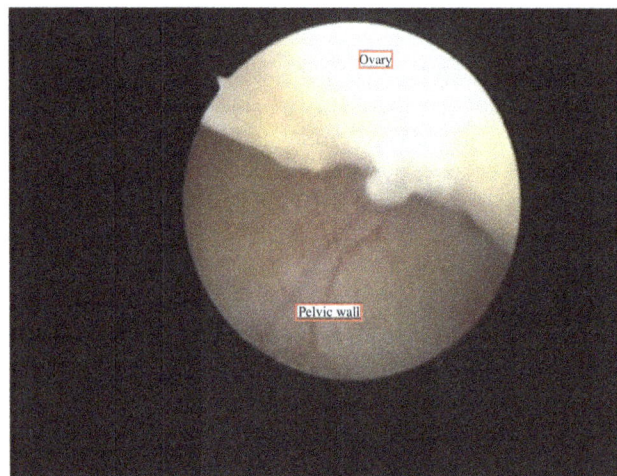

Fig. 2 Transvaginal hydrolaparoscopy follow-up

postoperative pain was evaluated using a pain visual analogue scale (VAS) ranging from 0 (absence of pain) to 10 (maximum pain). Per protocol, patients were discharged from the hospital 2 days after the procedure if no complication arose during the postoperative period. All patients were evaluated 60–90 days after surgery with transvaginal outpatient hydrolaparoscopy (THL). THL was not performed before because patients may not agree to undergo a second invasive procedure immediately after the initial surgery.

Transvaginal hydrolaparoscopy was performed by three surgeons: M.P. who performs approximately 100 procedures per year; U.C. and P.G. who perform about 25 procedures per year. Fertiloscopy was performed under local anesthesia with the patient in the lithotomic position. A Collin's speculum was placed in the vagina and a local anesthetic solution containing mepivacaine hydrochloride 3 % was injected in the posterior fornix, 1–2 cm below the cervix and on the posterior lip of the cervix which was grasped. A specially designed needle dilating trocar system with a total diameter of 3.9 mm (reusable system by Karl Storz Endoscopy—Tuttlingen, Germany) was placed 10–20 mm below the insertion of the posterior vaginal wall to the cervix. A 2.7-mm-diameter semi- rigid endoscope was used with an optical angle of 30°. The correct intra-abdominal trocar position was confirmed visually, and a slow continuous infusion of warmed saline solution was started [17, 18]. To keep the bowel and tubo-ovarian structures afloat the illumination was provided by a high-intensity cold-light source via fiber-optic lead. The images were viewed on high-resolution color monitor. The posterior wall of the uterus was inspected. Subsequently, by rotation and deeper insertion of the scope, the tubo-ovarian structures were visualized. Success was defined as the absence of any adhesion between the ovary and the ovarian fossa (Fig. 2). The vaginal fornix was left to close spontaneously, and antibiotic prophylaxis was prescribed.

The primary end-point was the proportion of women without ovarian adhesions as evaluated by THL 60-90 days after the primary surgical procedure. We hypothesized that women underwent ovarian suspension would develop ovarian adhesion in 30 % of cases as opposed to 70 % of women not undergoing this procedure. Considering these proportions, we calculated that we would need a sample size of 24 in group A and 24 in group B to give 90 % power to detect a significant difference between ovarian suspension and non ovarian suspension procedures with a one-sided type 1 error of 5 %. To account for loss to follow-up, we chose to enroll 31 patients in group A and 31 in group B. Secondary end-points were operative times, intra-operative blood loss, and intra- and postoperative complication rate.

Statistical analysis was performed using the Statistical Package for Social Science, version 15.0 (SPSS, Chicago, IL, USA). Data distribution for continuous variables was assessed with the Shapiro–Wilk's test. Difference in proportions between groups for the primary end-point was analyzed using the χ^2 test and the odds ratios were calculated. Student's t test for unpaired samples was used to compare parametric variables between groups. The Mann-Whitney test was used to analyze differences in non parametric parameters between groups. Analysis was performed both per protocol and on an intention-to-treat basis. Separate analysis was carried out considering all drop-outs as having formed adhesions (failures) or not having formed adhesions (successes) between the ovary and its fossa. Significance was set for a value of $p<0.05$.

Findings

Characteristics of patients are listed in Table 1. No statistical differences were observed in any variable between the two groups. In group A, three patients were excluded intraoperatively from the study for the presence of contralateral ovarian adhesions at laparoscopy and one patient for the presence of

Table 1 Characteristics of patients. Value are given as mean±SD or median [range], as appropriate p=NS for all comparisons

	Group A (n=31)	Group B (n=31)
Age (years)	26.5±16.5	28.2±15.8
Weight (kg)	63.1±8.9	62.2±10.5
Height (cm)	170.3±35.6	172.2±28.2
BMI (cm)	25.2±3.5	23.2±2.9
Primary infertility	21 (67.7)	23 (74.2)
Endometrioma diameter (cm)	5.2±1.1	6.1±2.1
Hb (g/dl)	12.3±1.5	13.1±2.1
Hospital stay (days)	2.2±2[2–4]	2.1±2 [2–3]
Operative time (min)	65.6±9.8	62.1±8.5

two ovarian cysts; in group B three patients were excluded for endometriosis stages III–IV (ASRM).

Five patients (three from group A and two from group B) dropped out of the study: one patient was pregnant to follow-up, two patients refused to undergo THL, and in two patients THL was not possible to perform for poor compliance (pain in the positioning of speculum or trocar in the posterior fornix).

Thus, a total of 24 women in group A and 26 women in group B were available for the analysis. In all the 50 procedures, it was possible to enter the pelvic cavity and visualize the pouch of Douglas.

At the THL control, a significant higher proportion of patients for group A were free of adhesions in comparison with patients from group B (Table 2; $p=0.001$). Analyses considering all patients as failures (i.e., with adhesions formation between the ovary and its fossa) or success (i.e., non adhesions formation) confirmed that ovarian suspension leads to a significantly higher proportion of patients who did not develop adhesions (Table 2).

We did not observe any difference in terms of postoperative pelvic pain between the two groups, according to VAS scale (4.78 ± 1.48 in group A vs 4.05 ± 1.67 in group B; $p<0.16$).

The operating time was similar between group A and group B ($p=0.11$). No major complications (rectum perforation) were reported in both groups. At follow-up, no ovary was still suspended to the round ligament; in all patients from group A, the ovary was found in its anatomical location.

Discussion

Endometriosis is a complex and heterogeneous condition characterized by a continuous state of inflammation that causes symptoms of pelvic pain and infertility. In this condition, fibrosis and adhesions are common. Some authors support that the inflammatory response may be the first cause of adhesion formation [19]. It leads to an upregulation of tissue factors by peritoneal cells and local macrophages. This causes activation of the extrinsic pathway of the coagulation cascade and the formation of an exudate rich in fibrin [19]. Adhesions can lead to infertility, dyspareunia, chronic pelvic pain, and complications at repeated surgery [20, 21]. Adhesions may produce disruption of the normal anatomy, thus altering normal tubal performance. Thus, follicular growth, pick-up of the oocyte after ovulation and spermatozoa or embryo transport may be impaired [20]. Several women develop postoperative adhesions after laparoscopy surgery. The most common site of postoperative adhesions formation is the ovary [12, 22]. Although several surgical measures and systemic pharmacologic treatments for adhesions prevention have been proposed, the rate of periovarian adhesion formation was not significantly reduced [13, 20–22]. The high incidence of postoperative adhesions in endometriosis patients and their clinical significance underline the importance of modifying surgical technique in order to reduce potential adhesion formation.

Adhesions may develop in locations previously unaffected (de novo) or in locations where adhesiolysis was performed (recurrence). The process of adhesions formation begins during surgery; the possible development of adhesions is determined within the first 7 days of the injury. In the injured area, a gel matrix of fibrin will form and macrophages recruit new mesothelial cells over the damaged surface which reaches the reconstruction of the mesothelial lining within 5–7 days. The adhesions will take place if the surfaces damaged remain in contact [23, 24]. This finding supports the idea of an ovariopexy.

Several authors previously proposed ovarian suspension techniques [25–30] (Table 3). The technique most frequently described has been temporary ovarian suspension to anterior abdominal wall [25–28]. This technique showed only limited results, with success rates ranging from 80 to 40 %. Moreover, this technique carries potential risks of infection due to the proximity of the ovary to the external abdominal wall. Only one author reported [26] an ovarian suspension to the round ligament, showing no dense adhesion of the ovary to the pelvic sidewall after definitive ovarian suspension to the round ligament. These results are in accordance with our

		Group A	Group B	OR (95 %CI)	p
Table 2 Rate of postsurgical adhesions between patients treated with ovarian suspension (group A) and patients treated without ovarian suspension (group B)	Analysis per protocol	$n=24$	$n=26$	0.119 (0.03–0.55)	0.001
	Postoperative ovarian adhesion formation	8 (33.3 %)	21 (80.8 %)		
	No postoperative ovarian adhesion	16 (66.7 %)	5 (19.2 %)		
	Considering all drop-outs as failures	$n=27$	$n=28$	0.149 (0.04–0.60)	0.002
	Postoperative ovarian adhesion formation	11 (40.7 %)	23 (82.1 %)		
	No postoperative ovarian adhesion	16 (59.3 %)	5 (17.9 %)		
	Considering all drop-outs as successes	$n=27$	$n=28$	0.140 (0.04–0.53)	0.001
	Postoperative ovarian adhesion formation	8 (29.6 %)	21 (75 %)		
	No postoperative ovarian adhesion	19 (70.4 %)	7 (25 %)		

Table 3 Ovarian suspension for adhesion prevention

	Number patients	Suspension	Suture type	Post operative removal stitch	Number second-look	No adhesion at second-look
Sedbon 1983	61	Pelvic rim outside the iliac artery	Catgut	No	17	76 %
Redwine 2001	3	Ipsilateral round ligament	Vicryl	No	3	100 %
Abuzeid 2001	20	Anterior abdominal wall	Prolene	Yes	5	80 %
Ouahba 2004	20	Anterior abdominal wall	Prolene	Yes	8	40 %
Mitwally 2006	59	Anterior abdominal wall	Prolene	Yes	–	50 %
Carbonnel 2011	218	Anterior abdominal wall	Prolene Mersuture	Yes	24	50 %

findings. The main drawback of previous analysis was the significant loss to follow-up. Indeed, in all previous studies, second-look surgery was performed only in a small number of patients (Table 3), since systematic laparoscopic second-look may be frequently refuted by patients. In this study, we used an office-based procedure performed under local anesthesia that should increase the compliance of patients in undergoing follow-up second-look.

Indeed, only five patients refused to undergoing second-look with THL, supporting this hypothesis. This is to our knowledge, the first study using Vycril Rapid to suspend the ovary to the round ligament. Because development of adhesion is determined within the first 5–7 days after surgery, we prefer to use Vicryl Rapid 2.0 suture for its characteristics loss of tensile strength in 5–7 days and fast reabsorption process. The ovary so remains separated from the peritoneum of the ovarian dimple for about 7 days, the time necessary for adhesions formation. In the present study, no significant difference was observed in terms of operative time.

Moreover, we did not observe a difference in terms of postoperative pain evaluated according to VAS scale. We believe that no difference in postoperative pain between the two groups is linked to the ovarian suspension technique used. We suspend the ovary approximately 1.5 cm from ovarian fossa with tension-free suture.

This study has several advantages. It can rely on effective blinding of the surgeon performing THL, so that a bias in determining adhesion formation is unlikely. Moreover, it was correctly powered to detect significant differences between the two groups. Finally, sensitivity analysis was performed to address differences in losses to follow-up in the two arms. A potential limitation of the study may be the nonrandomized design of the study that may lead to an allocation bias. Nevertheless, the population selected for the study was homogeneous, so that differences in the two groups are unlikely. Another potential limitation is the low external validity due to strict inclusion criteria. These criteria were chosen in order to evaluate the net effect of the proposed technique on adhesion formation rate due to the suturing of the ovary, avoiding interference of other factors.

Prospective comparative studies including more patients should be conducted to confirm our preliminary results.

In conclusion, this study seems to indicate that ovarian suspension to the round ligament with short-term resorbable suture may be a simple and effective surgical technique for the prevention of periovarian adhesion formation and could be included into the routine surgical procedure for single endometrioma. Moreover, THL can be considered to be a simple and minimally invasive technique with a good compliance for the postoperative follow-up, to evaluate adhesion formation.

Ethical standards All procedures followed were in accordance with the ethical standards of the responsible committee on human experimentation (institutional and national) and with the Helsinki Declaration of 1975, as revised in 2000. Informed consent was obtained from all patients for being included in the study.

References

1. Benschop L, Farquhar C, van der Poel N, Heineman MJ (2010) Interventions for women with endometrioma prior to assisted reproductive technology. Cochrane Database Syst Rev 10(11):CD008571
2. Gruppo italiano per lo studio dell'endometriosi (1994) Prevalence and anatomical distribution of endometriosis in women with selected gynaecological conditions: results from a multicentric Italian study. Hum Reprod 9(6):1158–62
3. Hart R, Hickey M, Maouris P, Buckett W, Garry R (2008) Excisional surgery versus ablative surgery for ovarian endometriomata. Cochrane Database Syst Rev 16(2):CD004992
4. Patrelli TS, Berretta R, Gizzo S, Pezzuto A, Franchi L, Lukanovic A, Nardelli Bacchi Modena A (2011) CA 125 serum values in surgically treated endometriosis patients and its relationships with anatomic sites of endometriosis and pregnancy rate. Fertil Steril 95:393–396
5. Raffi F, Metwally M, Amer S (2012) The impact of excision of ovarian endometrioma on ovarian reserve: a systematic review and meta-analysis. J Clin Endocrinol Metab 97(9):3146–3154
6. Alborzi S, Keramati P, Younesi M, Samsami A (2014) The impact of laparoscopic cystectomy on ovarian reserve in patients with unilateral and bilateral endometriomas. Fertil Steril 101(2):427–434

7. Donnez J, Lousse JC, Jadoul P, Donnez O, Squifflet J (2010) Laparoscopic management of endometriomas using a combined technique of excisional (cystectomy) and ablative surgery. Fertil Steril 94(1):28–32

8. diZerega GS (1994) Contemporary adhesion prevention. Fertil Steril 61:219–235

9. Mais V, Angioli R, Coccia E, Fagotti A, Landi S, Melis GB, Pellicano M, Scambia G, Zupi E, Angioni S, Arena S, Corona R, Fanfani F, Nappi C (2011) Prevention of postoperative abdominal adhesions in gynecological surgery. Consensus paper of an Italian gynecologists' task force on adhesions. Minerva Ginecol 63(1):47–70

10. Redwine DB (1991) Conservative laparoscopic excision of endometriosis by sharp dissection: life table analysis of reoperation and persistent or recurrent disease. Fertil Steril 56:628–634

11. Operative Laparoscopy Study Group (1991) Postoperative adhesion development after operative laparoscopy: evaluation at early second look procedure. Fertil Steril 55(4):700–704

12. Ahmad G, Duffy JM, Farquhar C, Vail A, Vandekerckhove P, Watson A, Wiseman D (2008) Barrier agents for adhesion prevention after gynaecological surgery. Cochrane Database Syst Rev 16:CD000475

13. Pellicano M, Bramante S, Guida M, Bifulco G, Di Spiezio Sardo A, Cirillo D, Nappi C (2008) Ovarian endometrioma: postoperative adhesions following bipolar coagulation and suture. Fertil Steril 89(4):796–9

14. Lower AM, Hawthorn RJ, Clark D, Boyd JH, Finlayson AR, Knight AD, Crowe AM, Surgical and Clinical Research (SCAR) Group (2004) Adhesion-related readmissions following gynaecological laparoscopy or laparotomy in Scotland: an epidemiological study of 24 046 patients. Hum Reprod 19:1877–85

15. Dunselman GA, Vermeulen N, Becker C, Calhaz-Jorge C, D'Hooghe T, De Bie B, Heikinheimo O, Horne AW, Kiesel L, Nap A, Prentice A, Saridogan E, Soriano D, Nelen W (2014) ESHRE guideline: management of women with endometriosis. Hum Reprod 29(3):400–412

16. Jacobson TZ, Duffy JM, Barlow D, Koninckx PR, Garry R (2009) Laparoscopic surgery for pelvic pain associated with endometriosis. Cochrane Database Syst Rev 7(4):CD001300

17. Verhoeven HC, Brosens I (2005) Transvaginal hydrolaparoscopy, its history and present indication. Minim Invasive Ther Allied Technol 14(3):175–180

18. Pellicano M, Catena U, Di Iorio P, Simonelli V, Sorrentino F, Stella N, Bonifacio M, Cirillo D, Nappi C (2007) Diagnostic and operative fertiloscopy. Minerva Ginecol 59(2):175–181

19. Imai A, Suzuki N (2010) Topical non-barrier agents for postoperative adhesion prevention in animal models. Eur J Obstet Gynecol Reprod Biol 149:131–135

20. Davey AK, Maher PJ (2007) Surgical adhesions: a timely update, a great challenge for the future. J Minim Invasive Gynecol 14:15–22

21. Robertson D, Lefebvre G, Leyland N, Wolfman W, Allaire C, Awadalla A, Best C, Contestabile E, Dunn S, Heywood M, Leroux N, Potestio F, Rittenberg D, Senikas V, Soucy R, Singh S (2010) Adhesion prevention in gynaecological surgery. J Obstet Gynaecol Can 32:598–60

22. Ahmad G, Duffy JM, Farquhar C, Vail A, Vandekerckhove P, Watson A, Wiseman D (2008) Barrier agents for adhesion prevention after gynaecological surgery. Cochrane Database Syst Rev 16:CD000475

23. Holmdahl L, Risberg B, Beck DE Burns JW, Chegini N, di Zerega GS, Ellis (1997) Adhesions: pathogenesis and prevention-panel discussion and summary. Eur J Surg Suppl 557:56–62

24. di Zerega GS, Campeau JD (2001) Peritoneal repair and post-surgical adhesion formation. Hum Reprod Update 7:547–55

25. Sedbon E, Madelenat P, Asher E, Palmer R (1983) Suspension temporaire des ovaires dans la prévention de la récidive adhérentielle après salpingostomie terminale. Gynecologie 34:421–4

26. Redwine D (2001) Laparoscopic ovarian suspension. Fertil Steril 76:105

27. Abuzeid MI, Ashraf M, Shamma FN (2002) Temporary ovarian suspension at laparoscopy for prevention of adhesions. J Am Assoc Gynecol Laparosc 9:98–102

28. Ouahba J, Madelenat P, Poncelet C (2004) Transient abdominal ovariopexy for adhesion prevention in patients who underwent surgery for severe pelvic endometriosis. Fertil Steril 82:1407–11

29. Mitwally MF, Palmer KG, Elhammady E, Eddib A, Diamond MP, Abuzeid MI (2006) Ovarian suspension during laparoscopic conservative surgery for endometriosis—associated infertility: a cohort of 59 consecutive cases. J Minim Invasive Gynecol 13:S50

30. Carbonnel M, Ducarme G, Dessapt AL, Yazbeck C, Hugues J, Madelenat P, Poncelet C (2011) Efficacy of transient abdominal ovariopexy in patients with severe endometriosis. European J Obstet Gynecol Reprod Biol 155:183–187

25

Comparison of dynamic MRI vaginal anatomical changes after vaginal mesh surgery and laparoscopic sacropexy

Hiromi Kashihara · Virginie Emmanuelli ·
Edouard Poncelet · Chrystèle Rubod ·
Jean-Philippe Lucot · Bram Pouseele · Michel Cosson

Abstract The aim of this study is to evaluate anatomical differences in vaginal length and axis between transvaginal mesh surgery (TVM) and laparoscopic sacropexy (LSC) by pelvic magnetic resonance imaging (MRI). Twenty-seven women with stage II or more symptomatic pelvic organ prolapse were involved in this study. Thirteen patients had undergone TVM, and fourteen had LSC. Preoperative and at 1 year postoperative clinical examination and dynamic MRI were performed. The angle between the vaginal axis and horizontal line or pubococcygeal line and the position of the Douglas pouch were evaluated on MRI. In clinical examination, all compartments (Aa, Ba, C, Ap, Bp, D) were significantly improved after both surgeries. Point C and D tended to be higher after LSC than TVM. In MRI assessment, the position of the Douglas was positioned significantly higher after LSC than TVM. There was no difference in postoperative vaginal axis at rest between the two surgical techniques, but the vaginal axis with maximal strain after TVM was more horizontal than LSC (LSC 143.7±6.3° vs. TVM 155.1±12.3°, $p=0.003$). As a result, the change of vaginal axis from at rest to maximal strain was also apparently greater after TVM.

(LSC 10.3±9.1° vs. TVM 20.7±11.3°, $p=0.014$). Both TVM and LSC significantly improved pelvic organ descent evaluated by clinical examination and MRI. LSC suspends the uterus, and Douglas pouch was significantly higher than TVM. The vaginal axis at rest leans horizontally after both surgeries, but the change of vaginal axis from at rest to maximal strain was significantly higher after TVM.

Keywords Pelvic organ prolapse · Vaginal mesh surgery · Laparoscopic sacropexy · MRI · Vaginal axis

Abbreviations

TVM	Transvaginal mesh
LSC	Laparoscopic sacropexy
MRI	Magnetic resonance imaging
POP	Pelvic organ prolapse
SUI	Stress urinary incontinence
POP-Q	Pelvic organ prolapse quantification
PCL	Pubococcygeal line
HL	Horizontal line
QOL	Quality of life

Brief summary Length and axis of the vagina at rest are comparable 1 year after TVM or LSC surgery for prolapse.

H. Kashihara · V. Emmanuelli · E. Poncelet · C. Rubod ·
J.-P. Lucot · B. Pouseele · M. Cosson
Department of Gynecologic Surgery, Hopital Jeanne de Flandre,
Centre Hospitalier Regional Universitaire de Lille, Lille Cedex,
France

H. Kashihara (✉)
Department of Obstetrics and Gynecology, Osaka Police Hospital,
10-31 Kitayama-cho Tennouji-ku Osaka, Osaka 543-0035, Japan
e-mail: hkathy_sky@yahoo.co.jp

B. Pouseele
Department of Obstetrics and Gynecology, OLV van Lourdes
Hospital, Waregem, Belgium

Introduction

Pelvic organ prolapse (POP) is one of the most common problems that can compromise women's quality of life. Women have a risk of 11% of undergoing surgery for pelvic organ prolapse or urinary incontinence [1]. There are two surgical routes for the treatment of POP: abdominal and vaginal. Traditional vaginal procedures using weak native tissue were reported to have a high recurrence rate and the reintervention rate is often up to 30% [1].

The transvaginal mesh (TVM) kit has been developed for the treatment of POP to overcome the high failure rate of traditional repair. This minimally invasive method consists of the fixation of a transvaginally introduced tension-free polypropylene mesh for the anterior and posterior compartment. The French Transvaginal Mesh group has established this standardized procedure. They reported a low operative morbidity and a high anatomical success rate [2]. Some randomized controlled trials that compare TVM with traditional vaginal repair suggest a better anatomical success rate, especially for anterior repair [3, 4]. However, there are some possible complications with TVM like mesh exposition and dyspareunia, which consequently lead to a high reoperation rate [4, 5]. In July 2011, the US Food and Drug Administration (FDA) declared the placement of surgical mesh for transvaginal repair for POP as an area of continuing serious concern because of its serious complications.

The abdominal sacrocolpopexy has been regarded as the gold standard procedure for treatment of vaginal vault prolapse [5, 6]. Nowadays, laparoscopic approach is introduced for this procedure with potential advantages in terms of reduced morbidity, shorter hospital stay, and faster recovery. According to some reports, laparoscopic sacrocolpopexy and sacropexy with conservation of the uterus seem to be safe and effective, with low recurrence and morbidity rates (comparable to laparotomy) [7–9]. There are discussions between laparoscopic and vaginal surgeons about the differences of vaginal length and axis after prolapse repair between these two surgical techniques, using different ligaments for the apex suspension (prevertebral ligament for sacropexy and sacrospinous ligament for TVM).

Magnetic resonance imaging (MRI) was introduced to facilitate the diagnosis of pelvic floor disorders because of its excellent soft tissue resolution. Dynamic MRI can detect pelvic organ prolapse with rapid scanning of the pelvis even with multiple compartments involved [10–12]. Several studies have already been conducted to evaluate pelvic reconstructive surgery. Some of them compare the anatomical results of different surgical procedures [13–21], but there is no study analyzing postoperative anatomical differences between transvaginal mesh repair and laparoscopic sacropexy (LSC) by using dynamic MRI.

The aim of this study was to compare anatomical results after two surgical methods, TVM and LSC, with MRI before and 1 year after operation.

Materials and methods

This is a prospective study comparing the anatomical results between TVM surgery and LSC by MRI before and after operation. After the institutional review board approval, patients with symptomatic POP who were introduced to our institution to undergo surgical intervention were recruited in the study. Inclusion criteria were stage 2 or more pelvic organ

prolapse in the pelvic organ prolapse quantification (POP-Q) system, subjective symptoms of POP, an age between 40 and 70 years, and the patients' agreement to participate in the study. Exclusion criteria were previous surgery for pelvic organ prolapse or previous hysterectomy for reasons of potential difficulties to assess the vaginal axis in such cases. Twenty-seven patients were involved in this study. Thirteen patients had undergone transvaginal mesh repair (TVM group) and 14 had undergone laparoscopic sacropexy (LSC group) between January and October 2010 in our university hospital. The choice of method of surgery depended on the surgeon's decision. In a first hand, prolapse surgery by laparoscopic sacropexy is used in our institution for younger patients under the age of 60 years and the vaginal approach for patients over 60 years old. All patients had a clinical interview, gynecological examination using the POP-Q system, and a MRI preoperatively and postoperatively. Postoperative assessment was scheduled at 1 year after operation. The surgical technique of TVM was the standardized transvaginal mesh procedure, which was previously described by the French TVM group [2, 22]. All mesh procedures involved use of the Prolift+M™ Total (Prolift Pelvic Floor Repair System; Ethicon Women's Health and Urology, Somerville, NJ), and the mesh was inserted in both anterior and posterior compartments without hysterectomy for all cases. In the LSC group, concomitant subtotal hysterectomy was performed initially and the same partially absorbable monofilament mesh (Ultrapro®, Ethicon Women's Health and Urology, Somerville, NJ) was adopted. Anterior dissection was performed up to the level of the bladder neck, and the mesh was fixed on the anterior vaginal wall using sutures. At the posterior side, dissection was performed bilaterally as for the levator ani muscles and the mesh was secured to the posterior vaginal wall or levator ani muscles using sutures. Both the anterior and posterior meshes were fixed to the uterine cervix with titanium helical fasteners. After dissection of the presacral space, anterior and posterior meshes were sutured to the presacral ligament at the level of promontory with a nonabsorbable suture. All operations were performed by two senior surgeons or under their supervision.

Nine patients (two of TVM and seven of LSC) who suffered from symptomatic stress urinary incontinence (SUI) preoperatively, underwent concomitant placement of a tension-free vaginal tape-obturator sling (TVT-O, Ethicon Women's Health and Urology, Somerville, NJ). In the LSC group, there was one patient who underwent both a rectopexy and culdoplasty at the same time, one patient had a rectopexy, one a culdoplasty, and one a myorraphy of the levator ani muscles concurrently.

MRI was performed with 1.5 T (GE Healthcare; Milwaukee, USA), with the patients lying in the supine position with their legs slightly flexed. Sonographic transmission gel was injected in the vagina and rectum, 50 and 250 mL, respectively. Images were obtained in sagittal, axial, and coronal orientation using body coil at rest, squeeze, and push with maximal strain [Fig. 1]. At first, imaging high resolution T2-weighted turbo spin-echo (TSE) sequences or 3 dimensional T2 was obtained to estimate pelvic anatomical structures. Then, the dynamic series of images were obtained in the midsagittal plane with very fast imaging (one image per second) in echo gradient (EG) T2. Last, three planes (sagittal, axial, and coronal) were performed in EG T2 with maximal strain. The evacuation and post-evacuation sequences with maximal strain were utilized for evaluation of the pelvic organ prolapse and the condition of the anal canal.

A preoperative and postoperative (1 year after surgery) clinical examination and MRI was executed in all patients. All MRI images were analyzed by one experienced radiologist, and measurements were done in a midsagittal plane. The vaginal axis was determined as the line connecting the posterior fornix and the vaginal introitus, and the distance between these two anatomical points at rest was measured as the position of the Douglas pouch on MRI. The position of the Douglas pouch was determined perpendicular to the vaginal axis at the highest part of the posterior fornix or at the level of a enterocele in case of a low enterocele. Both horizontal line (HL) and pubococcygeal line (PCL) were utilized as reference lines because it is still controversial which reference line is the most suitable to estimate pelvic floor disorders. PCL is defined as the line from the inferior part of the symphysis pubis to the last coccygeal joint. The HL is drawn between the inferior border of the symphysis pubis and the convex posterior margin of the puborectalis sling. The angle between the vaginal axis and the reference line were measured on the mid sagittal T2 image at rest and with maximal strain.

Statistical analysis was performed using the R 2.15.3®software, available freely online. The Mann-Whitney-Wilcoxon

Rank sum test was used to analyse POP-Q measurements and *MRI* datas. A *p* value below 0.05 was considered statistically significant.

Results

The LSC group was significantly younger than the TVM group (61.9±3.3 vs. 49.3±4.2 years, $p<0.05$). Median follow-up period was 47 weeks, and there was no difference between LSC and TVM.

The results of POP-Q examinations are shown in Table 1. Because of the missing data on POP-Q examination, three patients of the TVM group and two patients of the LSC group were excluded for evaluation by POP-Q. In the preoperative clinical examinations, no significant difference was detected between the TVM and LSC group, except for genital hiatus (GH). Postoperatively, point C and D tended to be higher in the LSC group than TVM, but there was no difference in TVL. In comparison of pre- and postoperation situation, all compartments (Aa, Ba, C, Ap, Bp, D) were significantly improved after both surgeries.

The result of the position of Douglas pouch measured by MRI is shown in Table 2. Point D and TVL in POP-Q are also listed to be compared. The position of the Douglas pouch was postoperatively significantly higher in the LSC group than TVM. As mentioned in the result of POP-Q, postoperative point D in the LSC group was also significantly higher compared to TVM. Both POP-Q and MRI observations suggest that LSC suspends the uterus and Douglas pouch higher than TVM, as preoperatively there was no difference between TVM and LSC in POP-Q point D and TVL.

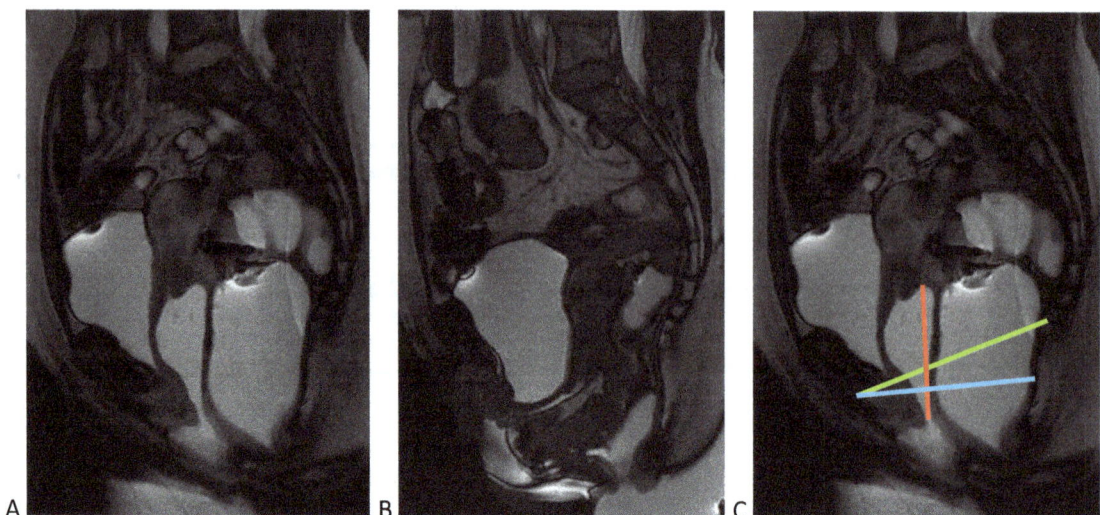

Fig. 1 Dynamic MRI with intravaginal and intrarectal gel. **a** At rest. **b** At maximal pushing. **c** Puboccyeal line (PCL, *green*), horizontal line (HL, *blue*), and vaginal axis (*red*)

Table 1 Comparison of POP-Q clinical measurements before and 1 year after operation for the TVM group and for the LSC group

	Preoperation			Postoperation		
	TVM $n=10$	LSC $n=12$	p value	TVM $n=10$	LSC $n=12$	p value
Aa	1.2±1.8	1.2±1.2	0.656	−1.2±1.2[a]	−1.8±1.4[a]	0.416
Ba	2.2±1.3	1.8±1.7	0.121	−1.5±1.3[a]	−1.7±1.4[a]	0.797
C	1.9±1.3	2.8±2.4	0.657	−5.0±3.2[a]	−7.6±1.7[a]	0.051
GH	5.2±1.0	4.0±0.6	0.040	4.6±1.3	4.3±1.1	0.443
PB	4.5±0.6	3.7±0.7	0.138	3.5±0.9	3.3±0.6	0.892
TVL	8.2±1.1	8.8±1.9	0.424	9.0±0.9	9.9±1.6	0.165
Ap	0.3±1.4	0.3±1.6	0.947	−2.7±0.9[a]	−2.4±1.0[a]	0.323
Bp	0.4±0.7	0.2±1.9	0.347	−2.2±1.8[a]	−2.3±1.1[a]	0.551
D	−1.0±2.5	−0.3±2.1	0.388	−6.2±2.3[a]	−8.8±1.0[a]	0.003

[a] Statistically significant

The results of MRI analysis are shown in Tables 3 and 4. All MRI images were of good quality, with all points necessary for measurement visible in each MRI analysis. Between TVM and LSC, there was no statistical difference of preoperative vaginal angle at rest and with maximal straining. Compared before and after each operation, the vaginal angle at rest tends to increase postoperatively, and it means that the vaginal axis leans horizontally in supine position after both operations (Table 3). It was statistically significant when PCL was adopted as a reference line (TVM: pre 126.5±9.0° vs. post 134.4±8.4°, p=0.026; LSC: pre 128.4±9.0° vs. post 133.4± 5.2°, p=0.036). The vaginal angle with maximal strain significantly changed to horizontal after TVM regardless of reference line (HL: pre 117.5±23.2° vs. post 134.0±16.9°, p= 0.048, PCL: pre 136.8±17.3° vs. post 155.1±12.3°, p= 0.007). On the other hand, the vaginal angle with maximal strain after LSC did not change from preoperation (HL: pre 124.3±17.2° vs. post 126.3±10.9°, p=0.991; PCL: pre 143.5 ±14.7° vs. post 143.7±6.3°, p=0.675).

As a result, the change of vaginal axis from at rest to maximal strain became greater after TVM and oppositely, this change became smaller after LSC (Table 4). In comparison of the change of vaginal axis from at rest to maximal strain between the two operations postoperatively, TVM had greater change than LSC. This difference was statistically significant

when PCL was used as a reference line (LSC 10.3±9.1° vs. TVM 20.7±11.3°, p=0.011).

Discussion

Our study confirmed a significant improvement of pelvic organ prolapse after TVM and LSC, respectively, and also detected by clinical examination and MRI that the position of the Douglas pouch was held up higher after LSC than TVM. MRI assessment revealed that the vaginal axis at rest leans horizontally after both surgeries, but the change of vaginal axis from at rest to maximal strain was significantly higher after TVM than LSC.

Many publications have described the feasibility of using dynamic MRI for diagnosis of pelvic organ prolapse preoperatively [10–12] and evaluate the effectiveness of surgery and recurrence postoperatively [13–21].

Pelvic organ prolapse usually consists of multiple pelvic compartments, even if patients may present with symptoms that involve only one compartment [10]. All involved compartments should be identified preoperatively or else, misdiagnosis may lead to surgical failure. But it is sometimes difficult to differentiate each compartment by clinical examination, especially for vaginal vault prolapse. Therefore, other

Table 2 Position of the Douglas pouch measured by MRI before and 1 year after operation for the TVM group and for the LSC group

		Preoperation			Postoperation		
		TVM	LSC	p value	TVM	LSC	p value
Position of Douglas	(mm)	70.3±6.9	78.2±6.8	0.014	69.9±10.0	81.0±7.3[a]	0.004
POP-Q D	(cm)	−1.0±2.5	−0.3±2.1	0.388	−6.2±2.3[a]	−8.8±1.0[a]	0.003
TVL	(cm)	8.2±1.1	8.8±1.9	0.424	9.0±0.9	9.9±1.6	0.165

[a] Statistically significant

Table 3 MRI measurement of the vaginal angle at rest and with maximal straining before and 1 year after operation for the TVM group and for the LSC group

		Preoperation	Postoperation	p value	Preoperation	Postoperation	p value
Vaginal angle (°)	Rest	101.5±9.2	108.4±9.7	0.142	97.1±8.9	105.3±4.7	0.008
HL	Valsalva	117.5±23.2	134.0±16.9	0.048	124.3±17.2	126.3±10.9	0.991
Vaginal angle (°)	Rest	126.5±9.0	134.4±8.4	0.026	128.4±9.0	133.4±5.2	0.036
PCL	Valsalva	136.8±17.3	155.1±12.3	0.007	143.5±14.7	143.7±6.3[a]	0.675

[a] Statistically significant

diagnostic tools such as perineal ultrasonography and dynamic MRI are newly introduced to help clinical examination. Gupta et al. evaluated 30 POP patients and suggested that the diagnosis of enterocele, which may be missed clinically, is efficiently made on dynamic MRI, and it can differentiate enterocele from high rectocele which can further classify the surgery needed [12].

It is still controversial which reference line is suitable to estimate pelvic floor disorders. For grading POP, we usually utilize horizontal line (HL) running the vaginal introitus horizontally. In order to grade pelvic organ prolapse, the distance from HL to the inferior margin of each pelvic organ is measured because we presume that it may correspond with the clinical examination. But seen the fact that this line can be moved with patient's strain, we had to choose another line fixed by bony landmarks seen on MRI to evaluate the vaginal axis. The pubococcygeal line (PCL) was adapted as a reference line for this purpose. In fact, PCL is the most commonly used reference line in the assessment of pelvic organ prolapse [10, 23]. We detected some differences in the results between the two reference lines. Since the HL could move with maximal strain and the change of vaginal axis may be masked, we suppose that the data of PCL are more reliable than those of HL.

There are several MRI studies that assess the effects of TVM and abdominal sacrocolpopexy. They found effectiveness of TVM and abdominal sacrocolpopexy, and positive correlations demonstrated between POP-Q and MRI findings [14–17].

Some MRI studies investigate anatomical changes after abdominal sacrocolpopexy and sacrospinous ligament suspension. Sze et al. [19] compared vaginal configuration on MRI after abdominal sacrocolpopexy and sacrospinous ligament suspension. They demonstrated that abdominal sacrocolpopexy with retropubic colposuspension more closely restored the vagina to its normal configuration, whereas sacrospinous fixation with transvaginal needle suspension creates an abnormal axis. Rane et al. [20] compared the vaginal configuration on MRI and found that significant improvements in the restoration of vaginal configuration were achieved in abdominal sacrocolpopexy, but that transvaginal sacrospinous fixation increases anatomical distortion of the vaginal configuration. Therefore, abdominal sacropexy seems to restore the normal vaginal axis rather than sacrospinous ligament suspension. The distortion of vaginal axis may result in a high recurrence rate after sacrospinous ligament suspension. In our current study, the vaginal axis leans to horizontal after TVM and LSC, but we could not conclude that the vaginal axis after the two operations differs or not from the normal axis, because we have no data compared with normal control.

There is only one report that compares clinical results of LSC and TVM. Maher et al. [24] compared LSC and TVM for vaginal vault prolapse at 2 years after operations. In their study, LSC had a significantly superior performance at POP-Q sites Aa, Ba, C, Ap, and Bp. TVL was unchanged after LSC but significantly shorter after TVM postoperatively. In our study, there was no difference in both anterior (Aa, Ba) and posterior (Ap, Bp) compartment between the two operations, but points C and D were positioned higher in LSC than TVM. TVL did not differ in both groups. Two reasons are considered to explain the different results. One is the presence of the

Table 4 Change of the vaginal axis from at rest to maximal strain, measured by MRI before and 1 year after operation for the TVM group and for the LSC group

		TVM			LSC			Between the two groups
		Preoperation	Postoperation	p value	Preoperation	Postoperation	p value	postoperation p value
Vaginal angle (°) HL	Valsalva-rest	16.1±21.2	25.8±15.5	0.269	27.1±15.2	21.0±10.0	0.048	0.215
Vaginal angle (°) PCL	Valsalva-rest	10.3±19.6	20.7±11.3	0.079	15.1±11.7	10.3±9.1	0.189	0.011

uterus or uterine cervix in our study. Vaginal length after hysterectomy becomes shorter. In addition to that, vaginal scar could cause vaginal shrinkage and lead to a shorter vagina. The other reason may be the shorter follow-up period in our study.

There is one study comparing abdominal sacrocolpopexy and TVM for vaginal vault prolapse by MRI before and after surgery [21]. Sixteen participants (six nulliparous control, five abdominal sacral colpopexy, five vaginal mesh kit repair) were involved in this study. They concluded that there are no differences in anatomical outcomes between abdominal sacrocolpopexy and TVM at 3 months by POP-Q examination and MRI analysis. They also described that the postoperative POP-Q point C and MRI parameters such as the vaginal axis were similar to nulliparous controls. On the other hand, points C and D after LSC were higher than TVM in our study. This different result may be due to the longer follow-up period of our study and the presence of the uterus or cervix. Our median follow-up was 37 weeks after surgery, whereas in the Ginath study, it was only 3 months. We also showed that the vaginal axis with maximal strain became more horizontal only after TVM, but they found no significant difference of the vaginal axis with maximal strain between the two procedures. Some reasons can be considered. They separated the vagina upper and lower part and measured the angle between the lower vagina and the PCL. But the upper part of the vagina has a more horizontal axis than the lower part, and it leans more horizontal by straining [25]. Their measurement of the vaginal axis may not reflect this vaginal axis change by straining. In our study, we measured the angle between the line connecting the vaginal introitus to the posterior fornix and the PCL, so we could reflect the movement of the upper vaginal part. Furthermore, we performed sacrocolpopexy by laparoscopic route but they did by abdominal approach, and paravaginal repair was concomitantly performed in all their cases. We also had four cases with concomitant surgery like rectopexy or culdoplasty in the LSC group, but their data were not far from the average. Those differences of surgical technique might affect the vaginal axis.

Balgobin et al. [26] measured the vaginal axis angle relative to a line between the lowest border of the pubic symphysis and the fourth sacral (S4) foramen at five lumbosacral mesh attachment sites in nine unembalmed cadavers. The mesh fixation point was situated from the lower border of S2 to the lower border of L5. Their result was a 3-fold increase in the vaginal axis angle from S2 to L5. The normal vaginal axis aims toward S3–S4 [25], so they concluded that fixation at the sacral promontory may result in significant anterior deviation of the vaginal axis. However in the living body, there is the abdominal pressure and the bowel compressing the mesh. As surgical technique, it is most important that the mesh should be placed without tension and not to be stretched. We suppose that the mesh after actual operation does not connect the vagina or uterine cervix to fixation point on promontory straightly but tries to hold the pelvic organs at their original position. As a result, the vaginal axis would not deviate excessively.

According to the current study, there was no difference of vaginal axis at rest between TVM and LSC. This may be the proof that both TVM and LSC could hold the vagina at the natural position without tension. The vaginal axis with maximal strain after TVM is more horizontal than LSC. This is because the fixation point of LSC, the sacral promontorium, is higher than that of TVM, the sacrospinous ligament. Though commonly believed that the vaginal axis after LSC becomes vertical, we found that LSC also makes the vagina horizontal at rest in comparison with the preoperative situation. However, it is also impossible to conclude that the vaginal axis after TVM and LSC is more horizontal than that of normal women because of the lack of normal control. At least we can suggest that LSC does not make the vagina deviate too much vertically.

Limitations of our study were the small sample size and the lack of a normal control group. Another weakness of our study is the lack of randomization and the surgical indication depending on surgeon's decision. We prefer the vaginal route in elderly patients and the laparoscopic route in patients younger than 60 years old. It leads to the difference in age between our two groups, and it could affect the anatomical results and the sexual quality of life (QOL). But there was no preoperative difference of POP-Q examination and MRI assessment in the two groups.

Furthermore, the group who underwent LSC is a rather heterogeneous group: 4 of the 14 patients had additional procedures. Procedures like rectopexy could possibly change the position of the Douglas or change the vaginal axis. But as we always implant a posterior mesh in LSC, we do not think that the vaginal axis is modified by an additional rectopexy.

The last limitation of the study is that we always have to keep in mind that any measurements done on dynamic MRI images of valsalva are dependent on the patient's ability to push reproducibly.

The strength of this report is that this is the first study to compare anatomical results of TVM and LSC by MRI measurement including dynamic evaluation. There are no reports about the vaginal configuration after LSC evaluated by MRI. We detected the new findings that the vaginal axis with maximal strain after TVM is more horizontal and that the change of vaginal axis from at rest to maximal strain is significantly greater after TVM than LSC. This anatomical difference might affect the positional relations of pelvic organs, and it can perhaps explain the differences of anatomical success rates or other clinical results such as de novo urinary incontinence or postoperative bowel dysfunctions of these surgical methods.

The necessity of LSC is increasing after the FDA public health notification which highlighted serious complications after transvaginal mesh prolapse surgery [27], but there are still few data about LSC. So, further rigorous evaluation of these procedures is required. There is also a need for standard criteria for estimation of pelvic floor disorders by dynamic MRI to help a correct clinical diagnosis of pelvic organ prolapse.

Conflict of interest M. Cosson is on the speaker's bureau, receives research support, and is a paid consultant for Ethicon Women's Health and Urology. He is a consultant for AMS and performs sponsored educational activities for Ethicon Women's Health and Urology, Olympus and Ipsen. Hiromi Kashihara, Virginie Emmanuelli, Edouard Poncelet, Chrystèle Rubod, Jean-Philippe Lucot, and Bram Pouseele declare that they have no conflict of interest. This study was entirely performed independently of manufacturer.

Informed consent All procedures followed were in accordance with the ethical standards of the responsible committee on human experimentation (institutional and national) and with the Helsinki Declaration of 1975, as revised in 2000 (5). Informed consent was obtained from all patients for being included in the study.

Authors contributions H. Kashihara wrote the manuscript and contributed to the data analysis. V. Emmanuell contributed to the project development and data collection. E. Poncelet contributed to the data analysis. C. Rubod contributed to the data collection. J.P. Lucot contributed to the data collection and manuscript editing. B. Pouseele contributed to the manuscript editing and rewriting. M. Cosson contributed to the project development, data collection, and manuscript editing.

References

1. Olsen AL, Smith VJ, Bergstrom JO, Colling JC, Clark AL (1997) Epidemiology of surgically managed pelvic organ prolapse and urinary incontinence. Obstet Gynecol 89:501–506
2. Fatton B, Amblard J, Debodinance P, Cosson M, Jacquetin B (2007) Transvaginal repair of genital prolapse: preliminary results of new tension-free vaginal mesh (Prolift technique)—a case series multicentric study. Int Urogynecol J Pelvic Floor Dysfunct 18:743–752
3. Altman D, Väyrynen T, Engh ME, Axelsen S, Falconer C, Nordic Transvaginal Mesh Group (2011) Anterior colporrhaphy versus transvaginal mesh for pelvic-organ prolapse. N Engl J Med 364:1826–1836
4. Nieminen K, Hiltunen R, Takala T, Heiskanen E, Merikari M, Niemi K, Heinonen PK (2010) Outcomes after anterior vaginal wall repair with mesh: a randomized, controlled trial with a 3 year follow-up. Am J Obstet Gynecol 203:235.e1–8
5. Maher C, Feiner B, Baessler K, Adams EJ, Hagen S, Glazener CM (2010) Surgical management of pelvic organ prolapse in women. Cochrane Database Syst Rev 14(4):CD004014, Review
6. Benson JT, Lucente V, McClellan E (1996) Vaginal versus abdominal reconstructive surgery for the treatment of pelvic support defects: a prospective randomized study with long-term outcome evaluation. Am J Obstet Gynecol 175:1418–1421
7. Sabbagh R, Mandron E, Piussan J, Brychaert PE, le Tu M (2010) Long-term anatomical and functional results of laparoscopic promontofixation for pelvic organ prolapse. BJU Int 106:861–866
8. Bacle J, Papatsoris AG, Bigot P, Azzouzi AR, Brychaet PE, Piussan J, Mandron E (2011) Laparoscopic promontofixation for pelvic organ prolapse: a 10-year single center experience in a series of 501 patients. Int J Urol 18:821–826
9. Freeman RM, Pantazis K, Thomson A, Frappell J, Bombieri L, Moran P, Slack M, Scott P, Waterfield M (2013) A randomised controlled trial of abdominal versus laparoscopic sacrocolpopexy for the treatment of post-hysterectomy vaginal vault prolapse: LAS study. Int Urogynecol J 24:377–384
10. Farouk El Sayed R (2012) The urogynecological side of pelvic floor MRI: the clinician's needs and the radiologist's role. Abdom Imaging. doi:10.1007/s00261-012-9905-3
11. Comiter CV, Vasavada SP, Barbaric ZL, Gousse AE, Raz S (1999) Grading pelvic prolapse and pelvic floor relaxation using dynamic magnetic resonance imaging. Urology 54:454–457
12. Gupta S, Sharma JB, Hari S, Kumar S, Roy KK, Singh N (2012) Study of dynamic magnetic resonance imaging in diagnosis of pelvic organ prolapse. Arch Gynecol Obstet 286:953–958
13. Goodrich MA, Webb MJ, King BF, Bampton AE, Campeau NG, Riederer SJ (1993) Magnetic resonance imaging of pelvic floor relaxation: dynamic analysis and evaluation of patients before and after surgical repair. Obstet Gynecol 82:883–891
14. Lienemann A, Sprenger D, Anthuber C, Baron A, Reiser M (2001) Functional cine magnetic resonance imaging in women after abdominal sacrocolpopexy. Obstet Gynecol 97:81–85
15. Brocker KA, Alt CD, Corteville C, Hallscheidt P, Lenz F, Sohn C (2011) Short-range clinical, dynamic magnetic resonance imaging and P-QOL questionnaire results after mesh repair in female pelvic organ prolapse. Eur J Obstet Gynecol Reprod Biol 157:107–112
16. Siegmann KC, Reisenauer C, Speck S, Barth S, Kraemer B, Claussen CD (2011) Dynamic magnetic resonance imaging for assessment of minimally invasive pelvic floor reconstruction with polypropylene implant. Eur J Radiol 80:182–187
17. Kasturi S, Lowman JK, Kelvin FM, Akisik FM, Terry CL, Hale DS (2010) Pelvic magnetic resonance imaging for assessment of the efficacy of the Prolift system for pelvic organ prolapse. Am J Obstet Gynecol 203:504.e1–5
18. Boukerrou M, Mesdagh P, Ego A, Lambaudie E, Crepin G, Robert Y, Cosson M (2005) An MRI comparison of anatomical changes related to surgical treatment of prolapse by vaginal or abdominal route. Eur J Obstet Gynecol Reprod Biol 121:220–225
19. Sze EH, Meranus J, Kohli N, Miklos JR, Karram MM (2001) Vaginal configuration on MRI after abdominal sacrocolpopexy and sacrospinous ligament suspension. Int Urogynecol J Pelvic Floor Dysfunct 12:375–379
20. Rane A, Lim YN, Withey G, Muller R (2004) Magnetic resonance imaging findings following three different vaginal vault prolapse repair procedures: a randomised study. Aust N Z J Obstet Gynaecol 44:135–139
21. Ginath S, Garely AD, Luchs JS, Shahryarinejad A, Olivera CK, Zhou S, Ascher-Walsh CJ, Condrea A, Brodman ML, Vardy MD (2012) Magnetic resonance imaging of abdominal versus vaginal prolapse surgery with mesh. Int Urogynecol J 23:1569–1576
22. Debodinance P, Berrocal J, Clave H et al (2004) [Changing attitudes on the surgical treatment of urogenital prolapse: birth of the tension-free vaginal mesh]. J Gynecol Obstet Biol Reprod (Paris) 33:577–588
23. Lienemann A, Sprenger D, Janssen U, Grosch E, Pellengahr C, Anthuber C (2004) Assessment of pelvic organ descent by use of functional cine-MRI: which reference line should be used? Neurourol Urodyn 23:33–37
24. Maher CF, Feiner B, DeCuyper EM, Nichlos CJ, Hickey KV, O'Rourke P (2011) Laparoscopic sacral colpopexy versus total vaginal mesh for vaginal vault prolapse: a randomized trial. Am J Obstet Gynecol 204(4):360.e1–7
25. Nichols DH, Milley PS, Randall CL (1970) Significance of restoration of normal vaginal depth and axis. Obstet Gynecol 36(2):251–256

26

A comparative study of Essure® hysteroscopic sterilisation versus laparoscopic sterilisation

Niblock Kathy · Connor Katie · Morgan David ·
Johnston Keith · Canadian Task Force Study of a Design-Category II-1

Abstract The purpose of this study is to compare success rate, patient satisfaction, discomfort, procedure time and intraoperative adverse events of hysteroscopic (Essure®) versus laparoscopic sterilisation. This study includes a retrospective case–control comparative study of 70 patients who had laparoscopic or hysteroscopic sterilisation performed. Systematic chart review for the documentation of preoperative counselling, operative time, intraoperative complications, documentation of correct application of Essure® and Filshie® clips and duration of hospital stay was also done. Patient follow-up was arranged and a questionnaire completed including details of postoperative pain, satisfaction of procedure, recovery time and compliance with confirmatory hysterosalpingogram attendance and associated pain. The main outcome measures were pregnancy rate following attempted tubal blockage, return to normal activity and patient satisfaction. Secondary outcome measures include patient discomfort, procedure time, device placement, compliance with hysterosalpingogram, postoperative complications and recovery time. There is a statistical difference in favour of Essure® for postoperative pain, operative time, return to work/normal activity and hospital stay with no difference in complications or pregnancy. As a conclusion, Essure® is a safe and effective alternative to laparoscopic sterilisation with significantly less procedure-related pain.

Keywords Hysteroscopic sterilisation · Essure® · Efficacy · Patient satisfaction · Recovery time · Coil placement · Laparoscopic sterilisation · Filshie Clips®

N. Kathy (✉) · C. Katie · M. David · J. Keith
Antrim Area Hospital, Derry, UK
e-mail: kathyniblock@doctors.org.uk

Introduction

The average woman in the UK spends over three decades of her life actively avoiding pregnancy [1]. Traditionally, laparoscopic sterilisation is the most accepted and widely used method of tubal sterilisation [2].

Approximately 50,000 laparoscopic sterilisations are performed annually in the UK; this number has remained surprisingly constant since the 1980s [3].

The purpose of this study is to compare well-established laparoscopic sterilisation with the newer hysteroscopic Essure® sterilisation. Primarily, we will analyse success in terms of pregnancy rate and patient satisfaction in terms of pain experienced, return to normal activity and acceptability. We will also compare device placement, patient demographics, appropriate preoperative counselling, use of general anaesthesia, intraoperative and postoperative complications, operative time, duration of hospital stay and compliance with postprocedure hysterosalpingogram.

Laparoscopic sterilisation is a well-established, relatively safe operation. Nevertheless, it does carry with it the risk of visceral damage, vascular injury, damage to retroperitoneal structures, risk of general anaesthesia and less serious complications such as postoperative wound infection and pain [4]. These risks are further increased in patients with large body mass index (BMI), patients with previous abdominal or pelvic surgery and patients with previous pelvic infection, conditions that gynaecologists are facing on an increasingly frequent basis.

In 2002, the Essure® hysteroscopic sterilisation system was approved by the US Food and Drug Administration [5]. It is a transcervical technique of tubal sterilisation. The Essure® system consists of two microinserts comprising a dynamic outer coil and an inner flexible coil which are placed hysteroscopically into the fallopian tubes under direct vision [5].

The Essure® system provokes a benign localised tissue response of inflammation and fibrosis leading to the obliteration and occlusion of the tubal lumen over a 3-month period [6].

Hysteroscopic sterilisation offers an alternative to traditional transabdominal approaches to tubal sterilisation; therefore, it is not associated with the same intraabdominal complications. It can also be performed successfully in the outpatient setting without the need for anaesthesia or sedation.

Methods

We retrospectively reviewed the charts of women who underwent sterilisation in the form of Essure® or laparoscopic sterilisation with Filshie Clips® between April 2008 and December 2011 in a district general hospital. The period of follow-up ranges from 6–50 months, mean follow-up of 19 months.

In this study, patients who underwent the Essure® procedure were placed in the lithotomy position; and where possible, the vaginoscopic technique was performed using a 30° hysteroscope 5 mm in diameter with continuous flow Bettocchi sheaths. Normal saline under low pressure was used to dilate the cervix and facilitate visualisation of the proximal portion of each fallopian tube lumen for the insertion of the microinserts. All procedures were performed by one of two trained minimal access consultant gynaecologists.

All patients who underwent Essure® sterilisation were identified from theatre database. Sixty patients were identified. Six charts were unable to be obtained from the records department and therefore not analysed. Nine charts had insufficient information to complete the study e.g. inaccurate patient contact details, no record of operative time.

A control group of 25 consecutive laparoscopic sterilisations performed over the same time period and by the same operators were also identified from theatre database.

Laparoscopic sterilisation was performed using the Hasson technique for the insertion of a 12-mm umbilical trocar. One 5-mm peripheral trocar was used. The procedure was performed using an intraabdominal pressure of 15 mmHg. Filshie clips were placed perpendicular to the isthmic portion of the fallopian tube 1–2 cm from the cornua under direct visualisation.

A total of 70 patients from one centre were involved in this study, of which 45 underwent Essure® and 25 underwent laparoscopic sterilisation.

The notes were analysed for patient demographics including age, parity and BMI. Documentation of appropriate counselling was analysed in terms of the following:

- discussion of other options available including male sterilisation
- failure rate of chosen procedure
- documentation of permanency and irreversibility

- in the cases of Essure®, the requirement for alternative contraception for 3 months followed by imaging in the form of hysterosalpingogram

Intraoperatively, we analysed type of anaesthesia, intraoperative complications, documentation or pictures of correct Filshie Clip® and microinsert placement. Correct placement is taken as 3–8 coils visible in the uterine cavity following the placement of the Essure® devise. In the laparoscopic sterilisation group, it is the placement of the Filshie Clips® at the proximal isthmus at 90° to the long axis of the fallopian tube as described by Hulka and Reich [7].

Duration of hospital stay was recorded along with operative time as documented for both groups. As this was taken from the anaesthetic database, it is the time from the patient is positioned on the table to the end of the procedure. Following the procedure, in the cases of Essure®, the number of patients attending for hysterosalpingogram and the results were recorded.

All 70 patients were then contacted by the investigators and a survey completed. This was performed after a mean of 19 months (range 6–50).

This survey included the following details:

- patients' awareness of alternative options of sterilisation
- in the case of Essure® were patients given the opportunity to have the procedure performed awake
- if not would they have chosen to be awake
- satisfaction of the procedure using a three-point scale (very, somewhat, not at all)
- pain following the procedure on a 10-point scale (10 being the worst pain ever experienced, 0 being pain-free)
- postoperative complications
- time before return to normal activities
- awareness of the requirement for contraception for 3 months followed by hysterosalpingogram in the Essure® cases
- pain associated with hysterosalpingogram on a three-point scale (mild, moderate, severe)
- success of procedure in terms of pregnancies

Results were analysed using SPSS 15.0. Normally distributed continuous data was analysed using two-tailed t test. Mann–Whitney U test was used for non-normally distributed data. Risk ratios were calculated with 95 % confidence intervals. Significance level has been taken as $P<0.05$.

Results

Demographics

The demographic characteristics of the Essure® and laparoscopic sterilisation groups are summarised in Table 1.

Table 1 The demographic characteristics of the Essure® and laparoscopic sterilisation groups

	Essure	Lap Filshie	*P* value
Mean age (range)	36.5 (27–44)	35.1 (25–46)	0.22
Mean parity (range)	2.8 (1–6)	2.3 (1–5)	0.12
Mean BMI (range)	28.6 (19–56)	26 (16–32)	0.10

The mean age, parity and BMI in both groups were comparable with *P* values of 0.22, 0.12 and 1.0, respectively.

The mean BMI in patients who underwent Essure® was 28.6 compared with 26.0 in the laparoscopic sterilisation group. In the Essure® group, however, six patients (13 %) had a BMI >40.

Preoperative counselling

Twenty-seven out of 45 patients (60 %) attending for Essure® had documented evidence of appropriate counselling including as follows:

- documentation of alternative contraception options including vasectomy
- failure rate of procedure
- permanency
- irreversibility
- need for on-going contraception until hysterosalpingogram

Procedure

Initially, 50 of the 70 patients were due to have Essure®; however, five of these cases were converted to laparoscopic sterilisation. Reasons included cervical stenosis and tubal spasm. Therefore, placement of Essure® was achieved in 45 cases, 82 % of patients compared with 100 % of placement in the laparoscopic sterilisation group.

Correct coil placement bilaterally, defined as between three and eight coils visible on both sides was documented in 53 % of patients (36 % of patients had documented less than three coils visible on at least one side, and 11 % of patients had more than eight coils visible on at least one side).

Ninety eight percent of Essure® patients had their procedure performed under general anaesthesia. This compared to 100 % of patients on the laparoscopic sterilisation group. This was the units' first experience with the Essure® technique; therefore, general anaesthesia was largely employed initially.

Operative time was recorded from the anaesthetic record. This was significantly less in the Essure® group, mean time of 15.6 mins, compared to the laparoscopic sterilisation group, mean time 35.2 mins, with a *P* value of <0.001. Procedure details for both groups are summarised in Table 2.

Postoperative tubal patency

Forty women (89 %) attended for hysterosalpingogram 3 months following their procedure. Correct placement and bilateral occlusion was confirmed in 100 % of hysterosalpingograms including cases where microinsert placement was suboptimal (i.e. not the desired 3–8 coils visible in the uterine cavity following device placement).

Patient reported outcome measures

Results of the retrospective follow-up survey are summarised in Table 3.

On a three-point scale of satisfaction, 42 patients (93 %) were "very" satisfied with the procedure, and the remaining three patients were "somewhat" satisfied.

In the laparoscopic sterilisation group, 92 % were "very" satisfied and 8 % "somewhat" satisfied.

The mean postoperative pain score in the Essure® group on a 10-point scale was 3.2 (range 0–9), this compared to 6.5 in the laparoscopic sterilisation group (range 1–10), making this difference statistically significant with a *P* value of <0.001. Mean return to normal activities also showed statistical significance, *P* value 0.02.

In patients undergoing hysterosalpingogram, 15 out of 40 (37.5 %) described the pain as severe on a scale of mild, moderate and severe. This resulted in three women claiming they would reconsider Essure® hysteroscopic sterilisation on the experience of hysterosalpingogram alone.

Complications in the Essure® group consisted of one patient (2 %) who required a course of oral antibiotics for a presumed case of endometritis. In the laparoscopic sterilisation group, three patients (12 %) reported complications. One patient required readmission for analgesia (this patient has been included in the overnight stay group), and two required oral antibiotics for wound infections.

Pregnancy

There have been no pregnancies in either group patients accounting for 104 woman years. Follow-up in the Essure® group ranged from 3–47 months (mean 18 months). This time has been taken from the time of confirmatory test (or 3 months postprocedure in patients who did not attend for hysterosalpingogram) to the completion of questionnaire. In the laparoscopic sterilisation group, follow-up ranged from 6–44 months (mean 20 months) and is taken from the date of the operation.

Discussion

This study evaluated multiple aspects of a new surgical technique from a clinician and, more importantly, patient

Table 2 Procedure details for both groups

	Essure	Lap Filshie	P value
Operative time	15.6(6–35)	35.2 (20–65)	P<0.001
Bilateral placement (%)	82	100	RR 0.83
			CI 0.72–0.96
			P=0.009
Overnight stay (%)	2	24	RR 0.09 [95 % CI 0.01–0.73]
			P=0.02

perspective. The majority of permanent sterilisations in the UK remain laparoscopic sterilisations.

Laparoscopic procedures require general anaesthesia, which increases the overall risk to the procedure. They are also associated with increased postoperative pain and prolonged hospital stay. Laparoscopic sterilisation requires instrumentation of the abdominal cavity; although it is generally safe, it does carry a risk of vascular and visceral injury ranging from 4.5 per 1,000 laparoscopies [8].

One of the major advantages of laparoscopic sterilisation is the opportunity it provides to inspect the pelvis and abdomen to exclude pathology. Patients enjoy the advantage of being able to rely on laparoscopic sterilisation as contraception immediately after the procedure without a need for a confirmation test. It also provides essential laparoscopic training opportunities to trainees in the specialty.

Similarly, the Essure® procedure offers gynaecologists skills in operative hysteroscopy and the patient the opportunity to have a diagnostic hysteroscopy performed.

Obesity is an ever-growing epidemic challenging the health service at present. It adds to the complexity of procedures and increases the associated risks.

Essure® is not suitable for every patient. Contraindications include patients with previous ablation procedures performed, certain gynaecological malignancies, abnormal uterine cavity and patients less than 10 weeks postpartum. It is particularly useful in patients with an increased BMI, previous pelvic and abdominal surgery and previous pelvic infection. Where intraoperative hurdles present during hysteroscopic sterilisation such as tubal spasm or cervical stenosis, laparoscopic sterilisation is a reasonable alternative. Although according to Bettocchi, these problems can often be overcome by improved training in hysteroscopy [9] and equipment such as fluid management systems to ensure optimal intrauterine pressure. As our study was carried out following the introduction

of Essure® into our unit, the conversion rate to laparoscopic sterilisation of 10 % may partially be attributed to operator inexperience.

Hysteroscopic sterilisation offers advantages to patients in terms of pain, hospital stay and recovery. In our study, there were less complications documented in the Essure® group; however, these were not statistically significant. From our study, the review of pregnancy rates has demonstrated that both procedures are comparable and reliable. Although the small number of cases prevents definitive conclusions, the follow-up period does provide reassurance that this new service is a safe alternative to laparoscopic sterilisation. Existing literature would further suggest that pregnancy rates are favourable for Essure® compared to laparoscopic sterilisation.

Hysterosalpingogram might be a source of considerable pain for some women. Thankfully, due to updated protocols, it is only indicated as a secondary confirmation test in special cases. Alternative modalities such as transvaginal ultrasound scan and plain x-ray have been recommended to be the best primary screening tests to demonstrate correct device placement and therefore increase the acceptability of Essure® [10].

A prospective multicentre cohort study carried out in the Netherlands in 2011 evaluating the use of transvaginal ultrasound in 1,145 women who underwent uncomplicated Essure® hysteroscopic sterilisation demonstrated that transvaginal ultrasound scanning was comparable to hysterosalpingogram in terms of diagnosing the adequacy of the procedure. As ultrasound is minimally invasive and avoids exposure to ionising radiation, the recommendation was that it should be considered as a first-line diagnostic test [11].

As with any retrospective study, there are obvious limitations. Firstly, six patients were unable to be included due to difficulties in the record department. Secondly, the operative time for Essure® patients should be documented as scope into vagina to scope out of vagina; however, as our time was

Table 3 Results of the retrospective follow-up survey

	Essure	Lap Filshie	
Return to work (days)	4.5 (1–17)	9.0 (1–35)	P=0.02
Postop pain score	3.2 (0–9)	6.5 (1–10)	P<0.001
Complications (%)	2	12	RR 0.19 [95 % CI 0.02–1.69] p=0.13
Pregnancy rate (%)	0	0	

recorded on the anaesthetic chart, this was not possible. However, by using times recorded by the anaesthetic staff, this does remove operator bias with regard to operative time. Thirdly, it is well-documented that patient recall of pain and satisfaction is less accurate and reliable with longer follow-up times.

The Crest Study previously demonstrated that one of the common beliefs regarding tubal sterilisation, that pregnancies were most common in the first year following the procedure, is in fact inaccurate. It demonstrated tubal sterilisation failures up to 10 years postprocedure [7]. This highlights the need for a longer follow-up period. The FDA recommends a 10 year follow-up postprocedure to monitor for additional pregnancies [10].

Several retrospective studies exist for pregnancy rates following hysteroscopic sterilisation such as "Hysteroscopic Sterilization: 10-Year Retrospective Analysis of Worldwide Pregnancy Reports" by Munro et al [12] which suggests that hysteroscopic sterilisation is 99.74 % effective against pregnancy at 5 years and smaller prospective studies such as "Hysteroscopic Sterilization Using a Microinsert Device: Results from a Multicentre Phase II Study" by Kerin et al [13] which reported no pregnancies after 6,015 woman months in 227 women. However, a large prospective study would be useful to further assess the reliability of Essure® such as exists for laparoscopic sterilisation in the Crest Study where >10,000 patients were followed up over 8–14 years for pregnancies [7].

Reviewing the outcome of Essure® in our unit has led to the introduction of this procedure being offered in our ambulatory outpatient hysteroscopy department using a vaginoscopic technique without anaesthesia or sedation. It is likely that by adopting the ambulatory approach to Essure®, outcome measures may become more favourable.

Conclusion

Essure® is a safe and effective alternative to laparoscopic sterilisation with significantly less procedure-related postoperative pain. Significantly shorter operative time, shorter hospital stay and faster return to normal activities make Essure® a superior procedure in many ways for women and health trusts.

This study has reinforced the need to thoroughly counsel women and document informed consent appropriately.

Consent All procedures followed were in accordance with the ethical standards of the responsible committee on human experimentation. Informed consent was obtained from all patients included in this study

References

1. Duffy S, Marsh F, Rogerson L et al (2005) Female sterilisation: a cohort controlled comparative study of ESSURE versus laparoscopic sterilisation. BJOG 112(11):1522–1528
2. Hurskainen R, Hovi SL, Gissler M et al (2010) Hysteroscopic tubal sterilization: a systematic review of the Essure system. Fertil Steril 94(1):16–19
3. Omnibus Survey. Office for national statistics 1999. Available: www.statistics.gov.uk
4. Kerin JF, Cooper JM, Price T et al (2003) Hysteroscopic sterilization using a micro-insert device: results of a multicentre phase II study. Hum Reprod 18(6):1223–1230
5. Cooper JM, Carignan CS, Cher D, Kerin JF (2003) Microinsert nonincisional hysteroscopic sterilization. Obstet Gynecol 102(1):59–67
6. Connor VF (2009) Essure: a review six years later. J Minim Invasive Gynecol 16(3):282–290
7. Peterson HB, Xia Z, Hughes JM et al (1996) The risk of pregnancy after tubal sterilization: findings from the U.S. Collaborative Review of Sterilization. Am J Obstet Gynecol 174:1161–1170
8. Jansen FW, Kapiteyn K et al (1997) Complications of laparoscopy: a prospective multicentre observational study. Br J Obstet Gynecol 104(5):595–600
9. Bettocchi S, Selvaggi L (1997) A vaginoscopic approach to reduce the pain of office hysteroscopy. J Am Assoc Gynecol Laparosc 4:255–258
10. Basinski CM (2010) A review of clinical data for currently approved hysteroscopic sterilization procedures. Rev Obstet Gynecol 3(3):101–110
11. Veersema S, Vleugels M et al (2011) Confirmation of Essure placement using transvaginal ultrasound. J Minim Invasive Gynecol 18(2):164–168
12. Munro M, Nichols J et al (2014) Hysteroscopic sterilization: 10-year retrospective analysis of worldwide pregnancy reports. J Minim Invasive Gynecol 21(2):245–251

27

Role of prophylactic antibiotics in endoscopic gynaecological surgery; a consensus proposal

Vasileios Minas · Nahid Gul · David Rowlands

Abstract Surgical site infection can result in increased morbidity for the patient, prolonged hospital stay and hospital readmission. Preoperative antibiotics reduce the incidence of such infections, particularly in open surgery. Universal use of antibiotic prophylaxis, however, is not recommended due to the risks of adverse reactions, generation of resistant bacteria and additional cost. Endoscopic procedures carry low risk of wound contamination and infection. Limited data suggest wide variability in antibiotic prophylaxis in gynaecological surgery and potential overuse of antibiotics in gynaecological endoscopic surgery. Bringing together the existing evidence allows for a consensus proposal for the use of preoperative antibiotics in gynaecological endoscopy.

Keywords Laparoscopy · Hysteroscopy · Gynaecological surgery · Prophylactic antibiotics

Background

Surgical site infection is a common postoperative complication and can result in increased morbidity for the patient, prolonged hospital stay and hospital readmission [1]. In gynaecological surgery, up to 8–10 % of patients develop surgical site infection [2]. The administration of preoperative antibiotics has been reported to be an important intervention to prevent such infections [3]. The aim is to achieve high levels of a broad-spectrum antibiotic at the surgical wound to avoid contamination by microorganisms. An intravenous dose is administered at induction of anaesthesia, whereas further doses do not appear to be beneficial [4]. Still, administration

of prophylaxis is not universally recommended, as not all surgical procedures carry a significant risk of wound contamination and infection [5]. Unnecessary administration of antibiotics may be detrimental as it can result in additional costs, adverse reactions and the emergence of resistant bacteria [6]. A recent survey performed in the USA showed wide variability in antibiotic prophylaxis in gynaecological surgery [7].

Laparoscopic procedures are performed via small abdominal incisions and trocars that isolate the operating site from the external environment. Hysteroscopic surgery is also minimally invasive surgery performed via the cervical orifice. It is therefore thought that the risk of contamination in endoscopic surgery is much lower compared to open surgery and the use of antibiotics may not confer any additional benefit [8]. Endoscopic gynaecological surgeons practicing in the United Kingdom currently have no available national recommendations on which to base their practice in relation to antibiotic prophylaxis; hence, practice is likely to differ between various hospitals and individual surgeons. Our group recently performed a relevant survey. Gynaecologists in the UK were asked to state whether they administer antibiotic prophylaxis for different endoscopic procedures. Although no solid conclusions could be drawn due to the low response rate the survey achieved, the responses were remarkably varied, thus enhancing our impression of varied practice (data not shown).

Classification of surgical wounds

Surgical wounds can be classified in four classes according to their potential for contamination and infection [9]. Class I/clean procedures are those where no inflammation is encountered and the respiratory, alimentary or genitourinary tracts are not entered. In laparoscopic gynaecological surgery, procedures such as diagnostic laparoscopy, laparoscopic sterilisation, excision of mild endometriosis, ovarian cystectomy and salpingo-oophorectomy fall into this category.

V. Minas (✉) · N. Gul · D. Rowlands
Minimal Access Centre, Department of Obstetrics and Gynaecology,
Wirral University Teaching Hospital, Arrowe Park Rd, Wirral,
Merseyside CH49 5PE, UK
e-mail: billminas@gmail.com

In class II/clean-contaminated procedures, the respiratory, alimentary or genitourinary tracts are entered but under controlled conditions and without unusual contamination or spillage, for example, a laparoscopic total hysterectomy or an excision of a rectovaginal nodule with a breech to the vagina. Class III/clean-contaminated procedures carry high risk of infection and involve operations where acute inflammation (without pus) is encountered, or where there is visible contamination of the wound. Examples include gross spillage from a hollow viscus during the operation or compound/open injuries operated on within four hours. Finally, class IV/dirty-infected operations are those performed in the presence of pus, where there is a previously perforated hollow viscus, or compound/open injuries more than 4 h old. Clearly, the majority of laparoscopic pelvic procedures performed in the UK (basic, intermediate and potentially some advanced laparoscopic procedures) are class I/clean operations, i.e. procedures with the lowest possible risk of contamination and infection.

Review of existing evidence and published recommendations

Guidelines on the use of antibiotic prophylaxis in gynaecological endoscopic surgery have been produced by the Society of Obstetricians and Gynaecologists of Canada (SOGC) [10], the American College of Obstetricians and Gynecologists (ACOG) [6] and the Surgical Infection Prevention Project [11]. In contrast, such official published guidance is lacking in most European countries. There exists one randomised controlled trial (RCT) which evaluated antibiotic use in benign gynaecological laparoscopic procedures (excluding hysterectomy) published to date [12]. The study found no statistically significant differences between prophylaxis

and no prophylaxis for any of the infectious outcomes, suggesting that in certain types of operations antibiotics do not offer any benefit compared to placebo. Based on the above data, the SOGC recommends against the use of prophylaxis for laparoscopic procedures that do not involve breach to the uterine cavity or vagina. A second RCT found no differences in infection rates between two different antibiotics (amoxicillin-clavulanic acid and cefazolin) used for prophylaxis in a variety of laparoscopic procedures that included total hysterectomy [13]. This RCT however involved no placebo-controlled group; therefore, no conclusions can be drawn regarding the actual benefit of prophylaxis. There are therefore no RCTs assessing the role of prophylactic antibiotics in any type of laparoscopic hysterectomy. A Cochrane review concluded that the rates of surgical site infection and febrile morbidity in laparoscopic hysterectomy are lower compared to abdominal hysterectomy and similar to vaginal hysterectomy [14]. Therefore, based on evidence from studies on vaginal hysterectomies, it is sensible to recommend antibiotic prophylaxis in laparoscopic hysterectomies [10]. Furthermore, total laparoscopic hysterectomy and laparoscopically assisted vaginal hysterectomy are class II/clean-contaminated procedures which carry a moderate risk of infection and can benefit from antibiotic prophylaxis. Subtotal (supracervical) laparoscopic hysterectomy may be considered a class I procedure, since the vagina is not entered. However, surgical site infection rates are again similar to vaginal hysterectomies, and therefore, antibiotics are likely to be beneficial based on the aforementioned rationale [10].

In terms of hysteroscopic surgery, an adequately powered prospective randomised study of 116 women undergoing hysteroscopic resection or laser ablation failed to produce conclusive evidence on the benefit of antibiotic prophylaxis [15]. A further pseudo-randomised study involving 631 women undergoing diagnostic hysteroscopy showed no difference

Table 1 Table summarizing the conclusions of available international guidelines [6, 10]. The quality of evidence assessment and classification of recommendations originate from the Canadian Task Force on Preventive Health Care [21]. The key to the evidence statements and grading of recommendations is shown below

Endoscopic procedure	Antibiotic prophylaxis	Level of evidence
Laparoscopic hysterectomy (total/subtotal/laparoscopically assisted vaginal hysterectomy)	Recommended	III-B
Laparoscopic procedures with no breach to the uterine cavity or vagina	Not recommended	I-E
Hysteroscopic surgery	Not recommended	II-2D

I—Evidence obtained from at least one properly randomized controlled trial. II-1—Evidence from well-designed controlled trials without randomization. II-2—Evidence from well-designed cohort (prospective or retrospective) or case–control studies, preferably from more than one centre or research group recommendation for or against use of the clinical preventive action; however, other factors may influence decision-making. II-3—Evidence obtained from comparisons between times or places with or without the intervention. Dramatic results in uncontrolled experiments (such as the results of treatment with penicillin in the 1940s) could also be included in this category. III—Opinions of respected authorities, based on clinical experience, descriptive studies or reports of expert committees. A—There is good evidence to recommend the clinical preventive action. B—There is fair evidence to recommend the clinical preventive action. C—The existing evidence is conflicting and does not allow to make a recommendation for or against use of the clinical preventive action; however, other factors may influence decision-making. D—There is fair evidence to recommend against the clinical preventive action. E—There is good evidence to recommend against the clinical preventive action. L—There is insufficient evidence (in quantity or quality) to make a recommendation; however, other factors may influence decision-making

in post-procedural infection between the prophylaxis and no prophylaxis groups [16]. In this study, patients either received or did not receive antibiotic prophylaxis based on the local protocol of the hospital they attended. The variable design and nature of the aforementioned studies does not allow a meta-analysis of their results, and a recent Cochrane review of prophylactic antibiotics for transcervical intrauterine procedures failed to identify any RCTs that met their criteria for inclusion in a meta-analysis [17]. Still, the data of the aforementioned studies were assessed as robust enough by the SOGC to recommend against the use of prophylaxis in hysteroscopic surgery [10]. Taken together, the conclusions of available international guidelines are shown in Table 1 below.

Certain special circumstances should be considered separately, for example, cases of prolonged surgery and pregnancy. Duration of surgery is positively associated with risk of wound infection. This risk is additional to that of the classification of the procedure [18]. Although no evidence exists for gynaecological laparoscopic or hysteroscopic surgery, it is sensible to consider prophylaxis in unusually prolonged procedures. Similarly, a pregnant patient who undergoes a class I gynaecological procedure (for example ovarian cystectomy) should be given prophylaxis in line with recommendations published for other types of surgery in pregnant women [18].

Discussion and conclusions

Preoperative antibiotics have the potential of reducing febrile morbidity and wound infection rates for a wide range of surgical procedures [19]. Their use comes with the disadvantages of additional cost, risk of anaphylactic reaction and potential contribution to the development of resistant bacterial strains. A large proportion of laparoscopic pelvic procedures performed in the UK are class I/clean procedures which carry low risk of infection.

We believe that in the absence of relevant national guidance, antibiotics may be overused in endoscopic surgery in the UK and potentially other European countries. That may be particularly true for class I/clean endoscopic procedures where some evidence against the use of antibiotics exists already. Further research is much needed on the subject. We recommend further randomised placebo-controlled trials to investigate the role of prophylaxis in hysteroscopic as well as advanced laparoscopic surgery and robotic gynaecological surgery. Such studies should be sufficiently powered and therefore likely multicentre to recruit the required numbers of patients.

Given the relative lack of robust data from studies investigating gynaecological procedures, evidence from other types of surgery may also be extrapolated to draw consensus [20]. For example, a Cochrane review looking at laparoscopic

cholecystectomy observed no statistically significant differences between antibiotic prophylaxis and no prophylaxis in the proportion of surgical site or extra-abdominal infections [8]. The meta-analysis involved 11 RCTs with 1,664 patients in total (900 in the prophylaxis group and 764 in the no-prophylaxis group). Surgical site infection rates were similar in the two groups; 2.7 % patients in the prophylaxis group had a surgical site infection against 3.3 % in the no-prophylaxis group. The odds ratio was 0.87, 95 % confidence interval (0.49 to 1.54). Overall, the review suggested that there is not sufficient evidence to support or refute the use of antibiotic prophylaxis to reduce surgical site infection. The results of the meta-analysis however have been adopted by the Scottish Intercollegiate Guidelines Network which recommends against prophylaxis for laparoscopic cholecystectomy unless other additional risk factors are present such as immunosuppression, pregnancy and existing infection [18].

In conclusion, review of published evidence suggests that laparoscopic procedures which do not involve entry to the vagina, uterine cavity or other viscera do not require antibiotic prophylaxis. The data on hysteroscopic surgery are weaker and although antibiotics may not appear to be beneficial, we suggest clinical judgment be used for each individual case. There is paucity of high-quality evidence and priority needs to be given to undertaking high-quality randomised controlled trials to address the subject of antibiotic prophylaxis in gynaecological hysteroscopic, laparoscopic and robotic surgery.

Informed consent statement   This article does not contain any studies with human or animal subjects performed by any of the authors.

References

1. Kirkland KB, Briggs JP, Trivette SL et al (1999) The impact of surgical-site infections in the 1990s: attributable mortality, excess length of hospitalization, and extra costs. Infect Control Hosp Epidemiol 20:725–730
2. Kamat AA, Brancazio L, Gibson M (2000) Wound infection in gynecologic surgery. Infect Dis Obstet Gynecol 8:230–234
3. Strachan CJ, Black J, Powis SJ, Waterworth TA, Wise R, Wilkinson AR et al (1977) Prophylactic use of cephazolin against antibiotic prophylaxis for patients undergoing elective laparoscopic cholecystectomy wound sepsis after cholecystectomy. BMJ 1:124–126
4. Weed HG (2003) Antimicrobial prophylaxis in the surgical patient. Med Clin North Am 87:59–75
5. Dellinger EP, Gross PA, Barrett TL et al (1994) Quality standard for antimicrobial prophylaxis in surgical procedures. Infectious Diseases Society of America. Clin Infect Dis 18:422–427
6. ACOG practice bulletin No. 104 (2009) Antibiotic prophylaxis for gynecologic procedures. Obstet Gynecol 113:1180–1189
7. Schimpf MO, Morrill MY, Margulies RU, Ward RM, Carberry CL, Sung VW (2012) Surgeon practice patterns for antibiotic prophylaxis

in gynecologic surgery. Female Pelvic Med Reconstr Surg 18:281–285

8. Sanabria A, Dominguez LC, Valdivieso E, Gomez G (2010) Antibiotic prophylaxis for patients undergoing elective laparoscopic cholecystectomy. Cochrane Database Syst Rev 12:CD005265

9. Mangram AJ, Horan TC, Pearson ML, Silver LC, Jarvis WR (1999) Guideline for prevention of surgical site infection. Centers for Disease Control and Prevention (CDC) Hospital Infection Control Practices Advisory Committee. Am J Infect Control 27:97–132, quiz 3–4; discussion 96

10. Van Eyk N, van Schalkwyk J (2012) Antibiotic prophylaxis in gynaecologic procedures. J Obstet Gynaecol Can 34:382–391

11. Bratzler DW, Hunt DR (2006) The surgical infection prevention and surgical care improvement projects: national initiatives to improve outcomes for patients having surgery. Clin Infect Dis 43:322–330

12. Kocak I, Ustun C, Emre B, Uzel A (2005) Antibiotics prophylaxis in laparoscopy. Ceska Gynekol 70:269–272

13. Cormio G, Bettocchi S, Ceci O, Nappi L, Di Fazio F, Cacciapuoti C, Selvaggi L (2003) Antimicrobial prophylaxis in laparoscopic gynecologic surgery: a prospective randomized study comparing amoxicillin-clavulanic acid with cefazolin. J Chemother 15:574–578

14. Johnson N, Barlow D, Lethaby A, Tavender E, Curr E, Garry R (2006) Surgical approach to hysterectomy for benign gynaecological disease. Cochrane Database Syst Rev 2:CD003677

15. Bhattacharya S, Parkin DE, Reid TM, Abramovich DR, Mollison J, Kitchener HC (1995) A prospective randomised study of the effects of prophylactic antibiotics on the incidence of bacteraemia following hysteroscopic surgery. Eur J Obstet Gynecol Reprod Biol 63:37–40

16. Kasius J, Broekmans F, Fauser B, Devroey P, Fatemi H (2011) Antibiotic prophylaxis for hysteroscopy evaluation of the uterine cavity. Fertil Steril 95:792–794

17. Thinkhamrop J, Laopaiboon M, Lumbiganon P (2013). Prophylactic antibiotics for transcervical intrauterine procedures. Cochrane Database Syst Rev. May 31;5:CD005637

18. Scottish Intercollegiate Guidelines Network (2008). Antibiotic prophylaxis in surgery. SIGN Guideline No. 104. http://www.sign.ac.uk/pdf/sign104.pdf

19. Brolmann FE, Ubbink DT, Nelson EA, Munte K, van der Horst CM, Vermeulen H (2012) Evidence-based decisions for local and systemic wound care. Br J Surg 99:1172–1183

20. Morrill MY, Schimpf MO, Abed H, Carberry C, Margulies RU, White AB, Lowenstein L, Ward RM, Balk EM, Uhlig K, Sung VW (2013) Antibiotic prophylaxis for selected gynecologic surgeries. Int J Gynaecol Obstet 120:10–15

21. Woolf SH, Battista RN, Angerson GM, Logan AG, Eel W (2003) Canadian Task Force on Preventive Health Care. New grades for recommendations from the Canadian Task Force on Preventive Health Care. CMAJ 169:207–208

28

Hysteroscopy findings and its correlation with latent endometrial tuberculosis in infertility

Subrat Kumar Mohakul · Venkata Radha Kumari Beela · Purnima Tiru

Abstract In India, 5 to 18 % of females attending infertility clinics are diagnosed to be suffering from genital tuberculosis. The present study was conducted to find out the prevalence of endometrial tuberculosis in infertility and its correlation with hysteroscopic changes. Patients attending infertility clinic with history of more than 2 years of unexplained infertility, failure to conceive in spite of successful ovulation induction in anovulatory infertility, and secondary infertility with a history of unexplained abortion or ectopic pregnancy were included in the study. In all the 105 cases, hysteroscopy was done, and the endometrium was subjected to DNA-PCR (polymerase chain reaction) testing for detection of *Mycobacterium tuberculosis* infection. Hysteroscopy features were compared in tuberculosis positive (39 %) and negative (61 %) cases for correlation. Tuberculosis was detected in 43.75 % of ostial and periostial fibrosis, 48.48 % of intrauterine fibrosis, and 66.67 % of the irregular cavity surface. A complete 6-month course of antitubercular treatment was given to the tuberculosis positive cases among which 39 % conceived without any additional treatment. The pregnancy rate of 64.7 % in secondary infertility and 20.8 % in primary infertility was very much promising. Tuberculosis is one of the major etiological factors in female infertility in developing countries. Preliminary assessment by hysteroscopy followed by PCR testing for *Mycobacterium tuberculosis* will detect it early. Subsequent antitubercular treatment may reverse the reproductive capability and prevent permanent damage to the female reproductive organs.

Keywords Hysteroscopy · Infertility · Latent endometrial tuberculosis · Female genital tuberculosis

S. K. Mohakul (✉) · V. R. K. Beela · P. Tiru
Visakha Steel General Hospital (RINL), Visakhapatnam, India
e-mail: skmohakulvizag@gmail.com

V. R. K. Beela
e-mail: bradhaaram@rediffmail.com

P. Tiru
e-mail: drpurnimatiru@vizagsteel.com

Introduction

Genital tuberculosis (TB) in females is by no means uncommon, particularly in communities where pulmonary or other forms of extragenital TB are common. TB can affect any organ in the body, can exist without any clinical manifestation, and can recur. Female genital TB is typically understood as a disease of young women, with 80 to 90 % of cases diagnosed in patients 20 to 40 years old, often during workup for infertility [1]. Genital tuberculosis in females is found in 0.75 to 1 % of gynecological admissions in India, with considerable variation from place to place [2]. The disease is responsible for 5 % of all female pelvic infections and occurs in 10 % of cases of pulmonary tuberculosis [3]. It is estimated that a third of the world's population is infected with tuberculosis and that a new infection occurs every second [4]. Most of these infections are asymptomatic and may not cause disease. However, TB remains a major health problem in many developing countries, and in these areas, genital TB is responsible for a significant proportion of female infertility [5].

It is often a secondary complication as a result of the reactivation of a silent bacillemia, primarily from the lungs, affecting most commonly the fallopian tubes (92–100 %), endometrium (50 %), ovaries (10–30 %), cervix (5 %), and the vagina and vulva (<1 %) [2, 6] but in some instances also from the kidney and intestines, etc. [7]. However, a few reports have found the endometrium to be the most commonly involved site [8, 9]. Direct inoculation of *Mycobacterium* can also take place over the vulva or vagina during sexual intercourse with a partner suffering from tuberculosis of the genitalia [10]. Establishment of the true incidence and prevalence of female genital tuberculosis is difficult because asymptomatic latent cases predominate over symptomatic ones [11].

This silent invader of the genital tract tends to create diagnostic dilemmas because of varied clinical presentations and diverse findings on imaging and endoscopy. Although the histopathologic evidence of mycobacterial infection is highly indicative of genital TB, its absence fails to exclude the infection. Identical lesions may also be seen in fungal and sarcoid diseases [12]. Similarly, culture methods, which have been considered a gold standard in proving genital TB, fail to exclude the infection. Furthermore, *Mycobacterium* is a temperamental bacillus that needs 4–5 weeks to grow on Lowenstein-Jensen (LJ) media and 2 weeks time to grow on radiometric BACTEC media [13]. The minimum *Mycobacterium* concentration at which histopathologic evidence appears is 10,000 bacilli/ml. For positive cultures, the required concentrations are 1,000 bacilli/ml for LJ and 10–100 bacilli/ml for BACTEC media. But by utilizing DNA-PCR (polymerase chain reaction) technique with high sensitivity of 96.4 % and specificity of 100 %, tuberculosis can be detected in the concentration as low as 10 bacilli/ml [14].

Therefore, the present study was conducted to identify the tubercular infection of the endometrium by TB-PCR analysis and correlate it with hysteroscopy features and posttreatment outcomes.

Materials and methods

This prospective study was conducted in Vishakha Steel General Hospital between November 2008 and December 2011.

Inclusion criteria

The couples presenting to the outpatient department for treatment of infertility meeting the following criteria were included in the study:

1) Couples with more than 2 years of unexplained infertility where all investigations were within normal limits.
2) Couples with diagnosed anovulatory infertility who failed to conceive even after 6 cycles of successful ovulation induction.
3) Couples with secondary infertility following a history of unexplained abortion or ectopic pregnancy.
4) Primary or secondary infertility with hypomenorrhea of the female partner (scanty flow defined by menstrual loss of 2 days or less).

Exclusion criteria

Couples with severe male factor or bilateral tubal damage were excluded from the study.

In all the cases, a detailed history was taken followed by clinical examination and basic hematological investigations. Specialized infertility investigations like hormonal assay, thyroid profile, follicular study, tubal factor assessment, including laparoscopy were performed wherever indicated before including in the study. Hysteroscopy with simultaneous TB-PCR testing of the endometrium was done for all the cases who qualified as per the inclusion criteria.

During diagnostic hysteroscopy, normal saline was used as the distension medium. A continuous flow double sheath hysteroscope was used to visualize the uterine cavity. The uterine wall and fundus were looked at for fibrosis, adhesion bands, ridges, and synechiae, indicating intrauterine fibrosis (Figs. 1, 2, 3, 4, and 5). Internal tubal ostia were checked for stenosis, a pinhole opening, blocks, and periostial fibrosis (Fig. 6). The surface of the uterine cavity was examined for irregularity (Fig. 7) or any other abnormality (Fig. 8). After the completion of hysteroscopy, a sample from the endometrium was collected by sharp curettage and stored in normal saline for TB-PCR testing.

Mycobacterium DNA was extracted from endometrial tissue using Qiagen DNA Mini Kit. DNA binds specifically to the silica-gel membrane while contaminants pass through. PCR inhibitors such as divalent cations and proteins are completely removed in two efficient wash steps, leaving purified DNA. The protocol mentioned by the manufacturer was exactly followed to obtain a final elute of 200 μl which was then subjected to *real time* PCR.

Oligonucleotides-designated Sp1 (5_-ACCTCCTTTCTA AGGAGCACC-3_) and Sp2 (5_-GATGCTCG CAACCA CTATCCA-3_) were used to amplify an approximately 220-bp fragment of the ITS (16S-23S rDNA internal transcribed spacer) sequence (European Bioinformatics Institute accession number L15623) from *Mycobacterium*. Amplified product was detected by using modified specific fluorescent probes. In order to specifically identify mycobacterium tuberculosis (MTB), paired fluorogenic hybridization probes were designed to recognize a region in the ITS fragment [15].

For each sample, 10 μl of template DNA was incorporated into a 50-μl PCR containing the amplification oligonucleotides and MTB-ITS hybridization probes using the QuantiTect Probe kit (Qiagen). The optimized PCR protocol included an initial denaturation step at 95 °C for 30 s and was followed by a three-step PCR cycle 95 °C for 30 s, 59 °C for 5 s, and 72 °C for 30 s for 40 cycles. Fluorescence measurements are made in every cycle. The threshold cycle (Ct) value is the cycle at which there is a significant increase in fluorescence, and this value is associated with an exponential growth of PCR product during the log-linear phase. Positive and negative controls were used in each run. A melt curve analysis performed on the Rotor-Gene 3000 confirmed the presence of ITS fragment amplification specific to mycobacterium tuberculosis complex (MTC) in all specimens.

Fig. 1 Normal hysteroscopy with normal left ostium and endometrial glands

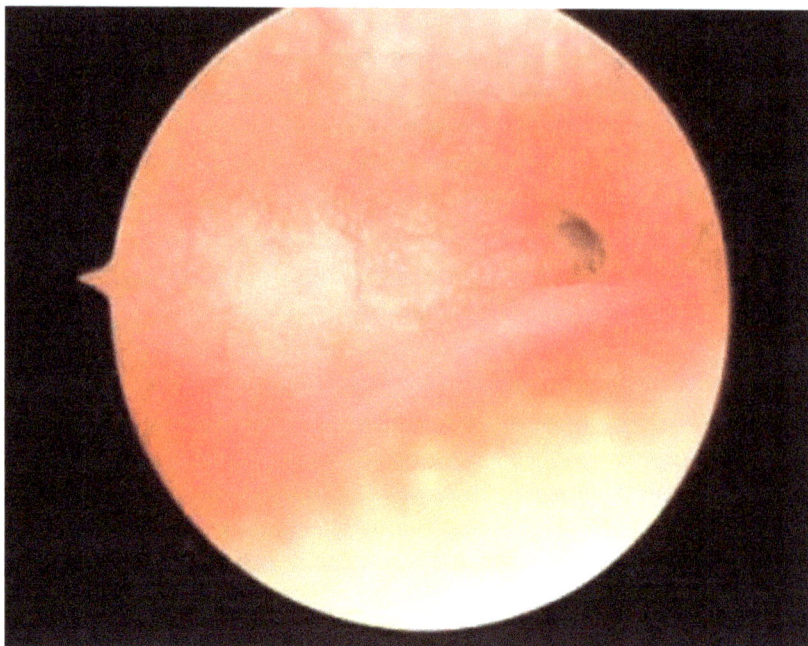

The hysteroscopy findings were analyzed and correlated with TB-PCR results. Those cases were found to be positive for TB-PCR were given a 6-month course of antitubercular treatment (ATT). The ATT consists of a four-drug regimen, i.e., rifampicin, isoniazid, ethambutol, and pyrazinamide for 2 months, followed by rifampicin and isoniazid for 4 months. Liver function test (LFT) was performed before starting ATT and repeated every month. Those showing common adverse effects like nausea and vomiting were managed with domperidone and ranitidine. Complaints of neuropathic symptoms were managed by a pyridoxine supplement.

Fig. 2 Fundal fibrosis

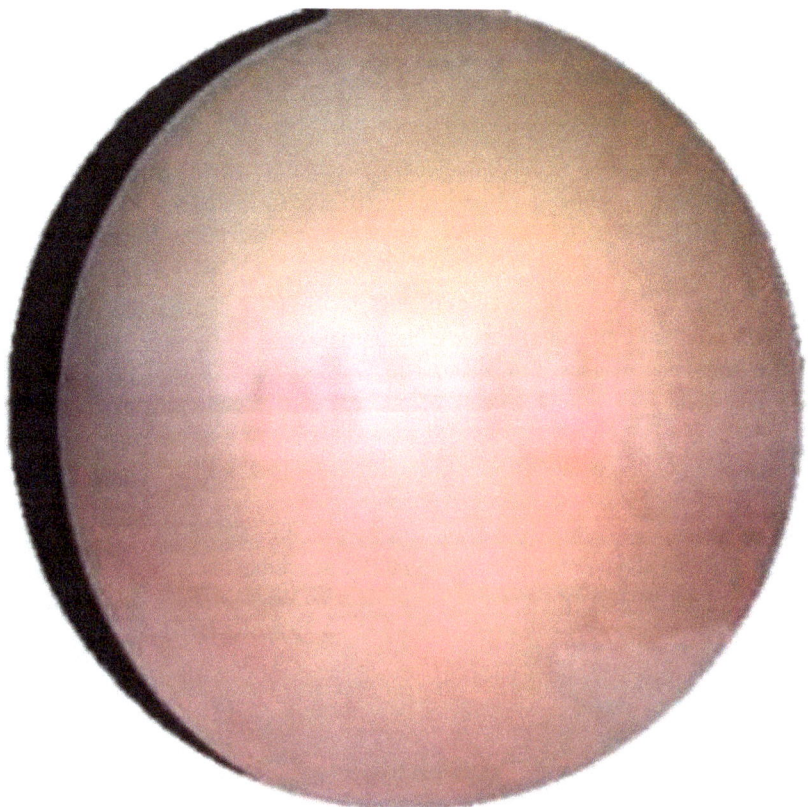

Fig. 3 Fibrotic band

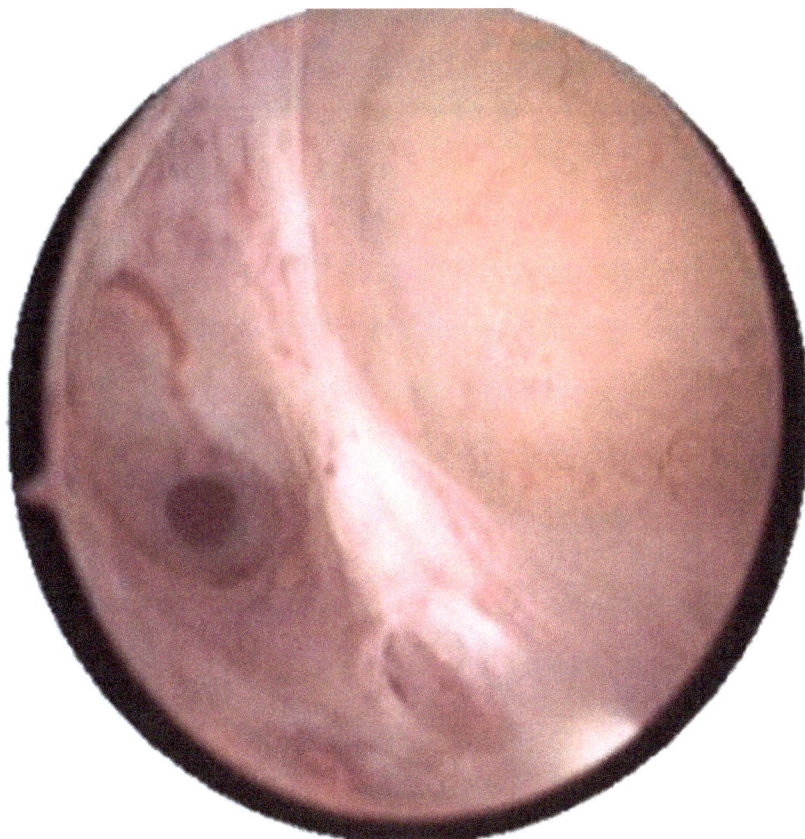

Fig. 4 Fibrotic ridge

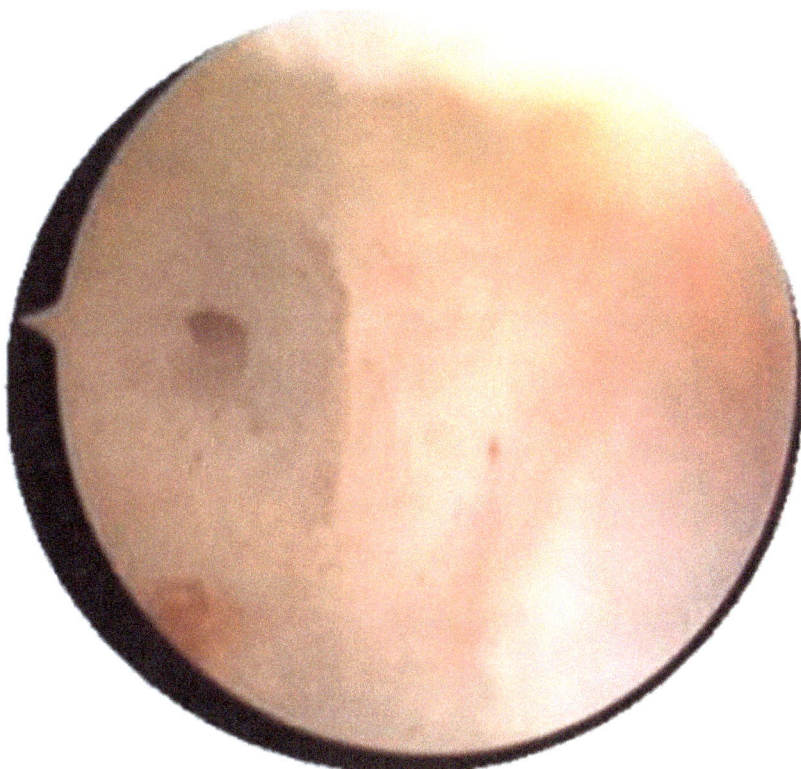

Fig. 5 Intrauterine synechiae

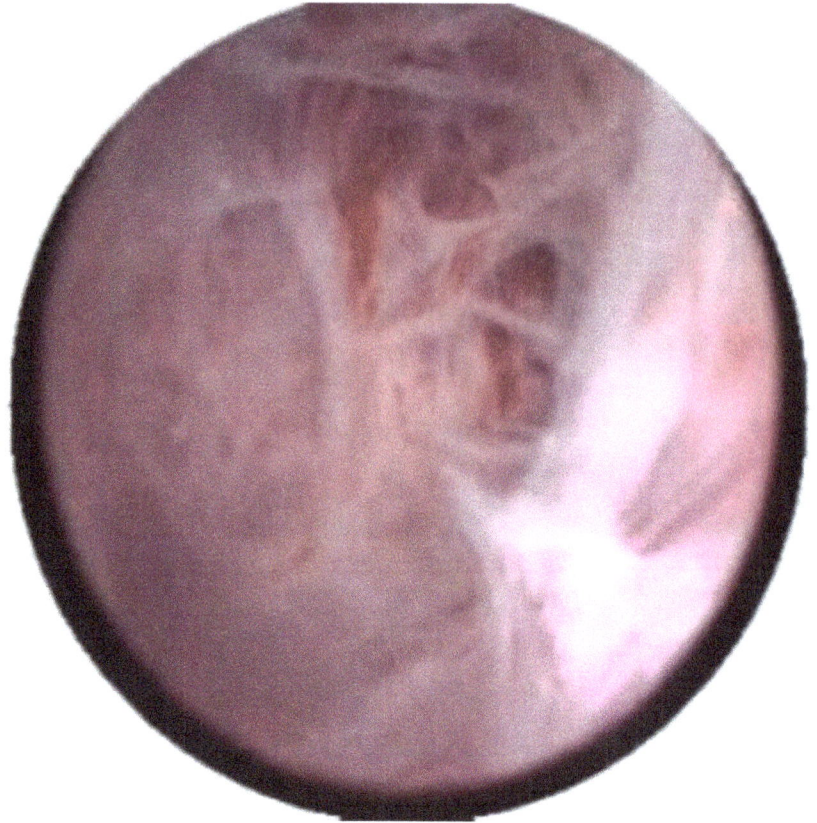

Results

In this study, a total number of 105 patients with complaints of infertility, meeting the inclusion criteria, were analyzed for the correlation of TB-PCR results with hysteroscopy findings. The treatment outcomes in terms of pregnancy rates were also analyzed. Majority (38 %) of cases presented between 26 and 30 years of age followed by the age group of 20 to 25 years

Fig. 6 Periostial fibrosis with pinhole left ostium

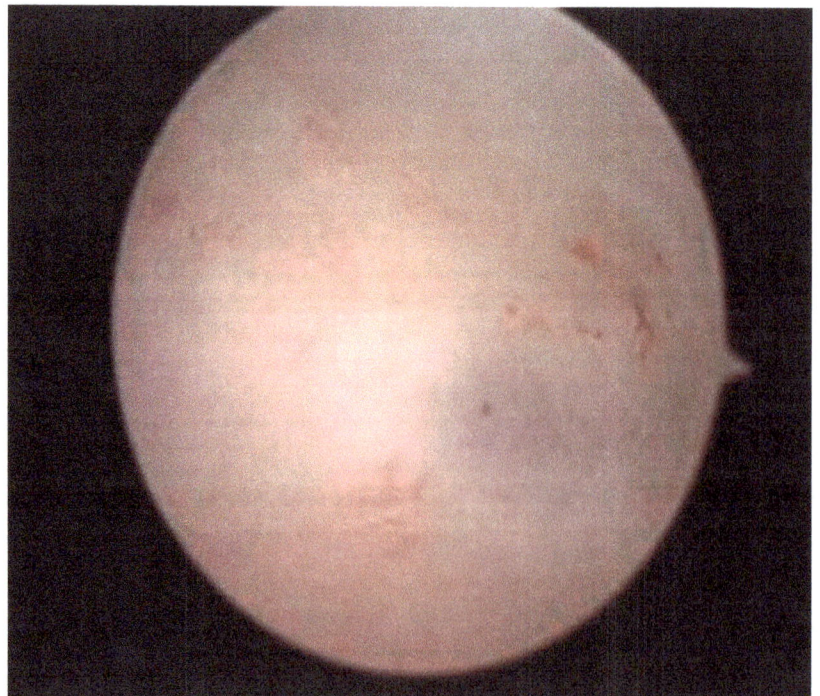

Fig. 7 Irregular endometrial surface

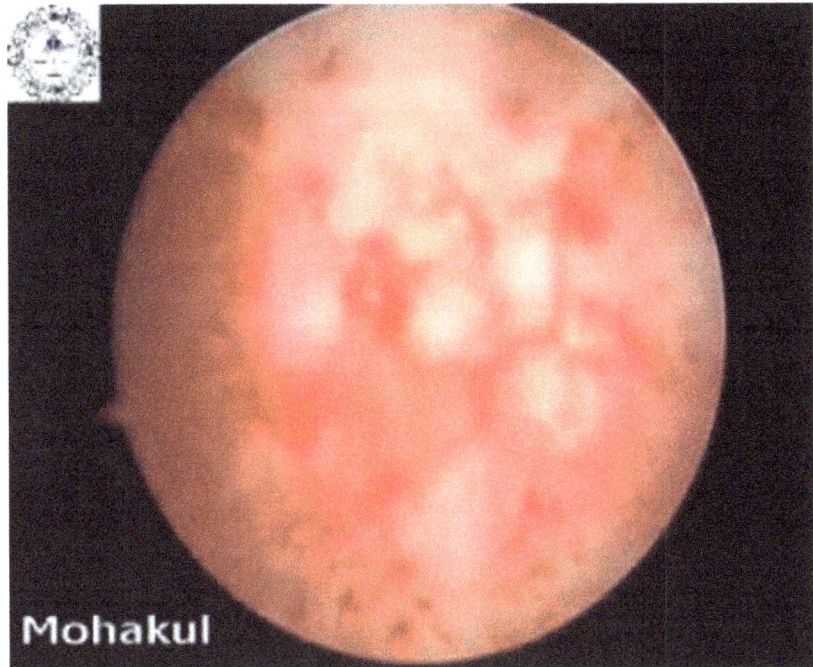

(35 %) (Table 1). Fifty-eight percent of the cases had primary infertility, and 42 % had secondary infertility. In 39 % of cases, the presence of *Mycobacterium tuberculosis* was detected in the endometrial tissue (TB-PCR positive) (Table 2).

Analyzing the hysteroscopy findings, it was found that among patients showing ostial and periostial fibrotic changes, there was 43.75 % of positive TB-PCR cases. Intrauterine fibrosis was associated with positive TB-PCR in 48.48 % of cases. Patients having irregular cavity wall was found to have 66.67 % of positive TB-PCR rate. At last, there was a single case of spotted endometrium and the same was positive for TB-PCR (Table 3).

Fig. 8 Spotted endometrium

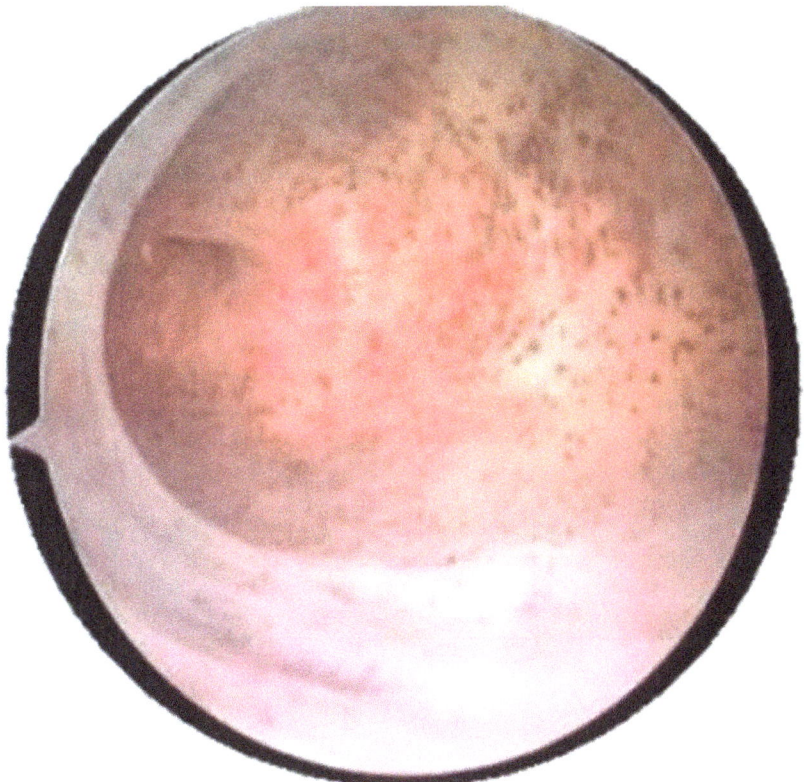

Table 1 Age distribution

Age (years)	No. of cases	Percentage (%)
20–25	37	35
26–30	40	38
31–35	13	13
>35	15	14

Out of all TB PCR positive cases, 39 % conceived with antitubercular treatment only without any surgical intervention (Table 2). A successful conception rate of 64.7 % was noted in secondary infertility whereas it was 20.8 % in primary infertility (Table 2).

The most common side effects of ATT were nausea and vomiting which was managed with domperidone and ranitidine. Neuralgia and tingling sensation were complained by very few patients and were managed successfully by 100 mg of pyridoxine supplementation per day. Abnormal liver function test with icterus and high values of liver enzymes leading to abandonment of treatment was observed in two patients during the initial 2 months of treatment and were hence excluded from the study.

Discussion

Female genital tuberculosis is a rare disease in developed countries but is a frequent cause of chronic pelvic inflammatory disease and infertility in underdeveloped and developing countries. Various studies show genital TB as a cause of infertility in 1–18 % of the cases, around 1 % in the developed countries and 18 % in India [1, 5].

Generally, *Mycobacterium* gains access through respiratory passage in lungs and then disseminates to different organs via the lymphatic drainage and blood circulation. The female genital tract is also an important site in this dissemination process. Once the immunity to *M. tuberculosis* contains and overrides the growth of small number of disseminated TB bacilli after primary infection, the infection may remain silent throughout life until lowered immunity or overwhelming reinfection precipitates the disease [16]. Increased circulation and hormone dependence of the female genital organs after

Table 2 Treatment results

Types of infertility	No. of cases	TB-PCR positive cases	Conception rate among PCR positive cases after ATT
Primary	61 (58 %)	24 (39.3 %)	5 (20.8 %)
Secondary	44 (42 %)	17 (38.63 %)	11 (64.7 %)
Total	105	41 (39 %)	16 (39 %)

*p=0.002

Table 3 Hysteroscopy findings and its correlation with TB-PCR

Hysteroscopic findings	No. of patients	TB-PCR positive
Ostial and periostial fibrosis	32 (30.48 %)	14 (43.75 %)
Intrauterine fibrosis	66 (62.86 %)	32 (48.48 %)
Irregular cavity wall	3 (2.86 %)	2 (66.67 %)
Spotted endometrium	1 (0.95 %)	1 (100 %)
Normal-looking cavity	3 (2.86 %)	0
Total no. of cases	105	41 (39 %)

sexual maturity may in part explain why the genital system is vulnerable to this infection after puberty [17]. The tuberculous process generally is localized to the endometrium, being most extensive in the fundus and decreases toward the cervix. The myometrium is not usually involved. In premenopausal patients, much of the infected tissue is shed during the menstruation, only to have the endometrium reinfected from the tubes with each cycle.

In genital TB, there is a high incidence of involvement of the endometrium. Schaefer reported an incidence of 50–60 % [1], Onuigbo, an incidence of 60 % [18], and Nogales-Ortiz and colleagues, an incidence of 79 % [8], whereas Sutherland estimated 90 % involvement of the endometrium in genital TB [9].

In endometrial tuberculosis, infertility is due to functionally altered endometrium or associated tuberculous salpingitis [19]. Tubercular infection greatly suppresses the sensitivity of the endometrium to ovarian hormones leading to deficient secretory phase and defective secretion of glycogen [20]. This results in defective implantation of an ovum, leading to infertility [21]. Therefore, if the infection could be diagnosed and treated early enough before permanent damage to the genital organs ensues, it may be possible to regain the reproductive capability.

Traditionally, the laboratory diagnosis of TB depends on demonstration of the causative organism, by acid-fast staining and/or growth of the organism on Lowenstein-Jensen (LJ) medium. The diagnosis of tubercular involvement of the endometrium is difficult because it is a paucibacillary infection, and infected endometrium is shed off during menstruation. Culture methods fail to exclude the infection, and it needs 4–5 weeks to show growth on LJ media and 2 weeks time on radiometric BACTEC media. The minimum *Mycobacterium* concentration at which histopathological evidence appears is 10,000 bacilli/ml. For positive culture, the required concentrations are 1,000 bacilli/ml for LJ and 10–100 bacilli/ml for BACTEC media [14]. Therefore, a more sensitive method is required for the early diagnosis of endometrial tuberculosis specifically in latent cases.

During the 1990s, nucleic acid amplification (NAA) techniques evolved and dramatically altered the way in which we can detect and identify *M. tuberculosis*. NAA technique is a

PCR-based test that amplifies *M. tuberculosis* DNA for the detection of *M. tuberculosis* from samples containing as low as 10 bacilli/ml [14]. Due to this reason, DNA-PCR techniques were utilized to identify *M. tuberculosis* directly from the clinical specimens, and the results were available in a day or two with high sensitivity (96.4 %) and high specificity (100 %) [22].

In our study, we tried to correlate the hysteroscopic changes to the presence of *Mycobacterium* in the endometrial tissue in cases of infertility where there were no other obvious causes detected. As we can understand that the major physical changes to the endometrium takes a long time to appear because of the repeated shedding, we have concentrated on the subtle as well as gross hysteroscopic changes that may suggest any low-grade inflammation. Therefore, minimal changes like pinhole ostium, periostial fibrosis and gross changes like fundal fibrosis, intrauterine fibrotic bands, and blocked ostia were all taken into consideration for assessing the possible involvement of the endometrium.

Because of targeting a very selective group of population and including subtle changes as abnormal, we found only 2.86 % of normal-looking endometrium. In our study, ostial and periostial fibrosis was associated with positive TB-PCR in 43.75 % and intrauterine fibrosis was associated with positive TB-PCR in 48.48 % of cases. This finding strongly suggests looking for the presence of *M. tuberculosis* in such types of hysteroscopic pictures in infertility. Although irregular cavity surface and spotted endometrium were associated with 66.67 and 100 % of positive TB-PCR, respectively, the number of patients was too minimal to derive any conclusion (Table 2). Baxi et al. reported 44.44 % positive TB-PCR in ostial fibrosis and 50 % positive TB-PCR in intrauterine fibrosis [23]. These reports were comparable to our study (*p*=0.47). The overall incidence of 32.18 % reported by Baxi et al. is also in close agreement with our report of 39 % (Table 4).

Out of all TB-PCR positive cases in our study, 39 % conceived with antitubercular treatment only, which is very a encouraging result. There was a drastic difference in conception rate between primary and secondary infertility. The conception rate of 64.7 % in secondary infertility as against 20.8 % of that in primary infertility (*p*=0.002) indicates a higher singular contributory role of tuberculosis toward infertility in the first group (Table 2). The lower pregnancy rate in primary infertility may indicate additional contributing factors apart from this acquired disease. Hence, subsequent IVF could be an ideal option for those who could not conceive after ATT.

Conclusion

Genital tuberculosis leading to tuberculous endometritis is one of the most intractable causes of infertility. Early diagnosis in the latent phase is possible by detecting the subtle hysteroscopic changes, supplemented by TB-PCR testing. A subsequent complete course of ATT may prevent the development of overt genital tuberculosis and reverse the reproductive capability. The results are very encouraging and more apparent in secondary than in primary infertility. Therefore, a large-scale study is recommended to establish the exact role of latent endometrial tuberculosis in infertility in developing countries where tuberculosis is endemic.

Informed Consent All procedures followed were in accordance with the ethical standards of the responsible committee on human experimentation (institutional and national) and with the Helsinki Declaration of 1975, as revised in 2000. Informed consent was obtained from all patients for being included in the study.

References

1. Schaefer G (1976) Female genital tuberculosis. Clin Obstet Gynecol 19:223
2. Varma TR (1991) Genital tuberculosis and subsequent fertility. Int J Gynaecol Obstet 35:1–11
3. Dawn CS (1998) Pelvic infections. In: Dawn CS 9th ed. Textbook of gynaecology and contraception: 9th ed. Calcutta: Arati Dawn p 321
4. Bartlett JG (2007) Tuberculosis and HIV infection: partners in human tragedy. J Inf Dis 196:S124–S125
5. Muir DG, Belsey MA (1980) Pelvic inflammatory disease and its consequences in the developing world. Am J Obstet Gynecol 138: 913–928
6. Arora VK, Johri A, Arora R et al (1994) Tuberculosis of the vagina in a HIV seropositive case. Tuber Lung Dis 75:239–240
7. Simon HB, Weinstein AJ, Pasternak MS et al (1977) Genitourinary tuberculosis: clinical features in a general hospital population. Am J Med 63:410–420
8. Nogales-Ortiz F, Tarancion I, Nogales FF Jr (1979) The pathology of female genital tuberculosis: a 31-year study of 1436 cases. Obstet Gynecol 53:422
9. Sutherland AM (1960) Genital tuberculosis in women. Am J Obstet Gynecol 79:486
10. Richards MJ, Angus D (1998) Possible sexual transmission of genitourinary tuberculosis. Int J Tuberc Lung Dis 2:439
11. Rom W, Garay S (1996) Tuberculosis, 1st edn. Little Brown, New York
12. Krishna UR, Sheth SS, Motashaw ND (1979) Place of laparoscopy in pelvic inflammatory disease. J Obstet Gynaecol India 29(3):505–510

Table 4 Comparison with the other study

Comparison with the other study	Our study	Baxi et al. study [23]
Total	*N*=105	*N*=174
Ostial fibrosis	43.75 %	44.44 %
Intrauterine fibrosis	48.48 %	50 %
Overall total PCR positive	39 %	32.18 %

*p=0.47

13. Katoch VM (2004) Newer diagnostic techniques for tuberculosis. Indian J Med Res 120:418–428

14. Bhanu NV, Singh UB, Chakraborty M et al (2005) Improved diagnostic value of PCR in the diagnosis of female genital tuberculosis leading to infertility. J Med Microbiol 54(Pt10):927–931

15. Kraus G, Cleary T, Miller N, Seivright R, Young AK, Spruill G, Hnatyszyn HJ (2001) Rapid and specific detection of Mycobacterium tuberculosis using fluorogenic probes and real-time PCR. Mol Cell Probes 15:375–383

16. Arora VK, Gupta R, Arora R (2003) Female genital tuberculosis—need for more research. Indian J Tuberc 50:9

17. Choudhary NN (1996) Overview of tuberculosis of the female genital tract. J Indian Med Assoc 94:345–361

18. Onuigbo WIB (1979) Genital tuberculosis and reproductive function. J Reprod Med 21:249

19. Falk V, Ludriksson K, Agnon C (1980) Genital tuberculosis in women. Am J Obstet Gynecol 138:933

20. Fox H, Buckely CH (1981) Histopathological study of endometrium in infertility cases. Recent advances in histopathology

21. Hughes EC (1945) Relationship of glycogen to problems of sterility and ovular life. Am J Obstet Gynecol 49:10–18

22. Rozati R, Roopa S, Naga Rajeshwari C (2006) Evaluation of women with infertility and genital tuberculosis. J Obstet Gynecol India 56: 423–426

23. Asha B, Hansali N, Manila K, Priti S, Dhawal B (2011) J Obstet Gynecol India 61(3):301–306

29

Closed entry technique for the laparoscopic management of adnexal mass during pregnancy

Alejandro Correa-Paris · Elena Suárez-Salvador ·
Antonia Gomar Crespo · Oriol Puig Puig ·
Jordi Xercavins · Antonio Gil-Moreno

Abstract Management of adnexal masses during pregnancy is challenging for most gynecologists. When surgery is needed, a minimally invasive approach should be preferred. The aim of this study was to evaluate the safety and feasibility of the closed entry technique for laparoscopic management of adnexal masses during pregnancy. We reviewed clinical records and videos of laparoscopic procedures performed during pregnancy. Seventeen pregnant patients with diagnosis of adnexal mass that required surgery underwent laparoscopic surgery using the closed entry or Veress technique. We searched for complications related to surgery and obstetrical and perinatal outcomes. Median gestational age at the moment of surgery was 17 weeks (range, 6–30^{+4} weeks). A total of 18 interventions were performed: 12 salpingo-oophorectomies, 3 cystectomies, 1 salpingectomy, and 2 ovarian detorsions. There were no major operative or entry-related complications. Median hospital stay was 2 days (range, 1–5). Perinatal outcomes were as follows: four preterm births (all of them induced), nine full-term deliveries, one early pregnancy loss at 7 weeks, one miscarriage at 18 weeks, and two ongoing uncomplicated pregnancies. Laparoscopic approach using closed entry technique with an individual selection of the puncture site is safe in the management of adnexal masses that require surgery during pregnancy. In our experience, the Veress technique is more versatile as it gives the surgeon more

freedom to choose the location of the first trocar in patients with important space limitations due to the size of the adnexal mass and/or the enlarged gravid uterus.

Keywords Laparoscopic surgery · Pregnancy · Adnexal mass · Closed entry technique · Veress needle technique

Background

In the past years, there has been an increase in the diagnosis of adnexal pathology during pregnancy. This is in part due to the advances in assisted reproduction techniques that achieve pregnancies in older women with higher risk and also due to the routine use of ultrasound during gestation.

Adnexal masses are found in 2–10 % of pregnant patients; the incidence ranges between 1 and 81 in every 8,000 pregnancies. Incidence is higher in the first trimester and declines progressively throughout gestation. Malignancy is found in 1–10 % of cases and is more frequent with increasing age [1–3]. The incidence reported in the literature includes the following differential diagnostics: dermoid cyst (25 %), corpus luteum cyst or functional cyst (17 %), serous cystadenoma (14 %), mucinous cystadenoma (11 %), endometriotic cyst (8 %), carcinoma (2.8 %), borderline tumor (3 %), and leiomyoma (2 %) [2].

Like in nonpregnant patients, suspicion of malignancy is based on ultrasound findings and individual clinical characteristics, for this the International Ovarian Tumor Analysis (IOTA) group criteria, and the use of an ultrasound-based risk of malignancy index (RMI) scoring system has been proven to be useful [4]. Traditional tumor markers for ovarian cancer are unreliable since they are physiologically elevated and vary according to gestational age. Spontaneous regression has been observed in 55–96 % of masses during gestation. Larger or more complex masses as well as those diagnosed later in gestation are more likely to persist.

A. Correa-Paris (✉) · E. Suárez-Salvador · A. Gomar Crespo ·
O. Puig Puig · J. Xercavins · A. Gil-Moreno
Servei de Ginecologia, Unitat de Ginecologia Oncològica, Hospital Universitari Vall d'Hebron, Universitat Autònoma de Barcelona,
Passeig de la Vall d'Hebron 119-129, Barcelona 08035, Spain
e-mail: correa.alejandro@gmail.com

A. Correa-Paris
e-mail: acorrea@vhebron.net

The most frequent complication is ovarian torsion, which appears in 7–15 % of cases. Some studies have found a higher rate of torsion in the first trimester and for masses larger than 5 cm [5].

Generally, surgery is only indicated in patients with adnexal masses suspicious of malignancy, persistent or enlarging (higher risk of torsion), ruptured cysts, or symptomatic cases that do not respond to medical treatment. Although traditionally, laparotomy was used in pregnant patients requiring surgery, multiple studies have demonstrated the safety and feasibility of laparoscopy during gestation [6–9]. Advantages of laparoscopy over laparotomy have been well established in the general population: reduced postoperative pain and use of analgesia, less adhesions and postoperative ileus, lower infection rate, early return to activities and less thromboembolic risk, shorter hospital stay, and lower costs. In parallel, all of these benefits have also been shown in pregnant patients [10].

In the present study, we present our experience in the laparoscopic management of adnexal masses during pregnancy using the closed entry (Veress) technique and determine its safety and convenience, evaluating maternal and fetal complications as well as perinatal outcomes.

Methods

A retrospective study was carried out in the Vall d'Hebron University Hospital, between January 2008 and January 2014. Data was collected by reviewing clinical records and videos of all laparoscopic procedures performed during pregnancy in the first, second, or third trimester. Inclusion criteria were as follows: all operative laparoscopies using the closed entry or Veress technique, scheduled or emergency, indicated by the presence of an adnexal mass, suspicious of malignancy on ultrasound, or associated with abdominal pain unresponsive to medical therapy, suspicion of torsion, or whose characteristics did not allow for clinical follow-up. Exclusion criteria were laparotomy or laparoscopy using the open technique (Hasson). All patients had an ultrasound (US) prior to surgery. When malignancy was suspected, the US was performed by a specialist with experience in gynecological ultrasonography. Each patient's individual risk was determined using the IOTA criteria and personal risk factors (i.e., age, family history of ovarian or breast cancer, history of malignancy or endometriosis). We analyzed the following variables: patient's age, gestational age at diagnosis and at the moment of surgery, findings on ultrasound, type of surgery, surgical time (from initial incision to wound closure), and postoperative histopathologic diagnosis. We searched for complications associated with the entry technique and intervention, including abdominal organ injury (bowel or bladder), vascular injury, and febrile and infectious complications

(e.g., postoperative fever, wound infection). We also recorded any complication that occurred throughout the gestation as well as obstetrical and perinatal outcomes. An ultrasound and/or fetal monitoring was made before and immediately after the operation to verify fetal well-being. No institutional review board approval was required at our hospital, given the characteristics of our study (chart review).

Abdominal access was achieved in all cases using the closed entry technique according to the classical procedure using the Veress needle (Lagis, Brussels) technique. On occasion, we alternatively used a Tuohy epidural needle (Smiths Medical, UK) as an alternative to the Veress needle. This type of needle is shorter (80 vs. 120 mm) and smaller in diameter (18 vs. 14 G). It is slightly curved at the end and has a blunted tip and little sharpness (Fig. 1).

The location for needle placement was chosen in the operating room by the surgeon according to patient's characteristics (e.g., previous surgery), uterine height, and size and the location of the mass (Fig. 2). All data were collected and analyzed in an Excel spreadsheet (Microsoft Corp., Redmond, WA, USA). We finally carried out a univariate statistical analysis for data presentation.

Findings

A total of 17 patients were included. The patients' median age was 34 years (range, 23–39 years). Median gestational age at diagnosis and at the moment of surgery was 12 weeks of gestation (range, $0-30^{+4}$ weeks) and 17 weeks (range, $6-30^{+4}$ weeks), respectively.

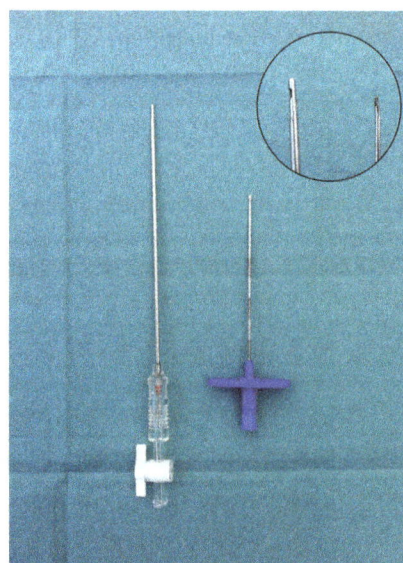

Fig. 1 Veress needle vs. Tuohy needle. Note the smaller dimensions of the epidural needle (*right*), being shorter and thinner than the Veress needle (*left*). A magnified image of each needle tip can be seen in the *top right corner*, showing the blunted tip of the Tuohy needle

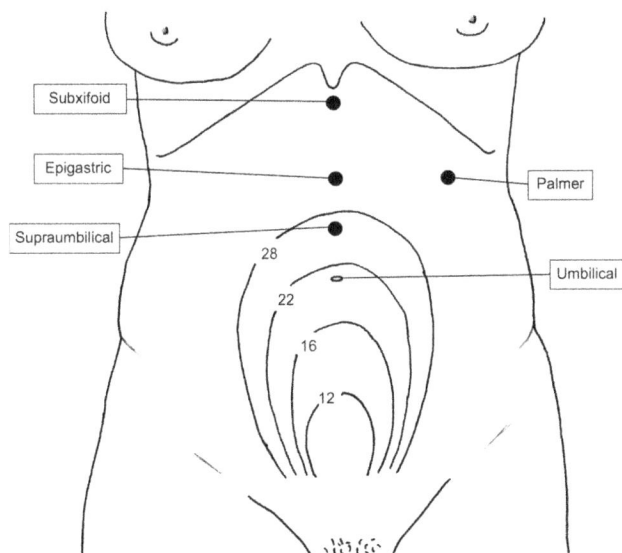

Fig. 2 Insertion sites of Veress needle according to gestational age and uterus size. The location for inserting the needle was determined by each surgeon in the operating room. *Numbers* indicate gestational age in weeks

Emergency surgery was necessary in six cases because of ovarian torsion. All cases are summarized in Table 1 including patient characteristics, complications, and obstetrical outcomes. Hospital stay was a median of 2 days (range, 1–5 days). The number of trocars used was decided in the operating room according to each case. Two to four trocars were used, with diameters of 5, 10, and 11 mm. Median surgical time was 60 min (range, 40–150 min). Only two surgeries required 150 min to be completed (cases nos. 2 and 10), one of them included peritoneal biopsies, and the other was an emergency laparoscopy under suspicion of ovarian torsion.

There were no conversions to laparotomy. No entry-related complications were observed. Only one case (no. 15) was complicated by postoperative anemia that required transfusion. This was the only twin pregnancy recorded in the cohort. An emergency laparoscopy was performed because of an ovarian torsion at 26^{+1} weeks, and difficult hemostasis because of venous bleeding from the ovarian pedicle was eventually achieved; the patient received a blood transfusion because of postoperative hemoglobin of 8 mg/dL. She was otherwise clinically stable and the rest of her postoperatory was uneventful.

Tocolytics were not routinely used. As for obstetrical outcomes, we recorded one dilation and curettage, four cesarean and ten vaginal deliveries (including one breech delivery), and two ongoing uncomplicated pregnancies, with a total of 18 healthy newborns (including one twin pregnancy). All cesarean deliveries were done because of obstetrical indications (two for acute fetal distress, one for severe preeclampsia in a twin pregnancy, and one because of umbilical cord prolapse). There were no perinatal complications. In four patients, labor was induced preterm, three of them for obstetrical

reasons and one for interval oncologic surgery in a patient with clear cell carcinoma who underwent neoadjuvant chemotherapy during pregnancy.

Gestational age at the moment of delivery was a median of 39 weeks (range, 18^{+2}–41 weeks). We observed two fetal demises in cases where emergency surgery was performed. One of them occurred almost 10 weeks after surgery, presenting with oligohydramnios at 18 weeks and ending by vaginal delivery of a 170-g fetus, following diagnosis of chorioamnionitis. The other was a miscarriage at 7 weeks of gestation after an emergency laparoscopy was performed 1 week earlier because of increasing pain and suspicion of heterotopic pregnancy (ultimately ruled out). Birth weights in the cohort were normal, with a median of 3,035 g (range, 170–3,870 g).

Histopathologic analysis reported two cases of malignancy: one borderline ovarian serous tumor and an ovarian clear cell carcinoma. All of them were treated according to our oncology protocols. The case of clear cell carcinoma underwent neoadjuvant chemotherapy beginning at 18 weeks of pregnancy and until the 34th week when labor was induced for interval surgery (14 days postpartum). Optimal surgery was achieved laparoscopically with complete surgical staging. All biopsies were negative except for the peritoneal lavage cytology. This patient continued chemotherapy with no evidence of disease for 9 months after surgery. Ultimately, she presented with peritoneal carcinomatosis resistant to platinum chemotherapy. The patient died of complications of advancing disease 26 months after the initial diagnostic surgery. As for the borderline serous tumor case, pathology confirmed a FIGO stage IA, grade 2 tumor, therefore not requiring any additional procedure or surgical staging according to our protocols. This patient continued controls every 6 months at our center with negative tumoral markers and is presently without evidence of disease.

Discussion

When facing an adnexal mass, as in nonpregnant patients, the most feared outcome is malignancy. The risk of malignancy during pregnancy is approximately 2–3 % [11–13]; however, most cases are diagnosed in early stages and usually have good maternal and fetal prognosis [14].

In the context of gestation, other important risks are a higher rate of torsion (associated with the enlarged mass and gravid uterus), rupture of the mass, or mechanical obstruction of labor. Some authors recommend follow-up of adnexal masses diagnosed during gestation, especially in asymptomatic patients diagnosed during a routine prenatal ultrasound

Table 1 Case description and outcomes of laparoscopy using closed entry (Veress) technique for adnexal masses during pregnancy

Case	US findings[a]	GE at surgery	Intervention	Entry site	Histopathologic Diagnosis	Complications	Outcomes
1	Complex mass[b], 56 mm	21^{+0}	RSO + peritoneal biopsy	SubX	Serous micropapillary borderline tumor	No	VD, 40 weeks, 3,870 g
2	Complex mass[b], 175 mm	16^{+3}	LSO + peritoneal biopsy	EpiG	Bilateral clear cell carcinoma	No	ABD, 34 weeks, 2,280 g
3	Simple cyst, 80 mm	16^{+1}	RSO	P	Mucinous cystadenoma	PROM + TPTL at 33^{+1} weeks	VD, 33^{+5} weeks, 1,870 g
4	Teratoma, 102 mm	14^{+1}	LSO	P	Mature cystic teratoma	No	VD, 39^{+1} weeks, 2,830 g
5	Teratoma, 60 mm	22^{+0}	RSO	SubX	Mature cystic teratoma	No	CS, 39^{+4} weeks, 3,100 g
6	Complex mass[b], 48 mm	19^{+6}	Bilateral cystectomy	EpiG	Bilateral serous cystadenoma	No	VD, 39 weeks
7	Simple cyst, 63 mm	8^{+4}	Unilateral cystectomy	Umb	Endometriotic cyst	Chorioamnionitis, fetal demise	VD, 18^{+3} weeks, 170 g
8	Teratoma, 74 mm	20^{+1}	RSO	P	Mature cystic teratoma	No	VD, 39^{+1} weeks, 3,300 g
9	Complex mass[b], 126 mm	13^{+5}	RSO	P	Mucinous cystadenoma + torsion	No	CS, 40 weeks, 3,700 g
10	Ovarian torsion, 55 mm	11^{+3}	LSO	Umb	Necrosis (torsion)	No	VD, 36 weeks, 3,100 g
11	Simple cyst, 100 mm	17^{+0}	LSO	SU	Endometriotic cyst	No	VD, 38 weeks, 3,260 g
12	Heterotopic pregnancy, 65 mm	6^{+0}	Cystectomy + detorsion	Umb	Corpus luteum	Miscarriage	Miscarriage
13	Adnexal torsion, 27 mm	30^{+5}	R salpingectomy	EpiG	Necrosis (torsion)	No	CS, 41 weeks, 3,815 g
14	Ovarian tumor (possibly malignant), 110 mm	20^{+1}	RSO	P	Mature cystic teratoma	No	Ongoing gestation
15	Ovarian torsion, 68 mm	26^{+1}	LSO	EpiG	Necrosis (torsion)	Blood transfusion	CS, 34^{+3} weeks, 1,740 and 1,540 g[c]
16	Simple cyst, 65 mm	13^{+3}	Ovarian detorsion	P	–	No	Ongoing pregnancy
17	Ovarian torsion, 73 mm	19^{+2}	RSO	P	Necrosis (torsion)	No	Ongoing pregnancy

GE gestational age given in weeks + days, *SubX* subxiphoid, *EpiG* epigastric, *P* Palmer's point, *Umb* umbilical, *SU* supraumbilical, *R/L SO* right/left salpingo-oophorectomy, *TPTL* threatened preterm labor, *VD* vaginal delivery, *ABD* assisted breech delivery, *CS* cesarean section

[a] Ultrasound (US) findings describe the mass characteristics or suspected diagnosis based on US and the maximum diameter of the mass (or in cases of ovarian torsion, maximal ovarian diameter)

[b] Refers to presence of septations and/or papillary projections with US suspicion of ovarian carcinoma

[c] CS delivery because of severe preeclampsia in a twin dichorionic diamniotic pregnancy

where a high percentage of masses found in the first trimester may spontaneously resolve.

Although torsion or rupture may be rare, there are no data regarding the ultrasonographic characteristics that could predict such risk. The risk of torsion appears to be greater in masses between 6 and 10 cm [5]. Surgical management is necessary for those masses suspicious of malignancy, at high risk of torsion, or symptomatic and nonresponsive to medical therapy.

Although laparoscopic management of adnexal masses during pregnancy is safe and feasible (when surgical management is warranted), most obstetricians/gynecologists are still reluctant and only well-trained and experienced endoscopic surgeons are at ease with this approach. An additional theoretical advantage of laparoscopy during gestation is the reduced manipulation of the uterus, which could minimize the potential risk of preterm birth.

In our hospital, over 10,000 routine prenatal ultrasound studies (first and second trimester) were performed between the study period; we found an incidence of adnexal mass of

1.1 %, similar to other published studies. Our practice results are also consistent with other series in rate of malignancy with an incidence of 1.7 % in pregnant patients (unpublished data). According to previously exposed criteria, only 20 % of pregnant patients with persistent adnexal mass underwent surgery in our hospital (unpublished results). In the present cohort, the elevated rate of malignancy (2/17) is due to a careful selection of patients that do require surgery.

Koo et al. have published the results of laparoscopic surgical management of 11 cases of adnexal complex benign masses during the first trimester of gestation. In their study, all laparoscopies were emergency operations, and they did not encounter any miscarriages and surgical or obstetric complications [15]. Another retrospective study described the results of 11 patients undergoing laparoscopy for adnexal mass in the second trimester also showing favorable outcomes and no complications [16].

In our present cohort, we performed elective surgery during the second and third trimester of pregnancy. The only five patients that underwent laparoscopy in the first trimester were emergency surgeries. The two fetal losses observed occurred after emergency surgery, one miscarriage after emergent laparoscopy performed at 6 weeks of gestation, and a late abortion due to chorioamnionitis 10 weeks after an emergency laparoscopy was performed at 8 weeks.

Approximately 50 % of complications during laparoscopic surgery are entry-related. This proportion has not changed in the last 20 years. According to recent guidelines for laparoscopy during pregnancy published by the Society of American Gastrointestinal and Endoscopic Surgeons (SAGES), entry can be performed with an open (Hasson) technique, Veress needle, or optical trocar, if the location is adjusted according to fundal height and previous incisions [17]. However, there is still much concern for the blind entry with the Veress needle because of its potential complications, namely, injury to the gravid uterus [18], hence the ongoing debate regarding abdominal access in the pregnant patient.

So far, no significant or clinically relevant differences have been found between any technique [19–22]. A meta-analysis published recently found no difference in major vascular or visceral complications. There was, however, a lower incidence of failed entry with the open technique, as well as less extraperitoneal insufflation and omental lesion [23].

As we lack enough evidence or even a unified consensus, the surgeon's experience and familiarization with any given technique are still more important. Most studies published regarding management of adnexal masses during gestation encourage the use of open or Hasson technique [19, 20, 22, 24], speculating that there is a higher risk of injury to the gravid uterus using the Veress needle method. Some studies have been published using the closed entry (Veress) technique [15, 16, 25], although there are no trials comparing the two in pregnant patients.

Because of the normal anatomical variations in pregnancy and the reduction of space due to the enlarged gravid uterus and adnexal mass, we must change our strategy for insertion of the trocars and insufflation of pneumoperitoneum. We believe that the closed entry technique permits more freedom in choosing the trocar insertion sites, since it allows a more accurate evaluation of the patient's abdomen once the CO_2 has been insufflated. Also, we evaluate the port site for presence of adhesions using Palmer's safety test and our "safety cone" technique (see video). With abdominal distention caused by pneumoperitoneum, it is easier to determine the best location for insertion of the first trocar according to the size of the gravid uterus and both size and location of the adnexal mass (Fig. 3). This is not possible with the open technique since the site chosen for insufflation will inevitably be the location of the first trocar (Hasson-type trocar), which usually is large in diameter (≥10 mm). Using the Veress needle technique also helps to reduce the use of large-diameter trocars to reposition the endoscope and therefore the possible complications associated with the use of such trocars, particularly the potentially

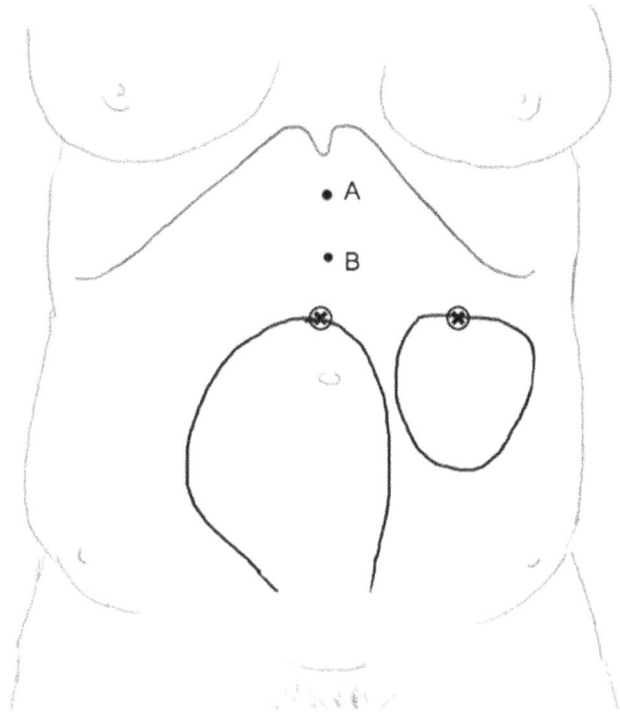

Fig. 3 Case of a left adnexal mass in a patient with a 17-week pregnancy. Abdominal entry at the supraumbilical or Palmer's point is not possible due to high risk of injury (X marks). Alternative entry points can be the subxiphoid (A) or epigastric (B) locations

increased risk of trocar site hernia with the use of these large trocars in pregnant patients.

In our present cohort, the use of the closed entry (Veress) technique proved to be safe and no complications occurred. It was never necessary to change the main trocar to reposition the endoscope. We also believe that the use of the Tuohy needle has the same advantages as the Veress needle, which are enhanced by its smaller dimensions, allowing for less potential risk of injury to the gravid uterus.

Conclusions

In summary, our findings support the safety of operative laparoscopy using the closed entry (Veress) technique in pregnant patients with adnexal masses diagnosed during pregnancy, with satisfactory maternal and perinatal outcomes. When managing adnexal masses in pregnant patients, we must take into account the risk of neoplasia and the risk of associated complications such as torsion, rupture, or obstetrical issues associated with such masses. Also, we must consider the risk of surgery at an early gestational age during the first trimester and the potential risks of emergency surgery with possibly worse obstetrical outcomes.

We believe that a closed entry technique using the Veress needle—or a similar needle (i.e., Tuohy needle)—is safe, useful, and convenient since it allows more freedom in choosing the location for inserting the first trocar in these specific cases. More large prospective trials are needed to establish if there is any difference between the open and closed technique for operative laparoscopy in pregnant patients diagnosed with adnexal mass.

Informed consent This article does not contain any studies with human or animal subjects performed by the any of the authors. Therefore, no additional informed consent was required by our institution's Ethics Committee.

References

1. Schwartz N, Timor-Tritsch IE, Wang E (2009) Adnexal masses in pregnancy. Clin Obstet Gynecol 52:570–585. doi:10.1097/GRF.0b013e3181bea9d7
2. Hoover K, Jenkins TR (2011) Evaluation and management of adnexal mass in pregnancy. Am J Obstet Gynecol 205:97–102. doi:10.1016/j.ajog.2011.01.050
3. Yazbek J, Helmy S, Ben-Nagi J et al (2007) Value of preoperative ultrasound examination in the selection of women with adnexal masses for laparoscopic surgery. Ultrasound Obstet Gynecol 30:883–888. doi:10.1002/uog.5169
4. Timmerman D, Ameye L, Fischerova D et al (2010) Simple ultrasound rules to distinguish between benign and malignant adnexal masses before surgery: prospective validation by IOTA group. BMJ 341:c6839
5. Lee GSR, Hur SY, Shin JC et al (2004) Elective vs. conservative management of ovarian tumors in pregnancy. Int J Gynaecol Obstet 85:250–254. doi:10.1016/j.ijgo.2003.12.008
6. Reedy MB, Källén B, Kuehl TJ (1997) Laparoscopy during pregnancy: a study of five fetal outcome parameters with use of the Swedish Health Registry. Am J Obstet Gynecol 177:673–679
7. Oelsner G, Stockheim D, Soriano D et al (2003) Pregnancy outcome after laparoscopy or laparotomy in pregnancy. J Am Assoc Gynecol Laparosc 10:200–204
8. Koo Y-J, KIM HJ, Lim K-T et al (2011) Laparotomy versus laparoscopy for the treatment of adnexal masses during pregnancy. Aust N Z J Obstet Gynaecol 52:34–38. doi:10.1111/j.1479-828X.2011.01380.x
9. Soriano D, Yefet Y, Seidman DS et al (1999) Laparoscopy versus laparotomy in the management of adnexal masses during pregnancy. Fertil Steril 71:955–960
10. Lee Y-Y, Kim T-J, Choi CH et al (2010) Factors influencing the choice of laparoscopy or laparotomy in pregnant women with presumptive benign ovarian tumors. Int J Gynaecol Obstet 108:12–15. doi:10.1016/j.ijgo.2009.07.040
11. Bernhard LM, Klebba PK, Gray DL, Mutch DG (1999) Predictors of persistence of adnexal masses in pregnancy. Obstet Gynecol 93:585–589
12. Whitecar MP, Turner S, Higby MK (1999) Adnexal masses in pregnancy: a review of 130 cases undergoing surgical management. Am J Obstet Gynecol 181:19–24
13. Ueda M, Ueki M (1996) Ovarian tumors associated with pregnancy. Int J Gynaecol Obstet 55:59–65
14. Leiserowitz GS, Xing G, Cress R et al (2006) Adnexal masses in pregnancy: how often are they malignant? Gynecol Oncol 101:315–321. doi:10.1016/j.ygyno.2005.10.022
15. Ko ML, Lai TH, Chen SC (2009) Laparoscopic management of complicated adnexal masses in the first trimester of pregnancy. Fertil Steril 92:283–287. doi:10.1016/j.fertnstert.2008.04.035
16. Stepp KJ, Tulikangas PK, Goldberg JM et al (2003) Laparoscopy for adnexal masses in the second trimester of pregnancy. J Am Assoc Gynecol Laparosc 10:55–59
17. Pearl J, Price R, Richardson W, Fanelli R (2011) Guidelines for diagnosis, treatment, and use of laparoscopy for surgical problems during pregnancy. Surg Endosc 25:3479–3492. doi:10.1007/s00464-011-1927-3
18. Friedman JD, Ramsey PS, Ramin KD, Berry C (2002) Pneumoamnion and pregnancy loss after second-trimester laparoscopic surgery. Obstet Gynecol 99:512–513
19. Yuen PM, Ng PS, Leung PL, Rogers MS (2004) Outcome in laparoscopic management of persistent adnexal mass during the second trimester of pregnancy. Surg Endosc 18:1354–1357. doi:10.1007/s00464-003-8283-x
20. Mathevet P, Nessah K, Dargent D, Mellier G (2003) Laparoscopic management of adnexal masses in pregnancy: a case series. Eur J Obstet Gynecol Reprod Biol 108:217–222
21. Moore RD, Smith WG (1999) Laparoscopic management of adnexal masses in pregnant women. J Reprod Med 44:97–100
22. Balthazar U, Steiner AZ, Boggess JF, Gehrig PA (2011) Management of a persistent adnexal mass in pregnancy: what is the ideal surgical approach? J Minim Invasive Gynecol 18:720–725. doi:10.1016/j.jmig.2011.07.002
23. Ahmad G, O'Flynn H, Duffy JMN et al (2012) Laparoscopic entry techniques. Cochrane Database Syst Rev 2, CD006583. doi:10.1002/14651858.CD006583.pub3
24. Rizzo AG (2003) Laparoscopic surgery in pregnancy: long-term follow-up. J Laparoendosc Adv Surg Tech A 13:11–15. doi:10.1089/109264203321235403
25. Koo Y-J, Lee J-E, Lim K-T et al (2011) A 10-year experience of laparoscopic surgery for adnexal masses during pregnancy. Int J Gynaecol Obstet 113:36–39. doi:10.1016/j.ijgo.2010.10.020

30

Ultrasound-assisted intraoperative localization and laparoscopic management of a previously missed unruptured retroperitoneal ectopic pregnancy

Athanasios Protopapas · Nikolaos Akrivos · Stavros Athanasiou · Ioannis Chatzipapas · Aikaterini Domali · Dimitrios Loutradis

Abstract Primary retroperitoneal ectopic pregnancy represents an extremely unusual entity with a rather obscure pathogenesis. Implantation in the retroperitoneal space has been reported to occur both spontaneously and with use of assisted reproduction techniques. The pelvic and the upper retroperitoneum have both been involved, and implantation in the most unusual anatomic sites has been reported. The majority of retroperitoneal gestations are located close to large blood vessels, and laparotomy is performed because of the high risk of massive hemorrhage. Few cases have been treated with laparoscopy so far. We report the case of an early first-trimester retroperitoneal broad ligament live pregnancy occurring after spontaneous conception in a patient who had a history of an ipsilateral tubal ectopic pregnancy, previously treated with laparoscopic right salpingectomy. Current gestation had been missed during initial laparoscopy, and was located and removed during a repeat laparoscopic procedure under intraoperative ultrasonographic guidance.

Keywords Retroperitoneal pregnancy · Abdominal pregnancy · Ectopic pregnancy · Laparoscopy

Introduction

Ectopic pregnancy occurs in 1.5–2 % of all gestations, and is one of the major causes of maternal mortality during the first trimester of pregnancy, accounting for 6 % of all pregnancy-related deaths [1]. Most ectopic pregnancies (95 %) are located in the fallopian tubes, whereas the ovary and abdominal cavity are less frequently involved [1]. Abdominal pregnancy is the rarest form of ectopic pregnancy with an incidence of 1.3 % amongst all ectopics, and mortality rates are seven times higher than in non-abdominal cases [2, 3]. Abdominal pregnancies have been classified as either primary or secondary. Most abdominal pregnancies originate as tubal or ovarian pregnancies that rupture into the peritoneal cavity, where they re-implant [4]. A small fraction of the reported cases occur as a result of primary implantation either in the peritoneal cavity or the retroperitoneum [4].

The occurrence of an ectopic pregnancy in a retroperitoneal location is very rare. In 1938, the incidence of this condition had been reported to be 1 in 183,900 pregnancies [5]. To date, less than 25 well-documented cases of primary retroperitoneal pregnancy implantation have been reported in the medical literature. Development of an ectopic pregnancy in a retroperitoneal location has been reported to occur in the most unusual anatomic sites, such as the rectovaginal space [6], the obturator fossa [7], between the leaves of the broad ligament [8], at the level of the right paracolic sulcus [9], above the inferior vena cava [10], in the upper retroperitoneum [11], and even attached to the head of the pancreas [12]. Both spontaneous conception and assisted reproductive technologies (IUI and IVF-ET) have been implicated in the retroperitoneal development of ectopic pregnancies [6, 12–14]. Gestational age at first diagnosis and clinical presentations may vary considerably, from the asymptomatic woman in her early first trimester of pregnancy to the hemodynamically unstable patient with an advanced ruptured ectopic gestation presenting with life-threatening retroperitoneal hemorrhage. As a result, management strategies should be tailored to the individual patient. Laparotomy, laparoscopy, and medical treatment with

A. Protopapas (✉) · N. Akrivos · S. Athanasiou · I. Chatzipapas · A. Domali · D. Loutradis
1st University Department of Obstetrics and Gynecology of the University of Athens, "Alexandra" Hospital, 80 Queen Sophie Ave., 11528 Athens, Greece
e-mail: prototha@otenet.gr

methotrexate have all been used in the treatment of retroperitonal pregnancies of various locations.

We report the case of an early first trimester retroperitoneal pregnancy occurring after spontaneous conception in a patient who had a history of an ipsilateral tubal ectopic pregnancy, previously treated with laparoscopic right salpingectomy. The current ectopic was developing between the leaves of the right broad ligament. The living retroperitoneal gestation had been missed during initial laparoscopy, and was located and removed during a repeat laparoscopic procedure under intraoperative ultrasonographic guidance.

Case report

A 31-year-old woman presented to our department with a 6-week history of amenorrhea and a positive pregnancy test for routine antenatal care. Her medical history was unremarkable. Her obstetric history included a right tubal ectopic pregnancy managed by laparoscopic salpingectomy, followed by a term normal vaginal delivery of a healthy infant.

At presentation, the patient was asymptomatic and hemodynamically stable. Transvaginal sonography at 6^{+3} weeks, showed an empty uterine cavity. A gestational sac with embryonic heart activity was demonstrated to the right side of the uterus and in contact with the uterine fundus. On clinical examination, no vaginal bleeding was observed, and no lower abdominal or adnexal pain was elicited during bimanual examination. β-hCG levels were 7,450 mIU/ml, whereas her hemoglobin levels were within normal limits.

With the possible diagnosis of a right cornual pregnancy, the patient was scheduled for laparoscopic evaluation and management. At laparoscopy, the uterus was found slightly enlarged. The fundus was of normal shape and contour. The left adnexa and right ovary were normal. The right tube was found amputated at the level of the isthmus. No evidence of an ectopic intraperitoneal pregnancy was found anywhere in the pelvis, and the procedure was completed without any further intervention.

The following day, a repeat pelvic ultrasound confirmed once more the presence of an ongoing live pregnancy in contact with the right uterine cornu. Furthermore, levels of β-hCG were rising (9,832 mIU/ml). Assuming that we had failed to locate the pregnancy during our previous laparoscopy, we decided for a second attempt, and the patient was taken again to the operating theater.

At first, hysteroscopy was performed, but no pregnancy sac was seen in the uterine cavity or near the right ostium. Laparoscopy, this time under ultrasound guidance, followed. Initial laparoscopic findings were again identical to those described above (Fig. 1). With the aid of the transvaginal ultrasound probe, we identified once more the fetal sac to the right of the uterine fundus and managed to locate its exact

position below and caudally to the right round ligament by carefully probing with a grasper the anterior leaf of the broad ligament, a maneuver that distorted the ultrasound image of the underlying pregnancy sac.

The round ligament and the anterior leaf of the broad ligament were opened above this area which was infiltrated with diluted vasopressin to reduce blood loss (Figs. 2 and 3). The reproperitoneal space was carefully dissected and a 3× 2.5×2 cm bulging mass was identified, arising from the right side of the uterine corpus (Figs. 4 and 5). Further dissection of the mass revealed the presence of a gestational sac (Figs. 6 and 7) through which an intact embryo could be clearly seen (Fig. 8). The sac was opened and the embryo along with the trophoblastic tissue were removed (Figs. 9 and 10). After evacuation of its trophoblastic contents, a fibrous capsule could be clearly identified. This structure had no communication with the uterine cavity (Fig. 11). Hemostasis was accomplished with bipolar diathermy and the broad and round ligaments were reconstructed with interrupted absorbable sutures (Fig. 12).

Our patient made an uneventful recovery and was discharged from our hospital on the second postoperative day. β-hCG levels were measured weekly and within 4 weeks they had returned to prepregnancy levels.

Discussion

Retroperitoneal ectopic pregnancy represents an extremely unusual entity with a rather obscure pathogenesis. Its incidence remains largely unknown mainly as a result of the frequent false reporting of abdominal intraperitoneal ectopic gestations with peritoneal invasion, as true retroperitoneal pregnancies. In the case of broad ligament ectopic pregnancy, according to Champion and Tessitore, the anatomical landmarks that surround the ectopic sac should include (a) the uterus medially, (b) the pelvic side walls laterally, (c) the pelvic floor inferiorly, and (d) the uterine tube or round ligament of the uterus superiorly [5]. These were exactly the boundaries in our case. To our opinion, the overlying peritoneum should also be found intact in order to confirm the diagnosis of a true retroperitoneal gestation.

Nevertheless, it is rather difficult to come up with a convincing explanation of how the embryo implanted in the retroperitoneal space in our case, as in others with similar locations. The patient conceived spontaneously and her only uterine surgery was a laparoscopic salpingectomy that preceded a normal-term vaginal delivery. The presence of a very small fistulous tract, resulting from past thermal injury during salpingectomy, cannot be entirely excluded as a causal factor. Nevertheless, the sac was found sufficiently distal to the tubal stump to support such a hypothesis. Another possible explanation, proposed by several investigators, is that the fertilized

Fig. 1–12 The film of
the procedure

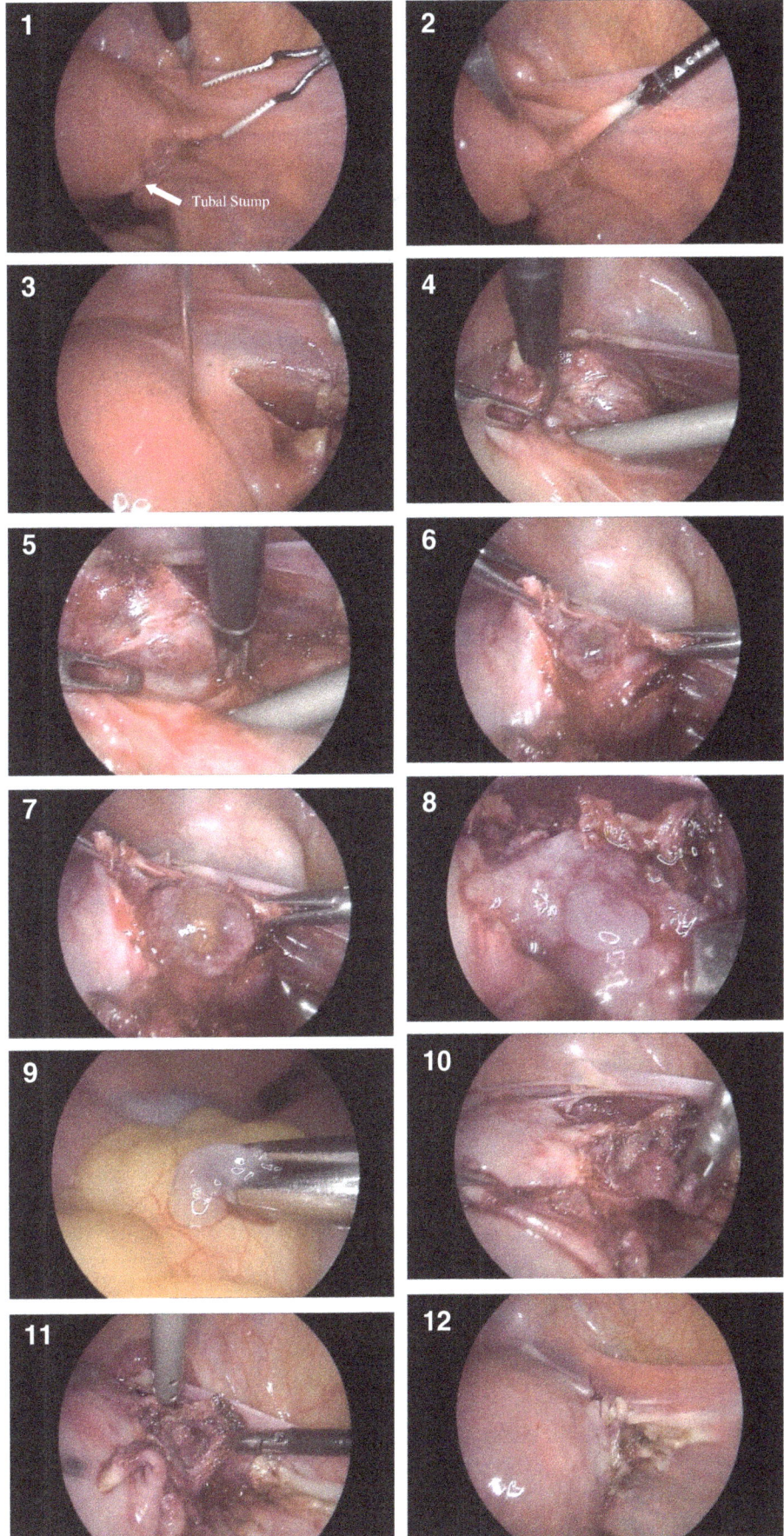

ovum may have reached the retroperitoneal space via the lymphatic system [7, 14, 15]. This hypothesis is supported by finding lymphatic tissue with the ectopic mass [15]. The transperitoneal route of implantation of the ectopic to the retroperitoneum through trophoblastic invasion provides a third yet not very convincing mechanism in our case, taking into account three factors: presence of an intact tubal stump, presence of healthy peritoneum above the sac, and conception occurring without use of assisted reproduction techniques.

Assisted reproductive techniques (both IVF-ET and IUI) appear to increase the risk of an ectopic pregnancy and thus implantation at unusual sites, which may be difficult to diagnose and have a high risk of life-threatening complications. Four mechanisms have been suggested for the abdominal location of an ectopic pregnancy in IVF-ET patients: spontaneous retrograde migration of the embryo after intrauterine transfer, iatrogenic placement of embryos in the retroperitoneal space at the time of transfer due to uterine perforation, retroperitoneal implantation through a fistulous tract, and transfer of the embryo from the uterine cavity to the retroperitoneal space through lymphatic channels [6, 7, 11].

Most of the reported cases of retroperitoneal pregnancies are located close to large blood vessels and the decision to dissect out the gestational tissue should not be taken without appropriate patient preparation and blood bank coverage. In the majority of such cases, laparotomy is performed because of the high risk of massive hemorrhage [11, 12, 16, 17]. The same applies naturally to cases with signs of acute and life-threatening intra-abdominal bleeding. Laparoscopic management has not been applied frequently, because of the risk of uncontrollable bleeding due to extensive trophoblastic invasion of the retroperitoneal vasculature. The incidence of deep trophoblastic infiltration of large retroperitoneal vessels has not been clearly reported in the existing literature. Nevertheless, there have been few reports of successful laparoscopic management of early retroperitoneal ectopic gestations, such as ours [3, 6, 10, 18], including a case with implantation of the sac on the inferior vena cava [19]. The laparoscopic approach is feasible and should be the treatment of choice, in hemodynamically stable patients without signs of rupture. Before attempting laparoscopic management of such cases, exclusion of large retroperitoneal vascular infiltration with the assistance of MRI may be necessary, especially in more advanced gestations. To our opinion, rupture of a retroperitoneal gestation is a contraindication for laparoscopic management as it results in a difficult to control, narrow operative field due to excessive bleeding from neovascularization. Injection of dilute vasopressin may assist in the dissection of the gestational sac, from surrounding structures, but one has to keep in mind that hemostasis should be meticulous, as the risk of a postoperative hematoma formation is high. Any gynecologist attempting such a procedure should be well-trained, have a thorough knowledge of the retroperitoneal anatomy, and be ready to convert to laparotomy in case of intraoperative complications or uncontrollable bleeding. Close cooperation with a general surgeon and/or an interventional radiologist may prove invaluable to safely conclude these procedures.

Adjuvant treatment with methotrexate, systemic or through selective arterial embolization has been suggested to control the risk of bleeding from the placental bed and to avoid the possibility of persistent trophoblastic tissue [3, 20]. Although surgery remains the mainstay of treatment for abdominal ectopic pregnancies, there are also case reports of early abdominal pregnancies being treated successfully with systemic methotrexate, leading to its resorption without the need for further surgery [21]. Factors that are associated with failure of medical management include initial β-hCG values greater than 5,000 mUI/mL, ultrasound detection of a moderate or large amount of free peritoneal fluid, the presence of fetal cardiac activity, and a pretreatment increase in the β-hCG level of more than 50 % over a 48-h period [1, 3, 5]. Our case presented with three out of four of the above-mentioned contraindications for medical management. Furthermore, the patient was hemodynamically stable, and this permitted the use of the transvaginal probe to assist in the exact localization of the ectopic gestation. Other preoperative imaging techniques, and in particular magnetic resonance imaging (MRI), may prove useful in guiding operative maneuvers but they are costly and not always readily available. It is very probable that the second laparoscopy would have been avoided if we had used intraoperative ultrasound during first surgery. We decided not to administer systemic methotrexate postoperatively, as removal of the trophoblastic tissue appeared complete. Indeed levels of β-hCG declined steeply postoperatively, indicating its complete excision.

In conclusion, although retroperitoneal pregnancy is an extremely rare condition, in a patient with clinical findings suggestive of ectopic pregnancy, if both the uterus and adnexa are normal during laparoscopic exploration, unusual locations such as the retroperitoneum should be carefully examined. Ipsilateral or bilateral salpingectomy does not exclude the occurrence of a parametrial pregnancy, and a clinician should be aware of such a possibility. Ultrasound should be used intraoperatively especially when we are dealing with a small and difficult-to-locate parametrial pregnancy

Informed consent All procedures followed were in accordance with the ethical standards of the responsible committee on human experimentation (institutional and national) and with the Helsinki Declaration of 1975, as revised in 2000. Informed consent was obtained from all patients for included in the study.

References

1. Barnhart KT (2009) Ectopic pregnancy. N Engl J Med 361:379–387
2. Chetty M, Elson J (2009) Treating non-tubal ectopic pregnancy. Best Pract Res Clin Obstet Gynaecol 23:529–538
3. Tsudo T, Harada T, Yoshioka H, Terakawa N (1997) Laparoscopic management of early primary abdominal pregnancy. Obstet Gynecol 90:687–688
4. Lee JW, Sohn KM, Jung HS (2005) Retroperitoneal ectopic pregnancy. Am J Reprod 184:1600–1601
5. Champion PK, Tessitore NJ (1938) Intraligamentary pregnancy: a survey of all published cases of over 7 calendar months, with the discussion of an additional case. Am J Obstet Gynecol 36:281–293
6. Martinez-Varea A, Hidalgo-Mora JJ, Paya V, Morcillo I, Martin E, Pellicer A (2011) Retroperitoneal ectopic pregnancy after intrauterine insemination. Fertil Steril 95:2433e1–e3
7. Lin JX, Liu Q, Ju Y, Guan Q, Wu YZ, Zheng N (2008) Primary obturator foramen pregnancy: a case report and review of literature. Chin Med J 121:1328–1330
8. Abdul MA, Tabari AM, Kabiru D, Hamidu N (2008) Broad ligament pregnancy: a report of two cases. Ann Afr Med 7(2):86–87
9. Chang YL, Ko PC, Yen CF (2008) Retroperitoneal abdominal pregnancy at left parcolic sulcus. J Minim Invasive Gynecol 15:660–661
10. Bae SU, Kim CN, Hwang IT, Choi YJ, Lee MK, Cho BS, Kang Y, Park JS (2009) Laparoscopic treatment of early retroperitoneal abdominal pregnancy implanted on inferior vena cava. Surg Laparosc Endosc Percut Tech 19(4):e156–e158
11. Ferland RJ, Chadwick DA, O'Brien JA, Granai CO (1991) An ectopic pregnancy in the upper retroperitoneum following in vitro fertilization and embryo transfer. Obstet Gynecol 78:544–546
12. Dmowski WP, Rana N, Ding J, Wu WT (2002) Retroperitoneal subpancreatic ectopic pregnancy following in vitro fertilization in a patient with previous bilateral salpingectomy: how did it get there? J Assist Reprod Genet 19(2):90–93
13. Apantaku O, Rana P, Inglis T (2006) Broad ligament ectopic pregnancy following in-vitro fertilisation in a patient with previous bilateral salpingectomy. J Obstet Gynaecol 26(5):474
14. Iwama H, Tsutsumi S, Igarashi H, Takahashi K, Nakahara K, Kurachi H (2008) A case of retriperitoneal ectopic pregnancy following IVF-ET in a patient with previous bilateral salpingectomy. Am J Perinatol 25:33–36
15. Rersson J, Reynisson P, Masback A, Epstein E, Saldeen P (2010) Histopathology indicates lymphatic spread of a pelvic retroperitoneal ectopic pregnancy removed by robot-assisted laparoscopy with temporary occlusion of the blood supply. Acta Obstet Gynecol Scand 89(6):835–839
16. Hall JS, Harris M, Levy RC, Walrond ER (1973) Retroperitoneal ectopic pregnancy. J Obstet Gynaecol Br Commonw 80:92–94
17. Siow A, Chern B, Soong Y (2004) Successful laparoscopic treatment of an abdominal pregnancy in the broad ligament. Singap Med J 45(2):88–89
18. Olsen ME (1997) Laparoscopic treatment of intraligamentous pregnancy. Obstet Gynecol 89:862
19. Bae SU, Kim CN, Kim KH, Hwang IT, Choi YJ, Lee MK, Cho BS, Kang YJ, Park JS (2009) Laparoscopic treatment of early retroperitoneal abdominal pregnancy implanted on inferior vena cava. Surg Laparosc Endosc Percutan Tech 19(4):e156–e158
20. Parant O, Sarramon MF, Laffitte A, el Ghaoui A, Reme JM (1999) Parametrial pregnancy. Report of a case of "paracervical" pregnancy treated by medico-surgical management. J Gynecol Obstet Biol Reprod (Paris) 28(1):69–72
21. Okorie CO (2010) Retroperitoneal ectopic pregnancy: is there any place for non-surgical treatment with methotrexate? J Obstet Gynaecol Res 36(5):1133–1136

31

Locoregional treatment of breast cancer during pregnancy

Antonio Toesca · Oreste Gentilini · Fedro Peccatori · Hatem A. Azim Jr. · Frederic Amant

Abstract The management of patients with breast cancer during pregnancy is very demanding and it should be better performed in highly qualified and experienced centers. Referral to institutes and physicians trained in this special clinical scenario allows reducing the risk of both overtreating and undertreating the patients. Moreover, patients can receive appropriate information regarding safety of treatments without old-fashioned *taboo*. The purpose of the current paper is to discuss the main issues concerning surgical management and in general locoregional treatment of patients diagnosed with breast cancer and treated during gestation, focusing on those women who chose to continue their pregnancy. We cover the issues regarding type of breast surgery, radiation therapy, immediate reconstruction during mastectomy, and management of the axilla.

Keywords Breast cancer · Pregnancy · Chemotherapy · Radiation therapy

A. Toesca (✉) · O. Gentilini
Division of Breast Surgery, European Institute of Oncology, Via Ripamonti 435, 20141 Milan, Italy
e-mail: antonio.toesca@ieo.it

F. Peccatori
Department of Gynecological Oncology, European Institute of Oncology, Milan, Italy

H. A. Azim Jr.
Department of Medicine, BrEAST Data Centre, Institut Jules Bordet, Université Libre de Bruxelles, 1000 Brussels, Belgium

F. Amant
Multidisciplinary Breast Center, Leuven Cancer Institute (LKI), UZ Gasthuisberg, Katholieke Universiteit Leuven, Leuven, Belgium

Introduction and general considerations

Breast cancer diagnosed during pregnancy (BCdP), defined as breast cancer which develops either during or within 1 year after pregnancy, is expected to become even more common, since women often delay childbearing to their thirties and forties when breast cancer rates tend to increase. Some studies have found that BCdP is more commonly diagnosed at an advanced stage because of increased breast density, making clinical examinations and mammography more difficult to interpret [1–3].

Prognosis is influenced by treatment options, either local or systemic, which might be limited by the concern of harming the fetus and conditioned by gestational age. Therefore, it is important to clarify that most part of therapies can be safely administered to pregnant patients as well giving the opportunity to the mother to receive optimal treatments [4–6]. Azim et al. [1] reported in their metaanalysis of pregnancy-associated breast cancer that there was a poorer breast cancer outcome for women diagnosed in the postpartum period compared with those diagnosed with breast cancer during pregnancy. This is not in contrast with Amant et al. [7] who reported on the prognosis of women with primary breast cancer diagnosed during pregnancy and note similar overall survival compared with general population of non-pregnant patients. Many studies in the past have considered the two groups (breast cancer during pregnancy and post-partum breast cancer) as part of the same condition, and this could be the reason for the controversial results on prognosis.

Though, the occurrence of BCdP represents a dramatic condition for the patient, her family, and sometimes her physician mostly if the lattest is not carefully and specifically trained on this special clinical scenario. In fact, the management of BCdP requires a collaborative team effort to provide the best medical options and most effective psychosocial support.

The purpose of the current paper is to discuss the main issues concerning surgical management and in general locoregional treatment of patients diagnosed with breast cancer during pregnancy (BCdP). As treatment of breast cancer during lactation does not imply special major problems in terms of availability of treatments, our paper will focus only on patients with breast cancer diagnosed and treated during gestation. Moreover, this special clinical scenario is still infrequent, and therefore, some of the recommendations may necessarily have only a low level of evidence (expert opinion). Before treatment, it is important to discuss and inform the woman and her family about the maternal prognosis and treatment options as well as the potential impact on pregnancy and delivery, according to different staging. As interruption of pregnancy give access to therapies as in a non pregnant woman, the multidisciplinary team have to discuss differences with the patients in case of continuation of the pregnancy.

Our considerations will be restricted to those women who choose to continue their pregnancy, and all the issues related to voluntary interruption of pregnancy will not be included. As a general statement, the patients should be made aware that interruption of pregnancy by itself does not seem to improve outcome of patients [8].

Breast conserving surgery and the problem of delaying radiation therapy

Historically, mastectomy was considered the standard surgical procedure in pregnant patients with breast cancer [9].

Actually, due to a frequent diagnostic delay, patients with BCdP often present with large tumors requiring radical surgery. Modern studies report a mean diagnostic delay during pregnancy and lactation ranging from 1 to 3 months with a median tumor size at diagnosis of 3.5 cm [9]. Nevertheless, in our opinion, it is important to inform the patient that mastectomy is not mandatory for the treatment of breast cancer just because of the presence of pregnancy by itself [10, 11].

The published experience on breast conservation is so far limited, but all the available data seem to go in the same direction supporting safety and feasibility of breast conservation with good prognostic results in terms of local control [12–14]. In the experience of European Institute of Oncology of Milan [12], tumor size and rate of axillary metastases in patients with BCdP were lower than in previous reports [13], probably because of the increased awareness among both patients and physicians. This earlier stage of presentation (median tumor size 2.4 cm) enabled a higher rate of breast-conserving procedures (15 of 21 patients) even though it has to be pointed out that all the six patients who were diagnosed during the first trimester opted for termination of pregnancy. After a short-term median follow-up (24 months), there were no intra-breast tumor recurrences. Kuerer et al. reported

similar survival rates between patients treated with breast-conserving surgery and those treated with mastectomy [14].

As a general recommendation, breast conservation can be safely performed, whenever possible, in women diagnosed during the third trimester, as radiotherapy can be postponed until after delivery without major concerns about a possible detrimental delay.

The concurrent diagnosis of breast cancer and an unexpected early pregnancy represents the most challenging treatment scenario. It is considered that abortion is not a therapeutic procedure in these cases [13], but termination of pregnancy can be considered in order to facilitate completion of treatment. For patients at the first trimester who desire to continue the pregnancy, treatment is possible but there is a limited number of options during the first weeks of gestation. In fact, chemotherapy is prohibited during the first trimester, and endocrine treatments are not feasible [13, 15]. Surgery is safe at any time and during the first trimester as well [16], but breast conservation performed during a very early gestational age is associated with a long delay in postoperative radiotherapy. Unfortunately, there is limited and retrospective experience published on the delayed radiotherapy after breast conservation and its effect on outcome. In a study evaluating 568 patients with T1–T2 N0 breast cancer who underwent lumpectomy and radiotherapy without systemic treatment, similar rate of recurrence was reported in node negative patients when radiotherapy starts up to 16 weeks after definitive surgery after a median follow-up of 11.2 years [17]. Another retrospective study reported on 13,907 patients aged 65 years or older with stage I–II breast cancer who underwent lumpectomy and radiotherapy taken from the Surveillance, Epidemiology, and End Results (SEER)–Medicare database. The authors concluded that delays of >3 months were associated with poor survival, even though older age, black race, advanced stage, more comorbidities, and being unmarried were associated with longer time intervals between surgery and RT, and therefore, it is not clear whether the association is causal or due to confounding factors [18]. Chen et al. [19] performed a systematic review on the relationship between waiting time for radiotherapy and clinical outcomes with special attention on local recurrence. In this meta-analysis considering 20 high quality studies that had adequately controlled for confounding factors, a significant increase of local failure was demonstrated with increasing waiting times. The authors subsequently converted the relative risks derived from the meta-analysis into estimates of the increment in risk attributable to 1 month of the waiting time for RT and this translated into an absolute increase in the risk of local recurrence of 1.0 % per month of delay of staring RT.

Trying to be practical despite these controversial data, it is very likely that pregnant patients with breast cancer will undergo adjuvant chemotherapy after surgery as this is the only adjuvant possible treatment during gestation. Actually, most part of nonpregnant patients undergoing adjuvant chemotherapy usually receive radiotherapy after more than 6 months, and in these patients, the delay of administration does not represent an issue of major concern.

Basically, we suggest that in patients at the second or third trimester, the surgical approach applied to women with BCdP should not significantly differ from the policy applied to nonpregnant women, and the delay in administering RT is probably similar to what happens to nonpregnant patients.

In a patient at the first trimester who wants to continue the pregnancy and also wishes to conserve the breast, all these issues have to be carefully discussed, and the patient has to be informed that a possible increased risk of local recurrence should be considered, even though this is difficult to quantify because of the lack of clear data. The patients should also be reassured that in nonpregnant patients receiving chemotherapy, radiotherapy is usually given 6 months after surgery.

External beam radiation therapy

Embryonic exposure resulting from breast radiotherapy with a dose of 0.1 Gy in the first trimester, during organogenesis, increases the risk of malformations and can cause mental retardation [20, 21].

The dose to a fetus resulting from tangential breast irradiation, measured using anthropomorphic phantoms simulating the geometry of a pregnant woman, has been calculated for the first, second, and third trimester of gestation [20]. The dose increased as the pregnancy became more advanced, because of the increased proximity of the fetus to the primary irradiation field. With shielding a 50–75 % dose reduction can be achieved [22, 23]. These data are applicable for all the X-ray energies from 4 to 10 MV used for breast radiotherapy. Thus, during the first and the second trimester of pregnancy, the fetal irradiation dose seems to be lower than the threshold values associated organ malformations. During the third trimester, however, the dose seems to exceed this threshold. In addition, in utero irradiation at all gestational ages may increase the risk of cancer during childhood [20]. A conservative estimate of the lifetime risk of radiation induced by fetal exposure to 0.01 Gy is about one in 1700 cases [22].

Successful radiotherapy of breast cancer during pregnancy and birth of healthy children has been reported [24–28]. The short-term fetal outcome following radiotherapy for BCdP has been recently documented. After a median follow up of 37 months, Luis et al. calculated 13/109 adverse outcomes, including spontaneous abortions ($n=2$), perinatal death ($n=5$), stillbirth ($n=1$), hypospadia ($n=1$), learning problem and scoliosis ($n=1$), sensory hearing loss ($n=1$), attention deficit disorder with delayed coordination ($n=1$), undescended left testicle, and an uncomplicated ventricular septal defect ($n=1$) [27]. Where available ($n=4$), the estimated fetal dose was

below the threshold dose (<0.1 Gy). Of the 24 patients treated for breast cancer, 3 had an adverse fetal outcome: 2 perinatal deaths were described after chest wall/axilla irradiation and one spontaneous abortion after lumbar spine irradiation (30 Gy) at 10 weeks of gestation for metastatic disease [29]. Overall, the fetal outcome is poorly documented and it is difficult to define the role of radiotherapy when an adverse outcome is noted.

Therefore, radiotherapy is considered relatively safe only during the first and second trimester of pregnancy but based on theoretical assumptions and few experiences. Better clinical data are needed and every single case should be discussed with a patient and by a multidisciplinary team, tailoring as much as possible every single case [11].

Is partial breast irradiation possible during pregnancy?

The strength and the attractiveness of accelerated partial breast irradiation (APBI) techniques for breast cancer are reducing the volume treated, with potential decrease of normal tissue toxicity, and reducing the treatment time [30]. In response to the increasing use of APBI off clinical trial several consensus statements from different panels have been published regarding the appropriate use of partial breast irradiation in nonpregnant breast cancer patients. The National Comprehensive Cancer Network (NCCN) guidelines published in 2011 [31] open the possibility to patients to be given APBI according to criteria identified by American Society for Radiation Oncology (ASTRO) consensus for the "suitable" group which includes only women aged >60 years. Therefore, the application of APBI remains controversial in young patients with breast cancer due to the increased local recurrence rate after breast conservation in this subset of patients. Nevertheless, the issues concerning on one hand safety and on the other hand the possible risks of delaying radiotherapy in pregnant patients with breast cancer make PBI theoretically attractive as an alternative option.

Electron beam intraoperative radiotherapy (ELIOT) is a new technique permitting breast radiotherapy to be completed in a single session. Since ELIOT is associated with much reduced irradiation to non-target tissues, Galimberti el at. carried out a study on nonpregnant breast cancer patients to estimate doses to the uterus during ELIOT [32].

The authors performed in vivo dosimetry with thermoluminescence radiation detectors (TLDs) in 15 premenopausal patients receiving ELIOT to the breast (prescribed dose 21 Gy) using two mobile linear accelerators. The TLDs were positioned subdiaphragmatically on the irradiated side, at the medial pubic position, and within the uterus. A shielding apron (2-mm lead equivalent) was placed over the viscera from the subcostal to the subpubic region. TLDs showed mean doses of 0.37 Gy (range 0.01–0.85 Gy) at subdiaphragm, 0.09 Gy (range 0.003–0.02 Gy) pubic, and 0.17 Gy (range 0.06–0.32 Gy) in utero, for beam energies in the range 5–9 MeV. These findings indicate that ELIOT with a mobile linear accelerator and shielding apron would be safe for the fetus, as doses of a few Gy are not associated with measurable increased risk of fetal damage, and the threshold dose for deterministic effects is estimated at 0.1–0.2 Gy.

Intraoperative radiotherapy could reduce fetal dose, and for this result so attractive for pregnant management, there are limitations and doubts about the efficacy of PBI in young patients with breast cancer. Nevertheless, we believe that this might be a further option to offer to pregnant patients with a small breast cancer diagnosed at a very early gestational age and who are motivated to continue the pregnancy after a thorough explanation of a possible increase in local recurrence if compared to WBRT. Always an estimation of the fetal exposure should be assessed by a physicist in order to assess fetal safety.

Mastectomy and immediate breast reconstruction

In the recent past, mastectomy has been considered the treatment of choice for pregnant patients with breast cancer [9]. To date, despite breast conservation can be considered, a considerable proportion of patients to date still require a mastectomy due to the large tumor size at presentation.

In 2010, a European Consensus on the management of breast cancer during pregnancy discouraged immediate breast reconstruction during pregnancy due to lack of data and recommended prosthetic implant-based reconstruction after delivery [11]. In fact, at the moment, there are no available data concerning immediate breast reconstruction (IBR) in pregnant patients undergoing mastectomy for breast cancer. Nevertheless, it is well known that IBR decreases the psychological impact of mutilation, provides superior esthetic outcome and better patient and physician satisfaction compared to delayed reconstruction [33–35].

Therefore, the obvious advantages of immediate breast reconstruction lead us to explore the possibility to consider an IBR whenever possible even in pregnant patients, and in our view, pregnant breast cancer patients should not be denied by definition the opportunity to undergo immediate breast reconstruction after mastectomy. At the European Institute of Oncology, we usually suggest a tissue expander which is a straightforward technique not significantly increasing operating time and risk of complications. Lohsiriwat et al. [36] reported the first analysis of 78 patients who underwent immediate breast reconstruction with expander following mastectomy for breast cancer diagnosed during pregnancy describing an excellent pregnancy outcomes without obstetrical complications after surgery. Moreover, the unpredictable

physiologic changes of the breast during and after pregnancy, makes not suitable IBR with definitive implant and contralateral reshaping. IBR by autologous tissue should not be considered for the long operative time and increased risk of blood loss and postoperative complications.

Sentinel lymph node biopsy

After initial concern for a safety issue, it is now widely agreed that sentinel lymph node biopsy (SLNB) for staging of the regional lymph nodes can be performed safely during pregnancy [37, 38].

In 2000, Nicklas and Baker [39] suggested that SLNB can be safely performed in pregnancy since the entire radioisotope injected (13.5 to16 MBq of double-filtered 99mTc sulfur colloid) remains trapped at the injection site on the breast or within the lymphatics. Morita et al. [40] stated that receiving a whole-body dose from activity 13.5 to 16 MBq in the breast, the dose of radiation exposure to the unborn child would be exceedingly low. Some authors [39, 41, 42] reported that the estimated absorbed dose to the fetus/embryo per unit activity of 99mTc-HSA administered intravenously to the mother is 5.1 mGy/MBq. Dosimetric evaluations reported in the literature as well as data from a simulation study gave evidence of negligible risks to the fetus [43]. Gentilini et al. performed a simulation in vivo study in order to investigate safety of lymphoscintigraphy in terms of radiation risk and estimate of the possible absorbed doses to the fetus with a single peritumoral injection of 99mTc-labeled human albumin colloid particles (99mTc-HSA nanocolloids) in a volume of 0.2 ml 16–18 h before the surgical intervention. The injected activity was found to be concentrated only in the injection site and in the lymph nodes, demonstrating negligible irradiation to other tissues, organs, and the absence of radiotracer uptake in the pelvis after 15 min. In 23 of 26 nonpregnant patients studied, all absorbed dose measurements were lower than the sensitivity of the thermoluminescent dosimeters used (<10 mGy); in the remaining three patients, the absorbed doses at the level of epigastrium, umbilicus, and hypogastrium ranged from 0.03 to 0.32 Gy. The total activity excreted in the urine within the first 16 h (time between injection and operation) was <2 % of the injected activity. The biological pharmacokinetic data showed that a very small amount of the injected activity is circulating in the blood pool and excreted by the urinary system confirming that the level of radioactivity in the body is absolutely negligible at each time point studied after the administration, proving that there is a negligible risk to the fetus [37]. This level is far less than the National Council on Radiation Protection and Measurements limit to pregnant women [44].

Experiences derived from treatment of melanoma or breast cancer who underwent lymphatic mapping during pregnancy have not shown birth defects or discernible malformations in born [38].

Gentilini et al. reported data from 12 pregnant patients with breast cancer who underwent lymphoscintigraphy and SLNB, focusing on the outcomes of the pregnancies. Eleven babies were born with normal weight and no malformations and after a median follow up of 32 months (6–83 months), were doing well. One baby had a diagnosis of ventricular septal defect (VSD) and was operated on at the age of 3 months because of the onset of cardiac failure. However, VSD was demonstrated with ultrasound before the lymphoscintigraphy procedure and therefore cannot be attributed to the injection of the radioactive tracer.

As a practical recommendation, it is advisable to inject colloid in the morning (1-day protocol) in order to reduce time and dose of radiation exposure.

Blue dye should not be used during pregnancy as its use has a possible risk of an allergic or anaphylactic maternal reaction, which can be harmful for the fetus [43]. Isosulfan blue has a possible risk (1 %) of an allergic and anaphylactic reaction, which can increase the risk of harm to the fetus. Methylene blue is contraindicated in the pregnant patients during first trimester because of known teratogenic effect of jejunal atresia due to of vasoconstrictive effects in blocking nitric oxide [43].

Concluding remarks

Surgery can be safely performed during pregnancy and during the first trimester as well. Mastectomy should not be recommended just because of the pregnancy itself, and breast conservation should be discussed whenever possible. In patients operated during the third or even the second trimester, radiation therapy can be safely postponed after delivery [11]. The risk of a possible too long delay of radiation therapy in case of surgery performed at a very early gestational age should be taken into account and all the options should be considered according to patient's preference. However, virtually, all patients need adjuvant chemotherapy, bridging the gap between surgery and radiotherapy. Partial breast irradiation, especially with electrons (ELIOT) might be an interesting option in the future even if at the moment there is lack of data and some doubts might be raised regarding treatment of young patients in terms of increased risk of local recurrence. For those patients requiring mastectomy, an immediate breast reconstruction with tissue expander can be performed as it does not excessively increase operative time and risk of complications. Lymphoscintigraphy and sentinel node biopsy by the use of 99mTc is safe in pregnant patients as well.

Informed consent statement   All procedures followed were in accordance with the ethical standards of the responsible committee on human experimentation (institutional and national) and with the Helsinki Declaration of 1975, as revised in 2000 (5). Informed consent was obtained from all patients for being included in the study.

References

1. Azim HA Jr, Santoro L, Russell-Edu W, Pentheroudakis G, Pavlidis N, Peccatori FA (2012) Prognosis of pregnancy-associated breast cancer: a meta-analysis of 30 studies. Cancer Treat Rev 38(7):834–842

2. Ishida T, Yokoe T, Kasumi F et al (1992) Clinicopathologic characteristics and prognosis of breast cancer patients associated with pregnancy and lactation: analysis of case–control study in Japan. Jpn J Cancer Res 83:1143–1149

3. Anderson BO, Petrek JA, Byrd DR, Senie RT, Borgen PI (1996) Pregnancy influences breast cancer stage at diagnosis in women 30 years of age and younger. Ann Surg Oncol 3: 204–211

4. Azim HA Jr, Botteri E, Renne G et al (2012) The biological features and prognosis of breast cancer diagnosed during pregnancy: a case–control study. Acta Oncol 51:653–661

5. Amant F, Loibl S, Neven P, Van Calsteren K (2012) Breast cancer in pregnancy. Lancet 379(9815):570–579

6. Amant F, Van Calsteren K, Halaska MJ, Gziri MM, Hui W, Lagae L, Willemsen MA, Kapusta L, Van Calster B, Wouters H, Heyns L, Han SN, Tomek V, Mertens L, Ottevanger PB (2012) Long-term cognitive and cardiac outcomes after prenatal exposure to chemotherapy in children aged 18 months or older: an observational study. Lancet Oncol 13(3):256–264

7. Amant F, von Minckwitz G, Han SN, Bontenbal M, Ring AE, Giermek J, Wildiers H, Fehm T, Linn SC, Schlehe B, Neven P, Westenend PJ, Müller V, Van Calsteren K, Rack B, Nekljudova V, Harbeck N, Untch M, Witteveen PO, Schwedler K, Thomssen C, Van Calster B, Loibl S (2013) Prognosis of women with primary breast cancer diagnosed during pregnancy: results from an international collaborative study. J Clin Oncol 31:2532–2539

8. Loibl S, Han SN, von Minckwitz G, Bontenbal M, Ring A, Giermek J, Fehm T, Van Calsteren K, Linn SC, Schlehe B, Gziri MM, Westenend PJ, Müller V, Heyns L, Rack B, Van Calster B, Harbeck N, Lenhard M, Halaska MJ, Kaufmann M, Nekljudova V, Amant F (2012) Treatment of breast cancer during pregnancy: an observational study. Lancet Oncol 13(9):887–896

9. Woo JC, Yu T, Hurd TC (2003) Breast cancer in pregnancy: a literature review. Arch Surg 138(1):91–98, discussion 99

10. Schwartz GF, Veronesi U, Clough K, Dixon JM, Fentiman IS, Heywang-Köbrunner SH, Holland R, Hughes KS, Margolese R, Olivotto IA, Palazzo JP, Solin LJ (2006) Proceedings of the Consensus Conference on Breast Conservation, April 28 to May 1, 2005, Milan, Italy Cancer; 107(2): 242–50

11. Amant F, Deckers S, Van Calsteren K, Loibl S, Halaska M, Brepoels L, Beijnen J, Cardoso F, Gentilini O, Lagae L, Mir O, Neven P, Ottevanger N, Pans S, Peccatori F, Rouzier R, Senn HJ, Struikmans H, Christiaens MR, Cameron D, Du Bois A (2010) Breast cancer in pregnancy: recommendations of an international consensus meeting. Eur J Cancer 46(18):3158–3168

12. Gentilini O, Masullo M, Rotmensz N et al (2005) Breast cancer diagnosed during pregnancy and lactation: biological features and treatment options. Eur J Surg Oncol 31:232–236

13. Berry DL, Theriault RL, Holmes FA et al (1999) Management of breast cancer during pregnancy using a standardized protocol. J Clin Oncol 17:855–861

14. Kuerer H, Gwyn K, Ames F et al (2002) Conservative surgery and chemotherapy for breast carcinoma during pregnancy. Surgery 131: 108–110

15. Cardonick E, Iacubucci A (2004) Use of chemotherapy during pregnancy. Lancet Oncol 5:283–291

16. Duncan PG, Pope WDB, Cohen MM, Greer N (1986) Fetal risk of anesthesia and surgery during pregnancy. Anesthesiology 64:790–794

17. Vujovic O, Cherian A, Dar AR, Stitt L, Perera F (2006) Eleven-year follow up results in the delay of breast irradiation after conservative surgery in node-negative breast cancer patients. Int J Radiat Oncol Biol Phys 64(3):760–764

18. Hershman DL, Wang X, McBride R, Jacobson JS, Grann VR, Neugut AI (2006) Delay in initiating adjuvant radiotheraphy following breast conservation and its impact on survival. Int J Radiat Oncol Biol Phys 65(5):1353–1360

19. Chen Z, King W, Pearcey R, Kerba M, Mackillop WJ (2008) The relationship between waiting time for radiotherapy and outcome: a systematic review of the literature. Radiother Oncol 87:3–16

20. Mazonakis M, Varveris H, Damilakis J et al (2003) Radiation dose to conceptus resulting from tangential breast irradiation. Int J Radiat Oncol Biol Phys 55(2):386–391

21. International Commission on Radiological Protection (1991) Recommendations of the International Commission on Radiological Protection, ICRP Publication 60. Pergamon Press, Oxford

22. Kal HB, Struikmans H (2005) Radiotherapy during pregnancy: fact and fiction. Lancet Oncol 6(5):328–333

23. Han B, Bednarz B, Xu XG (2009) A study of the shielding used to reduce leakage and scattered radiation to the fetus in a pregnant patient treated with a 6-MV external X-ray beam. Health Phys 97(6):581–589

24. Van der Giessen PH (1997) Measurement of the peripheral dose for the tangential breast treatment technique with Co-60 gamma radiation and high energy X-rays. Radiother Oncol 42:257–264

25. Ngu SL, Duval P, Collins C (1992) Foetal radiation dose in radiotherapy for breast cancer. Australas Radiol 36:321–322

26. Antypas C, Sandilos P, Kouvaris J et al (1998) Fetal dose evaluation during breast cancer radiotherapy. Int J Radiat Oncol Biol Phys 40: 995–999

27. Luis SA, Christie DR, Kaminski A et al (2009) Pregnancy and radiotherapy: management options for minimising risk, case series and comprehensive literature review. J Med Imaging Radiat Oncol 53(6):559–568

28. Kouvaris JR, Antypas CE, Sandilos PH, Plataniotis GA, Tympanides CN, Vlahos LJ (2000) Postoperative tailored radiotherapy for locally advanced breast carcinoma during pregnancy: a therapeutic dilemma. Am J Obstet Gynecol 183(2):498–499

29. Mulvihill JJ, McKeen EA, Rosner F, Zarrabi MH (1987) Pregnancy outcome in cancer patients. Experience in a large cooperative group. Cancer 60(5):1143–1150

30. Orecchia R, Leonardo MC (2011) Intraoperative radiation therapy: is it a standard now? Breast S3:S111–S115

31. NCC guidelines. http://www.nccn.org/professionals/physician_gls/PDF/breast.pdf

32. Galimberti V, Ciocca M, Leonardi MC et al (2009) Is electron beam intraoperative radiotherapy (ELIOT) safe in pregnant women with early breast cancer? In vivo dosimetry to assess fetal dose. Ann Surg Oncol 16(1):100–105

33. Morrow M et al (2009) Surgeon recommendations and receipt of mastectomy for treatment of breast cancer. JAMA 14:1551–1556

34. Al-Ghazal SK, Sully L, Fallowfield L, Blamey RW (2000) The psychological impact of immediate rather than delayed breast reconstruction. Eur J Surg Oncol 26:17–19

35. Fernandez-Delgado J, Lopez-Pedraza MJ, Blasco JA et al (2008) Satisfaction with and psychological impact of immediate and deferred breast reconstruction. Ann Oncol 19:1430–1434

36. Lohsiriwat V, Peccatori FA, Martella S, Azim HA Jr, Sarno MA, Galimberti V, De Lorenzi F, Intra M, Sangalli C, Rotmensz N, Pruneri G, Renne G, Schorr MC, Nevola Teixeira LF, Rietjens M, Giroda M, Gentilini O (2013) Immediate breast reconstruction with expander in pregnant breast cancer patients. Breast 22(5):657–660

37. Gentilini O, Cremonesi M, Trifiro G et al (2004) Safety of sentinel node biopsy in pregnant patients with breast cancer. Ann Oncol 15(9):1348–1351

38. Gentilini O, Cremonesi M, Toesca A et al (2010) Sentinel lymph node biopsy in pregnant patients with breast cancer. Eur J Nucl Med Mol Imaging 37(1):78–83

39. Du Bois A, Meerpohl HG, Gerner K et al (1993) Effect of pregnancy on the incidence and course of malignant diseases. Geburtshilfe Frauenheilkd 53(9):619–624

40. Morita ET, Chang J, Leong SP (2000) Principles and controversies in lymphoscintigraphy with emphasis on breast cancer. Surg Clin N Am 80:1721–1739

41. Russell JR, Stabin MG, Sparks RB, Watson E (1997) Radiation absorbed dose to the embryo/fetus from radiopharmaceuticals. Health Phys 73:756–769

42. Russell JR, Stabin MG, Sparks RB (1997) Placental transfer of radiopharmaceuticals and dosimetry in pregnancy. Health Phys 73:747–755

43. Khera SY, Kiluk JV, Hasson DM et al (2008) Pregnancy-associated breast cancer patients can safely undergo lymphatic mapping. Breast J 14(3):250–254

44. Pandit-Taskar N, Dauer LT, Montgomery L, Germain SJ, Zanzonico PB, Divgi CR (2006) Organ and fetal absorbed dose estimates from 99 mTc-sulfur colloid lymphoscintigraphy and sentinel node localization in breast cancer patients. J Nucl Med 47:1202–1208

32

A randomised trial of Medgyn Endosampler® vs Endocurette® in an outpatient hysteroscopy clinic setting

A. S. Khalid · C. Burke

Abstract Outpatient hysteroscopy and endometrial biopsy are increasingly being used in the investigation of abnormal uterine bleeding. In our unit, both Endocurette® and Endosampler® endometrial biopsy devices are available in the outpatient hysteroscopy clinic. Literature comparing these devices is lacking. This was a prospective, randomised trial involving women attending the outpatient hysteroscopy clinic at Cork University Maternity Hospital. Women were randomised to endometrial sampling with either Endosampler® or Endocurette® devices. A number of device insertions, pain scores, ease of handling and histological reporting of sample adequacy and tissue histology were recorded. One hundred and six women were recruited comprising 55 pre-menopausal and 51 post-menopausal women. A substantially higher rate of multiple device insertions to obtain a visually adequate sample was recorded using Endocurette® compared with Endosampler®. In the Endosampler® group, 10.7 and 12.5 % of women in pre- and post-menopausal categories had ≥ 2 device insertions compared to 88.8 and 58.3 %, respectively, with Endocurette® ($p=0.002$ and $p=0.0001$). There was no difference in the rate of histologically inadequate samples or difficulty with device handling between matched groups. Mean pain scores in the pre- and post-menopausal groups were 5.83 and 4.58 for Endosampler®, and 4.69 and 4.88 for Endocurette® ($p=0.02$). The rate of histologically inadequate samples was higher in post-menopausal compared to pre-menopausal women (27.4 vs 3.7 %, $p=0.0025$). A significantly lower rate of multiple device insertions for adequate histological sample was recorded with Endosampler®. No significant differences in operational difficulties, patient acceptability and sample adequacy were shown. Higher overall pain scores were reported with Endosampler®

with no difference in the rate of severe pain between groups' satisfaction with the procedure or willingness to undergo the procedure again.

Keywords Endometrial · Biopsy · Outpatient hysteroscopy · Post-menopausal bleeding · Menorrhagia

Introduction

Outpatient hysteroscopy and endometrial sampling are increasingly being favoured in the investigation of abnormal uterine bleeding. Whilst hysteroscopy, D&C requires general anaesthesia, endometrial sampling can be done without any anaesthetic, or with local anaesthetic. Fine-calibre rigid hysteroscopes and flexible fibre-optic hysteroscopes now allow hysteroscopy without general anaesthetic. This method is increasingly replacing hysteroscopy D&C due to its benefits of avoiding hospital admission and general anaesthetic complications, thus being cost-effective to the hospital [1].

A range of endometrial sampling devices has been developed over the years. The most commonly used endometrial sampling device is the Pipelle de Cornier® device which has shown comparable sensitivity to D&C, supporting its use in an outpatient setting [2]. An inadequate sample rate of 13–20 % with a mean pain score of 1–5 has also been reported [3–7]. Pipelle® has been compared to Vacurette®, Novak®, Vabra®, Accurette® and Explora® in different studies [8–11], which have shown comparable tissue yields, better if not comparable pain scores and shorter procedure time with Pipelle®.

At Cork University Maternity Hospital, women attending the outpatient hysteroscopy clinic are routinely investigated with transvaginal ultrasound followed by saline hysteroscopy and endometrial sampling. The sampling devices available in this setting are Endosampler® and Endocurette®. To date, no

A. S. Khalid · C. Burke (✉)
Cork University Maternity Hospital, Wilton, Cork, Republic of Ireland
e-mail: Cathy.burke@hse.ie

studies comparing these two devices have been reported in the literature. The aim of this study was to compare the Endosampler® and Endocurette® devices in terms of number of device insertions to achieve a visually adequate endometrial sample, pain scores using a visual analogue scale, patient acceptability and user acceptability.

Method

This was a prospective, randomised trial planned to involve around 100 women attending the outpatient hysteroscopy clinic at Cork University Maternity Hospital. All procedures followed were in accordance with the ethical standards of the responsible committee on human experimentation (institutional and national) and with the Helsinki Declaration of 1975, as revised in 2008. Ethics approval was obtained from the Clinical Research Ethics Committee of the Cork Teaching Hospitals. Women were given an information leaflet regarding the study prior to the procedure. Informed written consent was obtained from all women included in the study. Women were categorised into pre- and post-menopausal categories and were then randomised to Endosampler® or Endocurette® device use at the time endometrial biopsy. Stratified randomisation was used to ensure an approximately equal number of women in each group whilst minimising bias over time. Sealed opaque envelopes containing device allocation were randomly prepared in blocks of 10. Randomisation of device allocation was achieved using a random generator. Upon enrolment, an envelope was taken from the front of the relevant pack according to menopausal status. When 5 envelopes remained in a pack, an additional 10 envelopes were supplemented to the packs randomly. This method achieved blinded allocation at the point of enrolment, whist minimising bias over time.

All women had routine transvaginal ultrasound and saline hysteroscopy followed by endometrial sampling using the allocated device. Hysteroscopes used were diagnostic and not designed for directed biopsy, hence the need for blind endometrial sampling. Endocurette® is a straw-like structure with three radially arranged apertures at the tip of the device and an integrated piston which, when withdrawn, generates negative pressure within the cannula allowing endometrium to be drawn into the device as it is withdrawn from the uterus. Its appearance and mechanism of use are similar to the Pipelle® device. It measures 3.6 mm in diameter at the tip and 3.1 mm at the shaft. Endosampler® has a similar straw-like structure, slightly curved at the tip which contains a single aperture. The curette and shaft measure 3.0 mm and are attached to a 10 ml syringe prior to biopsy. The full withdrawn syringe becomes locked into position via a small stainless steel mechanism, generating a relatively strong vacuum effect. Radial curettage of the endometrium can thus be performed. The syringe can be removed from the cannula to expel residual saline from the

uterine cavity following saline hysteroscopy, without the need to reinsert the cannula. Two operators were involved in performing sampling. Women and pathologists were blinded to the sampling device used. Clinicians were obviously not blinded, but the devices were used according to manufacturers' instructions to minimise bias. Figures 1 and 2 show the design of both endometrial sampling devices.

Women were asked to rate discomfort during both the hysteroscopy and biopsy procedures separately using a visual analogue scale (VAS), and were asked to verbally rate the worst pain experienced during both procedures where the number 0 represented no pain and the number 10 represented the worst imaginable pain. A post-procedure questionnaire was completed by each participant. To assess the acceptability of outpatient hysteroscopy and endometrial biopsy, women were asked whether they would opt for outpatient hysteroscopy again in the future if required, and whether they would recommend others to undergo this procedure.

A datasheet was completed by clinicians on which information was gathered on the use of local anaesthetic, number of passes of the biopsy device, ease of handling and adequacy of the sample obtained. Ease of device handling was assessed in terms of insertion and operational function. Clinicians were asked to assess using a scale of 1–3 (1 unacceptable, 2 acceptable, 3 excellent) in order to make an objective assessment. Clinicians made a subjective assessment of sample adequacy after biopsy was complete using a scale of 1–3 (1 unacceptable, 2 acceptable, 3 excellent).

Histology reports were followed up post-procedure and were analysed in terms of percentage of adequate samples retrieved and sample volume, as well as the report on histological features. Data was stored in a password-protected file in the hospital computer and patient record number only will be used to identify patients, to ensure patient confidentiality and data protection. Statistical analysis was done using the SPSS statistical package 18 and GraphPad Prism statistical software. Fisher's exact test was used to test for statistical significance between groups.

Results

A total of 112 women consented to the study, of which data on 106 women was obtained, comprising 55 pre-menopausal and

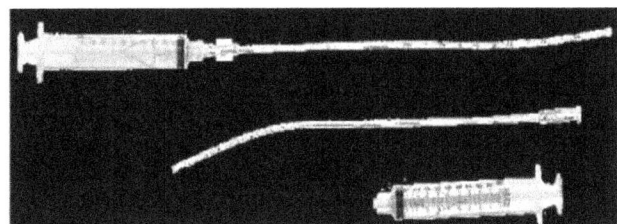

Fig. 1 Medgyn Endosampler®

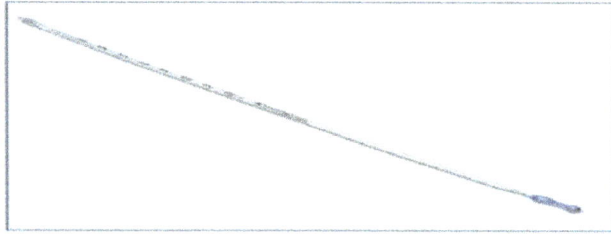

Fig. 2 Endocurette®

51 post-menopausal women. Six women were excluded from analysis due to intolerance of the outpatient hysteroscopy procedure. There were 54 and 52 women in the Endosampler® and Endocurette® groups, respectively. No differences in age or parity were observed between patients in the two groups. Figure 3 summarises the allocation of women in this study.

In terms of ease of device handling, no significant difference was observed between groups with regard to ease of insertion. Excellent insertion was recorded in 97 and 91 % with Endosampler® and Endocurette®, respectively ($p=0.61$). There were two occurrences of insertion difficulties which were both in the pre-menopausal group, one in the Endosampler® group and the other in the Endocurette® group. These were both associated with fibroid uteri. In terms of operational difficulties, there was no report of any difficulties in either groups and no significant difference was observed in both groups. Excellence in operational function was recorded in 90 and 85 % in the Endosampler® and Endocurette® groups, respectively ($p=0.43$).

The rate of repeated (≥ 2) device insertions was eight times higher in the Endocurette® than the Endosampler® group in

pre-menopausal women ($p=0.0001$), illustrated in Fig. 4. The percentage of patients requiring >2 device insertions to achieve a visually adequate biopsy sample with Endocurette® was 89 % and 58 % in the pre- and post-menopausal groups, compared with 11 and 12 % in respective groups where Endosampler® was used. ($p=0.002$ and $p=0.0001$). The overall inadequate sample rate according to the clinician performing the procedure was 17 % in the Endosampler® group and 14 % in the Endocurette® group. There was no significant difference in the rate of visually inadequate samples between groups. More inadequate samples were reported in post-menopausal women (27.4 % of post-menopausal women compared to 3.6 % of pre-menopausal women, $p= 0.0025$) due to the high level of endometrial atrophy in this group.

Mean pain scores of 5.8 and 4.6 were reported in the pre- and post-menopausal groups with Endosampler® use, compared with 4.7 and 4.9 in the Endocurette® group. The distribution of pain scores amongst all women is illustrated in Fig. 5. Whilst significantly more pre-menopausal women in the Endosampler® group reported pain scores ≥ 5 compared to the Endocurette® group ($p=0.02$), no significant difference was observed in post-menopausal women. When pain scores of ≥ 8 (severe pain) were analysed, no significant difference was observed between groups. Oral analgesics are routinely recommended prior to outpatient hysteroscopy, and were taken by 97 % of women in this study. Local anaesthetic was administered to 44 % ($n=47$) of women, 37 of which were post-menopausal and 10 pre-menopausal. Lignospan Special® (lignocaine hydrochloride 2 % and epinephrine 1:80,000) was the local anaesthetic used in all cases, two

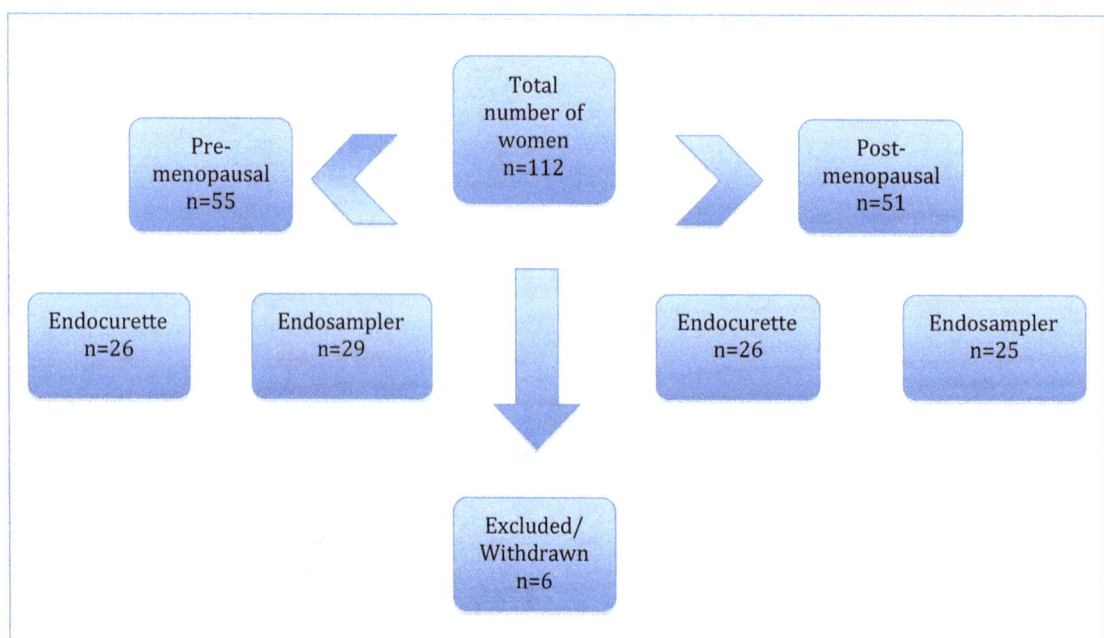

Fig. 3 Distribution of women who participated in our study

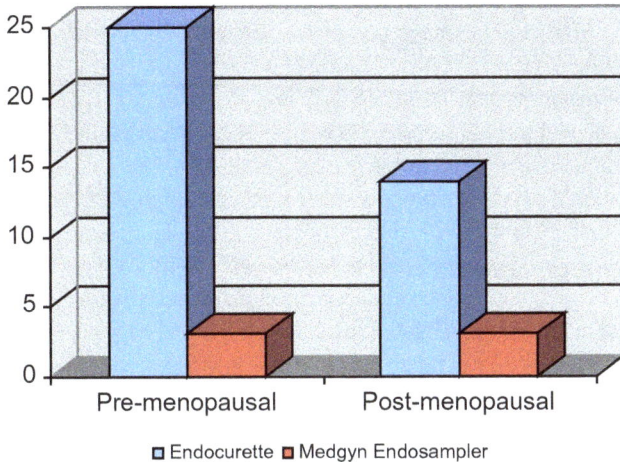

Fig. 4 Women with multiple (≥2) device insertions according to groups

Table 1 Histology sample sizes reported in aggregates

	Endosampler® (%)	Endocurette® (%)
Very scanty	3.7	5.7
0.1–1.0 cm	70.3	73.0
1.1–2.0 cm	18.5	15.4
>2.0 cm	9.3	3.8

ampoules of which were injected into four quadrants of the cervix prior to hysteroscopy. In cases where local anaesthetic was not used, mean pain scores were 3.39 and 2.30 in the Endosampler® and Endocurette® groups compared with scores of 5.0 and 4.3 in women given local anaesthetic. Significantly more women had pain scores ≥5 in the Endosampler® group (p=0.05). Side effects of local anaesthetic were not recorded in this study. Pain scores reported for hysteroscopy alone were recorded separately and found to be not significantly different between the two groups. In the Endosampler group, the mean was 3.17 (range 0–9), whereas in the Endocurette group, the mean pain score for hysteroscopy was 3.77 (range 0–8).

Histology reports commented on endometrial histology and tissue aggregate size. The aggregate size was subdivided into 'very scanty', 0.1–1.0 cm, 1.1–2.0 cm and >2.0 cm (Table 1). 'Very scanty' biopsy size was reported in 4 % in the Endosampler®, compared with 6 % in the Endocurette® group, all being in post-menopausal women. The difference in the yield of tissue of >2.0 and >1.0 cm in aggregate between devices was not statistically significant (p=0.43 and p=0.50), nor was the difference in 'very scanty' aggregates (0.67). In the Endosampler® group, one case of grade 2 endometrial cancer and two cases of endometrial hyperplasia were reported. In the Endocurette® group, one

case of grade 1 endometrial cancer was detected. In the post-menopausal group as a whole, 78.4 % were found to have atrophic or inactive endometrium on histology, 3.9 % (n=2) were found to have endometrial cancer, with the remaining 17.6 % having other benign pathology such as endometrial or cervical polyps (Table 2).

There was no difference between groups in terms of patient either willingness to undergo the same procedure in the future or recommendation of the procedure to an acquaintance. Only 4.7 % (n=5) of women reported they would not have the procedure again, 3 of whom were in the Endosampler® group, and 2 in the Endocurette® group with variable pain scores ranging from 1 to 9. Only 3.8 % (n=4) of women, 2 from each group, would not recommend the procedure to others, with pain scores ranging from 5 to 10. Fifteen women (14.1 %) found the procedure more uncomfortable than expected, with pain scores ranging from 0 to 10, of which 9 were in the Endosampler® group and 6 in the Endocurette® group. Sixty-five women (61.3 %) found it less uncomfortable than expected, again with non-correlating pain scores ranging from 0 to 9.

Discussion

Mean biopsy-related pain scores were higher in the Endosampler® group by a factor of around 1 unit. Significantly more women in the pre-menopausal Endosampler® group had pain scores ≥5. Interestingly, pain scores in post-menopausal women were not higher in the Endosampler group. This may be because of the high rate of local anaesthetic use in this group (72.5 %), or the need for fewer device insertions. There was a significantly lower rate of multiple device insertions with Endosampler® compared to Endocurette® in this study, with a consequently shorter procedural time. There was no difference in operational

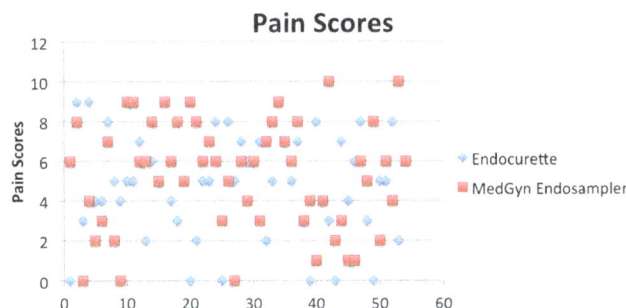

Fig. 5 Scatter plot of pain scores reported by women in all groups; x-axis representing the study number of participants

Table 2 Endometrial pathology in post-menopausal women

Histological findings	Post-menopausal women (%)
Atrophic endometrium	78.4
Benign pathology (endometrial polyps, simple hyperplasia)	17.6
Endometrial cancer	3.9

difficulties between the two devices. No difference in the number of inadequate samples was observed. There was no difference in the number of women consenting to a repeat procedure if required, or recommendation to others. The majority of women found the procedure to be less uncomfortable than expected, but this assertion did not correlate with low pain scores.

Pain scores were reported for the hysteroscopy and endometrial biopsy procedures separately using a visual analogue scale. As these were subsequent procedures, pain scores for both devices could have been affected. However, no significant differences between pain scores for hysteroscopy in both groups were seen. Significantly more women in the Endosampler® group had pain scores of ≥5. This could be explained by the degree of negative pressure generated within the uterine cavity with Endosampler® compared with Endocurette®, together with the technique of 'gentle radial curettage' similar to that done during a D&C. However no significant difference was found between devices when pain scores of ≥8 (severe pain) were examined. This could be limited by the sample size in this study, as only 22 women had pain scores of ≥8; 14 in the Endosampler® group and 8 in the Endocurette® group. The total number of insertions required to obtain a visually adequate endometrial sample was significantly higher in the Endocurette® group. This can be attributed to differences in the design of the two devices. Multiple device insertions theoretically pose a risk of subsequent postprocedural endometritis; however, this complication was not studied. There was no significant difference between the two devices in terms of ease of handling.

We believe that this study has good methodological strength. Women were randomised to either sampling devices in a manner allocating approximately equal numbers in each group according to menopausal status. Effort was also made to minimise potential bias in this study. Women and pathologists were blinded to the device used, allowing objective assessment of pain scores and histology samples. Only two operators were involved in performing sampling to ensure consistency in the technique used. The devices were used according to manufacturers' instructions. Although women and pathologists were blinded to the device used, it was impossible for the operator to be blinded due to the difference in the design and technique used for each device. A limitation of this study is that whilst repeated device insertions could potentially increase the risk of procedure-related endometritis, postprocedure complications were not recorded in the context of this study. Furthermore, the study was not designed to evaluate this risk, which would require a larger sample size, as the incidence of post-procedural endometritis is low. Time taken to obtain a visually adequate sample is likely to have been less in the Endosampler group, but this was not evaluated in our study.

Many studies have compared different endometrial sampling devices in recent decades; however, this is the first study which compares Endosampler® and Endocurette®. The adequacy of sample volume was assessed both subjectively by the clinician and objectively by the pathologist. The inadequate sample rate with both devices was comparable to that of Pipelle® in the published literature, and no significant difference was shown between the two devices in this respect [12]. The rate of diagnosis of endometrial malignancy was comparable to results of previous research [15]. The inadequate sample rate was much higher in post-menopausal women, which is to be expected given the high rate of endometrial atrophy in this group. Whilst some studies suggest further investigation [13–16], in the presence of a normal hysteroscopy, the need for further sampling is questionable. In terms of pain scores, similar visual analogue scoring systems were used in prior studies. Mean pain scores reported for the Pipelle vary between 1 and 6 [10, 11, 14], [17]. Studies comparing various sampling devices reported mean pain scores ranging from 1 to 6.9, comparable to our study [10, 11, 14, 17].

Comparison of different sampling devices is important in light of the increasing availability of outpatient hysteroscopy for the investigation of abnormal uterine bleeding. This study amongst others provides a comparison of two endometrial sampling devices used in an outpatient hysteroscopy setting. Whilst no significant difference in the handling of the devices and number of inadequate samples was observed, there was a significantly lower rate of multiple insertions recorded with Endosampler®, albeit at the expense of a higher mean pain score. In an outpatient hysteroscopy clinic setting where saline is used as the distension medium and a considerable amount of fluid may be present in the uterine cavity, it is particularly useful to use a device which minimises the number of device insertions. The higher pain scores experienced by patients in the Endosampler group, interestingly, did not translate into unwillingness to have the procedure again, or to recommend the procedure to others.

Future studies should seek to evaluate the performance of other available endometrial sampling devices in similar settings. Studies involving larger numbers should also be supported to compare and document the incidence of postprocedural endometritis.

Conclusion

No significant differences in operational difficulties, sample adequacy or acceptability to patients were shown between groups. Higher overall pain scores at endometrial biopsy were reported when Endosampler® was used, although not in the severe pain category and not translating into a reluctance to undergo a similar procedure in the future, or recommend the procedure to others. Significantly fewer device insertions were required with Endosampler® to obtain a visually satisfactory biopsy sample. The design of Endosampler® allows removal of the distension medium during saline outpatient hysteroscopy without the need for removal and reinsertion of the device catheter. On this basis, we conclude that Endosampler® may be superior to Endocurette® in an outpatient hysteroscopy clinic setting.

Acknowledgments Special thanks to nursing, midwifery and secretarial staff involved in the Outpatient Hysteroscopy Clinic, CUMH as well as all women who kindly volunteered to participate in the study.

Reference

1. Ghaly S, de Abreu Lourenco R, Abbott JA (2008) Audit of endometrial biopsy at outpatient hysteroscopy. Aust NZ J Obstet Gynaecol 48(2):202–206
2. Russell JB (1988) History and development of hysteroscopy. Obstet Gynecol Clin N Am 15:1–11
3. Huang GS, Gebb JS, Einstein MH et al (2007) Accuracy of preoperative endometrial sampling for the detection of high-grade endometrial tumors. Am J Obstet Gynecol 196(243):e1–e5
4. Madari S, Al-Shabibi N, Papalampros P, Papadimitriou A, Magos A (2009) A randomised trial comparing the H Pipelle with the standard Pipelle for endometrial sampling at 'no touch' (vaginoscopic) hysteroscopy. BJOG 116:32 37
5. Agostini A, Shojai R, Cravello L et al (2001) Endometrial biopsy during outpatient hysteroscopy: evaluation and comparison of two devices. Eur J Obstet Gynecol Reprod Med 97:220–222
6. Tanriverdi HA, Barut A, Gün BD, Kaya E (2004) Is pipelle biopsy really adequate for diagnosing endometrial disease? Med Sci Monit 10:CR271–CR274
7. Machado F, Moreno J, Carazo M, León J, Fiol G, Serna R (2003) Accuracy of endometrial biopsy with the Cornier pipelle for diagnosis of endometrial cancer and atypical hyperplasia. Eur J Gynaecol Oncol 24(3–4):279–281
8. Teale GR, Dunster GD (1998) The Pipelle endometrial suction curette: how useful is it in clinical practice? J Obstet Gynaecol 18:53–55
9. Stovall TG, Ling FW, Morgan PL (1991) A prospective, randomized comparison of the Pipelle endometrial sampling device with the Novak curette. Am J Obstet Gynecol 165:1287–1290
10. Naim NM, Mahdy ZA, Ahmad S, Razi ZR (2007) The Vabra aspirator versus the Pipelle device for outpatient endometrial sampling. Aust N Z J Obstet Gynaecol 47:132–136
11. Lipscomb GH, Lopatine SM, Stovall TG, Ling FW (1994) A randomized comparison of the Pipelle, accurette, and explora endometrial sampling devices. Am J Obstet Gynecol 170:591–594
12. Renaud MC, Le T, Le T et al (2013) Epidemiology and investigations for suspected endometrial cancer. J Obstet Gynaecol Can 35:380–383
13. Farrell T, Jones N, Owen P, Baird A (1999) The significance of an 'insufficient' Pipelle sample in the investigation of post-menopausal bleeding. Acta Obstet Gynecol Scand 78:810–812
14. Gordon SJ, Westgate J (1999) The incidence and management of failed Pipelle sampling in a general outpatient clinic. Aust N Z J Obstet Gynaecol 39:115–118
15. Renaud MC, Le T, Le T, et al (2013) Epidemiology and investigations for suspected endometrial cancer. J Obstet Gynaeco Can 35: 380–3
16. Gordon SJ, Westgate J (1999) The incidence and management of failed Pipelle sampling in a general outpatient clinic. Aust N Z J Obstet Gynaecol 39:115–8
17. Leclair CM, Zia JK, Doom CM, Morgan TK, Edelman AB (2011) Pain experienced using two different methods of endometrial biopsy: a randomized controlled trial. Obstet Gynecol 117: 636–641

33

Tailor-made proficiency curves in laparoscopic hysterectomy: enhancing patient safety using CUSUM analysis

A. R. H. Twijnstra · M. D. Blikkendaal · S. R. C. Driessen ·
E. W. van Zwet · C. D. de Kroon · F. W. Jansen

Abstract The objective of this study is to develop a risk-adjusted real-time quality control system in laparoscopic hysterectomy with respect to blood loss, operative time and adverse events in order to signal derailing surgical performance in a timely fashion. Based on prior research, uterus weight, body mass index, number of surgeons, prior abdominal surgery, and type of laparoscopic hysterectomy were identified as significant covariates predicting successful surgical outcome. Cumulative sum (CUSUM) analysis, a model based on dichotomous input (success or "failure"), was selected as a predictive tool for performance analysis. Cutoff values were set at blood loss <200 mL and operative time <120 min and no adverse event. Risk-adjusted CUSUM graphs were constructed. In order to detect progressive failure rates (odds ratio 2.0 compared to average) in surgical performance (for blood loss, operative time, and adverse events) within 20 procedures, as a result, surgeons with average clinical outcomes will be flagged once in every 70–75 procedures (median) without justified derailing performance. With proposed validated and risk-adjusted CUSUM graphs, gynecologists are able to continuously monitor their surgical performance in laparoscopic hysterectomy. Consequently, this identifies suboptimal factors, which allow improvement of their

surgical outcomes (by means of adjustment) and further enhancement of patient safety.

Keywords Hysterectomy · Laparoscopy · Quality control · CUSUM · Patient safety

Introduction

In order to enhance patient safety, it has become increasingly important to measure outcome in health care. Surgical outcomes such as blood loss, operative time, and the occurrence of adverse events are widespread applied instant measures. These measures, as well as skills and experience of the surgeon (usually expressed by the number of performed cases) are currently still used as quality predictors [1]. However, it is also established that surgical outcome, apart from surgical experience, is influenced by co-factors such as the makeup of the OR team and (inherently) patient factors (i.e., the case mix). These factors are not taken into account when the aforementioned crude and unadjusted parameters are used to measure and present the actual surgical outcome [2, 3].

With respect to patient-related factors, recent research in laparoscopic hysterectomy (LH) demonstrated five significant covariates predicting successful outcome: uterus weight, body mass index, number of surgeons present at surgery, prior abdominal surgery, and type of laparoscopic hysterectomy (i.e., total laparoscopic hysterectomy, supracervical laparoscopic hysterectomy, or laparoscopic-assisted vaginal hysterectomy) [4]. Moreover, experience is predicting successful surgical outcome in LH, with respect to blood loss and adverse events, up to at least a hundred procedures. This finding was also observed in the field of advanced colorectal laparoscopic surgery [5, 6]. Finally, recent research demonstrated a

A. R. H. Twijnstra · M. D. Blikkendaal · S. R. C. Driessen ·
C. D. de Kroon · F. W. Jansen (✉)
Department of Gynecology, Leiden University Medical Center, PO Box 9600, 2300 RC Leiden, The Netherlands
e-mail: f.w.jansen@lumc.nl

E. W. van Zwet
Department of Medical Statistics, Leiden University Medical Center, Leiden, The Netherlands

F. W. Jansen
Department of Biomechanical Engineering, Delft University of Technology, Delft, The Netherlands

significant experience independent and case mix-adjusted surgical skills factor (SSF) with regard to successful outcome in LH [4].

The aforementioned findings support that surgical outcomes in laparoscopic hysterectomy should be monitored consecutively, as both case mix and surgeon's skills may vary over time, and experience alone is not sufficiently predicting these outcomes. Parallel to the traditional outcome measures, the traditional single outcome learning curves in surgery, which were applied in order to assess surgical proficiency, do not take these findings into account [7–10]. Monitoring tools based on cumulative sum (CUSUM) analysis, already used in obstetrics and general surgery, overcome these shortcomings [11–16]. In the industrial setting, since 1974, CUSUM charts have been shown to be ideally suited to detect relatively small persistent changes in the event rates over time [3]. Traditional CUSUM approaches, however, make no adjustment for different risk profiles because machine inputs are usually relatively homogeneous. In contrast, patients undergoing a particular surgical intervention are often very heterogeneous in their clinical presentation. Additionally, the surgical approach may vary considerably due to the clinical presentation as well as the preference of the surgeon. As a result, the probability of successful outcome may vary considerably between patients. By using a likelihood-based scoring method, the cumulative sum procedure is adapted so that it adjusts for the surgical risk of each patient estimated preoperatively [2, 17, 18]. As a result, the user will be provided with a graphical representation of its surgical outcomes corrected for patient mix and instantly compared to the national average. Trends will be visualized, and significant deterioration in surgical outcome will be noticed.

In gynecology, nowadays, a shift in implementing more advanced surgical procedures is observed. However, several studies suggest that these advanced laparoscopic surgical procedures are characterized by a specific proficiency gaining curve due to the acquirement of unique operative skills [19]. Consequently, this learning curve is considered a barrier for widespread implementation of advanced laparoscopic surgery [5]. Other research already revealed that even in basic laparoscopy, nearly a fifth of surgeons never gain proficient skills to perform laparoscopic surgery adequately [20]. These insights, combined with the call for constant monitoring of patient safety, make us strive for risk-adjusted continuous quality assessments during mentorships and beyond in order to adjust performance when quality of surgery is at risk.

The aim of this study is to develop such a tool. In order to signal derailing surgical performance in a timely fashion, a risk-adjusted real-time quality control system for laparoscopic hysterectomy is analyzed, inquired, and launched.

Methods

A previously described data set of 1.534 LHs, performed by 79 surgeons, was used to validate and compose a risk adjusted CUSUM graph in LH [4]. Significant predicting covariates were included. These consisted of uterus weight, body mass index, number of surgeons present at surgery, prior abdominal surgery, and type of laparoscopic hysterectomy (Table 1).

The CUSUM score depends on four factors: the current average level of surgical performance, a chosen level of surgical performance deemed undesirable, the patient's surgical risk estimated preoperatively, and the actual surgical outcome in this patient. Preoperative surgical risk estimation was based on body mass index, uterus weight, and prior abdominal surgery. With respect to the continuous surgical outcomes, blood loss, and operative time, these were dichotomized using the rounded mean observed value. Consequently, successful surgical outcome was determined as blood loss <200 mL, operative time <120 min, and no adverse event. Because incidences of these outcomes varied, with accompanying

Table 1 Association between predictors and primary outcomes in laparoscopic hysterectomy

	Blood loss (>200 mL)	Operative time (>120 min)	Adverse event (yes)
Uterus weight increase per 100 g	*0.33 (P< 0.0001)*	*0.40 (P< 0.0001)*	*0.18 (P= 0.0002)*
Body Mass Index increase per 1 point (kg/m^2)	*0.28 (P< 0.0001)*	0.18 (P=0.0841)	0.02 (P=0.221)
Numbers of previous abdominal surgeries	0.19 (P=0.54)	0.78 (P=0.782)	*0.48 (P= 0.048)*
Two surgeons (vs. one)	−0.47 (P=0.072)	*0.64 (P= 0.028)*	0.05 (P=0.811)
LAVH vs. TLH	*0.91 (P= 0.0274)*	0.04 (P=0.915)	0.33 (P=0.306)
SLH vs. TLH	−0.14 (P=0.482)	*−0.47 (P= 0.032)*	−0.52 (P=0.079)

Positive predictors represent higher chance of suboptimal primary outcome, and negative predictors represent lower chance of suboptimal primary outcome. Italicized items are significant predictors

LAVH laparoscopic-assisted vaginal hysterectomy, *TLH* total laparoscopic hysterectomy, *SLH* supracervical laparoscopic hysterectomy

varying influences of covariates, we applied three risk-adjusted CUSUM graphs, one for each outcome.

With the chosen level of surgical performance deemed undesirable, we aimed to minimize the number of procedures before possible derailing performance is signaled, while minimizing "false alarms". For quality control, a lower boundary line is not used. To allow a sensitive and timely detection of "eventful" procedures, this model resets itself to 0, each time the x-axis is hit [18]. As a consequence, the median number of procedures needed to detect an unacceptable failure rate (in case a surgeon performs below an acceptable level) is based on the upper boundary ("out of control", odds ratio of 2 compared to average performance). Nevertheless, this model cannot prevent that also average clinical performance every once in a while is "flagged" as derailing (Fig. 2). The primary outcome of this study is the number of procedures after which surgeons are flagged, both true positive and false positive.

To apply a risk-adjusted (i.e., based on the patient's surgical risk estimated preoperatively) CUSUM analysis, we have to estimate the logistic regression model as described earlier [4]. Based on this model, we can compute the probability of an unfavorable outcome (failure) for each procedure. For ease of notation, suppose we use only uterus weight Ut as a predictor. Then, provided that the surgeon is performing exactly on the national average (i.e., is in control), the probability of failure in procedure i is:

$$p0(i) = 1/(1 + \exp(-\beta 0 - \beta 1 \times Ut(i)))$$

$\beta 0$ the intercept in the logistic regression model
$\beta 1$ log odds ratio for uterus weight

If the surgeon performs worse than average (OR=2 compared to the national average), the probability of failure becomes larger and is given by:

$$p1(i) = p0 = 1/(1 + \exp(-\beta 0 - \beta 1 \times Ut(i) - \log(2)))$$

Given the outcome of procedure i, we can compute the log likelihood ratio as

$$W(i) = \begin{cases} \log\ (p0/p1) & \text{if failure} \\ \log((1-p0)/(1-p1)) & \text{if success} \end{cases}$$

Now, we construct the CUSUM graph by plotting $X(i) = \max(0, X(i-1) + W(i))$

This X will provide the actual direction and weight of the outcome of procedure i on the CUSUM graph corrected for uterus weight. In our model, we included all covariates (uterus weight increase per 100 g, BMI increase per 5 points, numbers

of prior abdominal surgeries, 1 or 2 performing surgeons, and type of laparoscopic hysterectomy).

Results

Figure 1 provides an example of the principle of a risk-adjusted CUSUM graph of 21 consecutive LHs in one surgeon with respect to blood loss <200 mL. The horizontal axis represents the numbers of consecutive procedures. The vertical axis represents the cumulative sum of the risk-adjusted scores per procedure. As can be seen at "no. 1," the fourth procedure was complicated by blood loss >200 mL in a regular patient, followed by three regular procedures with blood loss <200 mL. The eighth procedure (no. 2) was performed uneventful in a "challenging patient" (e.g., high BMI and large uterus weight). At the 13th procedure (no. 3), blood loss >200 mL occurred; however, this occurred in a challenging case (high BMI and large uterus weight compared to no. 1). At the 15th procedure, another failure occurred (no. 4), however, because of average patient characteristics (see also Table 1); this procure was expected to be performed uneventful. A steep rise on the curve represents this discordance between the observed and expected outcome. At attempt number 21 (no. 5), the CUSUM graph goes out of control. Consequently, the chart signals.

For the defined outcomes of LH, respectively blood loss, operative time, and adverse events separate risk-adjusted CUSUM graphs that were constructed. In order to detect unacceptable failure rates (clinical performance OR 2.0 compared to average clinical performance) in surgical

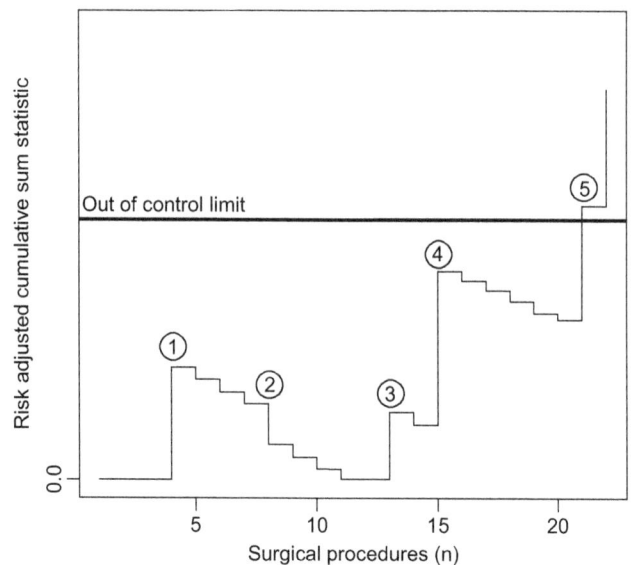

Fig. 1 Example of a cumulative summation analysis graph in one gynecologist with respect to blood loss <200 mL (see "Results" for explanation)

performance within 20 procedures, as a result, a surgeon with average surgical outcomes will be flagged without justified bad performance once in approximately every 70–75 procedures respectively (Fig. 2). Reference values are based on the previously described cohort of 1.534 procedures performed by 79 gynecologists.

Once one of the three CUSUM graphs signals, one should analyze at least 20 of its past performed procedures using a concise checklist, as depicted in Table 2. Five fields address possible causes. If one or more fields are ticked once ore more, this field should be studied and addressed in particular. This checklist is not validated yet.

Web-based non-commercial and protected application is available in order to process the proposed CUSUM graphs in the field of LH in order to provide the surgeon his/her performance statistics at a glance (https://www.qusum.org). The program is primarily designed for a national multicenter validation study; however, one is free to register and apply the application. This software should be easily integrated with (existing) data recording systems in the near future. The five characteristics (uterus weight in grams, body mass index (kg/m^2), number of previous abdominal surgeries, one or two surgeons, type of LH, and the three primary outcomes (operative time in minutes, blood loss in milliliters, and adverse event) can be entered immediately postoperatively or at any given moment.

Table 2 Check list after signaling of CUSUM graph

Factor	Example
Patient	Unexpected co-morbidity
Surgeon	Fatigue, stress, and inaccurate indication
Team	Communication and staff's experience
Equipment	Altered vision and new coagulation device
Logistic	Tight scheduled operation programs

Discussion

With proposed validated and risk-adjusted CUSUM graphs, gynecologists have the ability to continuously monitor their surgical performance in laparoscopic hysterectomy, consequently identifying suboptimal factors with respect to operative time, blood loss, and adverse events. As a result, they are able to enhance patient safety.

Despite correction for patient case mix (i.e., identified risk factors), this analysis model still inevitably yields flagging of surgeons with average clinical performance. This is due to the sensitivity of the model. If the CUSUM analysis has to identify derailing performance (OR 2 compared to average performance) in surgeons within a reasonable number of procedures (i.e., 20 laparoscopic hysterectomies), occasional flagging of surgeons with average clinical performance is inevitable.

Fig. 2 Threshold curves for blood loss, operative time, and adverse events. Horizontal axis represents amount procedures before flagging in case of out-of-control performance (OR 2.0 compared to average performance). When performing exactly on average, flagging will occur as frequent as depicted on the vertical axis

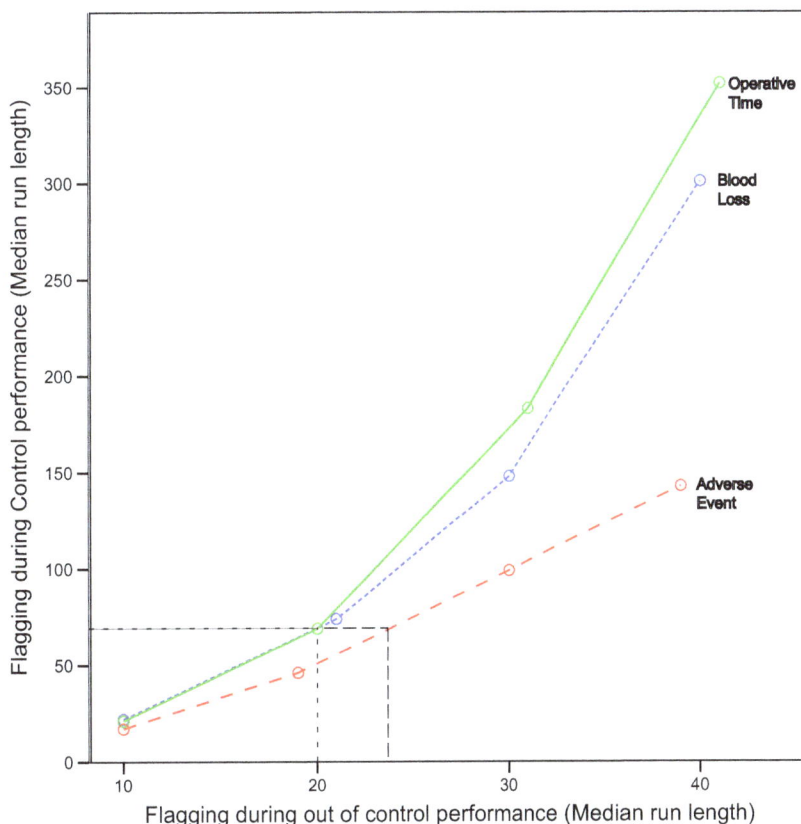

These proposed cutoff limits are set primarily to identify possible suboptimal situations and to enhance patient safety. The goal is twofold. Firstly, by alarming out of control limits in a timely fashion, the surgeon can evaluate his/her performance as well as of its surgical team and even its equipment and act if necessary. Secondly, by providing (national) averages as a standard of care, hypothetically at long-term, also suboptimal performing surgeons that do not cross the out-of-control line will improve their outcomes.

Although this proposed CUSUM system for laparoscopic hysterectomy is based on national averages of Dutch cohort in 2009, we suggest that the reference values are applicable to every gynecologist. The proposed cutoff values might appear "mild." However, if these values are raised, as a consequence, signaling will be delayed. This will result in less adequate flagging of potentially derailing performance.

If implemented in a straightforward digital registry tool (or stand alone computer program), this CUSUM for LH provides easy to understand and swift to apply insight into tailor-made proficiency curves. We suggest that out-of-control signaling should primarily be discussed internally and only after a certain acclimatizing period should be discussed with expert peers in order to identify suboptimal care and to provide "Best Practices."

A number of aspects of the proposed model should be addressed. Firstly, is the average signaling rate of one in 75 procedures in surgeons with average clinical performance acceptable? Yes, however, proper information and efficient evaluation are a prerequisite. Time-consuming evaluation will harm initial motivation. When a CUSUM chart goes out of control, one should be provided with a concise check box-based questionnaire in order to signal the origin of derailing performance (Table 2). This could be due to skills, technical issues, misjudging of a series of cases, problems with the OR team, etc. These issues should be directed. Secondly, ideally, the CUSUM chart (and preferably also its evaluation system) should be integrated and implemented in an already existing electronic patient file system. Registration of patient data in multiple sources will affect quality and quantity of data. Thirdly, the national averages set in this tool should be updated on a frequent basis, preferably every 5 years. Hypothetically, the cohort will improve its surgical outcomes over time. As a result, averages and out-of-control limits should be fine-tuned as well.

An example is found in the field of (surgical) oncology in which the value of continuous quality assurance is well studied [21–23]. However, these examples use evaluation of care on a yearly basis and often lack correction for patient case mix. Furthermore, most of these registries use adverse events as sole primary outcome and direct hospitals rather than surgeons personally. Some registries reflect hospital outcomes to national averages; however, most systems compare to (outdated) literature. CUSUM analysis addresses all abovementioned points of interest.

For a start, the CUSUM should be applied and compared indoors only. By means of a multicenter prospective cohort study, the proposed cutoff values are validated as well as the feasibility of this system should be researched. More information as well as the web-based CUSUM tool can be found on www.qusum.org. In conclusion, applying CUSUM charts as quality assurance for the surgical performance and clinical outcome measures in LH might enhance patient safety.

Informed consent All procedures followed were in accordance with the ethical standards of the responsible committee on human experimentation (institutional and national) and with the Helsinki Declaration of 1975, as revised in 2000. The Ethical Committee decided that no informed consent was mandatory in this observational study.

References

1. Hopper AN, Jamison MH, Lewis WG (2007) Learning curves in surgical practice. Postgrad Med J 83(986):777–779
2. Steiner SH, Cook RJ, Farewell VT, Treasure T (2000) Monitoring surgical performance using risk-adjusted cumulative sum charts. Biostatistics 1(4):441–452
3. Biau DJ, Resche-Rigon M, Godiris-Petit G, Nizard RS, Porcher R (2007) Quality control of surgical and interventional procedures: a review of the CUSUM. Qual Saf Health Care 16(3):203–207
4. Twijnstra AR, Blikkendaal MD, van Zwet EW, van Kesteren PJ, de Kroon CD, Jansen FW (2012) Predictors of successful surgical outcome in laparoscopic hysterectomy. Obstet Gynecol 119(4): 700–708
5. Park IJ, Choi GS, Lim KH, Kang BM, Jun SH (2009) Multidimensional analysis of the learning curve for laparoscopic colorectal surgery: lessons from 1,000 cases of laparoscopic colorectal surgery. Surg Endosc 23(4):839–846
6. Cheng JM, Duan H, Wang JJ, Zhang HT, Liu Y (2007) Clinical analysis of conversion from gynecological laparoscopic surgery to laparotomy. Zhonghua Fu Chan Ke Za Zhi 42(3):173–175
7. Perino A, Cucinella G, Venezia R, Castelli A, Cittadini E (1999) Total laparoscopic hysterectomy versus total abdominal hysterectomy: an assessment of the learning curve in a prospective randomized study. Hum Reprod 14(12):2996–2999
8. Wattiez A, Soriano D, Cohen SB, Nervo P, Canis M, Botchorishvili R et al (2002) The learning curve of total laparoscopic hysterectomy: comparative analysis of 1647 cases. J Am Assoc Gynecol Laparosc 9 (3):339–345
9. Leminen A (2000) Comparison between personal learning curves for abdominal and laparoscopic hysterectomy. Acta Obstet Gynecol Scand 79(12):1100–1104
10. Altgassen C, Michels W, Schneider A (2004) Learning laparoscopic-assisted hysterectomy. Obstet Gynecol 104(2):308–313
11. de Saintonge DM, Vere DW (1974) Why don't doctors use CUSUMs? Lancet 1:120–121

12. Schlachta CM, Mamazza J, Seshadri PA, Cadeddu M, Gregoire R, Poulin EC (2001) Defining a learning curve for laparoscopic colorectal resections. Dis Colon Rectum 44(2): 217–222

13. Bolsin S, Colson M (2000) The use of the Cusum technique in the assessment of trainee competence in new procedures. Int J Qual Health Care 12(5):433–438

14. Weerasinghe S, Mirghani H, Revel A, bu-Zidan FM (2006) Cumulative sum (CUSUM) analysis in the assessment of trainee competence in fetal biometry measurement. Ultrasound Obstet Gynecol 28(2):199–203

15. Boulkedid R, Sibony O, Bossu-Salvador C, Oury JF, Alberti C (2010) Monitoring healthcare quality in an obstetrics and gynaecology department using a CUSUM chart. BJOG

16. Lindenburg IT, Wolterbeek R, Oepkes D, Klumper FJ, Vandenbussche FP, van Kamp IL (2011) Quality control for intravascular intrauterine transfusion using cumulative sum (CUSUM) analysis for the monitoring of individual performance. Fetal Diagn Ther 29(4):307–314

17. Steiner SH, Cook RJ, Farewell VT (2001) Risk-adjusted monitoring of binary surgical outcomes. Med Dec Making 21(3):163–169

18. Grigg OA, Farewell VT, Spiegelhalter DJ (2003) Use of risk-adjusted CUSUM and RSPRT charts for monitoring in medical contexts. Stat Methods Med Res 12(2):147–170

19. Aggarwal R, Moorthy K, Darzi A (2004) Laparoscopic skills training and assessment. Br J Surg 91(12):1549–1558

20. Schijven MP, Jakimowicz J (2004) The learning curve on the Xitact LS 500 laparoscopy simulator: profiles of performance. Surg Endosc 18(1):121–127

21. Landheer ML, Therasse P, van de Velde CJ (2002) The importance of quality assurance in surgical oncology. Eur J Surg Oncol 28(6):571–602

22. Peeters KC, van de Velde CJ (2003) Surgical quality assurance in breast, gastric and rectal cancer. J Surg Oncol 84(3):107–112

23. Verleye L, Vergote I, Reed N, Ottevanger PB (2009) Quality assurance for radical hysterectomy for cervical cancer: the view of the European Organization for Research and Treatment of Cancer–Gynecological Cancer Group (EORTC-GCG). Ann Oncol 20(10): 1631–1638

34

Ovarian endometrioma in the adolescent: a plea for early-stage diagnosis and full surgical treatment

Stephan Gordts · Patrick Puttemans · Sylvie Gordts ·
Ivo Brosens

Abstract The incidence and severity of endometriosis in adolescent are comparable with the incidence in adult women. The mean delay between the onset of symptoms and the final diagnosis varies between 6.4 and 11.7 years. The longer the diagnosis is delayed, the more the endometriosis can progress to a more severe stage certainly in the group of patients with pelvic pain. The evolution of endometriosis and its progressivity are not predictable, and the severity of the disease is not directly related to the degree of pain. Endometriotic cysts have a detrimental effect on the ovarian reserve by the evolution in time and the surgical excision technique. Already, in small endometriotic cysts (<4 cm), loss of follicular reserve is present together with the formation of fibrosis in the cortex of the ovary. Early diagnosis of endometriosis in the adolescent deserves our full attention. Non-invasive imaging techniques like 2-D and 3-D ultrasound are helpful in the early diagnosis. Early ablative surgery is recommendable. Although laparoscopy is traditionally recommended, transvaginal laparoscopy has been shown to be most effective in ablating endometriomas with a maximum diameter of 3 cm. Early detection and intervention will contribute to a better quality of life in these adolescents and also to a lower damage of the ovarian tissue by a less invasive ablative surgery.

Keywords Ovarian endometriosis · Adolescence · Surgery · Transvaginal · Laparoscopy

S. Gordts (✉) · P. Puttemans · S. Gordts · I. Brosens
Leuven Institute for Fertility & Embryology, Tiensevest 168,
3000 Leuven, Belgium
e-mail: Stephan.gordts@lifeleuven.be

Introduction

Ovarian endometriosis, a disease similar to the Mona Lisa face, fails to be grasped and identified by current descriptions. At present, the diagnosis requires an invasive surgical technique, whether laparotomy or laparoscopy, to diagnose the presence of ectopic endometrium-like tissue. In the young woman, the symptoms may be suggestive, but vary greatly and elicit frequent compassion rather than investigation and treatment. Nevertheless, understanding endometriosis in the young woman may shed light on the more complex appearance in the adult woman and improve early-stage management [1]. This review will address the recent literature regarding premenarchal and adolescent endometriosis and discuss in particular the inherent risks of the delay in diagnosis and management of ovarian involvement.

Premenarchal and adolescent endometriosis

Endometriosis is described as premenarchal and distinguished from adolescent when symptoms and lesions occur during the phase of telarche before the menarche.

Premenarchal endometriosis

Marsh and Laufer [2] identified, in 2005, endometriosis as a cause of chronic pelvic pain in five premenarchal girls without an obstructive anomaly of the reproductive tract. Breast development in the patients ranged from Tanner I to Tanner III, and non-gynecological etiologies for pelvic pain were excluded. All subjects had laparoscopy with the identification of multiple clear and red lesions consistent with stromal endometriosis. Postoperatively, all of the girls had marked improvement of their pelvic pain based on self-reported pain scales. Two of the subjects had subsequent repeat laparoscopies 6 and 8 years after their initial surgery, which revealed classical endometriosis. More cases of endometriosis occurring before or around the time of menarche have been documented. Gogacz et al. [3] described an 11-year-old patient with a left ovarian endometrioma. Her menarche occurred spontaneously 6 months after surgery. Ebert et al. [4] reported on a 9-year-old premenarchal girl with cyclic pelvic pain since her 8th year of life. Multiple clear, red, and vascularized flame-like peritoneal lesions were observed. The resected lesions showed cytogenic stroma, small glands, and pigment-carrying macrophages.

Adolescent endometriosis

Originally described more than a century ago, endometriosis is thought of as a disease that affects adult women, but there is increasing awareness of its presence in young women. The disorder represents already in the young woman a vague and perplexing entity that frequently results in chronic pelvic pain, adhesive disease, and infertility. Differences exist between adolescent and adult types of endometriosis, but it is likely that diagnosis and treatment during adolescence decrease disease progression and prevent subsequent reproductive failure. The first study of adolescent endometriosis by Hanton et al. [5] covered the Mayo Clinic experience from 1935 until 1964 and included 68 young patients. The authors tried to determine the frequency, relation to menarche, and outcome. Sixty-three (93 %) out of the 68 patients experienced menarche 5 to 10 years before diagnosis, 9 could not date menarche but were 21 or younger at diagnosis, and 6 had congenital obstruction to menstrual flow. Usually, patients complained of dysmenorrhea or other pelvic pain, but 11 (16 %) had no pelvic complaints. Only three complained chiefly of infertility. Ten patients initially had procedures ablating menstrual function and 58 had conservative operations. One month to 25 years after conservative treatment, 15 patients required subsequent operation, radical in 12 cases. Subsequent fertility was about 50 % in this study. Parker and collaborators [6] recently investigated menstrual pain and other symptoms in teenagers to evaluate how many experience a degree of menstrual disturbance that needs to be further investigated. In a population of 1051 girls aged between 15 and 19 years, the authors concluded that menstrual pain and symptoms are common in teenagers. Girls indicating moderate to severe pain in association with a high number of menstrual symptoms, school absence, and interference with life activities should be effectively managed to minimize menstrual morbidity. Those girls who do not respond to medical management should be considered for further investigation for possible underlying pathology, such as endometriosis. In a study of Laufer et al. [7, 8], the prevalence of endometriosis in adolescents with chronic pelvic pain not responding to medical therapy was 69.6 %.

A recent Chinese study by Yang et al. [9] included 63 patients less than 20 years old with surgically diagnosed endometriosis at the Peking Union Medical College Hospital from 1992 to 2010. Mean age at diagnosis was 18.41 ± 1.84 years with a much earlier disease onset in adolescents with genital tract malformations. Of the 35 patients with follow-up time that ranged from 12 to 98 months, 9 in 15 patients discontinued medical treatment after operation and had a recurrence. Seven in 15 patients who took oral contraceptive pills or progestin only pills had recurrence, but none of the five patients receiving gonadotropin-releasing hormone agonist. Among the 15 cases without postoperative medical therapy, all five cases with lesions at multiple sites had recurrence, while only four of the other ten cases had relapse. The difference was of statistical significance (Fisher's exact test, $P=0.044$). The authors concluded that the presence of lesions at multiple sites is a risk factor of recurrence and that GnRHa can effectively prevent the recurrence.

Recent studies of endometriosis in adolescents show clearly that the disease is no longer characterized by subtle superficial lesions, but also by the presence of ovarian adhesions and endometriomas [1]. Comparison of the clinical features of the endometrioma in adolescent women to women of other age groups by Lee et al. [10] showed that adolescent females experienced menarche at a significantly earlier age and that the main symptom was pain (77 %). The proportion of incidental detection (23 %) was low in comparison with women older than 30 years. The authors concluded that, apart from pain, there were no other differences between the age groups. Apparently, adolescent endometriosis is a hidden, debilitating, and progressive disease that deserves greater attention for diagnosis and more appropriate management for the preservation of the integrity of reproductive life.

Views on the pathogenesis of premenarchal endometriosis

The presence of peritoneal and ovarian endometriosis in premenarchal girls without an obstructive anomaly has supported the concept that endometriosis may result from an etiology other than retrograde menses as proposed by Sampson in 1927 [11]. Batt and Mitwally [12] have argued for recognition of embryonic Mullerian rests as the pathogenesis in cases of early endometriosis not explained by accepted theories. Along with John Huffman, a founder of the subspecialty of pediatric and adolescent gynecology in North America, they proposed that telarche be recognized as a developmental benchmark, after which endometriosis is included in the differential diagnosis of chronic pelvic pain. In recent years, Signorile et al. [13, 14] demonstrated the presence of ectopic endometrium in human female fetuses at different gestational ages. They suggested that endometriosis is caused by dislocation of primitive endometrial tissue outside the uterine cavity during organogenesis. Also, Bouquet de Jolinière et al. [15] described the presence of misplaced endometrial glands and embryonic duct remnants in six of seven fetuses referring to the possible theory of involvement of Müllerian or Wolffian cell rests in the pathogenesis of endometriosis.

Following the current available evidence regarding stem/progenitor cells in the human endometrium, Oliveira et al. [16] suggested the possible involvement of these cells in the etiology of endometriosis. The identification of stem cells in animal and human tissues is, however, very complex, and the putative stem cells are supposed to be found through several assays such as clonogenicity, label-retaining cells, "side population" cells, undifferentiating markers, and cellular differentiation. Bone marrow-derived stem cells transplanted into humans and animals have also been identified in eutopic endometrium and endometriotic implants. The actual scientific knowledge obtained on the existence of somatic stem cells in the murine and human endometrium and the implication and biological pathways of these cells in endometriosis has been recently reviewed by Cervello et al. [17]. Recently, Brosens and Benagiano [18] formulated the hypothesis that perinatal uterine bleeding occurring in some newborns—a phenomenon that is routinely discounted as insignificant—may be a cause of premenarchal and adolescent endometriosis. The hypothesis is based on anatomical and functional observations. First, in the perinatal period, the fetal endometrium shows decidualization, shedding, and bleeding in some 5 % of the newborn girls [19, 20]. Secondly, the anatomical structure of the neonatal uterus favors, in contrast with menstrual bleeding, tubal reflux [21]. Thirdly, in premenarchal endometriosis, the sites of implantations have a similar pelvic pattern as in adolescent and adult endometriosis [2]. Fourthly, Arcellana has documented a case of neonatal endometriosis in 1996 [22]. Finally, neonatal and premenarchal lesions with scanty glandular development seem to reflect a stromal endometriosis that later develops into an adolescent and adult type of endometriosis. For these reasons, there is no reason to postulate a different origin and pathogenesis for premenarchal, adolescent, and adult endometriosis. Sampson's hypothesis can be modified by assuming the perinatal bleeding as the first uterine bleeding with reflux with the shedding of predominantly endometrial stem/niche cells [23].

Progression of endometriosis

Progression of the endometriotic lesion is characterized by two stages of morphological activities. In the first phase, the superficial endometriotic implant responds like eutopic endometrium to ovarian steroid hormones resulting in proliferation, secretory changes, and decidualization followed by superficial desquamation and bleeding. In the later phase, the interstitial implant is associated with smooth muscle metaplasia and formation of deep or adenomyotic nodules. In the ovary, progression of endometriosis leads to bleeding and adhesions resulting in endometrioma formation, while interstitial smooth muscle metaplasia and fibrosis affect the cortical zone and decrease the follicular reserve.

Ovarian endometrioma formation

Superficial endometriosis is characterized by adhesion formation. It is now well accepted that the typical ovarian endometrioma is caused by encapsulation of endometrial tissue between the ovarian cortex and the posterior leaf or the parametrium as originally described by Hughesdon in 1957 [24]. In an initial stage, Gordts et al. described the presence of small adhesions only upon the ovarian surface covering the early formation of an invaginating small endometrioma identified as a brownish vesicle [25].

Careful inspection by ovarioscopy [26, 27] allows identification of vascularization and pigmentation of the pseudocyst lining and to distinguish between the endometrioma with a pearl white or yellowish-pigmented cortex lined by a thin mucosa with prominent neoangiogenesis (red endometrioma) and the endometrioma with a dark, pigmented fibrotic tissue (black endometrioma). Occasionally, the endometrioma is connected to a corpus luteum that has a completely different surface, and early colonization by endometriotic surface epithelium can be observed. One can argue that full excision of the red endometrioma represents, in many cases, excessive surgery and that particularly in young adults, in whom fibrosis is absent, this invariably results in the resection of healthy ovarian cortex.

Cortical and interstitial changes in the endometriotic cyst

One of the subtle and poorly appreciated changes associated with ectopic endometrium is smooth muscle metaplasia (SMM). According to Anaf et al. [28], deep infiltrating endometriosis (deeper than 5 mm under the peritoneum) in adults often takes the form of a nodular lesion (or "adenomyotic nodule") consisting of smooth muscles and fibrosis with active glands and scanty stroma. They studied in adults 54 endometriotic lesions originating from four different pelvic locations (peritoneum, ovary, rectovaginal septum, and uterosacral ligaments) using a monoclonal antibody against muscle-specific actin for identifying the presence of smooth muscles and quantifying the smooth muscle content. They found that smooth muscles were frequent components of endometriotic lesions in pelvic locations and concluded that, in adults, the definition of distinct endometriotic entities based on the difference in the tissue composition of the lesions (endometriotic nodules versus adenomyotic nodules) is inconsistent with the very frequent presence of smooth muscle cells in endometriosis irrespective of their localization. In a study of ovarian endometriomas, Fukunaga [20] noted that SMM in ovarian endometriosis is not an uncommon phenomenon and assumed that smooth muscle may originate from either metaplastic endometrial stromal cells in endometriotic foci or metaplastic ovarian stromal cells in the rim of endometriosis.

At present, Sampson [11] and Hughesdon [24] are the only investigators to study systematically histological sections of ovaries with endometrioma in situ. Admittedly, the specimens were obtained in older women and, therefore, represent a later stage of the disease. The pathologist Hughesdon described the main features of disruption and disorganization of the cortical wall and loss of identity of the inner cortex by smooth muscle cell metaplasia occurring in any of its layer in 86 % of the chocolate cysts. As a result, the inner cortex may become quite unrecognizable by stretching and muscular metaplasia, and in addition, there is no cleavage plane. It is therefore likely that the main risk of late diagnosis and treatment of the ovarian endometrioma is the progressive structural disorganization of the inner cortex. In the absence of a cleavage plane, surgical reconstruction of the ovary is becoming critically difficult. The changes are not dependent on the size of the pseudocyst. In a study of cystectomy specimens, Scurry et al. [29] noted that the presence of oocyte in such specimens is influenced, in addition to age, by fibrosis, SMM, and stretching of the cortex making identification frequently unrecognizable. Clement [30] noted that a biopsy is required for histological diagnosis, but the diagnostic value is compounded by tissue that is limited to a small biopsy specimen.

Loss of follicle reserve

The question arises to which extent the SMM associated with the ovarian endometrioma affects the follicular reserve. In a recent study, Kuroda at al. [31] obtained a small amount of normal ovarian tissue during ovarian cystectomy in 61 women with ovarian endometrioma and 42 patients with non-endometriotic cysts. The density of follicles in the ovarian tissues correlated with the age of the patients in both groups, but in women aged <35 years, the relative density of follicles in healthy ovarian tissues was consistently lower in the endometriotic cyst group compared to the non-endometriotic cyst group. The resection rate of normal ovarian tissue in cystectomy specimen of the endometriosis group was significantly higher than in the non-endometriotic cyst group. The authors concluded that ovarian endometriomas have a detrimental impact on follicle reserve in younger patients, and furthermore, that laparoscopic cystectomy for endometriomas may accelerate the rate of oocytes loss associated with aging. This study is important for demonstrating that the impact of endometrioma on the follicular reserve is determined by both the evolution in time and the surgical excision technique. The data support the recommendation of early-stage ablation of the endometriotic implant and avoid both delay of surgery as well as excision technique.

The morphological data on follicle loss in women with endometrioma has been confirmed by the impact of endometrioma on serum anti-Mullerian hormone (AMH), which is proposed as a marker of ovarian reserve. In a retrospective study comparing serum AMH levels in 1642 infertility patients without endometrioma and 141 patients with endometrioma, Hwu et al. [32] found that both ovarian endometrioma and cystectomy are associated with a significant reduction on ovarian reserve. Moreover, the mean serum AMH level was significantly lower in patients with bilateral endometrioma compared to that of patients with unilateral endometrioma. A lower concentration of AMH in patients with ovarian endometriomas before any surgery compared to normal ovaries is also described by Pacchiaroti et al. [33].

Kitajima et al. [34] demonstrated that in ovaries with endometriomas less than 4 cm in diameter, follicular density is significantly lower than in cortex from contralateral normal ovaries. In their 2014 paper [35], a so-called "burnout" hypothesis has been described with an accelerated follicular recruitment and atresia in early follicles found in ovaries with endometriomas and not in the cortex of contralateral ovaries without endometriomas. Focal inflammation results in the structural alteration of the ovarian cortex, with massive fibrosis and loss of cortex-specific stroma. Focal loss of follicular density may be associated with a "vicious circle of dysregulated folliculogenesis that eventually results in a burnout of the stockpile of dormant follicles."

Fibrosis of the endometriotic cyst was also frequently observed (9/13) in the study of Schubert et al. [36] while this was not present in case of dermoid cyst and serous cyst where the ovarian cortex only seemed to be stretched by the cyst and not damaged.

Delay in diagnosis

According to the endometriosis literature, the two main reasons why medical advice is sought are chronic pelvic pain and infertility. However, several studies have shown that the onset of symptoms precedes by several years the diagnosis of endometriosis. In a study comparing demographic, epidemiological, and medical data, Dmowski et al. [37] noted that in the pelvic pain group, there was a negative correlation between the age at first symptom and the stage of endometriosis at the time of first diagnosis. Thus, the longer the diagnosis was delayed, the more the endometriosis was in an advanced stage at the time of diagnostic laparoscopy. The frequency of stage IV endometriosis at the time of initial laparoscopy was significantly higher in the pelvic pain group than in the infertile group (31 vs. 12 %). This suggests a more expedient diagnosis in infertile women as compared with those presenting pelvic pain symptoms.

The study also found that the majority of women with endometriosis and infertility had either mild or no pelvic pain symptoms, suggesting the possibility of asymptomatic endometriosis. According to previous studies, unsuspected endometriosis is found in multiparous women undergoing laparoscopic tubal sterilization with a prevalence ranging between 2 [38] and 3.7 % [39]. Hadfield et al. [40] recruited through endometriosis self-help groups a total of 218 women with surgically confirmed endometriosis. US women had a mean ±SD delay in diagnosis of 11.73±9.05 years, while in UK women, the delay of 7.96±7.92 years was significantly lower. Interestingly, American women reported their symptoms to commence some 5 years earlier than British women. Husby et al. [41] reported that the mean delay from the onset of symptoms to diagnosis included two phases of delay: first, a delay from the onset to a doctor visit of 1.4±2.9 years, and secondly, a delay from the doctor visit to establishing a surgical diagnosis of 5.2±5.6 years. It is noteworthy that 21 (6.4 %) of 328 patients with proven endometriosis were diagnosed without pain symptoms. When excluding this group, the mean diagnostic delay would be 6.5±6.3 years and the median delay 5.0 years. Factors influencing the delay in diagnosis included the IVF that can be performed without previously performing laparoscopy and that endometriosis can be present without pain. According to the study of Arruda et al. [42], the interval was dependent on the primary symptom since women with infertility took 4 years to be diagnosed with endometriosis, whereas 7.4 years elapsed from symptoms to diagnosis in patients with pelvic pain. A recent multicenter study performed principally in primary care found a delay of 6.7 years between the onset of symptoms and a surgical diagnosis of endometriosis [43]. The delay was longer in centers where women received predominantly state-funded health care (8.3 vs. 5.5 years) and positively associated with the number of pelvic symptoms (chronic pelvic pain, dysmenorrhea, and dyspareunia) and heavy periods and a higher body mass index. However, it has been documented that menstrual symptoms, while raising a high degree of suspicion for endometriosis, are not reliable as indicators of the severity of disease [44, 45].

Early-stage management

Early-stage management of endometriosis in the adolescent involves exclusion of reproductive tract anomaly, monitoring the response of pelvic pain to medical treatment and the early ultrasound diagnosis of an endometrioma and, in such cases, full ablative surgery of the ectopic endometrial tissue. The combined oral contraceptive pill has been used for the treatment of endometriosis-associated pain, such as dysmenorrhea

for several years. The treatment may also relieve deep dyspareunia, non-cyclic pelvic pain, and dyschezia. While adolescent endometriosis is a hidden, progressive, and severe disease, the medical and surgical tools for diagnosis and treatment should be effective, but minimally invasive.

Psychological benefits of early-stage diagnosis

Two studies have evaluated in detail the benefits of early diagnosis for the patient. Ballard et al. [46, 47] investigated the reasons why women experience delays in the diagnosis of endometriosis and the impact of this in a qualitative interview-based study of 32 women, 28 of whom were subsequently diagnosed with endometriosis. Delays in the diagnosis of endometriosis occur at an individual patient level and a medical level, as both women and family doctors normalize symptoms, symptoms are suppressed through hormones, and nondiscriminatory investigations are relied upon. Women benefited from a diagnosis because it provided a language in which to discuss their condition, offered possible management strategies to control symptoms, and provided reassurance that symptoms were not due to cancer. Diagnosis also sanctioned women's access to social support and legitimized absences from social and work obligations. They concluded that although recent guidelines for the management of chronic pelvic pain suggest that diagnostic laparoscopy may be considered a secondary investigation after the failure of therapeutic interventions, the present study highlights the importance of an early diagnosis for women who suffer at physical, emotional, and social levels when they remain undiagnosed.

Nnoaham et al. [43] assessed the impact of endometriosis on health-related quality of life (HRQoL) and work productivity in a multicenter cross-sectional study with prospective recruitment from 16 clinical centers in ten countries. Delay was positively associated with the number of pelvic symptoms (chronic pelvic pain, dysmenorrhea, dyspareunia, and heavy periods) and a higher body mass index. They concluded that endometriosis impairs HRQoL and work productivity across countries and ethnicities, yet women continue to experience diagnostic delays in primary care. A higher index of suspicion is needed to expedite specialist assessment of symptomatic women. Future research should seek to clarify pain mechanisms in relation to endometriosis severity.

It is clear that supportive and comprehensive treatment should be provided until the completion of childbearing.

Imaging diagnosis of ovarian endometrioma

Transvaginal ultrasound is the first choice for monitoring the ovaries for early-stage development of a uni- or bilateral endometrioma. In the study of Holland et al. [48], the sensitivity and specificity of preoperative ultrasound for the detection of ovarian endometrioma are, respectively, 84.0 (95 % CI

73.7–91.4) and 95.6 (95 % CI 92.8–97.6), although the diameter of the endometriotic cyst was not mentioned. In his paper, Raine-Fenning [49] reported that the results of the predictive value of 2-D ultrasonographic patterns for the detection of endometrioma were very discrepant with a variation of sensitivity and sensibility, respectively, ranging from 64–89 to 89–100 mostly due to inappropriate ultrasonographic diagnosis. In experienced hands, the technique allows reliably the diagnosis of an endometrioma with a size of more than 1–2 cm in diameter. With the use of B-Mode ultrasound and mean gray value, Alcazar et al. [50] reported a sensitivity of 80 (58–92) (95 % CI) and a specificity of 91 (77–97) (95 % CI) with a LR+ of 9.1 (3.0–27.3) and a LR− of 0.2 (0.1–0.5) (95 % CI). In most of the studies reporting the sensitivity and specificity of ultrasound in the differential diagnosis of the pathologic cysts, the mean diameter of the cyst is seldom mentioned, neither the relation of the diameter of the cyst and the accuracy of differential diagnosis. The lowest reported diameter varies between 18 and 24 mm [51–53]. In our consecutive series of 169 patients where endometriosis was diagnosed at transvaginal hydrolaparoscopy (THL), routine preoperative transvaginal ultrasound only detected 45 % of endometriomas smaller than 15 mm [25].

The place of transvaginal endoscopic surgery

Atraumatic ovarian surgery, to avoid loss of ovarian reserve, is based on early-stage diagnosis when cystectomy can be avoided. Although laparoscopy is traditionally recommended, transvaginal endoscopy has been shown to be safe and most effective in ablating ovarian endometriomas that are not larger than 3 cm in diameter [54, 55]. As the transvaginal laparoscopy is performed using a watery distension medium, it enables accurate visualization of the vascularization of superficial implants and adhesions covering the site of small endometriotic lesions. Apart from the watery distension medium, the supplementary advantage of the transvaginal approach is that it allows inspection of the tubo-ovarian organs in their natural position with easy exploration of the fossa ovarica without the need of manipulating instruments. Brownish vesicles present upon the ovarian surface are by closer inspection small invaginated hemorrhagic lesions in the ovarian cortex covered by thin adhesions. Adhesions can be ablated without extra manipulation. The site of invagination can clearly be identified. By the use of a bipolar needle, the pseudocystic invagination is opened. At the basis of these small invaginations, endometrial-like tissue is identified. After rinsing and identification of the endometrial-like tissue lining the wall, full ablation is easily performed using a 5-Fr. bipolar coagulation probe (Fig. 1). As the whole procedure is performed under hydroflotation, no carbonization occurs and the risk of surgical trauma and adhesion formation is minimal. By close inspection and in the presence of adhesions with the posterior leaf, areas of endometrium-like tissue in the lateral wall can be identified and coagulation is performed. The absence of an elevated intra-abdominal pressure due to the CO_2 pneumoperitoneum at standard laparoscopy enables not only a better visualization of superficial adhesions and vascularization, but the procedure is also performed in the absence of a status of intra-abdominal hypoxia present at standard laparoscopy. It is questionable if such a long time exposure to the hypoxia caused by the CO_2 pneumoperitoneum is finally not detrimental for the ovarian reserve and is a co-factor for the diminished AMH concentration after surgery.

In young patients with severe dysmenorrhea, we suggest the following decision tree: In a first step, presence of rectovaginal endometriosis and/or ovarian endometrioma should be excluded by a clinical examination and transvaginal

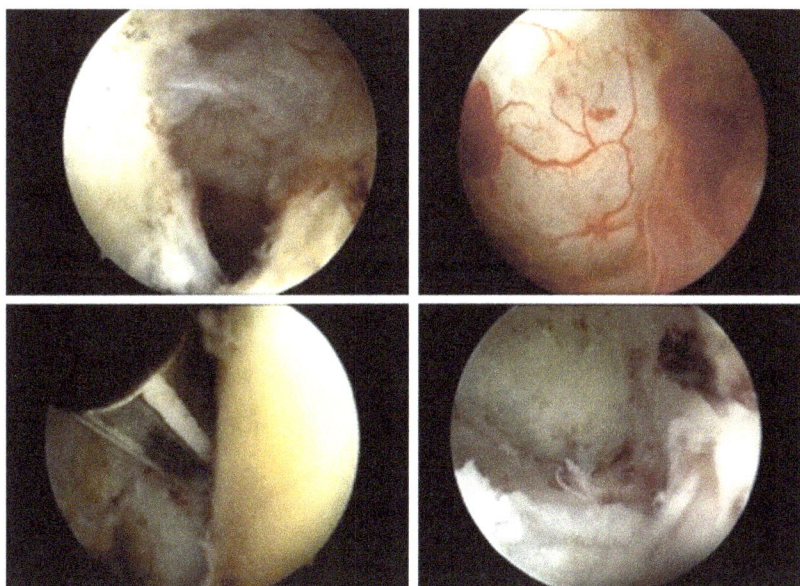

Fig. 1 Ablative surgery of small ovarian endometrioma by transvaginal hydrolaparoscopy. From *upper left* to *right under*. Opening of cyst with visualization of microvascularization at the base. Close-up (under water) of insight cyst: remark the pertinent vascularization and the presence of endometrial tissue on the right. Use of bipolar probe for ablative surgery. Final result after ablation: remark the absence of carbonization and the *white color* of the insight comparable with the ovarian cortex

ultrasound. In case of negative examination, patient can be put upon oral contraception and/or NSAID with yearly follow-up; in case of persistence or aggravation of pain, a transvaginal hydrolaparoscopy (THL) or in case of contraindication for a vaginal access standard laparoscopy (SL) should be performed and endometriotic lesions should be treated. In case of diagnosis of ovarian endometriosis in the absence of rectovaginal pathology at clinical examination, a six monthly follow-up under a contraceptive pill is advocated to exclude the increase of the ovarian endometrioma and to evaluate the regression of pain. In case of non-regression of the pain and/or increase of the size of the endometrioma, endoscopic exploration and treatment by THL or SL are mandatory. In the presence of rectovaginal endometriosis, the necessary exploration must be done before referring patient for an operative laparoscopic procedure (Fig. 2).

In the absence of contraindications for a vaginal access [55] and if the size of the endometrioma does not exceed 3 cm, a THL in our hands is preferable. Deep or adenomyotic lesions are rare in adolescents, and as long as there is no evidence, which peritoneal lesions will develop into adenomyotic or deep lesions, there is in our view no indication for "preventive" standard laparoscopy. At THL, the anterior cul de sac cannot be visualized. In asymptomatic patients, however, isolated lesions of the bladder are infrequent [56]. In patients with chronic pelvic pain and DIE, the incidence of bladder endometriosis is reported to be 1.58 % [57] until 6.6 % [58] and patients were complaining of frequent urination and dysuria. It is worth asking whether inspection of the anterior pelvis is necessary in infertility in the absence of tubo-ovarian pathology and in the absence of chronic pelvic pain or urinary complaints. In the presence of clinical symptoms suspicious for bladder endometriosis, appropriate investigation including MRI and standard laparoscopy is advocated. In Finland, the annual incidence, as evaluated from The Finnish Care

Register HILMO, increased from 3.6 to 9.4 cases/1,000,000 females aged 15–49 years per year during 1996–1999 and 2004–2007, respectively [59].

Can endometriosis in the adolescent be cured by full ablation?

At present, there is no evidence that in the adolescent all subtle peritoneal endometriosis can be visualized at laparoscopy. A variety of subtle lesions have been described [60], but the main visual criterion is the presence of microvascularization and cyclic bleeding. For this reason, GnRH agonist can cause disappearance of lesions, but they recur once the treatment is stopped and menstruations follow [61]. A major problem is that, at laparoscopy, the pneumoperitoneum causes collapse of the capillary blood flow inside and surrounding the implants, masking to a large extent the microvascularization in and towards the active subtle lesion. The recent study by Yeung et al. [62] suggested that complete laparoscopic excision of all areas of abnormal peritoneum with typical and atypical endometriosis has the potential to eradicate disease. This publication, however, was criticized by Laufer and Missmer [63] for the statement that the lack of visible endometriosis at second look laparoscopy in a relatively small number of patients was proof of the eradication of disease. As far as peritoneal endometriosis is concerned, the appearance may be variable and hormonal treatment may mask implants. Scanning electron microscopy can show the presence of invisible lesions in women with infertility and endometriosis [64]. Therefore, in the absence of the evidence that ablations of peritoneal endometriosis can cure the disease, the main issue is the full preservation of the ovarian function during reproductive life.

Discussion

From the early onset of female neonatal life, due to neonatal bleeding and retrograde menstruation, endometrial cells invade the pelvis and are possibly at the origin of the presence of premenarchal and adolescent endometriosis.

It is hard to understand why the diagnosis of endometriosis is so long delayed resulting in severe stages of endometriosis including a frozen pelvis. As health practitioners, we have to question ourselves why we are missing the development of this disease in individual women. Not only the patient herself is unaware of objective symptoms like severe dysmenorrhea and superfluous or frequent menstruation resulting in a late medical advice but also the general practitioners or gynecologist is not sufficiently sensitized for the importance of the symptoms. Furthermore, diagnosis is impaired as there is not a good correlation between the severity of the disease and the symptoms. All these results are a delay of an accurate diagnosis between the onset of symptoms and the final diagnosis.

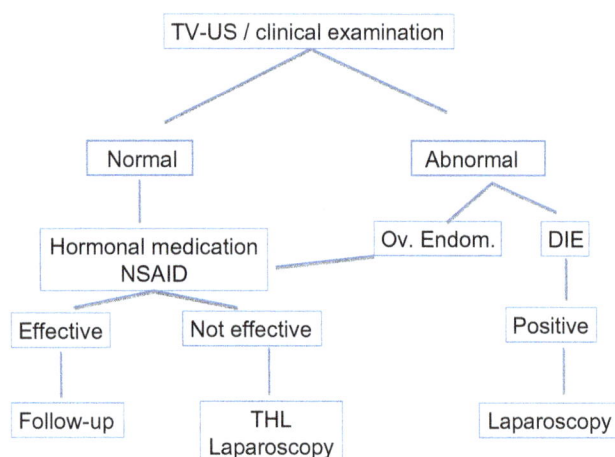

Fig. 2 Decision tree in young patients with severe dysmenorrhea. The necessary exploration must be done before referring patient for an operative laparoscopic procedure

Certainly, in adolescents with chronic pelvic pain such as dysmenorrhea resistant to medication, the incidence of endometriosis is around 70 % [7]. Early ultrasound diagnosis and meticulous follow-up are mandatory. Whether full ablative surgery should be envisaged in an early stage of the disease causing a minimal damage to the ovarian reserve is still debatable and requires further investigation. Long-standing presence of ovarian endometriotic cysts results in SMM and fibrosis of the ovarian cortex, impairing the ovarian reserve. Decisions to operate should be carefully balanced against the growing concern of potential damage of surgery upon the ovarian reserve [65, 66]. It is however questionable if the size of the ovarian endometrioma is of any importance in this decision process. The suggested diameter of 3 cm in the ESHRE guidelines is pure arbitrarily and not based upon any scientific evidence [67]. Alborzi et al. [65] demonstrated that the size of the cyst is inversely proportional with the ovarian reserve. The detrimental effect of the ovarian endometrioma on the follicle concentration and fibrosis, as described in the study of Kitajima et al. [34], was in ovarian endometrioma with a diameter smaller than 4 cm.

The purpose of an early intervention is the treatment of pain, prevention of the progression, and protection of the fertility [68]. As endometriosis is assumed to be a progressive disease, the ACOG recommends the early diagnosis and treatment in the adolescent [69]. In the editorial of Evers [70] evaluating the natural course of the disease in adults, the disease progressed in 29 %, while in the rest of the patients, the disease regressed or stayed stable. The issue of no progression and even disappearance involved mostly peritoneal endometriosis stages I and II, but not ovarian endometriosis [71]. In a prospective cohort study, Alcazar et al. [72] reported a spontaneous disappearance of endometriotic cysts in 30 % of the endometrioma diagnosed by ultrasound. In his study group, however, the mean age of the patients was 40.2±8.5 years and 33.7 % of the patients became menopausal during the follow-up period [mean follow-up time 45 months (9–109 months)]. It remains questionable first if these findings can be extrapolated to the adolescents, where the disease is more aggressive and, secondly, if no visualization at ultrasound means complete resolution of the disease as SMM and fibrosis can go on. In adolescents, the diagnosis is frequently postponed until several years after the onset of symptoms [37, 41, 42]. It is true that, at this moment, the progressivity of the disease cannot be predicted, but the frequent observation of severe stages of endometriosis, even in the absence of pain, is an indication of the progressivity of the disease in the adolescents and deserves our full attention. In a retrospective analysis of postoperative evolution of endometriosis in adolescents, Yang et al. [9] described a recurrence in 53 % of the adolescents, only in the small group of five patients receiving GnRha postoperatively in which no recurrence was observed. A more beneficial effect of acupuncture and Chinese medication in the

prevention of recurrence of endometriosis is mentioned in the study of Zhang et al. [73] compared to the use of gestrinone. A higher recurrence rate of endometriosis of 56 % in young women has been mentioned by Tandoi et al. [74], illustrating the degree of aggressiveness of the disease in adolescents.

As ablative surgery of small endometrioma intends to be more accurate and complete, reasonably, we could expect, although not proven, that this will result in a lower recurrence rate, being easier to perform and minimal invasive. Pados et al. [75] and Donnez et al. [76] advice to perform surgery for ovarian endometrioma larger than 5 cm in a two-step procedure enabling more accurate surgery on a smaller cyst in the second time and minimizing the risk of damaging the ovarian reserve.

The use of the transvaginal endoscopic approach adds to the minimally invasiveness of the procedure. The use of a watery distension medium allows an accurate visualization and early detection. Ablative surgery is done using a micro 5 fr bipolar probe causing minimal damage. In the absence of a panoramic view, the transvaginal endoscopic procedure is limited to the treatment of small endometrioma (<3 cm).

Endometriotic cysts differ from other benign cysts as they are extra-ovarian pseudocysts with the absence of a clear delineated capsule and not restricting the disease to the cyst itself but affecting the surrounding cortex by SMM and fibrosis. This explains the difference in ovarian reserve between patients with a dermoid cyst and an endometriotic cyst, with a negative impact on the latter.

Conclusion

Early diagnosis of endometriosis in the adolescent deserves our full attention. Early ablative surgery can contribute to a lower morbidity, a relief of symptoms, and a better quality of life. Treatment in early stage will result in less damage to the ovary caused by the disease itself and by a less invasive surgical procedure. Endometrial cells on the surface of the ovary carry the risk to affect the ovary in two ways: first by causing ovarian adhesions and pseudocysts and secondly by causing mesenchymal cell metaplasia in the interstitial ovarian tissue, sclerosis, and follicle loss. Similar as in oncology, there is no reason to wait.

Further research has to be done to elucidate if such early treatment will result in lower recurrence rates and less severe forms of the disease.

Informed consent This article does not contain any studies with human or animal subjects performed by any of the authors.

Contribution of authors   Patrick Puttemans revised the manuscript and searched for images. Gordts Sylvie revised the manuscript. Ivo Brosens provided scientific support of paper.

References

1. Brosens I, Gordts S, Benagiano G (2013) Endometriosis in adolescents is a hidden, progressive and severe disease that deserves attention, not just compassion. Hum Reprod 28:2026–31

2. Marsh EE, Laufer MR (2005) Endometriosis in premenarcheal girls who do not have an associated obstructive anomaly. Fertil Steril 83(3):758–760

3. Gogacz M, Sarzynski M, Napierala R, Sierocinska-Sawa J, Semczuk A (2012) Ovarian endometrioma in an 11-year-old girl before menarche: a case study with literature review. J Pediatr Adolesc Gynecol 25(1):e5–e7

4. Ebert AD, Fuhr N, David M, Schneppel L, Papadopoulos T (2009) Histological confirmation of endometriosis in a 9-year-old girl suffering from unexplained cyclic pelvic pain since her eighth year of life. Gynecol Obstet Investig 67(3):158–161

5. Hanton EM, Malkasian GD Jr, Dockerty MB, Pratt JH (1967) Endometriosis in young women. AJOG 98(1):116–120

6. Parker MA, Sneddon AE, Arbon P (2010) The menstrual disorder of teenagers (MDOT) study. Determining typical menstrual patterns and menstrual disturbance in a large population-based study of Australian teenagers. BJOG Int J Obstetr Gynaecol 117(2):185–192

7. Laufer MR, Goitein L, Bush M, Cramer DW, Emans SJJ (1997) Prevalence of endometriosis in adolescent girls with chronic pelvic pain not responding to conventional therapy. Pediatr Adolesc Gynecol 10(4):199–202

8. Laufer MR (1997) Identification of clear vesicular lesions of atypical endometriosis: a new technique. Fertil Steril 68:739–740

9. Yang Y, Wang Y, Yang J, Wang S, Lang J (2012) Adolescent endometriosis in China: a retrospective analysis of 63 cases. J Pediatr Adolesc Gynecol 25(5):295–299

10. Lee D-Y, Kim HJ, Yoon B-K, Choi D (2013) Clinical characteristics of adolescent endometrioma. J Pediatr Adolesc Gynecol 26(2):117–119

11. Sampson JA (1927) Peritoneal endometriosis due to the menstrual dissemination of endometrial tissue into the peritoneal cavity. Am J Obstet Gynecol 14:422–469

12. Batt RE, Mitwally MFM (2003) Endometriosis from telarche to midteens: pathogenesis and prognosis, prevention and pedagogy. J Pediatr Adolesc Gynecol 16(6):337–347

13. Signorile PG, Baldi F, Bussani R, D'Armiento M, De Falco M, Boccellino M, Quagliuolo L, Baldi A (2010) New evidence of the presence of endometriosis in the human fetus. RBM Online 21(1):142–147

14. Signorile PG, Baldi F, Bussani R, Viceconte R, Bulzomi P, D'Armiento M, D'Avino A, Baldi A (2012) Embryologic origin of endometriosis: analysis of 101 human female fetuses. J Cell Physiol 227(4):1653–1656

15. Bouquet de Jolinière J, Ayoubi JM, Lesec G, Validire P, Goguin A, Gianaroli L, Dubuisson JB, Feki A, Gogusev J (2012) Identification of displaced endometrial glands and embryonic duct remnants in female fetal reproductive tract: possible pathogenetic role in endometriotic and pelvic neoplastic processes. Front Physiol 3(444):1–7

16. Oliveira FR, Cruz CD, del Puerto HL, Vilamil QTMF, Reis FM, Camargos AF (2012) Stem cells: are they the answer to the puzzling etiology of endometriosis? Histol Histopathol 27(1):23–29

17. Cervelló I, Mas A, Gil-Sanchis C, Simón C (2013) Somatic stem cells in the human endometrium. Semin Reprod Med 31(1):69–76

18. Brosens I, Benagiano G (2013) Is neonatal uterine bleeding involved in the pathogenesis of endometriosis as a source of stem cells? Fertil Steril 100:622–3

19. Brosens I, Brosens J, Benagiano G (2013) Neonatal uterine bleeding as antecedent of pelvic endometriosis. Hum Reprod 28:2893–7

20. Fukunaga M (2000) Smooth muscle metaplasia in ovarian endometriosis. Histopathology 36:348–352

21. Fluhmann CF (1960) The developmental anatomy of the cervix uteri. Obstet Gynecol 15:62–9

22. Arcellana RC, Robinson TW, Tyson RW, Joyce MR (1996) Neonatal fellowship. McKusick-Kaufman syndrome with legal complications of hydrometrocolpos and congenital endometriosis. J Perinatol 16:220–3

23. Gargett CE, Schwab KE, Brosens JJ, Puttemans P, Benagiano G, Brosens I (2014) Potential role of endometrial stem/progenitor cells in the pathogenesis of early-onset endometriosis. Mol Hum Reprod 20(7):591–598

24. Hughesdon PE (1957) The structure of endometrial cysts of the ovary. J Obstet Gynaecol Br Emp 64(4):481–7

25. Gordts S, Puttemans O, Gordts S, Valkenburg M, Brosens I, Campo R (2014) Transvaginal endoscopy and small ovarian endometriomas: unraveling the missing link. Gynecol Surg 11:3–7

26. Brosens IA, Puttemans PJ, Deprest J (1994) The endoscopic localization of endometrial implants in the ovarian chocolate cyst. Fertil Steril 61(6):1034–1038

27. Darwish AMM, Amin AF, El-Feky MA (2000) Ovarioscopy, a technique to determine the nature of cystic ovarian tumors. J Am Assoc Gynecol Laparosc 7(4):539–544

28. Anaf V, Simon P, Fayt I, Noel J (2000) Smooth muscles are frequent components of endometriotic lesions. Hum Reprod 15(4):767–71

29. Scurry J, Whitehead J, Healey M (2001) Classification of ovarian endometriotic cysts. Int J Gynecol Pathol 20(2):147–54

30. Clement PB (2007) The pathology of endometriosis: a survey of the many faces of a common disease emphasizing diagnostic pitfalls and unusual and newly appreciated aspects. Adv Anat Pathol 14(4):241–60

31. Kuroda M, Kuroda K, Arakawa A, Fukumura Y, Kitade M, Kikuchi I, Kumakiri J et al (2012) Histological assessment of impact of ovarian endometrioma and laparoscopic cystectomy on ovarian reserve. J Obstet Gynaecol Res 38(9):1187–1193

32. Hwu YM, Wu FS, Li S-H, Sun F-J, Lin M-H, Lee RK (2001) The impact of endometrioma and laparoscopic cystectomy on serum anti-Müllerian hormone levels. Reprod Biol Endocrinol 9:80, art. no.1477

33. Pacchiarotti A, Frati P, Milazzo GN, Catalano A, Gentile V, Moscarini M (2014) Evaluation of serum anti-Mullerian hormone levels to assess the ovarian reserve in women with severe endometriosis. Eur J Obstet Gynecol Reprod Biol 172:62–4

34. Kitajima M, Defrere S, Dolmans MM, Colette S, Squifflet J, Van Langendonckt A, Donnez J (2011) Endometriomas as a possible cause of reduced ovarian reserve in women with endometriosis. Fertil Steril 96(3):685–91

35. Kitajima M, Dolmans MM, Donnez O, Masuzaki H, Soares M, Donnez J (2014) Enhanced follicular recruitment and atresia in cortex derived from ovaries with endometriomas. Fertil Steril 101:1031–7

36. Schubert B, Canis M, Darcha C, Artonne C, Pouly JL, Dechelotte P, Bouchera D, Grizard G (2005) Human ovarian tissue from cortex surrounding benign cysts: a model to study ovarian tissue cryopreservation. Hum Reprod 20:1786–1792

37. Dmowski WP, Lesniewicz R, Rana N, Pepping P, Noursalehi M (1997) Changing trends in the diagnosis of endometriosis: a comparative study of women with pelvic endometriosis presenting with chronic pelvic pain or infertility. Fertil Steril 67:238–43

38. Mathias SD, Kuppermann M, Liberman RF, Lipschutz RC, Steege JF (1996) Chronic pelvic pain: prevalence, health-related quality of life, and economic correlates. Obstet Gynecol 87(3):321–7

39. Matorras R, Rodíquez F, Pijoan JI, Ramón O, Gutierrez de Terán G, Rodríguez-Escudero F (1995) Epidemiology of endometriosis in infertile women. Fertil Steril 63(1):34–8

40. Hadfield R, Mardon H, Barlow D, Kennedy S (1996) Delay in the diagnosis of endometriosis: a survey of women from the USA and the UK. Hum Reprod 11(4):878–80

41. Husby GK, Haugen RS, Moen MH (2003) Diagnostic delay in women with pain and endometriosis. Acta Obstet Gynecol Scand 82(7): 649–53

42. Arruda MS, Petta CA, Abrão MS, Benetti-Pinto CL (2003) Time elapsed from onset of symptoms to diagnosis of endometriosis in a cohort study of Brazilian women. Hum Reprod 18(4):756–9

43. Nnoaham KE, Hummelshoj L, Webster P, d'Hooghe T, de Cicco Nardone F, de Cicco Nardone C, Jenkinson C, Kennedy SH, Zondervan KT (2011) Impact of endometriosis on quality of life and work productivity: a multicenter study across ten countries. Fertil Steril 96:366–373

44. Fedele L, Parazzini F, Bianchi S et al (1990) (1990) Stage and localization of pelvic endometriosis and pain. Fertil Steril 53:155

45. Mahmood TA, Templeton AA, Thomson L, Fraser C (1991) Menstrual symptoms in women with pelvic endometriosis. Br J Obstet Gynaecol 98(6):558–563

46. Ballard K, Lowton K, Wright J (2006) What's the delay? A qualitative study of women's experiences of reaching a diagnosis of endometriosis. Fertil Steril 86:1296–1301

47. Ballard KD, Seaman HE, de Vries CS, Wright JT (2008) Can symptomatology help in the diagnosis of endometriosis? Findings from a national case–control study—part 1. BJOG 115:1382–1391

48. Holland TK, Cutner A, Ertan Saridogan E, Mavrelos D, Pateman K, Jurkovic D (2013) Ultrasound mapping of pelvic endometriosis: does the location and number of lesions affect the diagnostic accuracy? A multicentre diagnostic accuracy study. BMC Women's Health 13:43

49. Raine-Fenning N, Jayaprakasan K, Deb S (2008) Three-dimensional ultrasonographic characteristics of endometriomata. Ultrasound Obstet Gynecol 31:718–24

50. Alcazar LJ, Leo NM, Galvan R, Guerriero S (2010) Assessment of cyst content using mean gray value for discriminating endometrioma from other unilocular cysts in premenopausal women. Ultrasound Obstet Gynecol 35:228–232

51. Mais V, Guerriero S, Ajossa S, Angiolucci M, Paoletti AM, Melis GB (1993) The efficiency of transvaginal ultrasonography in the diagnosis of endometrioma. Fertil Steril 60(5):776–680

52. Kurjak A, Kupesic S (1994) Scoring system for prediction of ovarian endometriosis based on transvaginal color and pulsed Doppler sonography. Fertil Steril 62:81–88

53. Guerriero S, Ajossa S, Mais V, Risalvato A, Lai MP, Melis GB (1998) The diagnosis of endometriomas using colour Doppler energy imaging. Hum Reprod 13:1691–95

54. Gordts S, Campo R, Brosens I (2002) Experience with transvaginal hydrolaparoscopy for reconstructive tubo-ovarian surgery. RBM Online 4(Suppl 3):72–5, Review

55. Gordts S, Campo R, Puttemans P, Gordts S, Brosens I (2008) Transvaginal access: a safe technique for tubo-ovarian exploration in infertility? Rev Lit Gynecol Surg 5:187–191

56. Jenkins S, Olive DL, Haney AF (1986) Endometriosis pathogenic implications of the anatomic distribution. Obstet Gynecol 67(3):335–8

57. Dai Y, Leng JH, Lang JH, Li XY, Zhang JJ (2012) Anatomic distribution of pelvic deep infiltrating endometriosis and its relationship with pain symptoms. Chin Med J 125(2):209–13

58. Chapron C, Chopin N, Borghese B, Foulot H, Dousset B, Vacher-Lavenu MC, Vieira M, Hasan W, Bricou A (2006) Deeply infiltrating endometriosis: pathogenetic implications of the anatomical distribution. Hum Reprod 21(7):1839–45

59. Vaarala MH, Hellstrom P, Santala M (2010) Is the incidence of urinary bladder endometriosis increasing? Figures from Finland. Gynecol Obstet Investig 70:55–9

60. Donnez J, Squifflet J, Casanas-Roux PC, Jadoul P, Vanlangendonckt A (2003) Typical and subtle atypical presentations of endometriosis. Obstet Gynecol Clin N Am 30(1):83–93

61. Evers JLH (1987) The second-look laparoscopy for evaluation of the result of medical treatment of endometriosis should not be performed during ovarian suppression. Fertil Steril 47:502–504

62. Yeung P Jr, Sinervo K, Winer W, Albee RB Jr (2011) Complete laparoscopic excision of endometriosis in teenagers: is postoperative hormonal suppression necessary? Fertil Steril 95(6):1909–12

63. Laufer MR, Missmer SA (2011) Does complete laparoscopic excision of endometriosis in teenagers really occur? Fertil Steril 96(3):145

64. Brosens IA, Vasquez G, Gordts S (1984) Scanning electron microscopic study of the pelvic peritoneum in unexplained infertility and endometriosis. Fertil Steril 41(Suppl):S21

65. Alborzi S, Keramati P, Younesi M, Samsami A, Dadras N (2014) The impact of laparoscopic cystectomy on ovarian reserve in patients with unilateral and bilateral endometriomas. Fertil Steril 101(2):427–34

66. Hirokawa W, Iwase A, Goto M, Takikawa S, Nagatomo Y, Nakahara T, Bayasula B, Nakamura T, Manabe S, Kikkawa F (2011) The postoperative decline in serum anti-Mullerian hormone correlates with the bilaterality and severity of endometriosis. Hum Reprod 26(4):904–10

67. Dunselman GAJ, Vermeulen N, Becker C, Calhaz-Jorge C, D'Hooghe T, De Bie B, Heikinheimo O, Horne AW, Kiesel L, Nap A, Prentice A, Saridogan E, Soriano D, Nelen W (2014) ESHRE guideline: management of women with endometriosis. Hum Reprod 29(3):400–412

68. Ozyer T, Uzunlar T, Ozcan N, Yesilyurt H, Karayalcin R, Sargin A, Mollamahmutoglu L (2013) Endometriomas in adolescents and young women. J Pediatr Adolesc Gynecol 26(3):176–179

69. ACOG Committee Opinion (2005) Number 310, April 2005. Endometriosis in adolescents. Obstet Gynecol 105:921–7

70. Evers JLH (2013) Is adolescent endometriosis a progressive disease that needs to be diagnosed and treated? Hum Reprod 28(8):2023

71. Brosens IA, Puttemans P, Deprest J, Rombauts L (1994) The endometriosis cycle and its derailments. Hum Reprod 9(5):770–771

72. Alcazar JL, Olartecoechea B, Guerriero S, Jurado M (2013) Expectant management of adnexal masses in selected premenopausal women: a prospective observational study. Ultrasound Obstet Gynecol 41:582–588

73. Zhang XY, Zhang CY (2014) Efficacy observation on the combination of acupuncture and Chinese medication in prevention of the recurrence of endometriosis after laparoscopic surgery. Zhongguo Zhen Jiu 34(2):139–44

74. Tandoi I, Somigliana E, Riparini J, Ronzoni S, Vigano P, Candiani M (2011) High rate of endometriosis recurrence in young women. J Pediatr Adolesc Gynecol 24(6):376–379

75. Pados G, Tsolakidis D, Assimakopoulos E, Athanatos D, Tarlatzis B (2010) Sonographic changes after laparoscopic cystectomy compared with three-stage management in patients with ovarian endometriomas: a prospective randomized study. Hum Reprod 25(3):672–7

76. Donnez J, Lousse JC, Jadoul P, Donnez O, Squifflet J (2010) Laparoscopic management of endometriomas using a combined technique of excisional (cystectomy) and ablative surgery. Fertil Steril 94(1):28–32

35

A mixture of 86% of CO$_2$, 10% of N$_2$O, and 4% of oxygen permits laparoscopy under local anesthesia

Philippe R. Koninckx · Jasper Verguts ·
Roberta Corona · Leila Adamyan · Ivo Brosens

Abstract The aim of this study is to verify that 10 % of N$_2$O in CO$_2$ sufficiently reduces pain to permit laparoscopy under local anesthesia. In nine patients undergoing laparoscopy under local anesthesia for tubal sterilization, a mixture of 86 % of CO$_2$, 10 % of N$_2$O, and 4 % of oxygen (the Gas Mixture) was used for the pneumoperitoneum. For CO2, N$_2$O, and for the Gas Mixture, the pain when blowing over the tongue tip and the pH changes of saline and Hartmann's solution were estimated. In all nine patients, discomfort was minimal and the intervention was well tolerated, similar to 100 % N$_2$O. Tongue tip pain ($n=15$), on VAS scale, was lower with 86 % CO$_2$+10 % N$_2$O+4 % O$_2$ (2.4 ± 1.4, $P=0.005$) and much lower with 100 % N$_2$O (0.3 ± 0.6, $P<0.0007$) than with pure CO$_2$ (3.6 ± 1.7). The pH of saline ($n=5$) decreased from 7.00 ± 0.07 to 4.18 ± 0.04 ($P=0.001$), 6.98 ± 0.08 (NS), and 4.28 ± 0.04 ($P=0.01$) with 100 % CO$_2$, 100 % N$_2$O and the Gas Mixture respectively. The pH of Hartmann's solution ($n=5$) decreased similarly from 7.00 ± 0.07 to 5.18 ± 0.04 ($P=0.01$), 7.02 ± 0.19 (NS), and 5.3 ± 0.4 ($P=0.01$), respectively. These data demonstrate that a mixture with 10 % of N$_2$O and 4 % of O$_2$ in CO$_2$ permits laparoscopy under local anesthesia. This result cannot be explained by direct irritation estimated by tongue tip pain or by pH changes.

Keywords Anesthesia · Conditioning · Gas · Laparoscopy · Pain · Pneumoperitoneum

P. R. Koninckx · J. Verguts · R. Corona · I. Brosens
UZ Gasthuisberg, Department of Obstetrics and Gynecology,
KULeuven, 3000 Leuven, Belgium

P. R. Koninckx (✉)
Gruppo Italo Belga, Vuilenbos 2, 3360 Bierbeek, Belgium
e-mail: pkoninckx@gmail.com

R. Corona
Centre for Reproductive Medicine, Free University Brussels, 101
Laarbeeklaan, 1090 Brussels, Belgium

J. Verguts
Department of Obstetrics and Gynecology, Jessa Hospital, Hasselt,
Belgium

L. Adamyan
Department of Reproductive Medicine and Surgery, Moscow state
University of Medicine and Dentistry, Moscow, Russia

Introduction

Laparoscopy under local anesthesia has never become popular notwithstanding the advantages of a short hospital stay without general anesthesia. Following the report in 1976 of salpingectomies for tubal sterilization using umbilical local anesthesia, slight sedation, and pure N$_2$O for the pneumoperitoneum [1], a Yoon ring tubal sterilization program under local anesthesia was started in 1976 in Leuven [2]. Although pure N$_2$O is less painful than CO$_2$ for the pneumoperitoneum [3–6], laparoscopy under local anesthesia using CO$_2$ pneumoperitoneum can be performed albeit with stronger sedation and/or microlaparoscopy [7–14].

That 100 % N$_2$O for the pneumoperitoneum causes less pain after surgery than 100 % CO$_2$, was demonstrated in randomized controlled trials [15, 16]. The mechanism through which a N$_2$O pneumoperitoneum causes little pain in comparison with CO$_2$ was believed to be a consequence of the absence of the irritation of CO$_2$. The use of other inert gases as helium and argon under local anesthesia was never reported to the best of our knowledge. The use of N$_2$O for the pneumoperitoneum is safe since the solubility of N$_2$O in blood and the exchange capacity in the lungs is comparable or better than CO$_2$. N$_2$O, in addition, avoids the metabolic effects of CO$_2$ resorption [17–21]. Nevertheless, the clinical use of N$_2$O for inducing the pneumoperitoneum during operative laparoscopy never became popular because of the explosion risk when using electrosurgery at concentrations of N_2O higher than 29 % [22, 23].

We recently demonstrated in our laparoscopic mouse model [24, 25] that the effect of as little as 5 % of N_2O in CO_2 had a similar effect in reducing postoperative adhesions as pure N_2O. In a randomized controlled trial (RCT) in the human [26], we subsequently demonstrated the virtual absence of adhesions and a strong decrease in pain following full-conditioning during surgery (i.e., 10 % of N_2O and 4 % of O_2 in CO_2 for the pneumoperitoneum, cooling of the peritoneal cavity to 30 °C, and absence of desiccation) and a barrier at the end of surgery in patients undergoing deep endometriosis excision.

We therefore planned an observational trial to test the hypothesis that 10 % of N_2O in CO_2 would reduce pain and permit laparoscopy under local anesthesia similar as 100 % of N_2O does.

Materials and methods

Tubal sterilization under local anesthesia

Since 1976, tubal sterilization under local anesthesia using 100 % N_2O for the pneumoperitoneum has been a routine procedure in the university hospitals of the Catholic University of Leuven (KULeuven) [2]. Following local anesthesia of the umbilicus with 10 ml of 2 % xylocaine, the pneumoperitoneum was induced with pure N_2O using a water valve limiting the pneumoperitoneum pressure to 15 mm of Hg, while all extra gas was permitted to escape freely [27] An insufflator CE marked to be used with N_2O indeed did not exist. The umbilical trocar was inserted with active pressure of the patient to distend the abdomen, thus increasing the distance between the peritoneal wall and the large vessels and the safety of insertion. Subsequently, using an operative laparoscope (initially the 12-mm KLI, USA single incision applicator; later the Storz AG, Tüttlingen Germany, operative laparoscope), 10 ml of an anesthetic gel (xylocaine gel, Astra Zeneca) was applied over the oviducts. Initially, only Yoon rings were applied; more recently, the department decided to use Filshie clips. The entire procedure of tubal sterilization under local anesthesia rarely exceeded 5 min. A short duration indeed is crucial for acceptability by the patient who becomes increasingly nervous when the procedure takes longer or when there is any sign of nonconfidence by the surgeon. Sedation before surgery consisted initially of Dipidolor (Janssens, Belgium). Later sedation was omitted if the patient was not too anxious. This technique had been used for 30 years in over 1000 patients without a single major complication and without a failure. Although the technique was almost systematically used in the late 1970s and early 1980s, general anesthesia became subsequently predominantly used in the department since the necessity of a short procedure and of a confident surgeon conflicted with the necessity of training the registrars.

Observational trial using 86% CO_2, 10% of N_2O, and 4% of O_2 (the Gas Mixture) for the pneumoperitoneum

In order to evaluate whether this mixture would be sufficient to permit laparoscopy under local anesthesia, this mixture was used instead of 100 % N_2O in all nine patients scheduled for laparoscopic sterilization under local anesthesia by PK from September 30, 2010, till September 30, 2011. The age of the women included ranged from 31 to 46 years and their weight from 61 to 85 kg.

Informed consent was obtained prior to the procedure with the explicit agreement that in case of pain, a general anesthesia would be performed immediately. All procedures were in accordance with the ethical standards of the responsible committee on human experimentation (institutional and national) and with the Helsinki Declaration of 1975, as revised in 2008. IRB approval had been obtained in September 2010 for the use of CO_2 with 10 % of N_2O and 4 % of O_2 for the pneumoperitoneum, e.g., for the randomized controlled trial on postoperative pain and adhesion formation [26].

The primary aim of the trial was to assess feasibility of the procedure without discomfort of the patient.

Tongue tip pain and pH

In order to measure the irritation by 100 % CO_2, 86 % CO_2+ 10 % N_2O+4 % O_2, and 100 % N_2O in 15 healthy volunteers (registrars between 23 and 31 years old), the severity of pain was assessed by a visual analog scale after directing through a Pasteur pipette a flow of 2 L/min to the tongue at 1 cm distance for 30 s. Also, the pH of saline and of Hartmann's solution was measured following equilibration with the three gases for 5 min.

Statistics

Means and standard deviations are given. For the pain dataset, overall statistical significance was calculated using Friedman's test (nonparametric paired ANOVA), while differences between groups was calculated by Wilcoxon matched pairs test. For the pH data, overall statistical significance was calculated using Kruskal–Wallis test (nonparametric unpaired ANOVA), while differences between groups was calculated by Mann–Whitney test. Analysis was done with GraphPad Prism (GraphPad software).

Results

In all nine patients, little or no pain was experienced during the induction of the pneumoperitoneum, and the procedures were comparable with previous interventions using 100 % N_2O for the pneumoperitoneum. All nine patients were discharged a few hours after the intervention and could return to their normal activity within a few days.

The tongue tip pain ($n=15$) on VAS scale (Friedman <0.0001), was lower with the Gas Mixture (2.4 ± 1.4, $P=0.005$) and with 100 % N_2O (0.3 ± 0.6, $P<0.0007$) than with pure CO_2 (3.6 ± 1.7). It was lower with N_2O than with the Gas Mixture ($P<0.0007$). The pH of saline ($n=5$) decreased (Kruskal–Wallis $P=0.007$) from 7.00 ± 0.07 to 4.18 ± 0.04 ($P=0.001$), to 6.98 ± 0.08 (NS) and to 4.28 ± 0.04 ($P=0.01$, NS versus CO_2) with 100 % CO_2, 100 % N_2O and the Gas Mixture. The pH of Hartmann's solution ($n=5$) decreased (Kruskal–Wallis $P=0.0008$) similarly from 7.00 ± 0.07 to 5.18 ± 0.04 ($P=0.01$), to 7.02 ± 0.19 (NS), and to 5.3 ± 0.4 ($P=0.01$, NS versus CO2), respectively.

Discussion

Although the numbers are small, these data demonstrate that the use of 10 % of N_2O and 4 % of O_2 in CO_2 for the pneumoperitoneum causes little peritoneal pain and permits laparoscopy under local anesthesia comparable to 100 % N_2O. Feasibility of laparoscopic sterilization under local anesthesia is close to a black and white result. If the procedure is short and the surgeon is confident and keeps intermittently eye contact with the patient, with or without showing the surgery on the screen, the procedure is uneventful and the patient tells afterwards that discomfort was minimal. If however, the patient looses confidence for whatever reason, e.g., because of pain, because the procedure takes longer than 5 to 7 min, because the surgeon starts sweating or displays any other signs of nervousness, because of a higher insufflation pressure, or more Trendelenburg positioning, the anxiety of the patient increases rapidly and the procedure becomes difficult and stressful for both, if not impossible. The patient afterwards describes this pain as anxiety. The procedure thus requires an experienced and fast laparoscopic surgeon. This was the main reason that laparoscopic sterilization under local anesthesia proved difficult to introduce as a routine while most of the registrars stopped to use the procedure after one minor but for them stressful incident with anxious patient.

The use of 10 % of N_2O has a major advantage in comparison with 100 % N_2O since the explosion risk is absent at a concentration below 29 % of N_2O, thus permitting eventual electrosurgery, e.g., to coagulate a bleeding. Another theoretical advantage is the reduced operating theater contamination in case of gas leaks and poor ventilation [28].

A mixture of 10 % of N_2O and 4 % of O_2 in CO_2 was chosen for the following reasons. Although in mice it had been demonstrated that 5 % of N_2O in CO_2 was as effective as 100 % of N_2O in reducing the acute inflammatory reaction and the subsequent enhanced adhesion formation caused by pure CO_2 [29], we preferred for this human experiment to use 10 % of N_2O since it remains far below the critical concentration of 29 % when explosions might occur. Although in the mouse model, no additive effect of 4 % oxygen could be demonstrated when 5 % of N_2O or more was used [25], we preferred to use also 4 % of O_2 for this exploratory trial since 4 % of oxygen when used alone had a small effect on postoperative pain in women [30].

The mechanism by which 100 % N_2O and 10 % N_2O+4 % O_2 in CO_2 cause much less pain than CO_2 during pneumoperitoneum is unclear. In our hands, insufflation with CO_2, as attempted during the 1980s, immediately causes a sharp pain and the procedure had to be interrupted. In order to understand the mechanism of reduced pain by using 100 % N_2O or the Gas Mixture, we measured the tongue tip pain and the pH changes caused by the different gases. CO_2 induces strong irritation of the tongue; 100 % N_2O was much less painful and the Gas Mixture with 10 % N_2O only slightly reduced the tongue tip pain. The effect on the tongue tip pain is comparable with the pH changes which are very pronounced with CO_2, almost inexistent with 100 % N_2O whereas the Gas Mixture decreased pH only slightly less than 100 % CO_2. Somatic pain of the tongue thus seems related to the irritative effect of CO_2 and the changes in pH. The mechanisms of visceral pain of the peritoneum are known to be different [31], and we do not have an explanation why 10 % of N_2O seems to be as effective as 100 % in reducing pain during laparoscopy under local anesthesia. This, however, is consistent with the effect of 100 % and 10 % N_2O upon adhesion formation and upon postoperative pain [26] and suggests an unknown drug-like effect of N_2O upon visceral pain.

It is unclear whether in the human that the addition of 4 % of oxygen has an additive pain-reducing effect. Unfortunately, we realize that the demonstration of an additive effect of 4 % of O_2 will require large series to reach statistical significance, while clinically not important. The same holds true for the use of 5 % of N_2O instead of 10 %. The only theoretical advantage of not using 4 % of O_2 is the lower risk of gas embolism since the solubility of O_2 in the blood is very low. With 4 % of O_2, the risk however is considered close to nonexistent.

In conclusion, the use of 10 % of N_2O in CO_2 is a preferred alternative to pure N_2O for laparoscopy under local anesthesia because of the absence of explosion risk by concentrations of N_2O lower than 29 %, thus permitting electrosurgery when needed. This mixture moreover is extremely safe since N_2O has an even higher solubility in water and exchange capacity in the lungs than CO_2. The effect cannot be explained by pH changes or a direct irritation as observed on the tongue.

Acknowledgments Dr. Karina Mailova (Moscow, Russia), Dr. med Mercedes Binda, Dr. Assia Stepanian (Atlanta, USA), and Dr. Anastasia Ussia (Rome, Italy) are thanked for the discussions and for reviewing this manuscript. We do thank eSaturnus NV (Haasrode, Belgium), for the practical help with these experiments.

Informed consent All procedures followed were in accordance with the ethical standards of the responsible committee on human experimentation (institutional and national) and with the Helsinki Declaration of 1975, as revised in 2000. Informed consent was obtained from all patients before being included in the study.

References

1. Aldrete JA, Tan ST, Carrow DJ, Watts MK (1976) "Pentazepam" (pentazocine + diazepam) supplementing local analgesia for laparoscopic sterilization. Anesth Analg 55:177–181

2. Debrock M, Brosens I (1979) Laparoscopic tubal ring sterilization under local anesthesia. Eur J Obstet Gynecol Reprod Biol 9:41–44

3. Minoli G, Terruzzi V, Spinzi GC, Benvenuti C, Rossini A (1982) The influence of carbon dioxide and nitrous oxide on pain during laparoscopy: a double-blind, controlled trial. Gastrointest Endosc 28:173–175

4. Crabtree JH, Fishman A, Huen IT (1998) Videolaparoscopic peritoneal dialysis catheter implant and rescue procedures under local anesthesia with nitrous oxide pneumoperitoneum. Adv Perit Dial 14:83–86

5. Sharp JR, Pierson WP, Brady CE III (1982) Comparison of CO_2- and N_2O-induced discomfort during peritoneoscopy under local anesthesia. Gastroenterology 82:453–456

6. Poindexter AN, Shattuck G (1990) Laparoscopic tubal sterilization under local anesthesia. Obstet Gynecol 75:1060–1062

7. Salah IM (2013) Office microlaparoscopic ovarian drilling (OMLOD) versus conventional laparoscopic ovarian drilling (LOD) for women with polycystic ovary syndrome. Arch Gynecol Obstet 287:361–367

8. DeQuattro N, Hibbert M, Buller J, Larsen F, Russell S, Poore S, Davis G (1998) Microlaparoscopic tubal ligation under local anesthesia. J Am Assoc Gynecol Laparosc 5:55–58

9. Risquez F, Pennehoaut G, McCorvey R, Love B, Vazquez A, Partamian J, Rebon P, Lucena E, Audebert A, Confino E (1997) Diagnostic and operative microlaparoscopy: a preliminary multicentre report. Hum Reprod 12:1645–1648

10. Bordahl PE, Raeder JC, Nordentoft J, Kirste U, Refsdal A (1993) Laparoscopic sterilization under local or general anesthesia? A randomized study. Obstet Gynecol 81:137–141

11. Poindexter AN III, Abdul-Malak M, Fast JE (1990) Laparoscopic tubal sterilization under local anesthesia. Obstet Gynecol 75:5–8

12. Mazdisnian F, Palmieri A, Hakakha B, Hakakha M, Cambridge C, Lauria B (2002) Office microlaparoscopy for female sterilization under local anesthesia. A cost and clinical analysis. J Reprod Med 47:97–100

13. Tiras MB, Gokce O, Noyan V, Zeyneloglu HB, Guner H, Yildirim M, Risquez F (2001) Comparison of microlaparoscopy and conventional laparoscopy for tubal sterilization under local anesthesia with mild sedation. J Am Assoc Gynecol Laparosc 8:385–388

14. Lipscomb GH, Dell JR, Ling FW, Spellman JR (1996) A comparison of the cost of local versus general anesthesia for laparoscopic sterilization in an operating room setting. J Am Assoc Gynecol Laparosc 3:277–281

15. Tsereteli Z, Terry ML, Bowers SP, Spivak H, Archer SB, Galloway KD, Hunter JG (2002) Prospective randomized clinical trial comparing nitrous oxide and carbon dioxide pneumoperitoneum for laparoscopic surgery. J Am Coll Surg 195:173–179

16. Aitola P, Airo I, Kaukinen S, Ylitalo P (1998) Comparison of N_2O and CO_2 pneumoperitoneums during laparoscopic cholecystectomy with special reference to postoperative pain. Surg Laparosc Endosc 8:140–144

17. El-Minawi MF, Wahbi O, El-Bagouri IS, Sharawi M, El-Mallah SY (1981) Physiologic changes during CO_2 and N_2O pneumoperitoneum in diagnostic laparoscopy. A comparative study. J Reprod Med 26:338–346

18. Ooka T, Kawano Y, Kosaka Y, Tanaka A (1993) [Blood gas changes during laparoscopic cholecystectomy–comparative study of N_2O pneumoperitoneum and CO_2 pneumoperitoneum]. Masui 42:398–401

19. Rademaker BM, Odoom JA, de Wit LT, Kalkman CJ, ten Brink SA, Ringers J (1994) Haemodynamic effects of pneumoperitoneum for laparoscopic surgery: a comparison of CO_2 with N_2O insufflation. Eur J Anaesthesiol 11:301–306

20. Hunter JG, Swanstrom L, Thornburg K (1995) Carbon dioxide pneumoperitoneum induces fetal acidosis in a pregnant ewe model. Surg Endosc 9:272–277

21. Schob OM, Allen DC, Benzel E, Curet MJ, Adams MS, Baldwin NG, Largiader F, Zucker KA (1996) A comparison of the pathophysiologic effects of carbon dioxide, nitrous oxide, and helium pneumoperitoneum on intracranial pressure. Am J Surg 172:248–253

22. Gunatilake DE (1978) Case report: fatal intraperitoneal explosion during electrocoagulation via laparoscopy. Int J Gynaecol Obstet 15:353–357

23. Robinson JS, Thompson JM, Wood AW (1975) Letter: laparoscopy explosion hazards with nitrous oxide. Br Med J 3:764–765

24. Mailova K, Osipova AA, Corona R, Binda MM, Koninckx PR, Adamian LV (2012) Intraoperative bleeding: adhesion formation and methods of their prevention in mice. Russian J Human Reproduct 2:18–22

25. Corona R, Binda MM, Mailova K, Verguts J, Koninckx PR (2013) Addition of nitrous oxide to the carbon dioxide pneumoperitoneum strongly decreases adhesion formation and the dose-dependent adhesiogenic effect of blood in a laparoscopic mouse model. Fertil Steril 100:1777–1783

26. Koninckx PR, Corona R, Timmerman D, Verguts J, Adamyan L (2013) Peritoneal full-conditioning reduces postoperative adhesions and pain: a randomised controlled trial in deep endometriosis surgery. J Ovarian Res 6:90

27. Koninckx PR, Vandermeersch E (1991) The persufflator: an insufflation device for laparoscopy and especially for CO_2-laser-endoscopic surgery. Hum Reprod 6:1288–1290

28. Meneghetti P, Scapellato ML, Marcuzzo G, Priante E, Bartolucci GB (1992) Pollution by nitrous dioxide during diagnostic laparoscopy interventions. G Ital Med Lav 14:59–61

29. Corona R, Verguts J, Schonman R, Binda MM, Mailova K, Koninckx PR (2011) Postoperative inflammation in the abdominal cavity increases adhesion formation in a laparoscopic mouse model. Fertil Steril 95:1224–1228

30. Verguts J, Vergote I, Amant F, Moerman P, Koninckx PR (2008) The addition of 4 % oxygen to the CO(2) pneumoperitoneum does not decrease dramatically port site metastases. J Minim Invasive Gynecol 15:700–703

31. Cervero F (1995) Visceral pain: mechanisms of peripheral and central sensitization. Ann Med 27:235–239

36

Transcervical, intrauterine ultrasound-guided radiofrequency ablation of uterine fibroids with the VizAblate® System: three- and six-month endpoint results from the FAST-EU study

Marlies Bongers · Hans Brölmann · Janesh Gupta · José Gerardo Garza-Leal · David Toub

Abstract This was a prospective, longitudinal, multicenter, single-arm controlled trial, using independent core laboratory validation of MRI results, to establish the effectiveness and confirm the safety of the VizAblate® System in the treatment of symptomatic uterine fibroids. The VizAblate System is a transcervical device that ablates fibroids with radiofrequency energy, guided by a built-in intrauterine ultrasound probe. Fifty consecutive women with symptomatic uterine fibroids received treatment with the VizAblate System. Patients had a minimum Menstrual Pictogram score of 120, no desire for fertility, and met additional inclusion and exclusion criteria. The VizAblate System was inserted transcervically and individual fibroids were ablated with radiofrequency energy. An integrated intrauterine ultrasound probe was used for fibroid imaging and targeting. Anesthesia was at the discretion of each investigator. The primary study endpoint was the percentage change in perfused fibroid volume, as assessed by contrast-enhanced MRI at 3 months. Secondary endpoints, reached at 6 months, included safety, percentage reductions in the Menstrual Pictogram (MP) score and the Symptom Severity Score (SSS) subscale of the Uterine Fibroid Symptom-Quality of Life questionnaire (UFS-QOL), along with the rate of surgical reintervention for abnormal uterine bleeding and the mean number of days to return to normal activity. Additional assessments included the Health-Related Quality of Life (HRQOL) subscale of the UFS-QOL, medical reintervention for abnormal uterine bleeding, and procedure times. Fifty patients were treated, representing 92 fibroids. Perfused fibroid volumes were reduced at 3 months by an average of 68.8±27.8 % (*P*<0.0001; Wilcoxon signed-rank test). At 6 months, mean MP and SSS scores decreased by 60.8±38.2 and 59.7±30.4 %, respectively; the mean HRQOL score increased by 263±468 %. There were two serious adverse events (overnight admissions for abdominal pain and bradycardia, respectively) and no surgical reinterventions. These 6-month results suggest that the VizAblate System is safe and effective in providing relief of abnormal uterine bleeding associated with fibroids, with appropriate safety and a low reintervention rate.

Keywords Fibroids · Radiofrequency ablation · VizAblate · Intrauterine sonography

Precis Transcervical radiofrequency ablation of uterine fibroids under intrauterine sonographic guidance is safe and effective in ameliorating fibroid-associated symptoms.

M. Bongers
Máxima Medisch Centrum, Veldhoven, The Netherlands

H. Brölmann
Vrije Universiteit Medisch Centrum, Amsterdam, The Netherlands

J. Gupta
Birmingham Women's Hospital, Birmingham, UK

J. G. Garza-Leal
Universidad Autónoma de Nuevo León, Monterrey, Nuevo Leon, Mexico

D. Toub (✉)
Gynesonics, Inc., Redwood City, CA, USA
e-mail: dtoub@gynesonics.com

D. Toub
Department of Obstetrics and Gynecology, Albert Einstein Medical Center, Philadelphia, PA, USA

Introduction

Uterine fibroids are the most prevalent benign uterine tumors and have an age-specific cumulative incidence in the United States that is nearly 70 % among white women and greater than 80 % among black women [1]. Despite the availability of several alternatives to hysterectomy, over 200,000 hysterectomies are performed annually for fibroids in the United States [1, 2]. More than 150 years after the first abdominal hysterectomy for fibroids, there remains a lack of consensus regarding what constitutes the "gold standard" treatment for fibroids against which all other treatment options may be compared [3]. Nonetheless, effective minimally invasive alternatives to hysterectomy exist to accommodate the growing preference of many women for uterine preservation.

Radiofrequency ablation (RFA) has been used as a fibroid treatment modality since the early 1990s, with multiple clinical studies confirming its safety and efficacy [4–10]. It has been shown that radiofrequency ablation produces thermal fixation and coagulative necrosis within the treated fibroids [9, 11]. Recent studies have been performed using RFA in conjunction with simultaneous, real-time sonography to enable volumetric ablations, resulting in volume reduction and symptom improvement [8, 9, 12].

The VizAblate System® (Gynesonics, Redwood City, CA) is a new medical device that has received CE Mark for distribution in the European Union. It combines radiofrequency ablation for the transcervical treatment of uterine fibroids with intrauterine sonography for real-time imaging [13]. The Fibroid Ablation Study-EU (FAST-EU) is a study designed to examine the safety and effectiveness of transcervical radiofrequency ablation of uterine fibroids under intrauterine sonography guidance with the VizAblate System. This report presents the 6-month endpoint results of 50 women treated under the FAST-EU study and is the first report of patient efficacy data after transcervical radiofrequency ablation of fibroids under intrauterine sonography guidance.

Materials and methods

Patient selection

This study is a prospective, non-randomized, single-arm, multicenter controlled trial using independent core laboratory validation of MRI results. Patients were enrolled from a total of seven sites in three nations: Mexico (one site), The United Kingdom (two sites), and The Netherlands (four sites). The protocol was approved by the Ethics Committees of the respective institutions as well as by the Federal Commission for Protection against Health Risks (COFEPRIS) in Mexico. All enrolled patients provided written informed consent for treatment with the VizAblate System prior to enrollment. The study overview was published on ClinicalTrials.gov (identifier—NCT01226290) and conducted in accordance with Standard ISO 14155 (Clinical investigation of medical devices for human subjects—Good clinical practice) of the International Organization for Standardization (ISO), the Helsinki Declaration of 1975, as revised in 2008, and in accordance with the ethical standards of applicable national

regulations and institutional research policies and procedures governing human experimentation.

Women were eligible for inclusion if they were 28 years of age or older and not pregnant, with regular predictable menstrual cycles and abnormal uterine bleeding for at least 3 months associated with one to five uterine fibroids measuring between 1 and 5 cm in maximum diameter. Fibroids were counted in this total if they had an edge within the inner half of the myometrium; these were termed "target fibroids," as they are believed to be more likely associated with heavy menstrual bleeding than myomata that are distant from the endometrial cavity. Target fibroids, which therefore were the only fibroids to be ablated, consisted of fibroids of FIGO types 1, 2, 3, 4, and 2–5 ("transmural"). At least one fibroid was required to indent the endometrium, as determined via hysterosonography and/or hysteroscopy and corroborated via contrast-enhanced MRI. All MRI studies were forwarded to a core laboratory (MedQIA, 924 Westwood Blvd., Suite 650, Los Angeles, CA 90024, USA) for quality control and interpretation to reduce variability in the measurements; the core laboratory also developed standardized imaging protocols for use at the individual study sites, credentialed the sites, and trained MRI technologists at each study site. A Menstrual Pictogram score ≥120 was required for inclusion along with a baseline UFS-QOL SSS score ≥20. The Menstrual Pictogram is a variant of the Pictorial Blood Loss Assessment Chart (PBAC) that patients complete to provide a visual assessment of menstrual blood loss during a single cycle [14, 15]. Unlike the original PBAC described by Higham and colleagues, the Menstrual Pictogram includes a greater range of icons representing different saturations of sanitary products, clots and losses in a toilet, and also distinguishes different absorbency levels of sanitary napkins and tampons [16].

Patients were willing to maintain the use or non-use of hormonal contraception from 3 months prior to the study through the 12-month follow-up period. Exclusions included a desire for future fertility, the presence of one or more type 0 myomata, cervical dysplasia, endometrial hyperplasia, active pelvic infection, clinically significant adenomyosis (>10 % of the junctional zone measuring more than 10 mm in thickness as measured by MRI), and the presence of one or more treatable fibroids that were significantly calcified (defined as <75 % fibroid enhancement by volume on contrast-enhanced MRI). Each patient underwent screening that included transvaginal sonography, hysteroscopy or hysterosonography, contrast-enhanced MRI, endometrial biopsy, and a pregnancy test.

Patients were assigned a unique identification number at the time that they provided informed consent for study screening. Patients were considered "enrolled" in the study once adherence with all inclusion and exclusion criteria had been verified and documented. All records were de-identified and only the range of each patient's age was documented, as per clinical trial requirements in The Netherlands. Women were followed at 7–14 days, 30 days, 3 months, 6 months, and at 12 months post-treatment.

The primary study endpoint was the percentage change in target fibroid perfused volume as assessed by contrast-enhanced MRI at baseline and again at 3 months. The patient success criterion was >30 % reduction in mean target fibroid perfused volume at 3 months in at least 50 % of patients.

Additional endpoints, reached at 6 months, included safety, percentage reductions in the Menstrual Pictogram (MP) score and the Symptom Severity Score (SSS) subscale of the Uterine Fibroid Symptom-Quality of Life questionnaire (UFS-QOL), the rate of surgical reintervention for abnormal uterine bleeding, and the mean number of days to return to normal activity. While there is no absolute level below which the SSS would be considered as "within normal limits," a population of 29 healthy women without uterine fibroids was demonstrated by Spies and colleagues to have an average SSS of 22.5±22.1 [17]. Additional assessments included the Health-Related Quality of Life (HRQOL) subscale of the UFS-QOL, medical reintervention for menorrhagia, and procedure times (as recorded from the start of transvaginal sonography to the end of RF ablation). Lower scores on the SSS subscale are desirable; conversely, higher scores on the HRQOL subscale are preferable. For the SSS, a 10-point reduction in the score is generally considered clinically significant [17–19].

Statistical analysis

The null hypothesis for this study endpoint is H_0: probability of success <50 % versus the alternative H_a: probability of success ≥50 %. Thus, the lower bound of the two-sided 95 % confidence interval on the observed probability of success must be greater than or equal to 50 %. We anticipated that at least 90 % of the patients would remain in the set of patients who were not excluded from analysis, and that the true probability of success for included patients would be 72.0 %. If this is the case, a sample of 40 patients is sufficient to detect this difference of 22 % in probability of success with a power of 82 % using a one-group chi-square test with a 0.05 two-sided significance level. Allowing for an expected dropout rate of 20 % at the 12-month follow-up visit, the minimum recommended sample size for the initial study protocol was 48. The primary study endpoint success criterion was achievement of >30 % reduction in mean target fibroid perfused volume in at least 50 % of patients. The primary endpoint analysis is performed on a per-fibroid basis, rather than using a subjective "dominant fibroid" in a given patient who could have multiple similar fibroids that were ablated.

The Full Analysis dataset includes all patients enrolled under the protocol who provided a baseline fibroid volume assessment and received treatment with the VizAblate System.

The Per-Protocol dataset includes all patients enrolled under the protocol who received treatment with the VizAblate System and provided both a baseline fibroid volume assessment and a 3-month assessment and/or who received a surgical reintervention. Patients who received a surgical reintervention were considered treatment failures. Any patients with major protocol deviations that were considered to influence a treatment evaluation were excluded (e.g., pregnancy, concomitant procedures, medical reintervention). The Per-Protocol dataset was used as the primary analysis set for the primary endpoint analysis.

All statistical analyses were performed with SAS 9.3 (SAS, Cary, NC). Values were considered significant at the level of $\alpha=0.05$. The Wilcoxon signed-rank test was used to test if a change was significantly different from 0. Missing data were not imputed for patients included in this Per-Protocol analysis.

Procedure

The VizAblate System consists of a reusable intrauterine ultrasound (IUUS) probe and a single-use, disposable articulating RF handpiece that are combined into a single treatment device (Fig. 1). Other integrated components of the VizAblate System include an RF generator and an ultrasound system with a custom graphical user interface. This graphical user interface provides the gynecologist with an image-guided treatment system that indicates the borders of the thermal ablation as well as the border beyond which thermal heating is not present (Fig. 2).

Pregnancy was excluded before the procedure by utilizing a urine pregnancy test. Anesthesia was chosen by each investigator in consultation with an anesthesiologist; options included general inhalational anesthesia, regional anesthesia, and conscious sedation with or without paracervical blockade. Two dispersive electrode pads were placed, one on each anterior thigh; the dispersive electrodes contain thermocouples positioned at each leading edge for skin temperature monitoring. Just before insertion of the VizAblate Handpiece, transvaginal sonography was employed at the discretion of each investigator to confirm the presence, location, and size of each fibroid.

Transvaginal sonography, if desired for fibroid mapping before insertion of the VizAblate Handpiece, was performed with a transvaginal ultrasound probe as provided with the

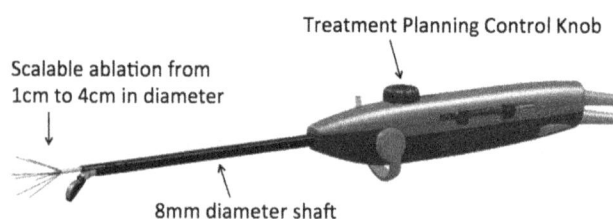

Fig. 1 The VizAblate treatment device

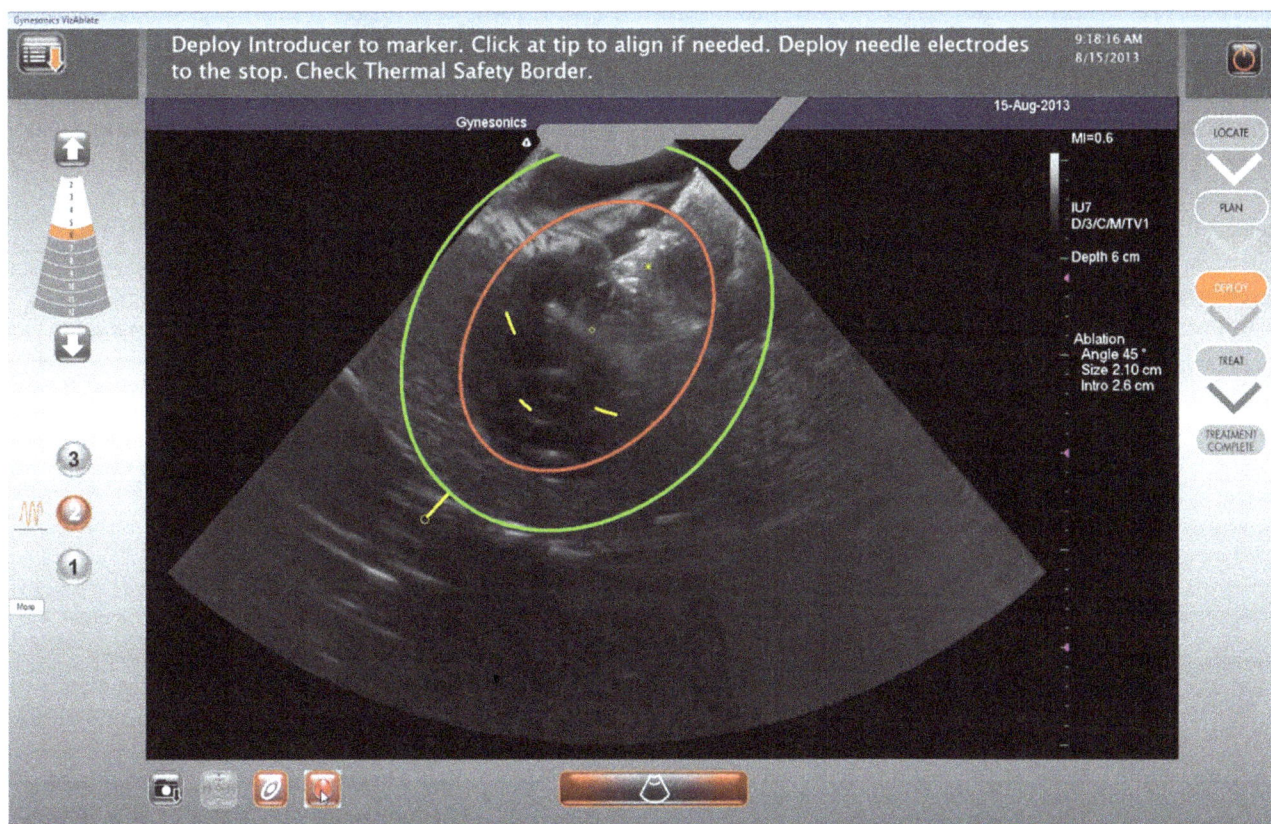

Fig. 2 Intrauterine sonogram of a submucosal fibroid with the VizAblate ablation guides visible (Ablation Zone in *red* and Thermal Safety Border in *green*). The Ablation Zone is a two-dimensional representation of the average region of tissue ablation for a selected treatment size. Tissue outside the Thermal Safety Border is at a safe distance from the Ablation Zone and will be preserved. The serosa is visible as an echogenic border around the uterus

VizAblate System. After achieving cervical dilatation to 8 mm, the integrated VizAblate Handpiece (containing the RF electrode array and the intrauterine ultrasound probe) was inserted transcervically into the uterus. A small volume (generally 10–15 mL) of hypotonic fluid such as sterile water or 1.5 % glycine was infused through the device for acoustic coupling. Leiomyomata were then visualized with IUUS and mapped in a systematic fashion within the uterus.

After articulating the ultrasound probe, the investigators used the graphical overlay to simulate various ablation widths, angles, and locations of the intended ablation. In this fashion, before introducing the RF electrodes into a fibroid, the investigator planned and optimized the ablation. Once the size, angle, and location of the ablation were established, the investigator advanced a trocar-tipped introducer into the fibroid under intrauterine ultrasound visualization. The investigator aligned the graphical overlay with the introducer tip and then rotated the VizAblate Handpiece about the introducer to assess the position of the Ablation Zone and Thermal Safety Border relative to the uterine serosa, as displayed on the graphical user interface, adjusting the size and/or position of the desired ablation if necessary. Depending on the width of the

ablation, the distance from the Ablation Zone to the uterine serosal margin will vary from 6.0 to 9.5 mm. When properly positioned, the introducer is located within the fibroid while the serosa is maintained tangent to or beyond the Thermal Safety Border. The investigator then deployed the electrodes, again rotating to ascertain the position of the Thermal Safety Border relative to the serosa. Once the Thermal Safety Border was confirmed to be within the uterine serosal margin in all adjacent ultrasound planes, RF energy was used to accomplish the ablation. Treated fibroids each received one or more ellipsoidal ablations, ranging from 1 to 4 cm in width and 2–5 cm in length. The number of ablations, along with their sizes, was at the discretion of the investigator. While usually only one ablation may sufficiently ablate up to a 5-cm myoma, two smaller ablations might be needed rather than one larger one, in order to ablate a greater aggregate volume when a fibroid is close to the serosa or where there is additional constraint on ablation volume and position (e.g., the cornu).

The VizAblate System delivers up to 150 W of RF energy for a preset duration. The RF generator controls energy delivery to maintain a constant temperature of 105 °C at the needle electrodes. Upon completion of RF treatment, the needle electrodes were retracted along with the introducer, the ultrasound articulation angle was reset to 0°, and the device was withdrawn.

Throughout this study, the investigator was asked to treat fibroids to maximize the ablated volume of each treated fibroid while maintaining the thermal safety border within the uterine serosal margin. In doing so, the investigator determined the best ablation size and location for each individual fibroid, and whether one or more ablations should be performed. The intent was to ablate all target fibroids (up to the eligibility limit of 5) present within a given patient. At each center, only a single physician would perform each procedure in the interests of consistency and quality.

Results

Patients

Fifty patients were treated in the FAST-EU study at seven sites. On average, each site treated 7.1 patients ±7.8 (median 5.0; range 1–23), with four centers treating five or more patients and the remaining three treating one to two patients. Baseline characteristics for all treated study patients are provided in Table 1. Anesthesia was provided as noted in Table 2.

Table 1 Baseline patient characteristics

Subjects treated	50
Most frequent age range	41–45 years[a]
Mean menstrual pictogram (MP) score	423±253 (range, 119–1582)
Mean UFS-QOL SSS score	61.7±16.9 (range, 28.1–100.0)
Mean UFS-QOL HRQOL score	34.3±19.0 (range, 0.0–73.3)
Total number of target fibroids identified on MRI	118
Mean number of target fibroids per patient	2.4±1.7 (range, 1–7)[b]
Mean diameter of target fibroids	2.9±1.4 cm (range, 1.0–6.9 cm)
Mean perfused fibroid volume	18.3±20.6 cc (range, 0.3–77.0 cc)
Mean total (perfused+nonperfused) fibroid volume	18.8±21.4 cc (range, 0.3–77.0 cc)

[a] Subject ages were specified as a range by each site to protect subject privacy

[b] Two small additional fibroids, beyond the upper limit of five target fibroids/patient, were identified on review of one MRI series after treatment

Table 2 Anesthesia provided to FAST-EU patients

Anesthesia option	Number of subjects
General anesthesia alone	15 (30.0 %)
Conscious sedation alone	15 (30.0 %)
Spinal anesthesia alone	8 (16.0 %)
Conscious sedation+epidural anesthesia	8 (16.0 %)
Epidural anesthesia alone	2 (4.0 %)
Paracervical blockade alone	1 (2.0 %)
General anesthesia+epidural anesthesia	1 (2.0 %)

The average procedure time (sonography time plus Treatment Device time) was 38.8±22.5 min (range, 11–95.5 min).

Exclusions from analysis

Two patients (four fibroids) were excluded from a Per-Protocol analysis of the primary endpoint, perfused fibroid volume. These two patients were deemed by the core MRI laboratory to have had unusable imaging for making precise fibroid measurements at the screening (one patient) and/or 3-month (both patients) MRI studies. Good faith efforts were made to obtain MRI studies for these patients that would meet the strict quality control requirements of the core MRI lab (MedQIA). As in the end, accurate fibroid contouring measurements could not be obtained in these two patients with any reasonable degree of reliability; their MRI data did not contribute to the data analysis. There were six (8 %) patients excluded from one or more of the patient-reported outcomes (MP, UFS-QOL). Two patients (4 %) underwent an ancillary fibroid or polyp resection at the time of RF ablation, and as a result, all of their patient-reported outcomes were excluded from a Per-Protocol analysis, including their baseline MP and UFS-QOL results. Three patients (6 %) underwent medical reintervention (e.g., tranexamic acid) for abnormal uterine bleeding within 6 months of the ablation procedure, resulting in exclusion of their patient-reported outcomes at 6 months. One patient reported a pregnancy at the time of her 6-month follow-up visit and was thus excluded from the 6-month analysis. One patient did not turn in her menstrual pictogram or complete the HRQOL portion of the UFS-QOL. Thus, at 6 months there were 43 patients who were included in the analysis of MP and UFS-QOL HRQOL and 44 who had data included in the UFS-QOL SSS analysis.

Mean percentage reduction in perfused and total fibroid volume

Characteristics of fibroids that were ablated are shown in Table 3 and ablation results at 3 months for both Per-Protocol and Full Analysis datasets are provided in Table 4.

Table 3 Characteristics of ablated fibroids

Total number of ablated target fibroids[a]	92
Mean number of ablated target fibroids per subject	1.8±1.1 (range, 1–5)
Total number of type 0 ablated fibroids	0
Total number of type 1 ablated fibroids	14
Total number of type 2 ablated fibroids	42
Total number of type 3 ablated fibroids	3
Total number of type 4 ablated fibroids	25
Total number of type 2–5 (transmural) ablated fibroids	8
Mean diameter of ablated fibroids	3.2±1.4 cm (range, 1.1–6.9 cm)

[a] Includes three fibroids that were ablated in a subject whose MRI data was not evaluable with regard to precise fibroid measurements

Fibroids are classified in Table 3 as per the International Federation of Gynecology and Obstetrics classification system [20]. While the Per-Protocol dataset is intended as the primary analysis source for the primary endpoint, the Full Analysis dataset is included for comparison. As noted in the ablation results, radiofrequency ablation with the VizAblate System was associated with statistically significant reductions in both total and perfused fibroid volumes at 3 months. This was true for both the Full Analysis dataset and Per-Protocol dataset. On a Per-Protocol basis, half of the fibroids experienced at least a 77.1 % reduction in perfused volume and at least a 63.1 % reduction in total volume (76.9 % and 62.5 %, respectively, for the Full Analysis dataset).

Seventy-nine of 88 treated fibroids (89.8 %), in 48 patients for which perfusion data was available at 3 months post-treatment, met or exceeded the primary study endpoint success criterion (achievement of >30 % reduction in mean target fibroid perfused volume in at least 50 % of patients).

Patient-reported outcomes

Patient-reported secondary endpoint data are provided in Table 5. A 50 % or greater reduction in MP was achieved in 33 of 43 patients (76.7 %) at 6 months. The median reduction in MP score at 6 months was 70.8 %. Reductions in the MP and SSS subscale of the UFS-QOL are desired, as are increases in the HRQOL subscale of the UFS-QOL.

As shown in Table 5, the reduction in the transformed SSS subscale of the UFS-QOL questionnaire at 6 months was statistically significant, as was the increase in the transformed HRQOL subscale. Patients experienced nearly a 60 % reduction in SSS at 6 months.

Device safety

All procedures were successfully completed. The adverse events attributable to the device or procedure consisted of dysmenorrhea (six patients), pelvic cramping (four patients), and abnormal uterine bleeding above the patient's baseline (seven patients). The abnormal uterine bleeding above baseline was seen in six of the seven patients at time points from 3 to 5 months post-ablation and were felt to have been consistent with fibroid sloughing based on their 3-month MRI studies and clinical presentation. At 6 months, there was a single bulk expulsion involving a 5.4-cm type 1 myoma at 12 days post-ablation. The patient did not initially mention it to her treating physician, noting only bulk passage of tissue (as opposed to gradual sloughing) in response to a physician query after the fibroid had been noted to have essentially disappeared on the 3-month MRI study. Given that it is unlikely that expulsion of a large fibroid could have been largely asymptomatic, presumably much of the fibroid had gradually sloughed off to the point where only a small portion was actually expelled.

Table 4 Reduction in mean perfused and total fibroid volumes at 3 months (Per-Protocol and Full Analysis datasets)

	Per-Protocol				Full Analysis set			
	Baseline	3 Months	% Reduction from baseline	P value[a]	Baseline	3 Months	% Reduction from baseline	P value[a]
Number of MRI-evaluable fibroids	89	88			89	89		
Number of subjects	49	48			49	49		
Perfused fibroid volume (cc)	18.3±20.6 9.5 (0.3–77.0)	5.5±9.2 1.6 (0.0–45.7)	68.8±27.8 % 77.1 % (−33.3–100 %)	<0.0001	18.3±20.6 9.5 (0.3–77.0)	5.8±9.6 1.6 (0.0–45.7)	68.1±28.6 % 76.9 % (−33.3–100 %)	<0.0001
Total fibroid volume (cc)	18.8±21.4 9.5 (0.3–77.0)	7.7±11.8 1.9 (0.0–56.3)	55.3±37.2 % 63.1 % (−85.7–100 %)	<0.0001	18.8±21.4 9.5 (0.3–77.0)	8.0±12.0 1.9 (0.0–56.3)	54.7±37.4 % 62.5 % (−85.7–100 %)	<0.0001

Data are mean±standard deviation; median; (range)

[a] Wilcoxon signed-rank test, null hypothesis of no change

Table 5 Improvement in patient reported outcomes at 6 months

	Baseline	6 Months	% Improvement from baseline	P value[a]
MP	48	43	43	<0.0001
	418±251	146±144	60.8±38.2 %	
	361	98	70.8 %	
	(119–1582)	(0–786)	(−73.1–100 %)	
UFS-QOL SSS	48	44	44	<0.0001
	62.1±16.8	23.5±17.8	59.7±30.4 %	
	60.9	18.8	66.7 %	
	(28.1–100)	(0.0–78.1)	(−22.2–100 %)	
UFS-QOL HRQOL	47	43	43	<0.0001
	34.5±18.7	82.5±17.8	263±468 %	
	30.2	86.2	126.0 %	
	(0.0–73.3)	(12.9–100)	(−28.6–2800 %)	

Data are number of subjects; mean±standard deviation; median; (range)

MP menstrual pictogram, *UFS-QOL SSS* uterine fibroid symptom and health-related quality of life symptom severity score subscale, *UFS-QOL HRQOL* uterine fibroid symptom and health-related quality of life health-related quality of life subscale

[a] Wilcoxon signed-rank test, null hypothesis of no change

There were two readmissions within 30 days of the procedure. One patient was admitted overnight on post-procedure day 9 to receive parenteral antibiotics for a urinary tract infection and was discharged on the following day. Another patient, who had no known history of cardiovascular disease or other medical disorders, developed bradycardia down to 38 bpm shortly after the procedure and was kept overnight in the hospital for treatment with atropine and observation; the patient was discharged the next morning in stable condition.

Reintervention

No patient underwent surgical intervention within 6 months of treatment. Three patients received medical reintervention with tranexamic acid after presenting at 3 months post-ablation complaining of persistent or increased abnormal uterine bleeding that was felt to have been secondary to fibroid sloughing based on the clinical presentation and 3-month MRI findings of markedly reduced submucous fibroid volume with partial extrusion into the endometrial cavity.

Pregnancy

There was a single pregnancy reported within the first 6 months after ablation with the VizAblate System. The patient presented with amenorrhea and a positive pregnancy test at her 6-month study visit and delivered a liveborn male

infant at term, weighing 3150 g and with Apgar scores of 9 and 9, via elective repeat Cesarean section [21].

Return to normal activity

A total of 47 patients completed a recovery diary relating to how long it took them to return to their normal activities of daily life. On average, return to normal activity took 4.4± 3.1 days (median 4.0 days; range 1–14 days).

Discussion

Since the 1990s, there have emerged several modalities to treat uterine fibroids, including uterine artery embolization (UAE) and magnetic resonance-guided focused ultrasound (MRgFUS). Uterine artery embolization is a treatment option, with a 20–28.4 % failure rate after 5 years [22, 23]. Of note, UAE is not considered generally applicable for women who desire future pregnancy, and has been associated with post-embolization syndrome and, occasionally in older women, premature ovarian failure [23–28]. Magnetic resonance-guided focused ultrasound, like radiofrequency ablation methods, ablates fibroids using energy to generate hyperthermic tissue temperatures. However, this modality is not widely available and requires up to 3 h per treatment.

The VizAblate System uses an incisionless, transcervical approach to treat symptomatic fibroids, including those that are not generally amenable to alternative intrauterine treatment approaches such as hysteroscopic resection or morcellation. Fibroid ablation takes place under real-time visualization provided by an intrauterine sonography probe that is integrated within the device. This built-in imaging removes the need for the physician to coordinate more than one device and more than one monitor. The graphical user interface delineates the boundaries of ablation and thermal spread outside the zone of ablation and enables the operator to avoid thermal injury to the serosa with its potential for adhesiogenesis and injury to adjacent viscera. Intrauterine sonography provides higher-resolution imaging than the more prevalent transvaginal sonography and has greater precision and accuracy for the measurement of fibroids near the endometrial cavity [29]. The use of intrauterine sonography has been demonstrated useful for the imaging of intratubal implants for sterilization after placement [30].

These 6-month results demonstrate that transcervical intrauterine sonography-guided radiofrequency ablation of fibroids can result in significant reductions in perfused fibroid volumes and fibroid-associated symptoms. In contrast with fibroid treatment modalities that often require 1–3 h to accomplish, mean treatment times with the VizAblate System were less than 40 min. Treatment did not require general anesthesia in nearly 70 % of patients and recovery time was relatively brief. The median time for the return to normal activity was 4.0 days, with a mean of 4.4±3.1 days (range, 1–14 days). This contrasts with laparoscopic radiofrequency ablation of fibroids, in which the largest published study to date reported a median time for returning to normal activities of 9 days (range, 2–60 days) [31].

Transcervical radiofrequency ablation avoids many of the potential complications associated with a laparoscopic or open procedure for the treatment of fibroids. There are no incisions and the uterine serosa is not penetrated or coagulated. There is no entry into the peritoneal cavity, so that intraperitoneal adhesiogenesis is unlikely. There is no overt risk of ureteral injury. In contrast to operative hysteroscopy, only a small quantity of hypotonic fluid is used for acoustic coupling, no large venous sinuses are exposed, and intrauterine pressure is not raised to levels above mean arterial pressure, avoiding significant fluid intravasation. The integral intrauterine sonography probe permits visualization of the myometrium and serosa, permitting a perspective of the myometrium and intramyometrial pathology that are not readily achievable with a hysteroscope.

At 6 months, there have been significant reductions in perfused and total fibroid volumes. Contrast-enhanced MRI demonstrated a significant reduction in the volume of perfused fibroid tissue at 3 months. The 3-month time point was selected in order to provide early data on the treatment impact on fibroid perfusion; it was not assumed prospectively that there would be a significant impact on total fibroid volume. It was suspected that reductions in total fibroid volume, caused by the process of coagulative necrosis, would require a longer time horizon to be demonstrated on contrast-enhanced MRI. As with MRgFUS, which is another form of hyperthermic ablation of uterine fibroids, it is known that sustained symptom relief may be accomplished by ablating as much of the fibroid volume as possible, although it is not necessary to ablate 90 % or more of the fibroid to reduce fibroid symptoms [32]. Nonetheless, there was an average 55.3 % reduction in total fibroid volume at 3 months, with some fibroids achieving 90–100 % reduction in total volume.

At 6 months, there were statistically significant reductions in menstrual blood loss, as evidenced by reductions in menstrual pictogram scores, as well as significant improvements in both subscales of the UFS-QOL questionnaire. No patients underwent surgical reintervention within 6 months. Based on the MP score, bleeding reduction was experienced by 76.7 % of patients at 6 months. It should be noted that Lukes and colleagues defined a reduction in menstrual blood loss of ≥36 cc, or a 22 %, reduction, to be the minimum level of improvement in bleeding that is meaningful to women [33, 34]. Thus, the majority of patients exceeded both standards.

In addition to clinical efficacy, device safety was also acceptable. No patient required emergency surgery and there

were no unscheduled returns to the operating room. Adverse events were generally minor and anticipated.

Seven patients experienced abnormal uterine bleeding above their baseline levels, generally around 3 months post-treatment. This was felt to be secondary to fibroid sloughing; MRI studies at 3 months typically revealed extrusion of ablated fibroids into the endometrial cavities with loss of total fibroid volume. As fibroids undergo coagulative necrosis after radiofrequency ablation, some patients may experience sloughing phenomena, particularly if the fibroid is already partially within the endometrial cavity or, as we speculate, the fibroid pseudocapsule has been ablated. As all patients are required to have at least one submucosal fibroid for entrance into the study, it is perhaps not surprising that 6 of 50 patients (12 %) had presumptive fibroid sloughing secondary to radiofrequency ablation. Consistent with reports of patient experiences after MRgFUS, gross expulsion of ablated fibroids was unusual, occurring in only one patient. Fibroid expulsion is more common after uterine artery embolization, in contrast to the experience of thermal ablation methods like MRgFUS and RF ablation [35–37].

Of the seven centers that treated patients in the FAST-EU study, half of the centers treated at least five patients. There was no unusual learning curve; the procedure time varied with the complexity of the case, with some first cases taking 14.5–18 min and others involving four to five larger fibroids requiring much longer.

This study has several advantages. Care was taken to exclude women with suspected anovulation through a strict inclusion criterion regarding the menstrual history, along with requiring the presence of at least one fibroid that indented the endometrial cavity. The latter requirement makes it more likely that a patient's bleeding symptoms are secondary to fibroids rather than another etiology. A core MRI facility was used to reduce variability and bias in MRI imaging quality, interpretation, and measurements relative to the primary study endpoint. In addition, the use of multiple clinical sites that include academic medical centers as well as community hospitals provides a more realistic assessment of the use of the VizAblate System than would a single site.

Nonetheless, there are some limitations to this study. The study is a nonrandomized single-arm study and does not include a sham or another fibroid treatment for comparison. It was not intended to examine outcomes for women with fibroids significantly larger than 5.0 cm, with the largest fibroid being 6.9 cm in diameter; additional study will be required to examine ablation outcomes in women with larger fibroid volumes. Finally, this report includes outcomes through the first 6 months after treatment with the VizAblate System; longer-term and comparative data are needed, are being acquired, and will be reported separately.

Conclusions

Based on the 6-month data from the FAST-EU study, radiofrequency ablation of uterine fibroids is an effective treatment modality that preserves the uterus. When performed transcervically with the VizAblate System, the integrity of the uterine serosa and abdominal cavity are not violated, concurrent intrauterine sonography provides a straightforward method for targeting myomata associated with abnormal uterine bleeding, and general anesthesia is not required.

Ethical standards All procedures followed were in accordance with the ethical standards of the responsible committee on human experimentation (institutional and national) and with the Helsinki Declaration of 1975, as revised in 2000. Informed consent was obtained from all patients for being included in the study.

Roles MB, HB, JG, and JGG-L were responsible for the conception and design of the study, data collection, patient recruitment, and were the responsible surgeons. DT was responsible for the conception and design of the study, data collection, data analysis and interpretation, statistical analysis, and drafting/preparation of this manuscript.

References

1. Baird DD, Dunson DB, Hill MC et al (2003) High cumulative incidence of uterine leiomyoma in black and white women: ultrasound evidence. Am J Obstet Gynecol 188(1):100–107
2. Dembek CJ, Pelletier EM, Isaacson KB et al (2007) Payer costs in patients undergoing uterine artery embolization, hysterectomy, or myomectomy for treatment of uterine fibroids. J Vasc Interv Radiol 18(10):1207–1213
3. Manyonda I, Sinthamoney E, Belli AM (2004) Controversies and challenges in the modern management of uterine fibroids. BJOG 111(2):95–102
4. Goldfarb HA (1992) Avoiding hysterectomy: Nd:YAG laser and bipolar coagulating needle. Clin Laser Mon 10(12):191–193
5. Goldfarb HA (1995) Bipolar laparoscopic needles for myoma coagulation. J Am Assoc Gynecol Laparosc 2(2):175–179
6. Bergamini V, Ghezzi F, Cromi A et al (2005) Laparoscopic radiofrequency thermal ablation: a new approach to symptomatic uterine myomas. Am J Obstet Gynecol 192(3):768–773
7. Carrafiello G, Recaldini C, Fontana F et al (2010) Ultrasound-guided radiofrequency thermal ablation of uterine fibroids: medium-term follow-up. Cardiovasc Intervent Radiol 33(1):113–119
8. Cho HH, Kim JH, Kim MR (2008) Transvaginal radiofrequency thermal ablation: a day-care approach to symptomatic uterine myomas. Aust N Z J Obstet Gynaecol 48(3):296–301
9. Ghezzi F, Cromi A, Bergamini V et al (2007) Midterm outcome of radiofrequency thermal ablation for symptomatic uterine myomas. Surg Endosc 21(11):2081–2085
10. Jones S, O'Donovan P, Toub D (2012) Radiofrequency ablation for treatment of symptomatic uterine fibroids. Obstet Gynecol Int 2012: 194839
11. Luo X, Shen Y, Song WX et al (2007) Pathologic evaluation of uterine leiomyoma treated with radiofrequency ablation. Int J Gynaecol Obstet 99(1):9–13
12. Iversen H, Lenz S (2008) Percutaneous ultrasound guided radiofrequency thermal ablation for uterine fibroids: a new gynecological approach. Ultrasound Obstet Gynecol 32(3):325
13. Garza-Leal JG, Toub D, León IH et al (2011) Transcervical, intrauterine ultrasound-guided radiofrequency ablation of uterine fibroids with the VizAblate System: safety, tolerability, and ablation results in a closed abdomen setting. Gynecol Surg 8(3):327–334
14. Wyatt KM, Dimmock PW, Walker TJ et al (2001) Determination of total menstrual blood loss. Fertil Steril 76(1):125–131
15. Higham JM, O'Brien PM, Shaw RW (1990) Assessment of menstrual blood loss using a pictorial chart. Br J Obstet Gynaecol 97(8):734–739
16. Warrilow G, Kirkham C, Ismail KMK et al (2004) Quantification of menstrual blood loss. Obstet Gynaecol 6(2):88–92
17. Spies JB, Coyne K, Guaou Guaou N et al (2002) The UFS-QOL, a new disease-specific symptom and health-related quality of life questionnaire for leiomyomata. Obstet Gynecol 99(2):290–300
18. Cho JY, Kim SH, Kim SY et al (2013) Efficacy and safety of daily repeated sonographically guided high-intensity focused ultrasound treatment of uterine fibroids: preliminary study. J Ultrasound Med 32(3):397–406
19. Hindley J, Gedroyc WM, Regan L et al (2004) MRI guidance of focused ultrasound therapy of uterine fibroids: early results. AJR Am J Roentgenol 183(6):1713–1719
20. Munro MG, Critchley HO, Broder MS et al (2011) FIGO classification system (PALM-COEIN) for causes of abnormal uterine bleeding in nongravid women of reproductive age. Int J Gynaecol Obstet: Off Org Int Fed Gynaecol Obstet 113(1):3–13
21. Garza-Leal JG, León IH, Toub D (2014) Pregnancy after transcervical radiofrequency ablation guided by intrauterine sonography: case report. Gynecol Surg 11(2):145–149
22. van der Kooij SM, Hehenkamp WJ, Volkers NA et al (2010) Uterine artery embolization vs hysterectomy in the treatment of symptomatic uterine fibroids: 5-year outcome from the randomized EMMY trial. Am J Obstet Gynecol 203(2):105 e1-13
23. Spies JB, Bruno J, Czeyda-Pommersheim F et al (2005) Long-term outcome of uterine artery embolization of leiomyomata. Obstet Gynecol 106(5 Pt 1):933–939
24. Homer H, Saridogan E (2010) Uterine artery embolization for fibroids is associated with an increased risk of miscarriage. Fertil Steril 94(1):324–330
25. Committee on Gynecologic Practice ACoO (2004) Gynecologists. ACOG Committee Opinion. Uterine artery embolization. Obstet Gynecol 103(2):403–4
26. Usadi RS, Marshburn PB (2007) The impact of uterine artery embolization on fertility and pregnancy outcome. Curr Opin Obstet Gynecol 19(3):279–283
27. Bradley LD (2009) Uterine fibroid embolization: a viable alternative to hysterectomy. Am J Obstet Gynecol 201(2):127–135
28. Katsumori T, Kasahara T, Tsuchida Y et al (2008) Amenorrhea and resumption of menstruation after uterine artery embolization for fibroids. Int J Gynaecol Obstet 103(3):217–221
29. Munro MG, Garza-Leal J, Grossman J (2007) Intrauterine ultrasound for the measurement of uterine fibroids: a comparative study. 1st AAGL International Congress in conjunction with SEGi Understanding and Treating Abnormal Uterine Bleeding. Palermo Italy
30. Veersema S, Varma R, Toub D (2011) Visualization of Essure implants with intrauterine sonography for confirmation of placement. Gynecol Surg 8(Supp 1):76
31. Chudnoff SG, Berman JM, Levine DJ et al (2013) Outpatient procedure for the treatment and relief of symptomatic uterine myomas. Obstet Gynecol 121(5):1075–1082
32. Stewart EA, Gostout B, Rabinovici J et al (2007) Sustained relief of leiomyoma symptoms by using focused ultrasound surgery. Obstet Gynecol 110(2 Pt 1):279–287

37

The trainees' pain with laparoscopic surgery: what do trainees really know about theatre set-up and how this impacts their health

Declan Quinn · James Moohan

Abstract Although it is clear that laparoscopic surgery is beneficial to the patient, such surgery brings with it unique challenges and possible injury to the surgeon. Firstly, we sought to investigate the prevalence of musculoskeletal distress experienced by trainees. Secondly, we sought to ascertain if the trainees had received appropriate instruction to optimise their operative environment during laparoscopic surgery. An anonymised questionnaire survey was distributed to all 89 trainees in obstetrics and gynaecology within Northern Ireland. Forty-four (83 %) trainees reported to having received formal instruction in theatre layout and operating body position. However, only 8 (15 %) were aware of the ideal operating surface height, and 6 (11 %) knew the ideal monitor position, while 11 (20 %) and 7 (13 %) knew the correct angles for grasping and suturing tissue, respectively. Eighty-five percent of trainees suffered some form of musculoskeletal distress with back, shoulder and neck pain the most common areas affected. Eyestrain was reported by 1/3 of trainees. Although no trainees required sick leave, one in three required regular analgesia, physiotherapy or alternative therapies. It is clear that current training has not addressed operating ergonomics sufficiently, and this is having a significant impact on trainees' health.

Keywords Laparoscopy · Ergonomics · Gynaecology · Training

D. Quinn (✉)
ST6 Antrim Area Hospital, 4 Bush Road, Antrim, NI, UK
e-mail: quinndeclan@hotmail.com

J. Moohan
Altnagelvin Area Hospital, Londonderry, UK
e-mail: James.moohan@westerntrust.hscni.net

Background

Among surgeons, musculoskeletal symptoms have been reported to increase in prevalence with increasing age [1]. In addition, Szeko et al., (2009) noted that the likelihood of musculoskeletal pain was closely related to the number of years worked in laparoscopic surgery [2]. In contrast, Sari et al. (2010) found that musculoskeletal symptoms were more prevalent in surgeons with less experience [3], while Soueid et al. (2010) found that such symptoms were often experienced at an early age [4]. Park et al. (2010) however found no relationship between musculoskeletal symptoms and age [5].

The elongated duration of the laparoscopic surgical procedure compared with the equivalent open procedure also appears to play a role in the prevalence of musculoskeletal distress among surgeons [6]

To date, little or no attention has been paid to the impact that the increasing proportion of surgery performed laparoscopically has had on the incidence of musculoskeletal distress among trainees.

The objectives of this study were to examine the prevalence of eyestrain and musculoskeletal distress among trainee gynaecologists and to ascertain whether instruction in theatre and surgical ergonomics had any impact on this.

Method

A survey in the form of a questionnaire was distributed to trainees in obstetrics and gynaecology of the Northern Ireland Deanery attending their monthly CME meetings between 1 September 2012 and 31 December 2012. A list of the email addresses of each trainee was obtained from the Northern Ireland Medical and Dental Training Agency, to enable a copy of the questionnaire survey to be sent electronically to any trainee who had either failed to complete a questionnaire at the

Table 1 Group demographics

	Male	Female	Between-group statistics
Age	33 (27–55)	29 (25–38)	<0.05
Height (cm)	178.3 (167–188)	164.5 (153–180)	<0.01
Weight (kg)	86.3 (68–110)	61.4 (47–49)	<0.01
Glove size	7.5 (5.5–8.5)	6 (5.5–7.0)	<0.01
Trainee ST level	3.0 (1–7)	3.0 (1–7)	ns
Years in specialty	5.6 (1–31)	3.9 (1–10)	ns

Data are presented as group mean values (range)

meeting or who had been unable to attend. Each questionnaire was accompanied by a letter explaining the aims of the study and included a consent form.

Survey design

The survey examined information in three categories:

1. Basic demographics of each trainee
2. The degree of instruction and knowledge on the ergonomics of gynaecological endoscopic surgery
3. The prevalence/frequency[1] and sites of possible musculoskeletal distress suffered and the requirement for treatment of such injury

Data analysis

The data obtained from the questionnaire were analysed using SPSS version 20. Basic demographics were assessed using descriptive statistics with male and female groups being compared using the independent sample t test. The chi-square test for independence was employed to compare the prevalence of musculoskeletal distress and eyestrain between the two sexes with the Yates correction for continuity being used to compensate for any overestimation in the chi value that results from a 2×2 table. Collinearity diagnostics were employed to exclude the possibility of high correlation between different variables before binary logistic regression was employed to determine whether different independent variables were able to predict the prevalence of musculoskeletal distress or eyestrain.

Findings

Fifty-three out of 89 trainees completed the questionnaire to give a response rate of 60 %. Nineteen of the trainees were male (36 %) with the remainder (64 %) being female, a ratio in keeping with the local medical school graduate output.

The median age for the group as a whole was 30 years (range 25–55) with males being somewhat older (median age 30 versus 29 years). As expected, male trainees were taller, heavier and had a larger hand size than their female counterparts (Table 1). In addition, although male and female trainees were at the same level of specialist training, male trainees had on average spent almost 2 years longer within the specialty (Table 1).

The majority of trainees experienced some degree of musculoskeletal distress with 1/3 suffering eyestrain (Table 2).

Although male trainees suffered a lower prevalence of both injuries when compared with females, a chi-square test for independence indicated no significant association between gender and injury (Yates correction for continuity=0.256, p=0.613 and 0.332, p=0.564 for musculoskeletal distress and eyestrain, respectively). All levels of trainees were found to suffer symptoms. Surprisingly, although one might have anticipated that senior trainees would perform a greater amount of laparoscopic surgery as well as more complex procedures than their junior colleagues and thus be more likely to experience injury, a chi-square test for independence revealed that they were no more likely to suffer symptoms (Pearson chi-square=4.575, p=0.599, phi=0.249).

Twenty-two trainees admitted to having received some form of instruction in the ergonomics of laparoscopic surgery with more than half of male trainees (11 of 19, 58 %) receiving instruction compared to only 1 in 3 female trainees (11 of 34, 32 %), but again, this difference was not significant (Yates

Table 2 Prevalence of pain and eyestrain between groups

	Male	Female	Total
Pain during laparoscopy	15 (78.9 %)	30 (88.2 %)	45 (84.9 %)
Eyestrain	5 (26.3 %)	13 (38.2 %)	18 (34 %)

---

[1] The frequency of musculoskeletal distress was rated on a Likert scale (always, frequently, occasionally, rarely and never).

Table 3   Ergonomic instruction and prevalence of pain

	Ergonomic instruction	Musculoskeletal pain	Eyestrain
Male	Yes	9	2
	No	5	3
Female	Yes	9	4
	No	21	9

Table 5   Prevalence of pain and direction of neck turning between the groups

	Neutral	Left	Right	Both	All directions
Male	1	1	3	1	0
Female	5	2	4	4	1
Total	6	3	7	5	1

correction for continuity=2.308, p=0.129, phi=0.249). The source of instruction on ergonomics was most often a course (11, 50 %), a senior colleague (3, 13.6 %) or both (7, 31.8 %).

Instruction on ergonomics however did not result in a significant reduction in the likelihood of musculoskeletal distress or eyestrain (Yates correction for continuity=0.019, p=0.889 and 0.327, p=0.567 for musculoskeletal pain and eyestrain, respectively, for the whole group of trainees). Indeed, 9 of 11 male trainees and 9 of 11 females who had received some degree of instruction still experienced musculoskeletal pain (Table 3).

Eighteen (33 %) trainees reported suffering eyestrain, with male trainees (5 of 19, 26 %) again being affected less often than their female counterparts (13 of 34, 38 %). Instruction on ergonomics does appear to reduce the incidence of eyestrain but not significantly, with only 27.3 % of trainees who had received instruction being affected compared to 38.7 % of those who had not. Among male trainees, the impact of instruction appears even greater with only 2 of 11 (18 %) suffering eyestrain compared to 3 of 8 (37.5 %) who did not receive such teaching. Four of 11 (36 %) female trainees suffered eyestrain despite having received instruction similar to the proportion of trainees who had received no instruction (9 of 23, 39 %). A chi-square test for independence did not reveal any significant difference between the sexes (Yates correction for continuity=0, p=0.72 and=0.055, p=0.815 for male and female, respectively). A larger study would hopefully confirm or refute these findings.

Pain occurred most commonly in the neck (42 %), back (72 %), shoulder (43 %) or leg (37 %), occurring less frequently in the elbow, wrist, thumb, fingers and foot (Table 4).

For each site of pain, there was no significant difference in prevalence between male and female trainees (Table 4).

Neck pain occurred most commonly on turning to the right (7 of 22, 31 %) followed by being in the neutral position (6 of 22, 27 %) with pain being reported as occurring frequently in 1/3 trainees and occasionally in 2/3 trainees, male and female alike. (Table 5)

With regard to back pain, this was just as likely to occur in the region of the lower as upper back, with female trainees being more likely to suffer pain in both areas when compared to their male counterparts (Table 6) although a chi-square test for independence did not detect any significant difference between the sexes (Pearson chi-square=2.724, p=0.256).

Male trainees suffered back pain frequently in three cases (21.4 %) compared to female trainees who experienced the pain frequently in eight cases (33.3 %), but again, this did not reach significance.

Shoulder pain occurred slightly more often on the right side (9 of 23, 39.1 %) with both shoulders being affected in more than 8 trainees (34.7 %). The dominance of right-sided injury was only apparent among female trainees (7/16, 43.8 %) with male counterparts actually experiencing pain more commonly in the left shoulder. However, this difference did not reach statistical significance (Yates correction for continuity=0.186, p=0.667). Pain was reported as occurring frequently in 5 trainees (21.7 %) and occasionally in the remainder with female trainees being twice (25 versus 14.2 %) as likely to be affected frequently as males, but again, this did not reach significance (Pearson chi-square=1.483, p=0.476).

Table 4   Site of pain between the groups and significance

Site of pain	Male	Female	Continuity correction	p	Phi	Approximate significance
Neck	6	16	0.650	0.420	0.151	0.279
Back	14	24	0.000	1.000	−0.033	0.810
Shoulder	7	16	0.186	0.667	0.099	0.472
Elbow	3	5	0.000	1.000	−0.015	0.916
Wrist	2	9	1.039	0.308	0.189	0.170
Thumb	5	7	0.018	0.892	−0.066	0.433
Finger	5	6	0.155	0.461	−0.103	0.456
Leg	7	13	0.000	1.000	0.014	0.920
Foot	5	6	0.155	0.461	−0.103	0.456

Table 6 Site of back pain between the groups

	Upper	Lower	Both
Male	6	7	1
Female	9	8	7
Total	15	15	8

Table 8 Number answering correctly

	Ergonomic training	Operating height	Monitor height	Manipulating angle	Suturing angle
Male	Yes	2	1	2	4
	No	2	1	3	2
Female	Yes	0	2	2	2
	No	3	2	5	4

Leg pain affected male and female trainees in similar numbers (36.8 and 38.2 %, respectively) and usually affected both legs (13/20). Furthermore, leg pain was usually only experienced occasionally (15/20, 75 %) rather than frequently (3/20, 9 %).

Two trainees, both female, had required sick leave as a result of the pain experienced, while one trainee, also female, had sought medical attention, but again, the difference between sexes was not significant (Yates correction for continuity=0.106, p=0.744 for sick leave and Yates correction for continuity=0.000, p=1.000 for medical attention). Seventeen trainees had however resorted to some form of treatment for their symptoms (Table 7).

Surprisingly, trainees who had received instruction in ergonomics were no more likely to answer correctly those questions (Table 8) pertaining to optimal ergonomics for gynaecological laparoscopy, such as the ideal height of the operating surface (Yates correction for continuity=3.191, p=0.784), ideal height of the centre of the monitor (Yates correction for continuity=7.393, p=0.117), ideal instrument angle for dissection/grasping (Yates correction for continuity=5.671, p=0.340) or suturing (Yates correction for continuity=6.892, p=0.199), than those trainees who had not received instruction (Table 8). Again, there was no significant difference between male (Pearson chi-square=2.943, 5.589, 8.573 and 4.369; p=0.709, 0.232, 0.073 and 0.358 for operating height, monitor position, ideal dissection/grasping and ideal suturing angle, respectively) and female trainees (Pearson chi-square=6.497, 1.526, 2.807 and 4.369; p=0.370, 0.676, 0.730 and 0.629 for operating height, monitor position, ideal dissection/grasping and ideal suturing angle, respectively).

After collinearity diagnostics had been performed to exclude high correlation between different variables within the model, direct logistic regression was performed to assess the

impact of a number of factors on the likelihood that trainees would report that they had experienced problems with pain or eyestrain following laparoscopic surgery. The model contained seven independent variables (age, sex, height, weight, hand size, years in specialty and ergonomic training).

The full model containing all predictors was not statistically significant, chi-square (7, N=47)=12.248, p=0.093, indicating that the model was not able to distinguish between trainees who reported musculoskeletal pain and those who did not. However, a Hosmer-Lemeshow goodness-of-fit test, chi-square=9.269, p=0.234, supports the model. The model as a whole explained between 22.9 (Cox & Snell R square) and 38.3 % (Nagelkerke R square) of the variance in pain status and correctly classified 83 % of cases. Only one of the independent variables made a uniquely statistically significant contribution to the model (height of trainee). The strongest predictor of reporting musculoskeletal pain was gender, recording an odds ratio of 2.19, indicating that females were over two times more likely to experience pain than their male counterparts. (Table 9)

Again for eyestrain, the full model containing all predictors was not statistically significant, chi-square (7, N=47)= 3.338, p=0.852, indicating that the model was unable to distinguish between trainees who suffered eyestrain and those who did not. A Hosmer-Lemeshow goodness-of-fit test however (chi-square=11.218, p=0.129) supports the model. The model as a whole explained only between 6.9 (Cox & Snell R square) and 9.5 % (Nagelkerke R square)

Table 7 Interventions required between the groups

	Male	Female	Total
Analgesia	3	8	11
Physiotherapy	1	0	1
Analgesia + physiotherapy	0	3	3
Analgesia + alternative	0	1	1
Physiotherapy + alternative	0	1	1

Table 9 Logistic regression predicting likelihood of reporting musculoskeletal pain

	B	S.E.	Wald	df	p	Odds ratio
Sex	.78	2.02	.15	1	.70	2.19
Age	−.08	.14	.33	1	.56	.92
Height	.28	.13	4.63	1	.03	1.32
Weight	−.07	.06	1.36	1	.24	.93
Glove size	−1.47	1.15	1.65	1	.20	.23
Years	−.11	.16	.47	1	.49	.90
Ergonomics	−.72	1.05	.47	1	.49	.49
Constant	−27.50	22.54	1.489	1	.22	.000

Table 10 Logistic regression predicting likelihood of reporting eyestrain

	B	S.E.	Wald	df	p	Odds ratio
Sex	.33	1.27	.07	1	.80	1.39
Age	−.18	.17	1.19	1	.28	0.84
Height	.04	.06	.44	1	.51	1.04
Weight	−.01	.04	.06	1	.80	1.00
Glove size	−.11	.91	.01	1	.91	0.90
Years	.14	.18	.62	1	.43	1.15
Ergonomics	.35	.69	.27	1	.61	1.42
Constant	−1.73	10.76	.03	1	.87	0.18

of the variance in eyestrain status and correctly classified 66 % of cases. None of the independent variables made a uniquely statistically significant contribution to the model. The strongest predictors for reporting eyestrain were training in ergonomics and gender, recording odds ratios of 1.38 and 1.42, respectively, indicating that females were over 1.4 times more likely to experience eyestrain than their male counterparts and that trainees who had received training in ergonomics were 1.4 times more likely to suffer eyestrain than those who had not received training (Table 10).

Binary logistic regression analysis was subsequently carried out for each individual region of the body using the same variables.

For the neck, although none of the independent variables made a uniquely statistically significant contribution to the model, female trainees were 7.9 times as likely to experience pain as their male counterparts, while for the back region, none of the independent variables made a uniquely statistically significant contribution to the model, with no variable being any more likely to predict pain than another.

With regard to the shoulder and elbow, none of the independent variables made a uniquely statistically significant contribution to the model.

Table 11 Logistic regression predicting likelihood of reporting wrist pain

	B	S.E.	Wald	df	p	Odds ratio
Sex	.25	2.22	.01	1	.91	1.28
Age	−1.31	.56	5.49	1	.02	.27
Height	−.36	.15	6.16	1	.01	.70
Weight	.40	.19	4.50	1	.34	1.49
Glove size	1.95	1.59	1.52	1	.22	7.04
Years	1.32	.62	.4.59	1	.03	3.75
Ergonomics	−2.70	1.64	2.71	1	.10	.07
Constant	62.52	27.22	5.28	1	.02	1.42E+27

However, for the wrist, the full model containing all predictors was statistically significant, chi-square=27.83, p=000, indicating that the model was able to distinguish between trainees who suffered wrist pain and those who did not. Three of the independent variables made a uniquely statistically significant contribution to the model (age, height and years in specialty). The strongest predictor of reporting wrist pain was years' experience recording an odds ratio of 3.75, indicating that each year spent in specialty led to an almost 4-fold chance of developing wrist pain. (Table 11)

For the thumb, the time that a trainee had spent in specialty was significantly related to the likelihood of suffering pain in that area (p=0.03). Indeed, for each additional year, the likelihood of developing injury rose 1.8 times. For the fingers, the likelihood of developing pain increased 3-fold for each rise in glove size.

For the leg and foot, although none of the independent variables made a uniquely statistically significant contribution to the model, males were 2.7 times more likely to suffer foot pain than their female colleagues.

Conclusions

This study reports on the prevalence of musculoskeletal distress and eyestrain among trainees in obstetrics and gynaecology.

Sari et al. (2010) reported that less experienced surgeons were more likely to experience injury with laparoscopy than their more experienced colleagues and suggested that this was the result of higher muscle tension and lack of ergonomic knowledge [3]. Indeed, Hemal et al. (2001) noted that surgeons with less than 2 years laparoscopic surgical experience suffered more discomfort than those with greater experience [7].

Thus, instruction in theatre and body ergonomics for laparoscopy early in the medical career should improve the surgical outcomes for both patient and surgeon alike.

Like Stomberg et al. (2010), we found that females were much more likely to suffer musculoskeletal distress than their male colleagues [1]. This difference in prevalence between the sexes has been attributed to the fact that women have a lower muscle mass in the upper extremities when compared with men. As the monitor is often placed on top of a trolley of fixed height, this would disadvantage a shorter surgeon, likely a female whose neck would be extended in viewing the monitor, leading ultimately to neck strain. In addition, as operating tables have traditionally been designed for open surgery, they are not optimal for laparoscopic procedures with the lowest height that most operating tables can be lowered to being only 725 mm, again disadvantaging the usually shorter female surgeon [8]. As our survey shows that female trainees are significantly shorter than their male counterparts, they will be automatically exposed to a greater risk of musculoskeletal injury during laparoscopic procedures.

It is somewhat concerning that only a minority of trainees were aware of how to optimise the theatre environment and equipment to minimise the risk of musculoskeletal injury or eyestrain during endoscopic surgery despite all being required to complete a course in Basic Surgical Skills. This would suggest that the current curriculum of the RCOG Basic Surgical Skills course devotes insufficient time and resources to this aspect of surgery and urgently needs to focus more on the ergonomics of both open and endoscopic surgeries if trainees are to minimise their risk of musculoskeletal injury or eyestrain with all the implications that this would have on the specialty.

Moreover, as the retirement age of healthcare workers continues to rise, it is likely that our current cohort of trainees will be forced to work much longer exposing them to an even greater risk of injury unless laparoscopic surgery and the theatre environment are made safer.

There is a potential for such musculoskeletal symptoms to escalate in the future with the increasing application of minimally invasive surgery.

Consent Informed consent was obtained from all participants included in the study. This article does not contain any studies with human or animal subjects performed by the any of the authors.

References

1. Stomberg MW, Tronstad S-E, Hedberg K, Bengsston J, Jonsson P, Johansen L, Lindvall B (2010) Work-related musculoskeletal disorders when performing laparoscopic surgery. Surg Laparosc Endosc Percutan Tech 20(1):49–53
2. Szeko GP, Ho P, Ting ACW, Poon JTC, Cheng SWK, Tsang RCC (2009) Work-related musculoskeletal symptoms in surgeons. J Occup Rehabil 19(2):175–184
3. Sari V, Nieboer TE, Vierhout ME, Stegeman DF, Kluivers KB (2010) The operation room as a hostile environment for surgeons: physical complaints during and after laparoscopy. Min Invasiv Ther 19:105–109
4. Soueid A, Oudit D, Thiagarajah S, Laitung G (2010) The pain of surgery: pain experienced by surgeons while operating. Int J Surg 8:118–120
5. Park A, Lee G, Seagull FJ, Meenaghan N, Dexter D (2010) Patients benefit while surgeons suffer: an impending epidemic. J Am Coll Surg 210:306–313
6. Cuschieri A (1995) Whither minimal access surgery: tribulations and expectations. Am J Surg 1:9–19
7. Hemal AK, Srinivas M, Charles AR (2001) Ergonomic problems associated with laparoscopy. J Endourol 15:499–503
8. Van Veelen MA, Kazemier G, Koopman J, Goossens RHM, Meijer DW (2002) Assessment of the ergonomically optimal operating surface height for laparoscopic surgery. J Laparoendosc Adv Surg Tech 12:47–52

38

Should medical students be given laparoscopic training?

Taner Shakir · Tae Lee · Jeffrey Lim · Kevin Jones

Abstract Undergraduate medical education does not usually involve training in laparoscopic skills despite the fact that minimal access surgery has become the norm in the developed world. We designed a study to evaluate the attitude of surgeons and medical students to formal teaching of these skills. Two surveys were sent; one to fourth year medical students at the University of Bristol and another to specialist laparoscopic surgeons. Student questions centred on whether they would find training in basic laparoscopic skills useful, whilst surgeons were asked whether it would be acceptable for medical students to assist with a laparoscopic case. Sixty percent [131/220] of students responded, with 60 % [79/131] of respondents stating that they would find assisting with laparoscopic surgery beneficial, despite 79 % [103/131] being undecided or having no interest in a surgical career, with 66 % [87/131] stating it would allow them to become more involved during theatre sessions. Eighty-three percent [83/100] of surgeons responded, and 74 % [62/83] said they would allow medical students to hold the camera. Seventy percent [65/83] felt that basic knowledge of the equipment was the most important aspect of training, and 66 % [55/83] felt that assisting was the second most important. This is the first study to look at both the student's and surgeon's views on laparoscopic training of medical students. The study highlights the benefits of acquiring laparoscopic skills such as camera holding and assisting. In response, we have set up a course for students prior to placements in surgical specialties.

Keywords Medical students · Laparoscopic skills training

Introduction

Medical student teaching in the operating theatre is often unsatisfactory [1]. The widespread introduction of laparoscopic surgery into clinical practice presents an opportunity to change this [2]. We believe that training in laparoscopic surgical techniques should start at medical school. Even if the student has no desire to pursue a surgical career after graduation, the opportunity to learn in the operating theatre will be enhanced if the student is taught basic laparoscopic techniques such as camera holding and the use of endoscopic graspers because they will be able to participate in the operation. In the past, students were asked to assist at operations by holding retractors so learning the basic techniques of laparoscopic surgery is no different in principle. Furthermore, being able to make a contribution in theatre will enhance the student's sense of belonging to the multidisciplinary team. They will no longer be asked to stand in a corner watching a TV monitor because they can once more "scrub in and join in".

In this study, we surveyed the attitude of medical students and experienced laparoscopic surgeons to the introduction of basic laparoscopic skills into the undergraduate medical curriculum. This is the first study of its kind in the UK.

Objectives and methods

We undertook a survey to investigate the attitude of surgeon's and students to introducing a laparoscopic training programme for medical students.

Two questionnaires were distributed electronically via email. The first (Appendix 1) questionnaire was sent to specialists in the UK and a second (appendix 2) questionnaire to

T. Shakir · T. Lee · J. Lim · K. Jones (✉)
University of Bristol Academy, Great Western Hospital, Marlbourgh Road, Swindon SN3 6BB, UK
e-mail: kevin.jones@gwh.nhs.uk

fourth year medical students at Bristol University, UK. The specialists were asked eight questions, and one free text box was included. Six of the questions required a single answer, while two contained multiple stems with a choice of answers to semi quantify the specialists answer. The students were asked nine multiple choice questions (one answer only for each question) and one optional written answer question. In some of the questions and answers, bracket descriptions had to be included for clarity and specificity; otherwise, different interpretations and therefore different answers might be given that could affect the results of the study.

Results

All the students who responded were in the fourth year of their medical degrees (The Bristol medical degree is divided into two pre-clinical years and three clinical years). Sixty percent [131/220] of students responded, with 60 % [79/131] of

respondents stating that they would find assisting with laparoscopic surgery beneficial, despite 79 % [103/131] being undecided or having no interest in a surgical career, with 66 % [87/131] stating it would allow them to become more involved during theatre sessions. Seventy-one percent [93/131] of students would like to be offered a basic course in laparoscopic skills.

In total, 83 % [83/100] of surgeons responded. Opportunities for student involvement are shown in Fig. 1a. There is an almost universal 98 % acceptance of student observation. Seventy-four percent of surgeons were comfortable with students holding the camera, and 61 % were comfortable with instrument holding whilst 51 % would support retraction of tissues. Thirty-seven percent felt comfortable with medical students performing blunt dissection whilst 56 % felt this should not be performed, and 65 % felt that sharp should never be undertaken by students.

The skill specialists thought students could acquire are shown in Fig. 1b. Surgeons stated that basic knowledge of

Fig. 1 **a** Responses to" How comfortable would you be with medical students…? Lay observing includes non-scrubbed observation. Scrubbed observing includes close observation whilst sterile. **b** Responses to "How important are the following factors in allowing medical student involvement on your laparoscopic list? Basic surgical skills include suturing, etc. Basic knowledge of equipment entails knowledge of the stack and camera trouble shooting, e.g. lens fogging. Basic skills exercises are retraction with graspers and simple stacking exercises. Advanced camera skills are the use of a 30° scope. Practice on a trainer includes active manipulation with graspers

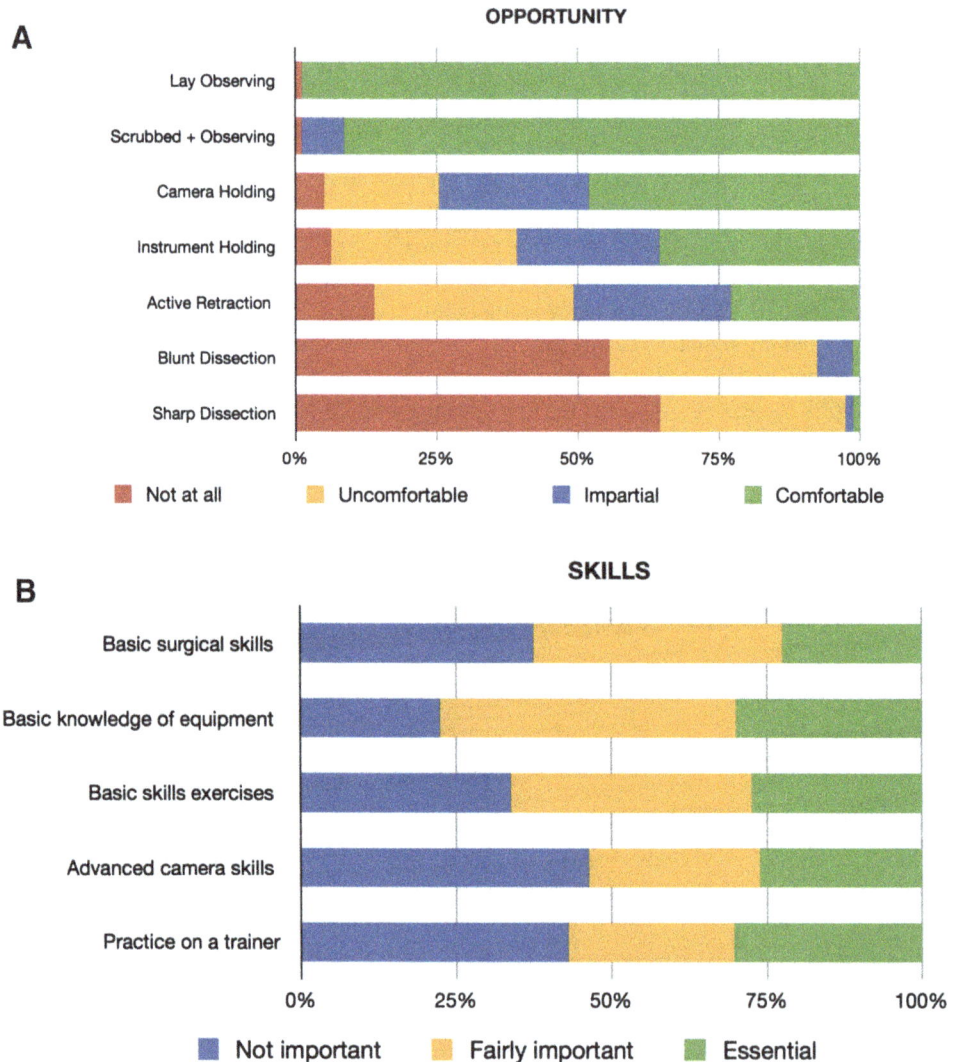

the equipment was the most important (78 %) [65/83], with basic laparoscopic skills being the second most important (66 %) [55/83] if such a course were to be offered to students.

Discussion

It is evident that an opportunity exists for medical students to be involved with laparoscopic procedures. This is not limited to camera holding, as over half were comfortable with instrument holding. A basic knowledge of the equipment in addition to basic skills exercises were the most important factors in allowing participation. This has implications for the development of a training programme.

Advantages to students are as follows:

1. *An Anatomy Lesson*

   A decline in dissection at medical school has resulted in the current trend of increased utilisation of prosection, plastic models and even digital (virtual) methods for learning anatomy. These techniques can help students understand the relationships of structures to each other. However, laparoscopic surgery allows the student to have a "surgeon's eye view", so it should be viewed as an adjunct to the more modern approach of anatomy teaching.

2. *Involvement*

   Medical students often feel as though theatre is not a favourable learning environment [1]. This translates into an uninspiring experience and may be a reason for the decline of interest in surgical careers [3]. Learning techniques such as camera and instrument holding offer the student an opportunity to participate in a low risk but essential task in theatre which in turn offers the chance for students to enhance their learning and enjoyment during undergraduate surgical placements.

Advantages to patients are as follows:

1. *Governance*

   Laparoscopic techniques are usually learnt on trainers in a skills laboratory unlike open techniques which are first done on patients undergoing operations. The ability to acquire surgical skills in a simulated situation enhances patient safety and underpins modern concepts of good governance because it offers students an opportunity to practice with scope for error. Scenarios can be repeated indefinitely until trainees are confident. Teaching laparoscopic surgery in a simulated setting also allows core skills to be tested and measured.

2. *The "Gameboy" generation*

   Patients can benefit from the changes already happening in society. Numerous systematic reviews have demonstrated a positive link between the acquisition of endoscopic skills and *some* video games [4–10]. Both laparoscopic surgery and video games require the translation of three-dimensional movement onto a two-dimensional screen. Concepts learned are "attentional weighting" (increased time spent on important aspects, whilst neglecting trivial features) as well as improving hand-eye coordination, dexterity and visuo-spatial abilities [4]. Video games are now so intrinsic to society (a norm even on mobile devices) that medical students may already possess these skills. Therefore, laparoscopy may be so intuitive to a modern-day medical student that it be natural. Observational studies have shown that age *may* also be a factor. In one study, there was a 77 % improvement in completion time of basic laparoscopic skills for undergraduate medical students compared to junior surgical trainees [11]. The younger the student, the fewer problems with technical issues such as the fulcrum effect or swiping left in order to move right on smartphones.

Possible limitations

1. *Surgical experience*

   We have assumed that basic and intermediate laparoscopic surgical techniques are part of every surgeon's skill set and that specialists have reached a level of competence where they can supervise a medical student to act as an assistant. We have also assumed that seniors are trained to give structured feedback. Where this is not the case, it will limit the involvement of students and post-graduate (PG) trainees in theatre. Furthermore, surgery is an apprenticeship which requires the acquisition of skills over time. This may be possible for a PG trainee, but medical students spend only short periods of time on surgical attachments.

2. *Training programmes*

   There are many PG programmes available in laparoscopic surgery which offer training on simulators, and similar courses are now available for medical student's, e.g. ICENI Centre at Colchester Hospital, UK (www.icenicentre.org). In order to deliver a structured training programme, it is necessary to have an evidence-based curriculum. The European Society of Gynaecological Surgery (ESGE) has, in collaboration with the European Academy of Gynaecological Surgery, developed such a curriculum [12–15]. The full programme is called Gynaecological Endoscopic Surgical Education and Assessment (GESEA, www.esge.org/education/guidlines/gesea). This training opportunity is accessible to everyone including medical students.

Conclusions

This is the first study to look at both the student's and surgeon's views on laparoscopic training of medical students. Both students and surgeons have highlighted the potential benefit of students acquiring basic skills such as camera holding. In light of these findings, we have set up a Self-Selected Component in Surgery. Students will take part in a laparoscopic training course before being placed in surgical specialties where these skills can be put into practice. We plan to evaluate the students' experience to determine whether they gain more from their time in the operating theatre having been on the course.

References

1. Fernando N et al (2007) Undergraduate medical students' perceptions and expectations of theatre-based learning: how can we improve the student learning experience? Surgeon 5:271–274
2. Green CJ, Maxwell R, Verne J, Martin RM, Blazeby JM (2009) The influence of NICE guidance on the uptake of laparoscopic surgery for colorectal cancer. J Public Health 31(4):541–545
3. Polk H (1999) The declining interest in surgical careers, the primary care mirage, and concerns about contemporary undergraduate surgical education. Am J Surg 178:177–179
4. Lynch J, Aughwane P, Hammond TM (2010) Video games and surgical ability: a literature review. J Surg Educ 67:184–189
5. Rosenberg BH, Landsittel D, Averch TD (2005) Can video games be used to predict or improve laparoscopic skills? J Endourol 19:372–376
6. Fanning J, Fenton B, Johnson C, Johnson J, Rehman S (2011) Comparison of teenaged video gamers vs PGY-I residents in obstetrics and gynecology on a laparoscopic simulator. J Minim Invasive Gynecol 18:169–172
7. Rosser JC et al (2007) The impact of video games on training surgeons in the 21st century. Arch Surg 142:181–186, Discusssion 186
8. Rosenberg BH, Landsittel D, Averch TD (2005) Can video games be used to predict or improve laparoscopic skills? J Endourol 19:372–376
9. Ou Y, McGlone ER, Camm CF, Khan OA (2013) Does playing video games improve laparoscopic skills? Int J Surg 11:365–369
10. Waxberg SL, Schwaitzberg SD, Cao CGL (2005) Effects of videogame experience on laparoscopic skill acquisition. Proc Hum Factors Ergon Soc Annu Meet 49:1047–1051
11. Salkini MW, Hamilton AJ (2010) The effect of age on acquiring laparoscopic skills. J Endourol 24:377–379
12. Campo R, Molinas CR, De Wilde RL, Brolmann H, Brucker S, Mencaglia L, Odonovan P, Wallwiener D, Wattiez A (2012) Are you good enough for your patients? The European certification model in laparoscopic surgery. Facts Views Vis Obgyn 4:95–101
13. Campo R, Reising C, Van Belle Y et al (2010) A valid model for testing and training laparoscopic psychomotor skills. Gynecol Surg 7:133–141
14. Molinas CR, Campo R (2010) Defining a structured training program for acquiring basic and advanced laparoscopic psychomotor skills in a simulator. Gynecol Surg 7:427–435
15. Campo R, Wattiez A, Leon De Wilde R, Molinas Sanabria CR (2012) Training in laparoscopic surgery: From the lab to the or. Slovenian. J Public Health. doi:10.2478/v10152-012-0032-x

Permissions

All chapters in this book were first published in GS, by Springer; hereby published with permission under the Creative Commons Attribution License or equivalent. Every chapter published in this book has been scrutinized by our experts. Their significance has been extensively debated. The topics covered herein carry significant findings which will fuel the growth of the discipline. They may even be implemented as practical applications or may be referred to as a beginning point for another development.

The contributors of this book come from diverse backgrounds, making this book a truly international effort. This book will bring forth new frontiers with its revolutionizing research information and detailed analysis of the nascent developments around the world.

We would like to thank all the contributing authors for lending their expertise to make the book truly unique. They have played a crucial role in the development of this book. Without their invaluable contributions this book wouldn't have been possible. They have made vital efforts to compile up to date information on the varied aspects of this subject to make this book a valuable addition to the collection of many professionals and students.

This book was conceptualized with the vision of imparting up-to-date information and advanced data in this field. To ensure the same, a matchless editorial board was set up. Every individual on the board went through rigorous rounds of assessment to prove their worth. After which they invested a large part of their time researching and compiling the most relevant data for our readers.

The editorial board has been involved in producing this book since its inception. They have spent rigorous hours researching and exploring the diverse topics which have resulted in the successful publishing of this book. They have passed on their knowledge of decades through this book. To expedite this challenging task, the publisher supported the team at every step. A small team of assistant editors was also appointed to further simplify the editing procedure and attain best results for the readers.

Apart from the editorial board, the designing team has also invested a significant amount of their time in understanding the subject and creating the most relevant covers. They scrutinized every image to scout for the most suitable representation of the subject and create an appropriate cover for the book.

The publishing team has been an ardent support to the editorial, designing and production team. Their endless efforts to recruit the best for this project, has resulted in the accomplishment of this book. They are a veteran in the field of academics and their pool of knowledge is as vast as their experience in printing. Their expertise and guidance has proved useful at every step. Their uncompromising quality standards have made this book an exceptional effort. Their encouragement from time to time has been an inspiration for everyone.

The publisher and the editorial board hope that this book will prove to be a valuable piece of knowledge for researchers, students, practitioners and scholars across the globe.

List of Contributors

Farr R. Nezhat
Division of Gynecologic, Oncology and Minimally Invasive Surgery, Department of Obstetrics and Gynecology, Columbia University, New York, NY 10019, USA
Department of Obstetrics and Gynecology, St. Luke's-Roosevelt Medical Center, 10th Floor, 1000 10th Avenue, New York, NY 10019, USA

Farr R. Nezhat, Susan S. Khalil and Tamara N. Finger
Division of Minimally Invasive Surgery, Department of Obstetrics and Gynecology, St. Luke's-Roosevelt Medical Center, New York, NY, USA

Farr R. Nezhat and Patrick F. Vetere
Division of Minimally Invasive Gynecologic Surgery, Department of Obstetrics and Gynecology, Winthrop University Hospital, Mineola, NY, USA

Vasileios Minas, Elizabeth Shaw and Thomas Aust
Minimal Access Centre, Department of Obstetrics and Gynaecology, Wirral University Teaching Hospital, Arrowe Park Rd, Wirral, Merseyside CH49 5PE, UK

Thierry Van den Bosch, Dominique Van Schoubroeck and Dirk Timmerman
Department of Development and Regeneration, KU Leuven, 3000 Leuven, Belgium

Thierry Van den Bosch
Department of Obstetrics and Gynecology, RZTienen, 3300 Tienen, Belgium
KU Leuven Department of Development and Regeneration, University Hospitals Leuven, Herestraat 49, 3000 Leuven, Belgium

José Gerardo Garza-Leal and Iván Hernández León
Universidad Autónoma de Nuevo León, Monterrey, Nuevo Leon, Mexico

David Toub
Gynesonics, Inc., 604 Fifth Avenue, Suite D, Redwood City, CA 94063, USA
Albert Einstein Medical Center, Philadelphia, PA, USA

J. A. Janse and S. Veersema
Department of Gynaecology and Obstetrics, St. Antonius Hospital, Koekoekslaan 1, 3430 EM Nieuwegein, the Netherlands

C. J. Tolman, F. J. M. Broekmans and H. W. R. Schreuder
Division of Woman and Baby, Department of Reproductive Medicine and Gynaecology, University Medical Center Utrecht, Utrecht, the Netherlands

Magdy Mohammed Moustafa
Frimley Park Hospital, Surrey, UK

Mohamed Abdel and Aleem Elnasharty
Cairo University Hospital, Cairo, Egypt

Antonio Perino, Francesco Forlani, Gloria Calagna, Stefano Rotolo and Gaspare Cucinella
Department of Obstetrics and Gynecology, University Hospital "P. Giaccone", Palermo, Italy

Antonio Lo Casto
Department of Radiological Sciences, DIBIMEF, University Hospital "P. Giaccone", Palermo, Italy

Giuseppe Calì
Department of Obstetrics and Gynecology, ARNAS Civico, Di Cristina e Benfratelli, Palermo, Italy

Jan Bosteels
Department of Obstetrics and Gynaecology, Imeldahospitaal
CEBAM, Centre for Evidence-based Medicine, the Belgian Branch of the Dutch Cochrane Centre, ACHG, Kapucijnenvoer 33, blok J bus 7001, 3000 Leuven, Belgium

Steven Weyers
Universitaire Vrouwenkliniek, University Hospital Gent, De Pintelaan 185, 9000 Gent, Belgium

Ben W. J. Mol
School of Paediatrics and Reproductive Health, The Robinson Institute, University of Adelaide, 5000 SA Adelaide, Australia

Thomas D'Hooghe
Leuven University Fertility Centre, KU Leuven, University Hospital Gasthuisberg, Herestraat 49, 3000 Leuven, Belgium

M. Possover
Center of Gynecologic Oncology and Neuropelveology, Possover International Medical Center, Hirslanden Clinic, Zurich, Switzerland

M. Possover and A. Forman
Dept of Gynecology and Neuropelveology, University of Aarhus, Aarhus, Denmark

G. Bigatti, S. Franchetti, M. Rosales and A. Baglioni
U.O. di Ostetricia e Ginecologia, Ospedale Classificato San Giuseppe Via San Vittore, 12, 20123 Milan, Italy

S. Bianchi
Direttore dell'Unità Opertiva di Ostetricia e Ginecologia Ospedale Classificato San Giuseppe Via San Vittore, Università degli Studi di Milano, 12, 20123 Milan, Italy

S. Gordts, P. Puttemans, Sy Gordts, M. Valkenburg, I. Brosens and R. Campo
Leuven Institute for Fertility and Embryology (L.I.F.E.), Tiensevest 168, 3000 Leuven, Belgium

S. Weyers
Department of Obstetrics and Gynecology, Ghent University Hospital, Ghent, Belgium

S. Van Calenbergh
Department of Obstetrics and Gynecology, AZ Turnhout, Turnhout, Belgium

Y. Van Nieuwenhove
Department of Surgery, Ghent University Hospital, Gent, Belgium

G. Mestdagh
Department of Obstetrics and Gynecology, Ziekenhuis Oost-Limburg (ZOL), Genk, Belgium

M. Coppens
Department of Anaesthesiology, Ghent University Hospital, Gent, Belgium

J. Bosteels
Department of Obstetrics and Gynecology, Imelda Hospital, Bonheiden, Belgium

Anita J. Merritt, Ilze Zommere, Richard J. Slade and Brett Winter-Roach
Department of Gynaecology, Salford Royal Hospitals NHS Trust, Stott Lane, Salford M6 8HD, UK

P. A. H. H. van der Heijden and M. P. M. L. Snijders
Department of Obstetrics and Gynaecology, Canisius-Wilhelmina Hospital, Nijmegen, The Netherlands

Y. P. Geels and L. F. A. G. Massuger
Department of Obstetrics and Gynaecology, Radboud University Nijmegen Medical Centre, Nijmegen, The Netherlands

S. H. M. van den Berg-van Erp
Department of Pathology, Canisius-Wilhelmina Hospital, Nijmegen, The Netherlands

P. A. H. H. van der Heijden
Department of Obstetrics and Gynaecology, Maxima Medical Centre, PO Box 777, Veldhoven 5500 MB, The Netherlands

Juliënne A. Janse and Sebastiaan Veersema
Department of Gynecology and Obstetrics, St. Antonius Hospital Nieuwegein, Koekoekslaan 1, 3435 CM Nieuwegein, The Netherlands

Emilie Hitzerd, Frank J. Broekmans and Henk W. R. Schreuder
Division of Woman and Baby, University Medical Center Utrecht, 3508 GA Utrecht, The Netherlands

Markus Wallwiener
Department of Obstetrics and Gynaecology, University of Heidelberg, Heidelberg, Germany

Philippe Robert Koninckx
University Hospital Gasthuisberg, Katholieke Universiteit, Leuven, Belgium

Andreas Hackethal
Queensland Centre for Gynaecological Cancer, Queensland Brisbane, Australia

Hans Brölmann
VU University, Amsterdam, The Netherlands

Per Lundorff
Gynecologic Clinic, Private Hospital Molholm, Vejle, Denmark

Michal Mara
Charles University, Prague, Czech Republic

Arnaud Wattiez
Hôpital de Hautepierre, Strasbourg, France

Rudy Leon De Wilde
Klinik für Frauenheilkunde, Geburtshilfe und Gynäkologische Onkologie, Universitätsklinik für Gynäkologie, Pius-Hospital, University Oldenburg, Oldenburg, Germany

Atef M. Darwish, Ahmad I. Hassanin, Mahmoud A. Abdel Aleem, Ibraheem I. Mohammad and Islam H. Aboushama
Department of Obstetrics and Gynecology, Woman's Health University Center, Assiut University, Assiut, Assiut 71111, Egypt

S. Gordts, R. Campo and I. Brosens
Leuven Institute for Fertility and Embryology, Tiensevest 168, 3000 Leuven, Belgium

Arpita Ghosh, Daniel Borlase, Tosin Ajala and Anthony James Kelly
Brighton and Sussex University Hospitals NHS Trust, Brighton, UK

Zaky Ibrahim
Western Sussex Hospitals NHS Trust, West Sussex, UK

P. G. Paul, Harneet Kaur, Dhivya Narasimhan, Gaurav Chopade and Dimple Kandhari
Centre for Advanced Endoscopy and Infertility Treatment, Paul's Hospital, Vattekkattu road, Kaloor, Cochin, Kerala 682 017, India

Ali M. El Saman, Mohamad T. Khalaf, Dina M. Habib, Omar M. Shaaban and Alaa M. Ismail
O. M. Shaaban A. M. Ismail Department of Obstetrics and Gynecology, Faculty of Medicine, Assiut University, Assiut, Egypt

Magdi M. Amin
Department of Obstetrics and Gynecology, Faculty of Medicine, Sohag University, Sohag, Egypt

Pietro Litta
Department of Gynecological Science and Human Reproduction, University of Padua, Padua, Italy

Luigi Nappi
Department of Medical and Surgical Sciences, Institute of Obstetrics and Gynaecology, University of Foggia, Foggia, Italy

Pasquale Florio
U.O.C. Obstetrics and Gynecology, "San Giuseppe" Hospital, Empoli, Italy

Luca Mencaglia
Section of Gynecology, Centro Oncologico Fiorentino, Sesto Fiorentino, Italy

Mario Franchini
Palagi Freestanding Unit, Florence, Italy

Stefano Angioni
Department of Surgical Sciences, Section of Obstetrics and Gynecology, University of Cagliari, Azienda Ospedaliero Universitaria, Blocco Q, SS554, Monserrato, Cagliari, Italy

Zhang Huanxiao, Chen Shuqin, Jiang Hongye, Xie Hongzhe, Niu Gang, Xu Chengkang and Yao Shuzhong
Department of Gynecology and Obstetrics, The First Affiliated Hospital of Sun Yat-sen University, No. 58 2nd Zhongshan Road, Guangzhou, Guangdong Province, China

Guan Xiaoming
Baylor College of Medicine, Houston, USA

Massimiliano Pellicano, Pierluigi Giampaolino, Giovanni Antonio Tommaselli, Ursula Catena, Carmine Nappi and Giuseppe Bifulco
Department of Obstetrics and Gynaecology, University of Naples, "Federico II", Via Pansini 5, 80131 Naples, Italy

Hiromi Kashihara, Virginie Emmanuelli, Edouard Poncelet, Chrystèle Rubod, Jean-Philippe Lucot, Bram Pouseele and Michel Cosson
Department of Gynecologic Surgery, Hopital Jeanne de Flandre, Centre Hospitalier Regional Universitaire de Lille, Lille Cedex, France

Hiromi Kashihara
Department of Obstetrics and Gynecology, Osaka Police Hospital, 10-31 Kitayama-cho Tennouji-ku Osaka, Osaka 543-0035, Japan

Bram Pouseele
Department of Obstetrics and Gynecology, OLV van Lourdes Hospital, Waregem, Belgium

Niblock Kathy, Connor Katie, Morgan David and Johnston Keith
Antrim Area Hospital, Derry, UK

Vasileios Minas, Nahid Gul and David Rowlands
Minimal Access Centre, Department of Obstetrics and Gynaecology, Wirral University Teaching Hospital, Arrowe Park Rd, Wirral, Merseyside CH49 5PE, UK

Subrat Kumar Mohakul, Venkata Radha Kumari Beela and Purnima Tiru
Visakha Steel General Hospital (RINL), Visakhapatnam, India

Alejandro Correa-Paris, Elena Suárez-Salvador, Antonia Gomar Crespo, Oriol Puig Puig, Jordi Xercavins and Antonio Gil-Moreno
Servei de Ginecologia, Unitat de Ginecologia Oncològica, Hospital Universitari Vall d'Hebron, Universitat Autònoma de Barcelona, Passeig de la Vall d'Hebron 119-129, Barcelona 08035, Spain

Athanasios Protopapas, Nikolaos Akrivos, Stavros Athanasiou, Ioannis Chatzipapas, Aikaterini Domali and Dimitrios Loutradis
1st University Department of Obstetrics and Gynecology of the University of Athens, "Alexandra" Hospital, 80 Queen Sophie Ave., 11528 Athens, Greece

Antonio Toesca and Oreste Gentilini
Division of Breast Surgery, European Institute of Oncology, Via Ripamonti 435, 20141 Milan, Italy

Fedro Peccatori
Department of Gynecological Oncology, European Institute of Oncology, Milan, Italy

Hatem A. Azim Jr.
Department of Medicine, BrEAST Data Centre, Institut Jules Bordet, Université Libre de Bruxelles, 1000 Brussels, Belgium

Frederic Amant
Multidisciplinary Breast Center, Leuven Cancer Institute (LKI), UZ Gasthuisberg, Katholieke Universiteit Leuven, Leuven, Belgium

A. S. Khalid and C. Burke
Cork University Maternity Hospital, Wilton, Cork, Republic of Ireland

A. R. H. Twijnstra, M. D. Blikkendaal, S. R. C. Driessen, F. W. Jansen and C. D. de Kroon
Department of Gynecology, Leiden University Medical Center, PO Box 9600, 2300 RC Leiden, The Netherlands

E. W. van Zwet
Department ofMedical Statistics, Leiden University Medical Center, Leiden, The Netherlands

F. W. Jansen
Department of Biomechanical Engineering, Delft University of Technology, Delft, The Netherlands

Stephan Gordts, Patrick Puttemans, Sylvie Gordts and Ivo Brosens
Leuven Institute for Fertility and Embryology, Tiensevest 168, 3000 Leuven, Belgium

Philippe R. Koninckx, Jasper Verguts, Roberta Corona and Ivo Brosens
UZ Gasthuisberg, Department of Obstetrics and Gynecology, KULeuven, 3000 Leuven, Belgium

Philippe R. Koninckx
Gruppo Italo Belga, Vuilenbos 2, 3360 Bierbeek, Belgium

Roberta Corona
Centre for Reproductive Medicine, Free University Brussels, 101 Laarbeeklaan, 1090 Brussels, Belgium

Jasper Verguts
Department of Obstetrics and Gynecology, Jessa Hospital, Hasselt, Belgium

Leila Adamyan
Department of Reproductive Medicine and Surgery, Moscow state University of Medicine and Dentistry, Moscow, Russia

Marlies Bongers
Máxima Medisch Centrum, Veldhoven, The Netherlands

Hans Brölmann
Vrije Universiteit Medisch Centrum, Amsterdam, The Netherlands

Janesh Gupta
Birmingham Women's Hospital, Birmingham, UK

José Gerardo Garza-Leal
Universidad Autónoma de Nuevo León, Monterrey, Nuevo Leon, Mexico

David Toub
Gynesonics, Inc., Redwood City, CA, USA
Department of Obstetrics and Gynecology, Albert Einstein Medical Center, Philadelphia, PA, USA

Declan Quinn
ST6 Antrim Area Hospital, 4 Bush Road, Antrim, NI, UK

James Moohan
Altnagelvin Area Hospital, Londonderry, UK

Taner Shakir, Tae Lee, Jeffrey Lim and Kevin Jones
University of Bristol Academy, GreatWestern Hospital, Marlbourgh Road, Swindon SN3 6BB, UK

Index